THE HANDBOOK OF PSYCHOLINGUISTIC AND COGNITIVE PROCESSES

THE HANDBOOK OF PSYCHOLINGUISTIC AND COGNITIVE PROCESSES

Perspectives in Communication Disorders

Edited by

JACKIE GUENDOUZI | FILIP LONCKE | MANDY J. WILLIAMS

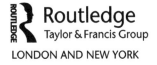

Routledge
Taylor & Francis Group

LONDON AND NEW YORK

First published in 2011 by Psychology Press

Published 2016 by Routledge
2 Park Square, Milton Park, Abingdon, Oxfordshire OX14 4RN
711 Third Avenue, New York, NY 10017

First issued in paperback 2015

Routledge is an imprint of the Taylor and Francis Group, an informa business

ISBN 13: 978-1-138-97568-2 (pbk)
ISBN 13: 978-1-84872-910-0 (hbk)

Library of Congress Cataloging-in-Publication Data

The handbook of psycholinguistic and cognitive processes : perspectives in communication disorders / edited by Jackie Guendouzi, Filip Loncke, and Mandy J. Williams.
    p. cm.
  Includes bibliographical references and index.
  ISBN 978-1-84872-910-0
  1. Psycholinguistics. 2. Cognitive psychology. 3. Communicative disorders. I. Guendouzi, Jacqueline. II. Loncke, Filip. III. Williams, Mandy J.

BF455.H26 2010
616.89'14--dc22   2010005129

Visit the Taylor & Francis Web site at
http://www.taylorandfrancis.com

and the Psychology Press Web site at
http://www.psypress.com

THE HANDBOOK OF PSYCHOLINGUISTIC AND COGNITIVE PROCESSES

Perspectives in Communication Disorders

Edited by

JACKIE GUENDOUZI | FILIP LONCKE | MANDY J. WILLIAMS

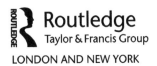

Routledge
Taylor & Francis Group

LONDON AND NEW YORK

First published in 2011 by Psychology Press

Published 2016 by Routledge
2 Park Square, Milton Park, Abingdon, Oxfordshire OX14 4RN
711 Third Avenue, New York, NY 10017

First issued in paperback 2015

Routledge is an imprint of the Taylor and Francis Group, an informa business

ISBN 13: 978-1-138-97568-2 (pbk)
ISBN 13: 978-1-84872-910-0 (hbk)

Library of Congress Cataloging-in-Publication Data

The handbook of psycholinguistic and cognitive processes : perspectives in communication disorders / edited by Jackie Guendouzi, Filip Loncke, and Mandy J. Williams.
    p. cm.
  Includes bibliographical references and index.
  ISBN 978-1-84872-910-0
  1. Psycholinguistics. 2. Cognitive psychology. 3. Communicative disorders. I. Guendouzi, Jacqueline. II. Loncke, Filip. III. Williams, Mandy J.

BF455.H26 2010
616.89'14--dc22
                                          2010005129

Visit the Taylor & Francis Web site at
http://www.taylorandfrancis.com

and the Psychology Press Web site at
http://www.psypress.com

Contents

SECTION I   Some Basic Considerations: Models and Theories

SECTION II *Developmental Disorders*

SECTION III   Acquired Disorders

SECTION IV   Language and Other Modalities

Editors

Jackie Guendouzi, PhD, is a linguist who received her undergraduate and graduate degrees from Cardiff University, United Kingdom, and is currently an associate professor at Southeastern Louisiana University. Her research interests include language processing in clinical populations and pragmatics.

Filip Loncke is associate professor at the University of Virginia. He has lectured, conducted research, and published in psycholinguistic processes involved in atypical communication and in their clinical applications. In 2003 and 2004, he was president of the International Society for Augmentative and Alternative Communication (ISAAC).

Mandy Williams, PhD, CCC-SLP, is an assistant professor in the Department of Communication Disorders at the University of South Dakota. Her research focuses on children and adults with fluency disorders.

Contributors

Lise Abrams is an associate professor of psychology at the University of Florida. Lise double majored in psychology and mathematics and then received a National Science Foundation Graduate Fellowship, earning her MA (1992) and PhD (1997) in cognitive psychology from the University of California, Los Angeles. She joined the faculty at the University of Florida in 1997, where she established the Cognition and Aging Laboratory to investigate memory and language processes in young and older adults, specifically the processes involved in retrieving words and the changes in these processes that occur with normal aging.

Herman Ackermann has a master's degree in philosophy and psychology, and a medical degree in neurology. He is Professor for Neurological Rehabilitation at the Medical School, University of Tübingen, and head of the Research Group Neurophonetics at the HERTIE-Institute for Clinical Neurosciences, University of Tübingen. He is also head of the Department of Neurological Rehabilitation at the Rehabiliation Center Hohenurach, Bad Urach.

Sharon Armon-Lotem finished her PhD in linguistics (syntax and language acquisition) at Tel-Aviv University in 1997. After three years as a visiting researcher at the University of Maryland, she moved to Bar-Ilan University, where she holds a position as senior lecturer. She studies the language of English–Hebrew and Russian–Hebrew in typically developing bilingual preschool children and bilingual children with specific language impairments (SLI) focusing on syntax and morphosyntax.

Dana Arthur, MS, EdM, is a doctoral student in the Department of Communication Sciences at the University of Connecticut. Her research interests include the language literacy connection in language-disordered populations, particularly in children with SLI. She holds an MS in speech pathology from Boston University and an EdM from Harvard University.

Hadeel Ayyad is a doctoral student funded by the Kuwait University working on Arabic phonological acquisition in the School of Audiology and Speech Sciences at the University of British Columbia.

Martin J. Ball is a Hawthorne-BoRSF Distinguished Professor and director of the Hawthorne Research Center at the University of Louisiana–Lafayette. He is co-editor of the journal *Clinical Linguistics and Phonetics*. His main research interests include sociolinguistics, clinical phonetics and phonology, and the linguistics of Welsh. He was president of the International Clinical Phonetics and Linguistics Association from 2000 to 2006. His most recent books are *The Handbook of Clinical Linguistics*, and *Phonetics for Communication Disorders*.

Jennifer Barnes is a Fulbright Scholar and a recent graduate of both Yale and Cambridge. She is currently working on a PhD in developmental psychology, and she doubles as a multipublished novelist whose books have been translated into eight languages worldwide.

Simon Baron-Cohen is professor of developmental psychopathology at the University of Cambridge and director of the Autism Research Centre at Cambridge. He is the author of *Mindblindness and the Essential Difference*.

Teri James Bellis, PhD, is professor and chair of the Department of Communication Disorders at the University of South Dakota. She has published extensively on the subject of auditory neuroscience and central auditory processing disorders. Dr. Bellis is a Fellow of the American Speech-Language-Hearing Association.

Ursula Bellugi is professor and director of the Laboratory for Cognitive Neuroscience, and is a pioneer in the study of the biological foundation of language. She is regarded as the founder of the neurobiology of American Sign Language, because her work was the first to show it is a true language, complete with grammar and syntax, and is processed by many of the same parts of the brain that process spoken language. Her work has led to the discovery that the left hemisphere of the human brain becomes specialized for languages, whether spoken or signed, a striking demonstration of neuronal plasticity. Bellugi is currently studying individuals with Williams Syndrome.

B. May Bernhardt is a professor in the School of Audiology and Speech Sciences at the University of British Columbia. Her area of specialization in research and teaching are child language acquisition and impairment, particularly protracted phonological development, most recently with a cross-linguistic focus.

Hiram Brownell received a BA in psychology from Stanford University and the MA and PhD in psychology from The Johns Hopkins University. He is currently a professor of psychology at Boston College and is also an adjunct faculty member in the Department of Neurology at the Boston University School of Medicine and an investigator affiliated with the Harold Goodglass Aphasia Research Center. Brownell's primary research interests are the effects of right hemisphere injury on language, communication, and social cognition.

Martha Burns serves on the faculty of Northwestern University, Department of Communication Sciences and Disorders, and has served on the medical staff of Evanston-Northwestern Hospital for 30 years. Dr. Burns is the author of a book on aphasia, right hemisphere dysfunction, and the *Burns Brief Inventory of Communication and Cognition*. She has published over 100 peer reviewed articles and book chapters on the brain and language.

José G. Centeno, PhD, CCC-SLP, is an associate professor in the Department of Communication Sciences and Disorders at St. John's University, New York City. His teaching and research focus on stroke-related impairments and aspects of service delivery in monolingual Spanish/bilingual Spanish–English adults.

Beverly Collisson, MS, is a doctoral student in the Department of Communication Sciences at the University of Connecticut. Her clinical and research interests lie in the area of semantic development in typical and atypical language learners.

Nelson Cowan obtained his PhD in 1980, from the University of Wisconsin. He is Curators' Professor of Psychological Sciences at the University of Missouri. His research on working memory, its relation to attention, and its childhood development has recently demonstrated a capacity limit in adults of only three to five items, unless the items can be rehearsed or grouped together. His books include *Attention and Memory: An Integrated Framework* and *Working Memory Capacity*.

Clotilde Degroot is a student in master of biomedical sciences at the University of Montreal. She also works as a research assistant at the Centre de Recherche of the Institut Universitaire de Gériatrie de Montréal.

Gary Dell obtained his PhD in psychology from the University of Toronto in 1980, and is currently professor of psychology at the University of Illinois at Urbana–Champaign. He is also chair of the Cognitive Science Group of the Beckman Institute.

Katherine DeLong completed her MS and is working toward her PhD in cognitive science at the University of California, San Diego. She primarily uses event-related potentials to explore issues of semantic language comprehension, particularly questions relating to the anticipatory nature of such processing.

Susan Duncan is a psycholinguist and has published widely on the topic of gesture.

Meagan T. Farrell is a second-year graduate student in the PhD program in Psychology, Neurobehavioral, and Cognitive Sciences at the University of Florida, and was a psychology major at Appalachian State University where she earned her BS in 2006. She is currently a member of the NIA-funded predoctoral research training program in aging at the University of Florida, where her research is focused on the cognitive processes that enable the production and comprehension of language in young and older adults, and identifying the source of age-related changes to these processes.

Manuela Friedrich has a PhD from the Institute for Psychology, Humboldt-University, Berlin and also a diploma in mathematics from the University of Rostock. She has worked at the Institute for Psychology, Humboldt-University, Berlin; the Centre for General Linguistics (ZAS), Berlin; the MPI for Human Cognitive and Brain Sciences, Leipzig; the department of Neuropsychology at the Max Planck Institute for Human Cognitive and Brain Sciences, Berlin; and is currently involved with the research program Cluster of Excellence "Languages of Emotion" at the Free University Berlin.

Bernard Grela, PhD, CCC-SLP, is an associate professor in the Department of Communication Sciences at the University of Connecticut whose area of expertise is children with specific language impairment. His research focuses on the impact of linguistic complexity on grammatical errors in this population of children.

Gregory Hickok is professor of cognitive sciences and director of the Center for Cognitive Neuroscience at the University of California, Irvine. Hickok's research centers on the neural basis of both signed and spoken language as well as human auditory perception.

Peter Howell is professor of experimental psychology at University College London. His long-term interests are on the relationship between speech perception and speech production. This motivated his interest in stuttering.

William Hula, PhD, CCC-SLP, is a research speech pathologist at the VA Pittsburgh Healthcare System. His research interests include measurement of language performance and health outcomes in aphasia and the use of dual-task methods and theories to help identify specific points of breakdown in word production and comprehension in aphasia.

Yves Joanette is professor at the Faculty of Medicine of the Université de Montréal and Lab Director at the Centre de Recherche of the Institut Universitaire de Gériatrie de Montréal. His work has focused on the relative contribution of each cerebral hemisphere to language and communication, as well as on the neurobiological determinants of successful aging for communication abilities. He was honored by a Doctorat Honoris Causa by the Université Lyon 2.

Karima Kahlaoui is a postdoctoral fellow in cognitive neurosciences at the Montreal University, Canada and a clinical neuropsychologist. Her topics include the semantic processing of words across the hemispheres, the semantic memory, and the aging. She holds a PhD in psychology from Nice University, France.

Juliane Kappes is a trained speech–language pathologist and has a diploma in patholinguistics, from the University of Potsdam. Since 2006, she has a research grant at the Clinical Neuropsychology Research Group (*From dynamic sensorimotor interaction to conceptual representation. Deconstructing apraxia.* German Fed. Ministry of Research and Education).

Michael Kiang, MD, PhD, is assistant professor in the Department of Psychiatry and Behavioural Neurosciences at McMaster University in Hamilton, Ontario, Canada.

Audrey Kittredge received a BA in linguistics from Brown University in 2004 and was awarded a National Science Foundation Graduate Research Fellowship in 2006. She obtained a MA in cognitive psychology from the University of Illinois at Urbana–Champaign in 2007.

Marta Kutas is director of the Center for Research in Language, University of California, San Diego, and a distinguished professor in the Departments of Cognitive Science and Neurosciences, University of California, San Diego.

Eeva Leinonen is a professor of psycholinguistics and deputy vice-chancellor at the University of Hertfordshire and private docent in clinical linguistics at the University of Oulu, Finland. She has published two books and various articles, focusing particularly on clinical pragmatics and pragmatic language comprehension difficulties in children.

John Locke is interested in the biology of human communication. He is currently working on a selection-based account of various aspects of language and speech.

Catherine Longworth obtained her PhD in cognitive neuroscience at the Centre for Speech and Language in the Department of Experimental Psychology at Cambridge University, where she then went on to hold the Pinsent Darwin Research Fellowship in Mental Pathology before obtaining a doctorate in clinical psychology. Her clinical and research interests include the cognitive and neural basis of morphological impairments in aphasia and psychological adjustment to acquired language disorders.

Kristine Lundgren, ScD, is associate professor in the Department of Communication Sciences and Disorders, University of North Carolina Greensboro and assistant professor in the Neurology Department, Boston University School of Medicine. Her areas of interest include cognitive-linguistic disorders in adults with acquired brain injury and the use of complementary/alternative approaches to treating communication disorders.

Brian MacWhinney is a professor of psychology, computational linguistics, and modern languages at Carnegie Mellon University and has developed a model of first and second language acquisition and processing called the Competition Model. He has also developed the CHILDES Project for the computational study of child language transcript data and the TalkBank System for the study of conversational interactions.

Chloë Marshall, PhD, is a researcher at the Centre for Developmental Language Disorders and Cognitive Neuroscience, at University College London. Her research interests include language and literacy development; developmental disorders of language, speech, and literacy (SLI, dyslexia, stuttering); phonology and its developmental relationship to morphology, syntax, and the lexicon; the cognitive skills underlying typical and atypical language/literacy acquisition in hearing and deaf children; and the phonology of English and British sign language.

William Marslen-Wilson is director of the MRC Cognition and Brain Sciences Unit in Cambridge, England, and honorary professor of language and cognition at the University of Cambridge. He is an influential and prominent figure in the cognitive science and neuroscience of language, studying the comprehension of spoken language in the mind and the brain. His work is interdisciplinary and cross-linguistic, aimed at identifying the neural processing streams that support the immediate interpretation of spoken utterances. His current research brings together behavioral, neuropsychological, and neuroimaging data from contrasting languages (such as Arabic, Polish, and English) to determine the underlying general properties of human language systems.

Malcolm McNeil, PhD, CCC-SLP, BC-NCD, is distinguished professor and chair of the Department of Communication Science and Disorders at the University of Pittsburgh and Research Career Scientist, VA Pittsburgh Healthcare System. His research interests are in the cognitive mechanisms underlying the language behaviors in aphasia, aphasia test development, and in the mechanisms and treatment for apraxia of speech.

David McNeill has published several books on gesture, thought, and language. His 1992 book, *Hand and Mind*, received the Laing Prize in 1994 from the University of Chicago Press.

Gareth Morgan is pursuing his PhD in speech and hearing sciences and his MS in educational psychology in the Measurement Statistics and Methodological studies program at Arizona State University. He is interested in integrating the most current methods in measurement theory (construct representation) and psychometrics (item response theory) to design assessments to detect language disorders in predominately Spanish-speaking and bilingual (Spanish–English) speaking children.

Katherine Morton studied biopsychology at the University of Chicago, Illinois and linguistic phonetics at University of California, Los Angeles. Her current research is in modeling how speaking and understanding speech might be mediated by biological and cognitive systems.

Nora Presson is a doctoral student in cognitive psychology at Carnegie Mellon University. Her work focuses on second language acquisition and the use of cognitive psychology principles to improve second language instruction.

Maria Adelaida Restreppo is an associate professor in the Department of Speech and Hearing Science at Arizona State University. She is a bilingual speech–language pathologist and obtained her PhD from the University of Arizona. Dr. Restrepo's research deals with differentiating language differences from language disorders, assessment in culturally diverse children, especially those from Spanish-speaking homes; further, she studies language maintenance, loss, and intervention in children developing language typically and those with language disorders. She currently is a principal investigator on a grant to provide intervention for Spanish-speaking kindergarten children to improve literacy skills in English and the principal investigator on a grant to develop a screener for Spanish speakers. She is also the co-investigator of a grant providing intervention to children in preschool who are bilingual and present with language disorder and the principal investigator on professional development for Head Start teachers. She has published in a range of national and international journals in Spanish and English and collaborates with international investigators on matters relating to language disorders and children with attention deficit and hyperactivity disorders.

Ardi Roelofs is a senior researcher at the Donders Institute for Brain, Cognition and Behaviour of Radboud University Nijmegen, the Netherlands. His research is on attention and language performance. He investigates attention for listening, reading, and speaking using response time, eye tracking, electrophysiological, hemodynamic neuroimaging, molecular genetics, and computational modeling approaches.

Ben Rutter is an assistant professor in the Department of Communication Sciences and Disorders at the University of Oklahoma Health Sciences Center. He holds a BA (Hons.) in linguistics from the University of York and a PhD in communication disorders from the University of Louisiana–Lafayette. His research interests include clinical phonology, acoustics phonetics, and the sound patterns of human interaction.

Nuala Ryder is a research fellow in the Psychology Department at the University of Hertfordshire and a founder member of the distributed language group at the University. Her research focuses on children's development of language, the assessment of pragmatic comprehension in clinical populations and the relationship between cognition and pragmatics in communication.

John Shelley-Tremblay is the founding director of the Experimental Event-Related Potentials Laboratory at the Department of Psychology at the University of South Alabama. His research investigates the interaction between visual attention and the cognitive processes that underlie reading. He employs psychophysiological, neuropsychological, and educational methodologies combining basic and applied research interests. Current projects involve assessing neural plasticity as a function of visual training for persons with reading disability.

Terri Shive is an assistant professor of audiology at the University of South Dakota with research interests in implantable devices, telemedicine, and counseling.

Bernadette Ska obtained her PhD in cognitive psychology at the University of Leuven, Belgium. She went on as a postdoctoral fellow in neuropsychology. She is a researcher at the Institut Universitaire de Geriatrie de Montréal and associate professor at the École d'Orthophonie et Audiologie, Faculty of Medecine, Université de Montréal, Québec, Canada.

Ekaterina Smyk is a doctoral student in the Department of Speech and Hearing Science at Arizona State University. Her current research interests focus on developing language proficiency measures for English language learners, exploring specific language impairment in bilingual populations, and investigating syntactic development of Russian–English bilingual children.

Joseph Stemberger is currently head of the Department of Linguistics at the University of British Columbia. His research focuses on mental representations and the processing of phonological and morphological information during language production, addressing implications for both psychological models and linguistic theories. Much of his research focuses on the errors that occur in language production, both the infrequent nonsystematic errors of adult (and child) production and the frequent systematic errors of child production. While he began with research on English, his current major projects address Zapotec and Slovene and other languages to a lesser extent.

Holly Storkel is an associate professor in the Department of Speech-Language-Hearing: Sciences and Disorders at the University of Kansas in Lawrence. Her research focuses on sound and word learning by typically developing children and children with phonological or language impairments.

Jee Eun Sung gained her PhD from the University of Pittsburgh and is currently at Ewha Women's University, Seoul, Korea. Her research interest is sentence processing and its underlying cognitive mechanism in normal elderly adults and persons with aphasia.

Mark Tatham has worked at the University of Essex (where he is emeritus professor), Ohio State University, and University of California, Los Angeles. His current research is in building computationally adequate models of speech production and perception.

Leanne Togher is an associate professor and principal research fellow and senior NHMRC research fellow at The University of Sydney, Australia. Her primary interest is in developing empirically based assessments and treatments for people, and their families, who have communication disorders following traumatic brain injury.

Angela Ullrich is working both as a research associate at the University of Cologne and as a speech language pathologist in private clinics since 2005. For her dissertation project she focuses on the clinical application of nonlinear phonological theories in German-speaking children.

Heather van der Lely is professor and director of the Centre for Developmental Language Disorders and Cognitive Neuroscience, at University College London. Her research in communication disorders has focused on specific language impairment (SLI) and she has published extensively in this field.

Mieke Van Herreweghe is professor of English language and linguistics in the Department of English at Ghent University. Her PhD dissertation dealt with the acquisition of Dutch by Flemish deaf children and adolescents. Since then, her research has shifted toward grammatical, lexicographical, and sociolinguistic aspects of Flemish sign language. Furthermore, she is a certified sign language interpreter, co-founder and board member of the Vlaams GebarentaalCentrum (Flemish Sign Language Centre) and chair of the Advisory Committee on Flemish Sign Language, recently installed by the Flemish government.

Diana Van Lancker Sidtis has published widely on a variety of research topics in communicative disorders. She teaches at New York University and is a research scientist at the Nathan Kline Institute.

Rosemary Varley is a professor of cognitive neuroscience at the University of Sheffield and in 2006 was awarded an ESRC Professorial Fellowship. Her research seeks to develop neurobiological plausible models of speech and language functions. Current projects explore word production impairments in apraxia and aphasia, and the impact of severe language impairment on domains of nonlanguage cognition such as math and reasoning.

Myriam Vermeerbergen is assistant professor of Flemish sign language at the Department of Applied Language Studies, Lessius University College (Antwerp, Belgium) and affiliated researcher at the Katholieke Universiteit Leuven. She has been researching the linguistic structure of sign languages for 20 years. She is also co-founder and current president of the Vlaams GebarentaalCentrum (Flemish Sign Language Centre) and member on the board of the Sign Language Linguistics Society.

Joel Walters trained in applied psycholinguistics at Boston University, where he worked on pragmatics in bilingual children. His book *Bilingualism: The Sociopragmatic and Psycholinguistic Interface* was published in 2005. His current work focuses on language impairment in bilinguals and implications for social integration and language policy.

Mark Yates obtained his PhD from the University of Kansas. Currently, he is an assistant professor at the University of South Alabama. His latest research has focused on the influence of phonological similarity on visual word recognition and reading, with recent publications on this research appearing in *Quarterly Journal of Experimental Psychology,* and the *Journal of Experimental Psychology: Human Perception and Performance, and Cognition.*

Jing Zhao received her MS for medical science from Shanghai Second Medical University in 1996 and practiced as a developmental pediatrician for almost seven years before undertaking a MS in speech language pathology from the School of Audiology and Speech Science, University of British Columbia in 2007. She worked as a research assistant at UBC Bilingualism Research Centre during her studies and was involved in five research projects relating to bilingualism and cross-linguistic study. She is currently a certified and registered speech–language pathologist in Canada.

Wolfram Ziegler has a diploma and doctoral degree in mathematics. He worked as a research assistant at the Max-Planck-Institute for Psychiatry and is now head of the Clinical Neuropsychology Research Group (EKN), City Hospital Munich, and a lecturer of phonetics and neurophonetics at the Phonetics Department and at the Speech Pathology School, University of Munich.

Introduction

Jackie Guendouzi, Filip Loncke, and Mandy Williams

WHY THIS BOOK? SOME BASIC CONSIDERATIONS

This book is not intended to provide a definitive or extensive survey of the field of psycholinguistics; indeed, it would be impossible in a single book to cover this area comprehensively. Due to restrictions of time and space there are invariably research areas that we have not been able to include. Although this book does not require a background in psycholinguistics it does assume a basic knowledge of language and some familiarity with the field of communication disorders. Section I provides an overview of some of the theoretical approaches that have been influential in the field of psycholinguistics and cognitive processing. Although some chapters in this section focus on language processing in "normal" language, many of the authors consider what such theories and models have to teach us about communication disorders. Sections II and III of this book provide a selection of chapters that have drawn on theories from psycholinguistics and directly applied them to the context of specific communication disorders. Section IV considers theoretical approaches to language and cognitive processing in modalities (e.g., gesture) that have not traditionally been included in a book on psycholinguistics.

The field of psycholinguistics has yielded many diverse and competing theories over the years; some have dominated language research more than others. This book, however, does not take a particular stance in relation to any one theoretical framework, rather it is intended that readers draw their own conclusions as to the robustness of specific models or theories. It should be noted that many of the chapters in this book focus on Specific Language-Impairment (SLI) (Hayiou, Bishop & Plunkett, 2004) and aphasia. Both SLI and aphasia provided ideal populations for exploring language processing, because while impacting the individual's ability to use language in the past it was thought that they left other cognitive systems untouched (e.g., intelligence in SLI and comprehension in Broca's aphasia). However, as our knowledge of language processing increases this perspective is changing and, as work in this book will show, researchers in both aphasia and SLI are focusing on the role of other cognitive systems for more extensive explanations of how language develops and is processed within the brain.

It is important for the readers to approach this book with a critical eye; it is not the intention to provide answers or avoid conflicting theoretical positions. Research that explores theoretical issues or attempts to establish models is a continuing project that rarely arrives at a definitive answer. When asked why his theory had undergone so many changes (i.e., from Transformational Generative Grammar through to Minimalism), Chomsky noted that he considered his research an on-going project (personal correspondence). Chomsky's point was that research does not necessarily reach a final conclusion, and can only improve through continual debate and revision if we are to produce robust theories.

PSYCHOLINGUISTICS: A HISTORICAL PERSPECTIVE

Psycholinguistics has always involved the art of finding models to help us understand why and how people speak, listen, read, and write. In some of the earliest reflections on language and speech, questions are raised that have kept the interest of scholars to this day. *Plato's Cratylus* (Sedley, 2003) discusses the relationship between words and their referents, an issue that has remained central both in developmental accounts of language (Piaget, 1929/1997) and its disorders and in the field of cognitive semantics (Evan & Green, 2006).

A general fascination with language, where it came from, its plasticity, and its disorders is reflected in discussions from the time of the Enlightenment on. Twentieth-century linguists explicitly trace back their line of thinking to Descartes's reasoning on the nature of ideas and mental functioning (Chomsky, 1966).

The 19th century was the time of the precursors of our understanding of the neurolinguistic underpinnings of language, starting with Gall's speculation of the brain's mental areas to Broca's and Wernicke's description of types of aphasia. Theories about localization have led to a rudimentary psycholinguistic theory, most notably reflected in the Wernicke/Lichtheim model (Caplan, 1987). This model assumed the existence of an (anatomically based) system of connections between brain centers. Problems in processing language were described as a breakdown, a deletion, or a distortion in the communication system. The Wernicke/Lichtheim classification may be considered the earliest model of internal linguistic processing, combining a brain localization approach with an information processing approach. The study of aphasia also led to the first classifications and distinctions between subcomponents of language and language processing. The terms motor aphasia, conduction aphasia, receptive aphasia, transcortical aphasia reflect an attempt to grasp both the internal organization of language and its interaction with the brain. For a century and a half, these distinctions have been a basis on which intervention rationales have been built. At the same time, already in the early twentieth century, the accuracy of these approaches was challenged and criticized.

These early neurolinguistic models served as a framework to understand language disorders in children: Until the 1970s childhood language problems were often referred to as *developmental dysphasia* (Wyke, 1978), a clear reference for a purported neuropsychological explanation of the phenomenon. These approaches initially have helped to conceptualize the relationship between language and brain.

Language as a system was the object of study of De Saussure's *Cours de Linguistique Générale*, published in 1916, This influential work marks the beginning of a strong structuralist view in language theory. Although De Saussure described language as rooted in historical "diachronic" development, he also thought that a "panchronic" (p. 134) approach would be possible. This latter concept corresponds with today's "universal" view on language, a view that implies that explanatory models of language, language disorders, and language intervention should be valid and applicable across languages.

Today's schools of thought on language acquisition are often categorized in empiricism, rationalism, and pragmaticism (Russell, 2004). The influence of the empiricists in speech–language intervention was the most obvious in the 1950s and 1960s but remains powerful and obvious to this day. The empiricist approach apparently offers a framework that easily lends itself into concept of trainability and modifiability, which are central for interventions.

Rationalism tends to consider language as a semiautonomous self-developing system. An underlying hypothesis is that understanding the rules of languages helps to grasp language functioning and will lead to most effective interventions. In the period of linguistic structuralism, we find an interest in patterns that learners would use as reference frames to build language structures. One example here is the Fitzgerald key (1954), meant to make syntactic structures transparent and to help the student to "build" sentences according to visually laid out patterns.

In the past 20 years, the influence of linguistics on language intervention has waned. Its place is taken by a more cognitivist, emergentist, and information-processing oriented focus, as is the case for much of the entire field of psycholinguistics (Harley, 2008).

Interestingly, for a long time, the pragmaticists did not become a dominant factor in theory of speech, language, and their disorders until the 1970s, a time when interest in research areas such as early development, social interaction, and sociolinguistics started to rise. It changed the field of speech–language pathology, with a stronger emphasis on early and functional intervention, and especially involvement of communication partners.

The developments in the first decade of the twenty-first century maintain some of the old debates. However, many of the therapeutic approaches integrate and motivate multiple approaches. For example, Nelson (2000) proposes the "tricky mix approach," which strives to create multiple conditions that converge to increase learning. Nelson suggests that attention, motivation, and the right contrastive examples work together to make learning possible in typically developing children. Knowing this, the clinician's task is to recreate similar favorable conditions.

Throughout history, psycholinguistic theory and intervention have always benefited from clinical research, starting with Broca, to today's genetic studies, syndrome studies, and neuroimaging studies.

THE LANGUAGE DEBATE

In relation to the language debate, two theories had major effects on language research in the 1950s, Skinner's behaviorist model emphasizing the effects of reinforcement and environmental input (1957), and Chomsky's nativist (cognitive) approach (1957). Chomsky's work stimulated a search to discover what was going on in the mind of the *ideal speaker* when forming a sentence. Thus the emphasis of research in linguistics shifted toward the study of a speaker's *competence* (rather than their *performance*) and the pursuit of uncovering the underlying mechanisms of language. Chomsky's work also highlighted the role of biological factors in language by suggesting a language acquisition device (LAD) innate to humans. Chomsky's subsequent critique of Skinner's *Verbal Behaviors* (1959) led to nativist approaches becoming the agenda of most linguistic programs during that period. Chomsky's work was also highly influential in driving language acquisition research at that time.

However, despite the primacy of Chomsky's work during the 1970s and 1980s, work in language acquisition has continued to explore both biological factors and environmental influences. Indeed, most current theories draw on the interaction between biological factors and socioenvironmental factors when considering how language develops across the life span. Furthermore, advances in neurosciences and computational modeling have resulted in a research agenda focusing on the notion of language as an emergent property of competing systems. However, the debate is far from over in the field of communication disorders and, as will be shown below, there is still a case in SLI for a more modular approach (see van der Lely & Marshall, Chapter 20).

THE STRUCTURE OF LANGUAGE

When studying language it is typically dissected into its component parts. However, it is important to note that this is an artificial construct; that is, the degree to which any language system (e.g., morphosyntactic, semantic) is independent of other systems is debatable. Perhaps a good analogy is that of driving in a car; in order for the car to move all the component parts and systems of the car need to be operating. In addition, a driver is required to coordinate the exercise; thus one event "driving down the road" is the sum of many interrelating and synchronized systems. However, if the car breaks down and stops moving we need to establish what system or part failed in order to repair the damage. A global failure may be due to a minor failure in the electrical system rather than engine damage itself, but in order to diagnose the problem, the mechanic has to have a working knowledge of each individual system and how it interacts with other systems.

A similar situation occurs with language; in order to produce an utterance, a variety of cognitive systems are brought into play. For example, when hearing an acoustic stimulus (e.g., a request for coffee) a listener initiates several cognitive systems; first he or she has to focus on the speaker (attention), retain the information heard (working memory), interpret the acoustic signal (auditory discrimination), parse the utterance (morphosyntactic system), and then comprehend the message (semantic and conceptual systems). In addition, there is a need to coordinate visual stimuli such as gesture and facial expressions into the interpretation of the utterance. And yet this simple action takes place in a split second of time as a holistic event and listeners are not aware of the separate systems operating to process the utterance. One is only aware that someone requested a cup of coffee.

In academic programs focusing on communication disorders, language has traditionally been studied in a way that is modular in its approach. For example, language processing is often taught within courses relating to specific disorders (e.g., motor speech disorders or child language disorders) and is typically divided up into the following areas: neurobiological correlates of language, the motor system, the phonological system, the grammatical system (morphosyntax), the semantic system (the lexicon), and pragmatics. However, as the chapters within this book will demonstrate, other equally important systems may play a major role not only in language processing, but in how we view interventions. These systems include attention, working memory, auditory discrimination, visual processing, gestures, paralinguistic features, and facial expressions. If there is a central theme to this book, it is the notion of language as an emergent property of dynamic interacting systems.

SECTION I: MODELS AND THEORIES

Models and theories drive research, yet as noted above, language processing is not often an integral part of many communication disorders programs. This may be because it is not often easy to see the connection between theory and practice, particularly in relation to psycholinguistic models. However, as Stackhouse and Wells (1997) have noted, although traditional linguistic approaches offer very detailed descriptions they do not always offer adequate explanations for the development of linguistic systems in individuals with disorders. A psycholinguistic approach to intervention in speech and language disorders "embraces the goal of explaining speech impairment" (Baker, Croot, McLeod & Paul 2001, p. 686). In their review of both Box-and-Arrow models and Connectionist models, Baker and colleagues consider the implications of such models to clinical practice and suggest that psycholinguistic approaches to understanding communication disorders will ultimately help identify more effective treatments.

As can be seen from Locke's work (Chapter 1), explanations that integrate biological factors with social and environmental factors are currently more common than the either/or explanations of the last century. Locke examines the evolution of language and raises questions relating to both social and biological needs and their role in the process of language acquisition. He suggests it may be hard to disentangle these two driving forces in the development of human language and offers explanations for gender and cultural differences within and across language use.

Interactionist approaches such as Locke's consider both the biological bases of language, and the role the child's environment plays in sculpting the brain for language. MacWhinney and colleagues (1982) suggest a functional account of language learning that proposes alternative interpretations compete online during language processing. In Chapter 2, Presson and MacWhinney elaborate on the Competition Model and show how it can offer explanations in the cases of SLI and aphasia.

Abrams and Farrell (Chapter 3) consider both age-related biological factors and social aspects of language to discuss the underlying differences in language use in later life. They review research that has explored both comprehension and production of language in older adults and conclude with a discussion on directions for future research that might improve functional communication with older interlocutors.

Other cognitive systems such as attention and working memory play an important role in the process of both acquiring and processing language. In Chapter 4, Cowan offers an overview of both his own work and that of Baddeley (1986) to show how attention and working memory interact both with each other and with other language systems such as verbal syntax. He also raises questions relating to work (Caplan, Waters, & DeDe, 2007) that might be considered as deriving from a Chomskyan paradigm that links working memory specifically to syntax.

Advances in brain imaging techniques have led to the study of neurobiological aspects of language processing moving beyond merely describing structures that are thought to correlate with specific areas of language. In Chapter 5, Kahlaoui, Ska, Degroot, and Joanette first review imaging methods and then consider what each method can tell us about the neurobiological bases of semantic processing. Kutas, DeLong, and Kiang (Chapter 6) note that, when compared to other neuroimaging methods, electrophysiological studies are not only economical but they can provide a potential "window" on the brain's language related processing operations. Kutas and colleagues provide an overview of studies that have used Event Related Potentials (ERPs) and then consider what such paradigms reveal about normal and abnormal language processing. In Chapter 7, Friedrich compares mathematical models and artificial neural networks (connectionist models) to brain imaging techniques. In particular, she reflects on what ERP studies can contribute to our knowledge of early word learning.

As noted above, current models and theories in psycholinguistics consider how language functions as a system, particularly how individual language systems influence and, are influenced by, other systems. Many theories have drawn on what we know about neural networks and artificial intelligence to develop new models of language processing. Such research has moved away from trying to link individual centers (or modules) of the brain to specific aspects of language (e.g., lexicon, syntax), to suggest that language is subject to parallel processing within interconnected networks. Thus, rather than associating a lesion in a specific region of the brain with a particular language deficit, a connectionist approach would consider the extent to which a disturbance in one area of the network might affect other levels of the language system.

Research based on connectionist approaches have been very influential in the field of communication disorders, particularly when considering acquired disorders of language and cognition such as aphasia. In Chapter 8, Dell and Kittredge apply a connectionist approach to the context of aphasia and other communication impairments and suggest a cooperative view of language that argues for models based on interaction between processing parts. Roelofs (Chapter 9) considers vocal utterance production from the standpoint of Wernicke's classical model to the current version of the WEAVER++ model. He suggests that future research should draw on such models to develop intervention methods.

In Chapter 10, Shelley-Tremblay reviews some of the more influential and widely researched theories of semantic representation. He focuses attention on models of semantic memory, word identification, and semantic priming to assess the efficacy of local theories, feature-based theories, and distributed models.

Longworth and Marslen-Wilson (Chapter 11) examine language comprehension from the perspective of what occurs within the milliseconds it takes the brain to recognize individual words. They explore this aspect of connectivity and language processing through a clinical example and go on to suggest a neurocognitive model that contrasts with the classic model of a single processing pathway. As they suggest their model forms part of the current "Words and Rules" debate in cognitive science.

Another form of language use that has been noted in people with aphasia and other neurogenic disorders, such as dementia, is the use of formulaic language (fixed phrases). As Van Lancker Sidtis (Chapter 12) point out formulaic language has been both neglected and misunderstood. However, she claims, it has finally come into its own and they cite a growing body of recently published research studies. Van Lancker Sidtis notes that formulaic expressions operate differently to the rules of grammar for novel expressions, suggesting such forms are reliant on instantaneous rather than incremental memory processes. The study of formulaic language has implications and relevance to models of language competence, language learning, and language loss in neurological disorders.

In Chapter 13, Yates notes that single word recognition and similarity in phonological and orthographic forms are issues of cognitive psychology that have been widely studied. This area of language processing is highly relevant when we consider the issue of literacy and language processing. Yates considers models of Interactive Activation and Competition (IAC) that have been influential in examining the effects of inhibition by words that have orthographic or phonological competitors.

Phonology has been an area of psycholinguistics that has been in the foreground of research in communication disorders for some time. Given that articulation therapy has often been seen as the "bread and butter" work of speech pathology, it is hardly surprising that theories of phonology have been of interest to researchers in communication disorders. The move away from linear phonetics and phonology to nonlinear approaches (e.g., autosegmental, feature geometry, and optimality theory) has led to a great deal of research in constraint-based phonology. However, this area of psycholinguistics has been highly debated in the research arena, particularly in relation to the issue of phonological representation. Tatham and Morton (Chapter 14) consider classical phonetic approaches to speech production in comparison to a cognitive approach and examine theories that see speech as a continuous dynamic process.

In contrast, Rutter and Ball (Chapter 15) overview theoretical approaches in phonology that have moved away from the traditional notion of considering that a child stores a representation of his/her ambient language's system of sounds. Such theories suggest that we have exemplars of each sound that enables processing of speech sounds to be carried out online. Ziegler, Ackermann, and Kappes (Chapter

16) draw on neurophonetics and brain imaging to examine the processing chain from abstract phonological representations to intended motor acts (articulation). As Ziegler and colleagues note, there is considerable disagreement about the separation of phonological and phonetic encoding and therefore further research incorporating a neurological approach is needed.

SECTION II: DEVELOPMENTAL DISORDERS

Chapters in this second section draw on many of the theoretical paradigms that have emerged from psycholinguistics and apply them to specific communication disorders. The authors of these chapters develop their own current work to exemplify the relevance of using theoretical constructs to better understand particular disorders and to provide evidence-based practice.

(Central) Auditory Processing Disorder (C)APD is a highly contentious area in the field of communication disorders. No researcher would deny the existence of a central area of the brain where auditory information is processed. However, whether or not an individual can have a disorder that is specific to the central auditory processing system and thus affects language development is hotly debated issue. In Chapter 17, Shive and Bellis examine current conceptualizations of Auditory Processing Disorder and the controversy surrounding (C)APD. They discuss the diagnosis of (C)APD and the neurobiological sequalae associated with the disorder. Burns (Chapter 18) considers this issue in a broader sense focusing on temporal processing in children with language disorders. She draws on the work of Tallal and colleagues (1981) to explore the issues of bottom-up and top-down processing and their role in language interventions.

In Chapter 19, Grela, Collisson, and Arthur provide a comprehensive review of theories that attempt to explain SLI. As they suggest, the classification of SLI was originally intended to differentiate between other language related conditions (e.g., mental retardation). Grela and colleagues suggest that children with SLI are a heterogeneous population with different underlying causes to their language deficit. In contrast, the work of van der Lely and Marshall (Chapter 20) make the case for a subgroup of children with specific problems in the morphosyntactic and phonological systems. Van der Lely has labeled this group Grammatical Specific Language Impairment (G-SLI). In a book that deals with current research into language processing there will invariably be an emphasis on connectionist approaches, but there is still a need to consider research such as van der Lely's because it points to a domain specific aspect of disorders such as G-SLI.

Storkel (Chapter 21) examines a subset of properties of lexical items that are typically incorporated within both adult and child models of spoken language processing. She considers several models of the lexicon in relation to normal development before applying these theories to the case of SLI.

Howell (Chapter 22) addresses the question of whether fluency disorders can be seen as a phenomenon that is caused by a breakdown in the motor system, which is assumed to operate independently of the language system, or whether the language system is involved. His research suggests that the problem could result from the processes by which language and speech are coupled. His theory of stuttering contrasts with two alternate theories, the covert repair hypothesis (Kolk & Postma, 1997) and the vicious cycle (Bernstein Ratner & Wijnen, 2007), theories that both draw on Levelt's model of speech production (1983, 1989).

The final three chapters in this section of the book apply theories of language processing to bilingual contexts. Armon-Lotem and Walters (Chapter 23) consider bilingual processing models before applying their approach to the contexts of bilingual SLI and schizophrenia. They suggest a way to approach assessment in cases of bilingual communication disorders and offer a way to analyze data from individual profiles to group patterns.

Bernhardt, Stemberger, Ayyad, Ullrich, and Zhao (Chapter 24) outline major characteristics of nonlinear phonology and consider the implications for clinical applications across four languages (English, Arabic, German, and Chinese). In Chapter 25, Restrepo, Morgan, and Smyk consider how SLI and bilingualism are at the crossroads of linguistic and psycholinguistic accounts of language. They discuss how bilingualism interfaces with SLI from the theoretical position of Dynamic Systems Theory and review research evidence of SLI in bilingual populations.

SECTION III: ACQUIRED DISORDERS

Chapters in this section focus on acquired disorders of language. Varley (Chapter 26) notes the historical divide between generative approaches and more diverse work in cognitive and neurobiological approaches to language disorders. She explores conceptualizations of the processes involved in speech programming, in particular, a dual mechanism model and its implications for acquired apraxia of speech.

McNeil, Hula, and Sung (Chapter 27) suggest that the traditional approach to researching and classifying aphasia has been framed within the anatomically based *centers* and *pathways* paradigm; a direct descendent of the Wernicke/Lichtheim model. They outline many attributes of aphasia that are untenable with this model and they discuss the role of working memory and particularly the executive attentional component of working memory as the source of the language impairments in persons with aphasia—constructs that are consistent with general attributes of aphasia and that are supported by the research directed toward these alternative cognitive mechanisms.

Lundgren and Brownell (Chapter 28) show how theory can be applied to clinical practice by reviewing a training program for brain injured adults that is based on Theory of Mind (see also Chapter 35). Lundgren and Brownell suggest that theory of mind performance can be differentiated from performance in other cognitive domains. In contrast, Togher (Chapter 29) examines the issue of cognitive disorganization in people with brain injuries and its effects of communication. She focuses on the heterogeneous nature of communication breakdown in brain injury and notes that theoretical advances in language processing are being translated into novel treatment approaches.

In Chapter 30, Shelley-Tremblay draws on his previous chapter outlining theories of semantic processing to provide further support for the hypothesis that many of the problems in dementia and aphasia are related not only to the representation of semantic information but also with the allocation of attention resources. He reviews ERP studies of dementia and relates their findings to the Center Surround Model (CSM). Finally in Chapter 31 of this section, Centeno examines the case of aphasia in bilingual individuals. In particular, he explores whether the monolingual and bilingual brains are organized differently.

OTHER MODALITIES

Last, but no means least, we have included a section on nonverbal aspects of communication processing, an area that has often been regarded as outside the field of language processing. This includes aspects of communication such as gesture, face processing, sign language, and augmentative and alternative communication (AAC). As McNeill and Duncan argue in Chapter 32, gesture is an integral part of the language system and should be treated as such. Indeed, gesture was likely the primary system of human communication to which later verbal forms were added.

Sign language is another area of language processing that should be included in any book relating to communication disorders. In Chapter 33, Hickok and Bellugi examine evidence from sign language to theorize on the neural organization of language, while in Chapter 34, Vermeerbergen and Van Herreweghe review the structure of sign language and examine research that explores the way in which sign language is processed.

In Chapter 35, Barnes and Baron-Cohen review theories that look at narrative in terms of the ability to ascribe mental states to others in the social world (Theory of Mind). They then present the results of a study that examined the way that individuals with and without Autism Spectrum Conditions (ASC) view film clips and produce narratives about what they have seen.

Although psycholinguists have been investigating the area of pragmatics since the 1970s, it is only recently that researchers have begun to explore this topic experimentally (see Novek & Sperber, 2004). Ryder and Leinonen (Chapter 36) draw on Relevance Theory (Sperber & Wilson, 1995) to explore the communication of children with language disorders. Although emerging from work in pragmatics, Relevance Theory is a psychological theory of communication that lends itself to experimental design.

Finally, we have also included an overview (Loncke, Chapter 37) of an area that is often overlooked in texts covering language processing, the psycholinguistics of AAC. The AAC is an area of communication that raises many questions for further research into how AAC users incorporate the language system to process other modalities of communication.

We hope this book will introduce students and new researchers in the field of communication disorders to an area we feel is an important area of language study. More importantly, we hope it will stimulate debate and encourage further research into the topics presented here. We have tried where possible to include contributors who are leaders in their field or who have grounded their work in theory to investigate questions relating to communication disorders. It is deliberate that many of the chapters in this book have overlapping interests and we encourage readers to cross-reference the different perspectives of the authors in pursuing an understanding of this fascinating field.

REFERENCES

Baddeley, A. D. (1986). *Working memory.* Oxford, England: Clarendon Press.

Baker, E., Croot, K., McLeod, S., & Paul, R. (2001). Pyscholinguistic models of speech development and their practice in clinical practice. *Journal of Speech, Language, & Hearing Research, 44,* 685–702.

Bates, E., & MacWhinney, B. (1982). Functionalist approaches to grammar. In E. Wanner & L. Gleitman (Eds.), *Language acquisition: The state of the art* (pp. 173–218). New York, NY: Cambridge University Press.

Bernstein Ratner, N., & Wijnen, F. (2007). The vicious cycle: Linguistic encoding, self monitoring and stuttering. In J. Au-Yeung & M. M. Leahy (Eds.), *Research, treatment and self help in fluency disorders: New horizons* (pp. 84–90). Proceedings of the Fifth World Congress on Fluency Disorders Dublin: The International Fluency Association.

Caplan, D. (1987). *Neurolinguistics and linguistic aphasiology.* New York, NY: Cambridge University Press.

Caplan, D., Waters, G., & DeDe, G. (2007). Specialized verbal working memory for language comprehension. In A. R. Conway, C. Jerrold, M. J. Kane, A. Miyake, & J. N. Towse (Eds.), *Variation in working memory.* New York, NY: Oxford University Press.

Chomsky, N. (1957). *Syntactic structures.* The Hague, Netherlands: Mouton.

Chomsky, N. (1959). Review of Skinner's verbal behavior. *Language, 35,* 26–58.

Chomsky, N. (1966). *Cartesian linguistics.* New York, NY: Harper and Row.

Evan, V., & Green, M. (2006). *Cognitive linguistics. An introduction.* Mahwah, NJ: Lawrence Erlbaum Associates.

Fitzgerald, E. (1954). *Straight language for the deaf: A system of instruction for deaf children.* Washington, DC: Volta.

Harley, T. A. (2008). *The psychology of language: From data to theory* (3rd ed.). New York, NY: Psychology Press.

Hayiou-Thomas, M. E., Bishop, D. V. M., & Plunkett, K. (2004). Simulating SLI: General cognitive processing stressors can produce a specific linguistic profile. *Journal of Speech, Language, and Hearing Research, 47*(6), 1347–1362.

Kolk, H., & Postma, A. (1997). Stuttering as a covert repair phenomenon. In R. F. Curlee & G. M. Siegel (Eds.), *Nature and treatments of stuttering: New directions* (pp. 182–203). Needham Heights, MA: Allyn & Bacon.

Levelt, W. (1983). Monitoring and self-repair in speech. *Cognition, 14,* 41–104.

Levelt, W. (1989). *Speaking: From intention to articulation.* Cambridge, MA: Bradford Books.

Nelson, K. (2000). Methods for stimulating and measuring lexical and syntactic advances. Why fiffins and lobsters can tag along with other recast friends. In L. Menn & N. Bernstein Ratner (Eds.), *Methods for studying language production* (pp. 115–148). Mahwah, NJ: Lawrence Erlbaum Associates.

Novek, I. A., & Sperber, D. (2004). *Experimental pragmatics.* Hampshire, UK: Palgrave Macmillan.

Piaget, J. (1997). *The child's conception of the world: Jean Piaget: Selected works* (A. Tomlinson & J. Tomlinson, Trans.). London: Routledge. (Original work published 1929.)

Russell, J. (2004). *What is language development? Rationalist, empiricist, and pragmaticist approaches to the acquisition of syntax.* Oxford, UK: Oxford University Press.

Saussure, De, F. (1916). *Cours de linguistique générale.* Paris, France: Payot.

Sedley, D. N. (2003). *Plato's Cratylus.* New York, NY: Cambridge University Press.

Skinner, B. F. (1957). *Verbal behavior.* New York, NY: Appleton, Century & Croft.

Sperber, D., & Wilson, D. (1995). *Relevance: Communication & cognition.* Oxford, UK: Oxford University Press.

Stackhouse, J., & Wells, B. (1997). *Children's speech and literacy difficulties: A psycholinguistic framework.* London, UK: Whurr.

Tallal, P., & Stark, R. E. (1981). Speech acoustic-cue discrimination abilities of normally developing and language-impaired children. *Journal of the Acoustic Society of America, 69*(2), 568–574.

Wyke, M. (1978). *Developmental dysphasia.* London, UK: Academic Press.

Section I

Some Basic Considerations: Models and Theories

1 The Development of Linguistic Systems: Insights From Evolution

John Locke

INTRODUCTION

About a year ago I encountered a statement that, on the surface, appeared to be eminently reasonable. It expressed the idea that linguistics may be able to grapple with evolutionary questions—a matter that has drawn new scholars at an exponential rate over the last 20 years—but not until linguists have come to a decision about what language is. One might suppose that similar thinking applies with equal force to development. How, according to the logic, can we possibly understand the development of language until we find out precisely what it is that develops?

There are at least two problems with this. The first is that it ignores the considerable merits of "reverse engineering." According to this methodology, we improve our understanding of language, and any other complex behavior, when we take it apart. Since language is a biological trait, this means, among other things, seeing how it was put together in evolution and comes together in development.

Reverse engineering contrasts sharply with the traditional approach. From the dawn of research on language development, the *leitmotif* has been to document the appearance of behaviors that seemed relevant to language or were actually linguistic. It was never clear what we might gain from knowing what these behaviors do for infants at the time of their appearance, if anything, nor was there an obvious way to find out. As a consequence, development was seen, by default, as something that "happens" to infants, not as an unfolding of new functions that contemporaneously benefit the infant and might, to some extent, be under the infant's own control.

There is, as mentioned, a second problem with the primacy of formal definition. It is a classic confrontation between internal evidence and external evidence. What if language met a series of discipline-internal tests but was later found to resist all attempts to characterize its emergence in the species and the child? Would we reject the principles of evolutionary and developmental change that have worked, with some success, for other traits, purely on the basis of the language experience; or would we argue that language is so unlike other complex traits that it emerged according to entirely different principles—ones unknown to biologists? Where evolution is concerned, one could argue that, to some extent, this has been happening for some time and is still taking place (e.g., Chomsky, 2002).

If we are more likely to understand language by looking at its evolution and development, I think we will be unusually advantaged if we look at the interactions that have occurred, and that still occur, between these processes (Locke, 2009). Evolution and development are collaborative. They feed each other. If we treat them independently, the result can only be distortion of each process and of the faculty of language itself.

I will begin here with a brief summary of evidence that, in its totality, indicates that language is a biological trait, as Steven Pinker (1994) famously declared, not a cultural trait or the product of some form of instruction. The emergence of "language" in the infant will be seen as the development of adaptive mechanisms that take in socially and linguistically relevant behaviors—among other "duties" that they might have—store this material long enough to extract organizing principles, and use the principles to generate novel utterances. This much relates to the code of language, but development also includes the activation of rather different mechanisms that oversee the application of linguistic knowledge by, and for the benefit of, the speaker in a variety of biosocial contexts. In the next section, I will examine a view of language that is widely shared in the linguistic community, one that has been unhelpfully influenced, paradoxically, by a factor that plays no role in its development—formal instruction—and by the cultural variables responsible for instructional institutions. In the succeeding section, I will ask what actually evolved, or could have evolved, according to a selection-based account in which observable behaviors enhanced fitness. The emergence of *these evolved traits*, I will submit, requires a new theoretical framework, one that provides a biological context for the development of neurological, cognitive, and social functions, as well as linguistic ones. Life history provides such a framework, partly because it enables one to trace critical effects of evolution on development, and partly because it is receptive, in principle, to reciprocal effects of development on evolution. In the end, what is needed is a strict evolutionary ↔ developmental ("evo-devo") approach or, better, evo-devo-evo-devo ...

LANGUAGE IS A BIOLOGICAL TRAIT

Language evolved in humans uniquely and develops in the young universally. A strong biological endowment was suspected a half-century ago when it was noted that infants acquire linguistic material rapidly in view of the seeming inadequacy of ambient models and the rarity of teaching or corrective feedback (Chomsky, 1959, 1980). Later, it was observed that infants appear to invent aspects of linguistic structure, as when pidgins are transformed into creoles (Bickerton, 1984) and deaf children reconstruct sign languages that have been awkwardly modeled by their nonnatively signing parents (Senghas & Coppola, 2001; Senghas, Kita, & Ozyurek, 2004). If only a portion of the language known to these individuals originated outside of their heads, then the rest, it has been assumed, must have come from the inside.

One consequence of the strong role played by *internal* factors is a course of development that appears relatively uneventful to observers, who tend to think that language, given its size and complexity, should require more *effort* than is actually witnessed. In some societies, of course, parents do direct a great deal of talk to their infants, and speak more slowly, or with exaggerated prosody; and they usually supply the names of particularly salient objects, actions, and concepts. These practices, or the disposition to engage in them, may not facilitate language learning (Hart & Risley, 1995; Nelson, Carskaddon, & Bonvillian, 1973), and may be no more helpful than merely modeling speech (Akhtar, 2005). But they cannot be essential, since infant-directed speech is rare in some societies (Ochs, 1982), and it is unusual—in any culture—for caregivers to do much that is specifically tutorial. Chomsky saw this disparity between knowledge and experience as "the most striking fact about human language." Accounting for it, he wrote, "is the central problem of linguistic theory" (Chomsky, 1967, p. 438).

For Chomsky, "knowledge" is linguistic grammar, the primary function of which is cognitive (2002). But "speech," as de Laguna advised, "must be envisaged ... as performing some objective and observable function, before one can hope to discern the factors which have led to its development" (1927, p. 10). Whether she meant to exclude "language" is unclear, but the distinction is salient, for speech does things that language does not do, and cannot do. These observable functions, we may assume, relate to the ways that people *use* language.

Some might consider questions of use to be outside the purview of language scientists. Others would surely rebut this contention, claiming that pragmatics, conversation rules, and other principles of usage are among the critical components of language. This division between lexical and grammatical knowledge on the one hand, and the social and communicative applications of language on the other, is one of the issues about which evolution and development have something important to say. But there is another issue here. Since we are dealing with an evolved trait, we must assume that the function of language determined its form in evolution, and to some extent continues to do so in development (Studdert-Kennedy, 1991). Since language evolved, it should be possible to locate cases where function was responsible for something about the physical nature of speech or ways of speaking.

LANGUAGE IS WHAT LINGUISTS SAY IT IS

Speaking is one of the more dynamic forms of human action that one can imagine, one so dynamic that critical elements fade as rapidly as they appear (Hockett, 1960). Linguistics, however, has encouraged its followers to regard language as an object, a stable cache of knowledge about grammar that is stored in the brains of all normal individuals who are socially reared. Although Chomsky (2002) is a strong proponent of this view, one can hardly blame him for the objectification of language. He was born four years after Jespersen complained that language was being viewed as a collection of "things or natural objects with an existence of their own" (Jespersen, 1924/1963, p. 17). Later, objectification troubled Lakoff and Johnson (1980), who commented that words and sentences were being seen as "objects that have properties in and of themselves and stand in fixed relationships to one another, independently of any person who speaks them or understands them" (p. 204). This depersonalized view of language also concerned Linell (2005), who commented that when linguists consult their intuitions on matters of linguistic practice, they encounter "an inventory of forms, and rules for generating forms" (p. 4). Recently Hermann (2008) called the language-as-thing metaphor a "systematically misleading expression." He suggested that it is time for a better metaphor, one that captures the fleeting and subjective nature of speech.

How did language come to be seen as an object? Most scholars blame literacy training (Goody, 1977; Jespersen, 1924/1963; Lakoff & Johnson, 1980; Linell, 2005; Olson, 1994). When people learn to read, they experience a cross-modal phenomenon that is on a par with hearing a taste or touching an odor. They *see words*. They also see spaces between the words in a sentence. If the language is alphabetic, they are conditioned to notice the sound symbols—hence the sounds—that make up words, and they additionally discover the spaces between these symbols. From capitalization and punctuation, their attention is further drawn to sentences and phrases.

It is instructive, I think, to consider the things that readers do *not* encounter on the printed page. They see no prosody, no voice quality, no tone of voice, no rate of speaking, no loudness, no vocal pitch, and no formant structure. As a consequence, they get little or no reliable information about the sender's identity, temperament, emotionality, attitude, social class, place of birth, height, age, sex, physical status, or hormonal status. These personal factors relate to important fitness variables such as social dominance and reproductive status, and therefore provide the raw material for evolutionary accounts of vocal communication and spoken language.

With speech literally off the page, it is not surprising that language would come to be conceptualized as whatever is left behind. But there is more, for literacy training is usually followed by 5 or 6 years of language arts instruction. Students learn the parts of speech. They are taught to recognize and correct sentences that are ungrammatical. They learn about topic sentences and paragraph structure and the importance of making sense. They become conscious of rules that they inferred in infancy and memorize others. It is a festival of linguistic prescription.

Predictably, literacy training affects the way individuals process linguistic material. In a study carried out in Portugal, subjects who were literate or culturally illiterate were enrolled in a lexical decision task. Concurrent brain scans revealed unequal activation of the right frontal opercular-anterior insular region, left anterior cingulate, left lentiform nucleus and anterior thalamus and hypothalamus in the two groups. In a separate repetition task, the illiterate subjects substituted real words for nonsense constructions 25 times more often than the literate subjects (Castro-Caldas, Petersson, Reis, Stone-Elander, & Ingvar, 1998; also see Ostrosky-Solís, Ramirez, & Ardila, 2004).

This work relates to the ways people think about and process language, but there are also huge measurement issues. Language is learned in one modality and tested in another. The result is a personal problem for good speakers who are poor readers, and a theoretical problem for scholars who wish to find out what the evolved trait of language actually entails (Locke, 2008a).

But it is not just a matter of conflicting modalities. Most standard measures of language are, in fact, evaluations of the ability to use linguistic knowledge *to solve cognitive problems* (e.g., anagrams). The relevant skills are usually classified as "metalinguistic." Individuals with metalinguistic ability are able "to deliberately reflect on and manipulate the structural features of spoken language" (Tunmer & Cole, 1991, p. 387). This ability does not naturally emerge from the biological trait of language. If untrained in literacy, normally speaking adults tend to perform poorly on metalinguistic tests (Morais, 2001; Navas, 2004; see Locke, 2008a for other references).

It is serious enough that academic training affects the way people process and use language and that scientists measure it, but instructed material forms a significant portion of the language that is *tested*. Recently, I analyzed some data collected over 90 years ago on an unusual population—the canal boat children of early 20th century England (Locke, 2008a). These children lived on boats, in constant interaction with their parents and siblings, but rarely went ashore or set foot in a classroom. Governmental concern brought about the evaluation of a number of the canal boat children using a standardized intelligence test. This instrument revealed that at 6 years, when all tests were necessarily oral, the canal boat children scored in the normal range on language measures. But as the years went by, they sank further and further below the norms on four oral subtests— language comprehension, vocabulary knowledge, sentence construction, and verbal fluency—while displaying age-appropriate abilities on nonverbal subtests. The children were not forgetting what they had learned about language, they were simply not improving at the same rate as their academic peers in the areas affected by instruction. At 12, their scores on the oral subtests approached zero. The results thus dramatized the fact that language, as tested, is heavily influenced by what children learn in schools.

All of these assessment, neuropsychological, and linguistic problems are significant, but they converge upon a hugely important biological issue. For it appears that formal training transforms language from a trait that was selected to a talent that is instructed (Locke, 2008a). A talent, according to Simonton (1999), is "any innate capacity that enables an individual to display exceptionally high performance in a domain that requires special skills and training" (p. 436). Competitive chess is considered a talent. No language scientist would assert that the faculty of human language *requires* instruction—we have already seen that it does not—but my claim here is that language, as it has come to be defined, *reflects* it. Formal instruction makes a talent out of a trait.

Having said all of this, I would not be particularly worried about these issues if my focus were the development of language in preschool children, as it once was (Locke, 1993a). But why stop studying the development of language (or anything else) just because the child starts school? Of course we know the answer—at this age, they know enough language and are cognitively mature enough to learn to read and take classroom instruction. But an evolutionary approach is necessarily blind to cultural inventions. We will see below and in the section on life history that the trait of language continues to develop well into adolescence.

LANGUAGE IS WHAT EVOLVED

There are some 6,912 natural languages in the world (Gordon, 2005). All of them are spoken. If just one of these languages was produced in a different modality, the incidence of nonvocal languages would be about 0.0001%, but the true incidence is zero. We do not know why the vocal modality is so robust, possibly because few scholars have taken the question seriously, or even recognized that this is a question that needs to be answered (Locke, 1998a). But it is possible that when we know what caused our ancestors to "go vocal" we will be a step closer to an explanation for language itself.

In the past, the higher primates have seemed to give us very little to work with. For some time, it appeared that apes were more gestural than vocal (Locke, 2001a). Even in recent years, linguists have looked at the ape literature and found little more than "a few calls and grunts" (Newmeyer, 2003). How, under the circumstances, could language-as-mental-code have entered the heads of their successors? If we are tacitly discouraged from addressing the modality of language, the medium that contains all of the physical cues, how do we get to the object? Framed in this way, the problem seems insoluble.

Fortunately, we have about six million years to work with—the time elapsed since the *Homo* line diverged from that of the apes. In that period, there were significant environmental changes that brought about a number of different adaptations. As we will see, two that were heavily deterministic were the shift to bipedalism and increased social complexity. It is also the case that the cognitive and communicative abilities of our last common ancestors were closer to those of humans than has generally been thought. For one thing, the functional value of ape vocalization has been greatly underestimated. While linguists were busily noting the vocal poverty of apes, animal behaviorists were conducting field studies that revealed unsuspected vocal riches. It is now clear that apes' calls and grunts carry a great deal of information about the age, size, and sex of individuals, as well as their location. They also carry information about the motivational state of the individual, and his intentions with respect to aggression and sex (Seyfarth & Cheney, 2003; see review in Locke, 2009). In its totality, this literature makes it less strange to ask where the human affection for vocal communication came from, even if we are left wondering how our species, and not the apes, evolved the capacity to control and process particulated vocalization (Oller, 2004; Studdert-Kennedy, 2005).

At the other end of the evolutionary spectrum—the theoretical endpoint—it is not psychologists' and linguists' ability to use and think about language that needs to be explained, but the ability of traditionally living individuals. For them, speaking seems to be more important than speech, the ability to joke, riddle, and tell stories more highly appraised than phonological (and grammatical) knowledge. The task, then, is to find links between the "more vocal than previously suspected" apes and the verbally artful members of traditional societies, and to ask how environmental changes produced fitness-enhancing behaviors that edged our evolutionary ancestors closer to spoken language.

In preliterate societies, language is heavily situational. This allows individuals to speak in a relatively inexplicit way (Linell, 2005). Some have difficulty thinking about the concept of "word" (Goody, 1977). Others act puzzled when asked what a word "means," possibly because words take their meaning from the context in which they are used (Malinowski, 1923). In some societies, words are thought to possess a "magical" quality (Tambiah, 1983). In none of these preliterate societies can a word's meaning be "looked up," nor can one know a word but wonder how it is pronounced.

In these societies, there are few if any schools, and no standardized language tests. Thus, what we know is what anthropologists have mentioned in their accounts. These descriptions make it clear that the communicative practices of traditionally living individuals appear neither as *language* nor *speech*. They appear as *speaking*. In these societies as with the apes, there is a special relationship between speaking and status. In a range of human societies anthropologists have noted unusual linguistic knowledge and rhetorical skill in individuals, invariably men, who have risen to positions of authority and power (Burling, 1986; Locke, 2001a; Locke & Bogin, 2006). I have speculated elsewhere that selection for vocal extravagance expanded the capacity to coordinate and control longer sequences of phonetic material, and that listeners who were able to evaluate these sequences received fitness information that others did not (Locke, 2008a,b, 2009).

There are links between speaking and sex, too. Miller's (2000) claim is that sexual selection shaped human language directly, through mate choice, and indirectly, through its effects on social status.

> Verbal courtship can be viewed narrowly as face-to-face flirtation, or broadly as anything we say in public that might increase our social status or personal attractiveness in the eyes of potential mates. Sexual flirtation during early courtship accounts for only a small percentage of language use, but it is the percentage with the most important evolutionary effects. This is the time when the most important reproductive decisions are made, when individuals are accepted or rejected as sexual partners on the basis of what they say. (Miller, 2000, pp. 356–357)

Spoken language may also have played a role in sexual selection outside of courtship by advertising various male qualities. It was through public speaking and debate that individuals were able

> to advertise their knowledge, clear thinking, social tact, good judgment, wit, experience, morality, imagination, and self-confidence. Under Pleistocene conditions, the sexual incentives for advertising such qualities would have persisted throughout adult life, in almost every social situation. Language put minds on public display,

where sexual choice could see them clearly for the first time in evolutionary history. (Miller, 2000, p. 357)

I agree that language helped to exhibit these qualities, but it could only do so when people spoke. Then, I propose, the variables facilitative of status and sex had less to do with grammar than various aspects of speaking, including prosody, fluency, rhythm, tone of voice, rate, loudness, and humor (Locke, 2001a). But these elements would have exerted no effect had they not enjoyed some relationship to fitness variables such as dominance and attractiveness for mating.

Below, in the section on life history, I will offer proposals as to how our ancestors evolved the capacity for controlled vocalization and speech at a level of complexity that prepared them for modern language, and suggest some functions of various events or milestones in the development of language.

LANGUAGE IS WHAT DEVELOPS

Purely by cataloguing the world's languages, we find out about the range of linguistic elements that can be handled by the nervous system of young humans. But what *is* language from the *infant's* point of view? Over 40 years ago, George Miller made a simple but provocative statement. The child, he wrote, "learns the language because he is shaped by nature to pay attention to it, to notice and remember and use significant aspects of it" (1965, p. 20). When I first thought about this I wondered what "it" was from the infant's perspective (Locke, 1993a). My reaction was that "it" must refer to the things people do while talking. This vocal, facial, and gestural activity, and associated situational cues, comprise the totality of linguistically relevant stimulation (Locke, 1993b, 1994).

The process gets off to an early start. Because fetuses eavesdrop on their mother's voice, infants are born with a preference not only for her voice, but for the language she spoke during this period, even when the speaker is someone else (DeCasper & Fifer, 1980; Moon, Cooper, & Fifer, 1993). But in an astonishingly short time, the mother's tongue lays the physical groundwork for what will become the infant's mother tongue. The most obvious function at this point is indexical learning—learning about people—but it incidentally produces linguistic learning.

So does what I have called "vocal communion," a continuous state or feeling of connectedness that is maintained largely by the vocalizations of infants and caregivers (Locke, 2001b). As we will see, infants place certain kinds of vocal behaviors in this channel, and are rewarded with physical approach, handling, and other forms of care. Several of the social behaviors that predict lexical learning, including joint attention and vocal imitation, may also be associated with maternal attachment. Since quality of attachment predicts language development (van Ijzendoorn, Kijkstra, & Bus, 1995), research is needed to determine those behaviors that are functionally related to language learning and that are only symptomatic of a relationship that is independently influential.

But of course infants do not merely listen. There is a call–response aspect to vocal signaling. When mothers vocalize, infants tend to respond and vice versa. This sort of communications link resembles what Schleidt (1973) called tonic communication. When they respond, there is a tendency on the part of caregivers and infants to do so "in kind"; that is, to produce like behaviors (Locke, 1993a). One might suppose that infants are "attempting" to learn to speak. But if that is the purpose, how do we explain mothers' frequent imitations of their infants (Pawlby, 1977; Veneziano, 1988)?

It is beginning to appear that vocal imitation may be an important way of demonstrating pacifistic intent and willingness to relate, possibly even to establish the identity of the other. Several years ago, Meltzoff and Moore (1994) published a relevant paper on 6-week-old infant's imitation of an adult's facial gestures. Each of several assistants came into the lab at various times and made a distinctive gesture, then left. When they returned to the lab the next day, the same assistants entered the room. Infants responded by reproducing the gesture that the assistants had made the day before, even if they merely saw the person on the second occasion. The results thus suggested that the infants were attempting to relate to, and possibly to identify, individuals on the basis of characteristic behaviors.

These results make it possible to see the function of a particular behavior—imitation—that would otherwise merely pass as something that infants do at certain ages. If the adult were to speak instead of gesture, there is nothing here to suggest that the infant would not reproduce aspects of his speaking voice as a means of relating to or identifying him. This would make it appear that the infant was learning language, and might suggest to some observers that the infant was aware of the existence of language, and was attempting to learn it.

Infants who traffic in *speech* are likely to be credited with progress in the acquisition of *language*. But perhaps this is not altogether inappropriate. In a prospective study of normally developing children, Nelson et al. (1973) found a relationship between the sheer number of utterances recorded in a session held at 20 months and the age at which a 50-word expressive vocabulary was attained. The number of utterances also was correlated with the age of children at their 10th phrase, and with their rate of lexical acquisition and mean length of utterances. Other work indicates that lexically delayed infants exhibit fewer vocally communicative intentions per minute than normally developing children (Paul & Shiffer, 1991), and produce far fewer utterances, independent of their quality (Paul & Jennings, 1992). Similar findings have been reported by others (Rescorla & Ratner, 1996; Thal, Oroz, & McCaw, 1995).

This is consistent with a paradox about language development. Infants rarely vocalize at normal levels of frequency and complexity during the babbling stage, imitate aspects of their mother's speech, and produce isolated words—behaviors that ostensibly require no grammatical ability at all—and later stumble as they enter the domains of morphology and syntax (Locke, 1998b). Whatever problems arise at the grammatical level of language are typically forecast by deficiencies in early lexical development (Bates & Goodman, 1997), just as the rate of word learning is predicted, to some degree, by the level of vocal sophistication and control revealed in the babbling stage (Oller, Eilers, Neal, & Schwartz, 1999).

But it gets better. Grammatical development is also linked to personality factors. Slomkowski, Nelson, Dunn, & Plomin (1992) found that a measure of introversion and extroversion at the age of 2 years was highly predictive of scores on eight different standardized language measures at the age of seven. Infants who were extraverted learned language with unusual speed. Thus, it appears that sociability and volubility—measures that are neither linguistic nor cognitive—predict the development of language even when it is defined as code.

How do we make sense of these links between volubility and the lexicon, and between personality and grammar? Earlier I referred to species-specific linguistic mechanisms. Language development involves the activation of these mechanisms, but there is no evidence that the mechanisms are turned on solely by maturation or exposure to people who talk. It makes more sense to suppose that they, like other neural systems, are *pressured* to turn on. I have suggested elsewhere that the precipitating event is a storage problem, created by the accumulation of utterances that are appropriately analyzed prosodically, but underanalyzed phonetically (Locke, 1997). It has been suggested that children must have a "critical mass" of words in their expressive lexicon—perhaps as many as 70 verbs, and 400 words overall—before they discover and begin to apply the rules of linguistic morphology (Bates, Dale, & Thal, 1994; Marchman & Bates, 1994; Plunkett & Marchman, 1993).

With language presupposing the operation of mechanisms that do other things, there is naturally a question about what the language faculty can be said to include. Hauser, Chomsky, & Fitch (2002) solved this problem, to their satisfaction, by positing a broad and a narrow faculty, the former including social and cognitive mechanisms, the latter excluding them. This is a reasonable way of thinking about linguistic systems, in a logical sense, but when it comes to development a different kind of "sense" creeps in. If social factors are critical to language, then they are *critical components* in the *developmental system* that is responsible for language. Here we begin to see the problem—the difference between a developmentally and a theoretically based definition of language.

We have seen that evolution plays a role in development. It supplied the mechanisms that, with appropriate experience, carry out linguistic operations. But it has been overlooked until recently that evolution also supplied the *developmental stages in which language develops*, so that when evolution produced new and modified developmental stages, they fed back new candidate behaviors for selection.

THE EVOLUTION OF DEVELOPMENT

To evolve, genetically supported traits must offer a selective advantage. Pinker and Bloom (1990) argued that natural selection is the only way to explain the origin of language and other complex abilities. In doing so, they said little about any role that selection might have played in development. But as Hogan (1988) has pointed out, natural selection "should operate at all stages of development, and not only on the adult outcome, since any developmental process that reduces the probability of reaching adulthood will be very strongly selected against" (p. 97). Thus, in this section I offer several new proposals relating to vocal and verbal selection as it may have operated in infancy and childhood.

There are lots of theories (or pseudotheories) of evolution in which language, like a *deus ex machina*, enters the hominin scene in the nick of time, supplying our ancestors with just the communicative tool they need to solve some pressing environmental problem. But evolution is a tinker who works from available parts. No species can manufacture a new part just because having it would come in handy.

Nor can an adult member of any species do this. No trait can evolve unless precursory forms appear during a stage of development, and *this is the only time that they can appear.* St. George Mivart hinted at this well over a century ago when he suggested that new species emerged from "affections of their generative system" (1871, p. 267). A half-century later, Walter Garstang wrote that ontogeny "creates" phylogeny. It is "absurd," he said, to think that a new trait could evolve in adults (Garstang, 1922).

In the interim, a number of respected biologists have embraced and elaborated upon Garstang's claim (Gottlieb, 2002; Gould, 1977; Northcutt, 1990; West-Eberhard, 2003; see other references in Locke, 2009). It is now understood that evolution is a two-step process (West-Eberhard, 2003). In the first step, a plastic phenotype responds to environmental variation—in development—producing novel forms that vary genetically. In the second step, selection acts on the variants. A selection-based account of language cannot be complete unless it identifies the linguistically favorable genetic variations that arise in ontogeny and the processes of selection that reinforced and expanded those variations.

If development occurs in stages, then behaviors that develop owe their existence to some feature of those stages. This implores us to look beyond the development of mechanisms that evolved and explore the *evolution of development.* I believe the case can be made that in evolution, some type of selection occurred for language—or what was to become language—at every stage of development from infancy to sexual maturity—and that each new behavior that develops serves a distinct function. I have suggested elsewhere that selection in infancy helped produce the vocal complexity and social functionality that were later reselected in the rather different biological contexts supplied by childhood, juvenility, and adolescence (Locke, 2006). But even if selection had initially applied in adolescence, the behaviors reinforced at that stage would already have to have "been there" in some form, even if they had never functioned in the new way.

To be prepared for a socially complex adulthood, there must be appropriately structured intervals for development and learning. Humans have four such stages—two more than the other primates. We also have two stages that were remodeled (Bogin, 1999a). I propose that all four of these new and remodeled stages were needed for language to evolve, and that all four are needed for the young to acquire knowledge of language and to become fully proficient in its use (Locke, 2009; Locke & Bogin, 2006).

The approach to human life history that will be used here was developed by Barry Bogin (1988; 1999a). Much of what will be said about the individual stages is adapted from a paper coauthored with Bogin several years ago (see Locke & Bogin, 2006 for details and references).

INFANCY

Infancy begins at or before birth and ends at about 30 to 36 months when, in traditional societies, weaning takes place. This stage is characterized by rapid physical growth, provision of nourishment by maternal lactation, and eruption of deciduous dentition. Human infants are more helpless than ape and monkey infants, a "deficiency" that requires a long period of continuous care.

It is thought that the initial change that produced greater helplessness was bipedal locomotion, which realigned the spine and narrowed the pelvis. This produced problems at birth for the mother and her large-headed fetus. There being a range of variation among infants, some had smaller heads at the time of birth, and these infants—and their mothers—were more likely to survive the delivery. Over time, differential rates of survival caused a shift in skull and brain development from the prenatal to the postnatal period. This increased infant dependency and need of care.

These changes *remodeled* the premodern human infancy. In doing so, they positioned it for language and other complex behaviors. For, in a number of important respects, the conditions above—in danger of being seen as design flaws—offered more and better opportunities for social, vocal, lexical, and symbolic learning (Bjorklund, 1997; Locke, 1993a, 1999).

This tendency to view helplessness and heightened care as socially and cognitively beneficial is supported by anthropological accounts, which indicate that most hunter–gatherer mothers rarely put their babies down, and then do so for no more than a few seconds. Separation cries usually evoke pick up and breast feeding. When infants cannot be carried, they are often left in the care of others (Hrdy, 2006).

Beginning prenatally, infants learn aspects of the prosodic and segmental characteristics of the ambient language. By 6 months, most infants have heard enough speech to recognize a few words and stereotyped phrases, and to experience some perceptual reorganization, a process that continues in succeeding months.

From a variety of developments in the first year or life, parents and language scientists alike conclude that infants are learning speech or acquiring language. Undoubtedly they are, but in some sense, these advances are unintended consequences. There are many reasons why helpless individuals might benefit by attending to, storing, and reproducing caregiver speech, most of which have a great deal to do with the negotiation of their own care (Locke, 1996).

In our species, weaning comes earlier than it does in the apes. It is generally held that earlier weaning would have shortened the interbirth interval, enabling women to have more infants in their reproductive lifetime. I have proposed that this produced an increase in the number of siblings—competitors for care. This heightened competition, combined with unprecedented levels of helplessness, forced infants to explore clever new ways of using the voice to secure and maintain maternal proximity, and to monitor and "read" maternal feedback; and that, therefore, some of the vocal ability presupposed by spoken languages was asserted initially by hominin infants and reinforced by successful interactions with their parents.

According to the proposal, infants who issued more effective care-elicitation signals received more care, and were marginally more likely to live on to reproductive age (Locke, 2006). The *parental selection* hypothesis proposes that some of the vocal ability presupposed by spoken languages emerged from infancy, having been asserted initially by hominin infants and supported by interactions with their parents. This hypothesis holds that infants who issued more effective care-elicitation signals (e.g., measured or strategic levels of cry) were better positioned to receive care than infants who issued stress vocalizations noxiously or inconsolably—behaviors that invite neglect and abuse in primates generally, and forecast language-learning problems in humans. The hypothesis also envisions that infants who cooed and babbled at appropriate intervals were more likely to engage with adults, to be liked by them, to receive more sophisticated forms of care as infancy progressed, and to generate and learn complex phonetic patterns. Infants who were able to monitor adult reactions to their behaviors would have been able to discover those vocalizations that had the most beneficial effects, and thus could use structured vocalization to maximum effect.

It is also possible that syllabic and articulatory activity played a "decoupling" role (Oller, 2004), making available for recombination the discrete movements, hence the phonetic segments that make phonological systems possible (Studdert-Kennedy, 1998; 2005; Studdert-Kennedy & Goldstein, 2003). I propose that further elaboration of vocal repertoires would have occurred later in development under different pressures, potentially enhancing fitness in one or more of these stages, particularly adolescence. The result is a system flexible enough to be used for speech, and there is evidence that vocal abilities presupposed by variegated babbling are in fact adequate for infants' initial words (Vihman, Macken, Miller, Simmons, & Miller, 1985).

It is generally recognized that development is continuous, but continuity would also have played a role in evolution. I have proposed that new levels of vocal complexity, flexibility, and control that emerged from infancy were carried into later ontogenetic stages where—development being continuous and cumulative—they were reinforced and elaborated (Locke & Bogin, 2006). In the new childhood that evolved (see below), these signaling capabilities would surely have proved beneficial, for if children are to avoid hazardous aspects of their environment, they must be warned if not "instructed."

It is at this point that we begin to see the first of several sets of discontinuities. In the typical case, the close of intimacy is co-timed with evidence that the mechanisms responsible for each of the recognized components of language-as-code—the lexicon, phonology, morphology, and syntax—are operating at some level of efficiency.

CHILDHOOD

Childhood is a uniquely human stage that is thought to have entered the *Homo* line about two million years ago (Bogin, 2001, 2003). Since chimpanzees wean at about five years, it is assumed that earlier weaning liberated about two years from infancy. This is what created childhood (Bogin, 1990). It has been suggested that the extension of childhood to its present length—which extends from about three to nearly seven years—was due, at least in part, to the increasing functionality of communicative behaviors in this stage (Locke & Bogin, 2006).

The childhood stage is peculiar to humans, having been evolutionarily inserted between the infant and juvenile stages that characterize social mammals. Childhood, according to Bogin, is defined by several developmental characteristics including: a deceleration and stabilization of the rate of growth, immature dentition, dependence on older people for food, and immature motor control. The evolutionary value of childhood is associated with the mother's freedom to stop breast-feeding her 3-year-old, enabling her to become pregnant again. This enhanced reproductive output without increasing the risk of mortality for the mother or her infant or older children, for in cooperatively breeding societies, others were available to help care for the young.

Childhood is largely defined by the long period, extending from 3 to 7 years, in which food must be provided. By seven, dentition is becoming adult-like, and with parallel increases in jaw control, it becomes possible for children to eat adult foods. Socially, childhood produces new friendships outside of the home as well as increased disenchantment with siblings. In some modern societies, 5-year-olds have social hierarchies. In these hierarchies, low-status children behave positively toward their higher status peers, without reciprocity. Children with good communication skills are likely to be popular (Asher & Renshaw, 1981; Putallaz & Gottman, 1981), whereas children with speech and language disorders are typically unpopular, and may even be victimized (Conti-Ramsden & Botting, 2004). Children with pragmatic or higher-level language processing disorders are likely to experience serious peer interaction problems (Botting & Conti-Ramsden, 2000). Delayed language predicts poor quality of friendship in adolescence; it may independently impair friendship or do so in conjunction with poor social cognition (Botting & Conti-Ramsden, 2008; Durkin & Conti-Ramsden, 2007).

As childhood draws to an end, a second set of discontinuities in native language learning occurs. One relates to the fact that languages acquired after the age of six are often produced with an accent that reflects interference from previously learned languages (Flege & Fletcher, 1992). In large epidemiological samples of midwestern American children, 6 years of age was also treated as the approximate age of native language mastery, based on standardized tests that are oriented to school performance (Shriberg, Tomblin, & McSweeny, 1999; Tomblin et al.,

1997). Thus, in one modern society, and undoubtedly far more, much of the childhood period is needed to master the basic structure and elementary vocabulary of a knowledge-based linguistic system.

But there is more to be accomplished in childhood. One advance involves verbal fluency, which continues to improve throughout this stage (Starkweather, 1987). Other developments relate to automaticity and rate of speaking (Smith, 2006). If something goes wrong with the sensory system that guides ambient learning during childhood, there is likely to be significant deterioration of speech. Clinical studies indicate that all of childhood is needed to achieve a speaking ability that can tolerate the discontinued stimulation entailed by acquired deafness (Waldstein, 1990; also see Locke & Bogin, 2006).

Some of the communicative skills arising in childhood do so in tandem with certain cognitive advances. One such development is the "theory of other minds," which typically emerges between 2 and 4 years of age (Baron-Cohen, Tager-Flusberg, & Cohen, 1993), enabling children to take the perspective of others. There is also an improvement in autobiographical memory, which usually occurs between 3 and 8 years of age (Nelson, 1996), enabling children to describe sequential events and to share memories of their own experience. This comports with the fact that childhood also sees improvement in discourse and narration (Girolametto, Wiigs, Smyth, Weitzman, & Pearce, 2001).

In recent years, there has been increased attention to pragmatics, but there are few if any accounts of language development that seriously address verbal performance. Some of the developments that occur in childhood relate to verbal competition and performance. These include joking (McGhee, 1979; Shultz & Horibe, 1974) and the use of "off the shelf" verbal routines (Gleason & Weintraub, 1976). In many cultures, jokes and riddles mark the beginning of various sorts of verbal competition (Gossen, 1976a,b; Sanches & Kirshenblatt-Gimblett, 1976).

During childhood, males tend to speak assertively to get and maintain attention and to make evident their desires, and girls tend to speak softly in order to promote interpersonal closeness and harmony (see review in Locke & Bogin, 2006). The linguistic acquisitions of infancy are thus joined, in childhood and succeeding stages, by other factors that elevate the quality of verbal expression and facilitate development of communicative skills (e.g., Sherzer, 2002).

Since it begins with weaning, childhood liberated the young from continuous maternal restraint. Naïve children's exploration of their physical environment presumably increased the need for parents to warn and instruct, giving them and other kin self-serving reasons to send honest signals. But childhood also positioned the young to know about, thus to convey information about, events occurring in the absence of others. I would suggest that childhood handed the young and their families a key ingredient of human language—displacement—in the form of new opportunities and needs to talk about things not physically present (Fitch, 2004; Hockett, 1960). It is possible that the swing period in development of native-like language abilities—6 to 8 years of age—is related to changing pressures associated with the transition to a more independent and autonomous stage of development.

In development, childhood would have given the young opportunities to integrate and automate linguistic operations, to introspect on language and to analyze it, and to develop an appreciation of rhyme, alliteration, fluency—all of which would be needed in juvenility.

Juvenility

Juvenility is the next stage of human development. In mammals generally and primates more specifically, juveniles are sexually immature but independent of others for survival. It is not unusual in traditional human societies for juveniles to find much of their own food, avoid predators, and compete with adults for food and space (see Locke & Bogin, 2006).

Juvenility begins at 7 years, with the onset of adrenarche and associate cognitive and social advances. This stage ends at 10 and 12 years in females and males, respectively. Juveniles are sexually immature but more independent of older individuals than children. Since it comes after a remodeled infancy and new childhood, the juvenile stage of our evolutionary ancestors could hardly have remained unchanged. In various species of mammals, juvenility provides additional time for the brain growth and learning that is required for reproductive success (Janson & van Schaik, 1993; Joffe, 1997). In complex human societies, it takes all of juvenility and adolescence for the development of social and linguistic skills that are needed in sexual maturity.

Although there is increased independence from family members in childhood, juvenility would have given the young opportunities to prepare themselves, while still sexually immature, for a stage in which vocal and verbal performance would play a prominent role in the competition for precious resources—particularly sex and dominance (Locke, 2001a; Locke & Bogin, 2006). Many of the language developments that occur in modern juvenility take place beyond the sentence level, in the quality of extended discourse and narratives. New abilities in pragmatics and verbal performance contribute to a variety of socially relevant activities, from gossiping to joking and storytelling.

Juvenility also accommodates additional syntactic advances (cf. Nippold, 1998), but many of the new developments affect *performance*. These include an increase in respiratory capacity, which continues into adolescence (Engström, Karlberg, & Kraepellen, 1956; Hoit, Hixon, Watson, & Morgan, 1990), and further increases in fluency and speaking rate. Changes occur beyond the sentence level too, in the quality of extended discourse and narratives (Bamberg, 1987; Burleson, 1982; Karmiloff-Smith, 1985). These advances facilitate a number of socially relevant activities, including gossip and storytelling, and contribute to successful competition and courtship as sexual maturity approaches.

Around 10 to 12 years, riddles and jokes become more important. In Turkey, boys engage in verbal duels—ritualistic insults and replies that require "skill in remembering and selecting appropriate retorts to provocative insults" (Dundes, Leach, & Özkök, 1970, p. 135). These duels occur between 8 and 14 years, bracketing the transition from juvenility to adolescence.

In a sense, juvenility parallels infancy. Whereas the linguistic knowledge and structure gained in infancy helps to satisfy the informational needs of childhood, juvenility provides opportunities to perfect the persuasive and attractive use of speech, and the ability to manipulate elaborate and socially appropriate utterances, which will be valued in adolescence.

ADOLESCENCE

Adolescence is the fourth stage of life history, and the second stage that is uniquely human, since the other primates proceeding directly from juvenility to adulthood (Bogin, 1999b). This stage begins at the end of juvenility and extends to 19 years, when adulthood commences. In modern humans, adolescence is announced by puberty and a simultaneous surge in skeletal growth, strengthening of friendships, and development of new relationships.

In humans, uniquely, there is a distinct skeletal growth spurt in both sexes after several years of gently decreasing juvenile growth. The onset of this spurt, along with puberty or gonadarche marks the onset of adolescence (Bogin, 1999a). Neuroendocrinological changes differentially affect the vocal tract of the two sexes, females revealing negligible changes, males displaying a significant increase in tract length and decrease in fundamental frequency, with further drops in the transition from adolescence to adulthood (Fitch & Giedd, 1999; Lieberman, McCarthy, Hiiemae, & Palmer, 2001; Pedersen, Moller, Krabbe, & Bennett, 1986; Pedersen, Møller, Krabbe, Bennett, & Svenstrup, 1990; Vuorenkoski, Lenko, Tjernlund, Vuorenkoski, & Perheentupa, 1978). The critical variable, testosterone, increases the size of the vocal folds, lowers the fundamental frequency, and changes the vibratory characteristics of the vocal folds (Abitol, Abitol, & Abitol, 1999; Beckford, Rood, & Schaid, 1985; Titze, 1989).

In adolescence—if not sooner—and certainly in adulthood, males also display lung and respiratory superiority over females (Becklake, 1999; Cook & Hamann, 1961; Hibbert, Lannigan, Raven, Landau, & Phelan, 1995; Higgins & Saxman, 1991; Schrader, Quanjer, & Olievier, 1988; Thurlbeck, 1982). Although this variable is often neglected in developmental accounts of language, even in accounts of speech, it undoubtedly has a great deal to do with speaking in a public and competitive way. In humans and a range of other species, respiratory capacity is positively correlated with body size (Engström et al., 1956; Helliesen, Cook, Friedlander, & Agathon, 1958; Stahl, 1967; Tenney & Remmers, 1963), and in the context of mate selection, this ability is likely to have been of considerable interest to ancestral females.

In men, status and dominance are linked to testosterone (Mazur & Booth, 1998), which tends to be higher in men with low vocal pitch (Dabbs & Mallinger, 1999; Pedersen et al., 1986). It comes as no surprise, then, that men with low-pitched voices are judged by female listeners, from vocal samples, to be more dominant and attractive (Collins, 2000; Collins & Missing, 2003; Feinberg, Jones, Little, Burt, & Perrett, 2005; Puts, Gaulin, & Verdolini, 2006). Women also *prefer* male voices that are low in pitch (Collins, 2000; Oguchi & Kikuchi, 1997), a preference that appears to be enhanced by estrogen (Feinberg et al., 2006; Puts, 2005). Male university students with low voices report slightly more sexual partners than other men (Puts et al., 2006), and baritone opera singers report having more affairs than tenors (Wilson, 1984). In hunter–gatherer societies, men with low voices report fathering more children than men with higher voices (Apicella, Feinberg, & Marlowe, 2007). These findings could be taken to mean that vocal pitch is a fixed trait, but of course men are able to manipulate their voices, and do so when it could alter their perceived dominance (Puts et al., 2006).

Earlier I mentioned rising group size and rising social complexity as a spur to increased brain size and linguistic behavior. If these pressures applied with unusual force during any one of the stages of life history, adolescence—when the draw of the group is especially strong—would surely be that stage. It is therefore interesting that recent imaging research is now indicating that adolescence, to a surprising degree, is a time of renewed brain development. The volume of cerebral gray matter sharply decreases from childhood to adolescence, evidently due to dendritic pruning, and there are large increases in white matter, caused by myelination, increases in axonal size, and glial proliferation (De Bellis et al., 2001; Giedd, 2005; Giedd et al., 2001; Shaw et al., 2006). This pattern of exuberant growth and pruning is relevant to arguments that adolescence conferred reproductive advantages on our ancestors, partly by giving the young additional opportunities to acquire social and sexual skills before reproducing (Bogin, 1999a,b).

Adolescence provides opportunities to learn the pragmatic and performative skills that are needed to converse and to narrate (Dorval & Eckerman, 1984; Nippold, 1998). It also offers opportunities to learn slang, idioms, and other formulaic expressions, which contribute to group solidarity and enhance the ability to perform, possibly by increasing fluency and rate of speech for that material (Kuiper, 1996). Other performance skills that develop in adolescence include refinements in gossiping, joking, arguing, negotiating, and persuading; and in the rate of speaking (Walsh & Smith, 2002). All these skills stand to impress peers and facilitate the achievement and maintenance of social relationships.

I have emphasized adolescence as an innovative stage with reproductive advantages. The reason, in part, relates to the benefits and pressures associated with group life. Dunbar (1993) has argued that group pressures played a role in the evolution of language. It is reasonable to suppose that the benefits of group affiliation, and the achievement of personal identity and autonomy, have motivated adolescents to invent vocal and verbal behaviors, thereby reinforcing any improvisational abilities carried forward from previous stages. Modern adolescents do not merely learn additional linguistic features and rules of usage. They also modify material learned earlier, and invent new words and constructions. But the changes are not merely lexical. "The relatively high degree of phonological innovation in the adolescent age group," wrote Eckert (1988), "is an indication that the development of adolescent social structure provides a major impetus for phonological change" (p. 197).

Development of other secondary sexual characteristics, and a sharp increase in height and weight, also occur in adolescence. These physical changes are paralleled by an intensification of preexisting friendships, and the development of new relationships. The new affiliations, and membership in peer groups, facilitate intimacy and mutual support (Whitmire 2000). Adolescence draws to a close with the attainment of adult stature and the biosocial skills needed for successful reproduction. Typically, this occurs at about 19 years of age in women and 21 to 25 years in men (Bogin 1999a, 2001).

CONCLUDING REMARKS

If development occurs in stages, then behaviors that develop owe their existence to some feature of those stages. This implores us to look beyond the development of mechanisms that evolved and explore the evolution of the developmental stages themselves, asking which of many biological factors are responsible for the induction of linguistic systems.

The stages of life history have unique and coherent properties. These properties provide the context for a range of social and cognitive developments, including language. This suggests that there are linguistic discontinuities at stage boundaries. Several have been identified here, but there are likely to be a great many others.

In research on language development, there is a tendency to focus on infancy and childhood, probably because it is during these stages that knowledge of words and grammatical rules is acquired. This accords well with implicit views of language as an object. But knowledge of language enables one to speak, thus to act in social situations, and to express oneself in social groups. By adopting human life history as our theoretical framework, one is encouraged to ask about the contribution of each developmental stage, from infancy and childhood through juvenility and adolescence, and it is during these later stages that this second (social) view of language becomes more salient.

It is for these reasons that developing individuals who speak in accepted ways should experience far more social success than those who do not, and there is no shortage of evidence that this is so. However, the causes of social acceptance (and rejection) at sexual maturity are not as closely linked to linguistic knowledge and structure as to vocal and verbal performance. Clearly, the relevant *speaking skills*—the perceptible and, from a causal standpoint, proximate behaviors—presuppose prior accomplishment in all areas of language, however inconspicuous these accomplishments might be initially.

Until now, research on language development has emphasized acquisition of a lexicon and linguistic grammar, but other advances in maturation, learning, and consolidation are necessary for the young to speak informatively, attractively, and persuasively, thus competitively. If in evolution, as now, these developments occurred during a stage that follows childhood, communicative ability in *preceding* stages would have been important. In a treatise on the embryological development of the chick, Caspar Friedrich Wolff wrote, "each part is first of all an effect of the preceding part, and itself becomes the cause of the following part" (Wolff 1764, in Hall 1999, p. 112). Since development is continuous, one supposes that infants and children who achieved effective use of sound-meaning signals precociously carried some form of the relevant control behaviors into juvenility and adolescence. The result, on a continuity hypothesis, would have been other exceptional skills in the use of spoken language. These would have facilitated attainment for status, sex, and additional resources, enhancing reproductive success while strengthening the precursory behaviors that had persisted, in some form, from earlier stages.

I have suggested that studies of language development can benefit from a new model—one that explores synergies between evolution and development. Such a model encourages us to think in new ways about development and to explore new issues. These include the fitness-cue value of various components of spoken language. If elements of speech were selected, they may now be supported by special-purpose mechanisms. To the degree that they are, the behaviors enabled by these mechanisms may enjoy a different developmental course than other behaviors.

It is clear that we need a functional account of vocal imitation, one that parallels work on facial and manual activity, and its necessity to develop greater understanding of the proximal mechanisms that are at work in infants' learning of vocal and symbolic activity. Before infants become aware of the communicative value of linguistic material, they absorb and accommodate to it, but on what motivation?

Where the faculty of language is concerned, the biological trait that evolved was the ability to speak, and yet there are no standardized tests of speaking. As a consequence, we have no way to measure the relationship of language-as-code and the ability to speak, where speaking is sensitive to performance variables of the sort mentioned above. There is room for a great deal of research here.

REFERENCES

Abitol, J., Abitol, P., & Abitol, B. (1999). Sex hormones and the female voice. *Journal of Voice, 13*, 424–446.

Akhtar, N. (2005). The robustness of learning through overhearing. *Developmental Science, 8*, 199–209.

Apicella, C. L., Feinberg, D. R., & Marlowe, F. W. (2007). Voice pitch predicts reproductive success in male hunter-gatherers. *Biology Letters, 3*, 682–684.

Asher, S. R., & Renshaw, P. D. (1981). Children without friends: Social knowledge and social-skill training. In S. R. Asher & J. M. Gottman (Eds.), *The development of children's friendships.* Cambridge, UK: Cambridge University Press.

Bamberg, M. (1987). *The acquisition of narratives.* Berlin, Germany: Mouton de Gruyter.

Baron-Cohen, S., Tager-Flusberg, H., & Cohen, D. J. (Eds.). (1993). *Understanding other minds: Perspectives from autism.* New York, NY: Oxford University Press.

Bates, E., Dale, P. S., & Thal, D. (1994). Individual differences and their implications for theories of language development. In P. Fletcher & B. MacWhinney (Eds.), *Handbook of child language.* Oxford, UK: Basil Blackwell.

Bates, E., & Goodman, J. C. (1997). On the inseparability of grammar and the lexicon: Evidence from acquisition, aphasia and real-time processing. *Language and Cognitive Processes, 12*, 507–584.

Beckford, N. S., Rood, S. R., & Schaid, D. (1985). Androgen stimulation and laryngeal development. *Annals of Otology, Rhinology, and Laryngology, 94*, 634–640.

Becklake, M. R. (1999). Gender differences in airway behaviour over the human life span. *Thorax, 54*, 1119–1138.

Bickerton, D. (1984). The language bioprogram hypothesis. *Behavioral and Brain Sciences, 7*, 173–188.

Bjorklund, D. F. (1997). The role of immaturity in human development. *Psychological Bulletin, 122*, 153–169.

Bogin, B. (1988). *Patterns of human growth*. Cambridge, UK: Cambridge University Press.

Bogin, B. (1990). The evolution of human childhood. *BioScience, 40*, 16–25.

Bogin, B. (1999a). *Patterns of human growth* (2nd ed.). New York, NY: Cambridge University Press.

Bogin, B. (1999b). Evolutionary perspective on human growth. *Annual Review of Anthropology, 28*, 109–153.

Bogin, B. (2001). *The growth of humanity*. New York, NY: Wiley-Liss.

Bogin, B. (2003). The human pattern of growth and development in paleontological perspective. In J. L. Thompson, G. E. Krovitz, & A. J. Nelson (Eds.), *Patterns of growth and development in the Genus Homo*. Cambridge, UK: Cambridge University Press.

Botting, N., & Conti-Ramsden, G. (2000). Social and behavioural difficulties in children with language impairment. *Child Language Teaching & Therapy, 16*, 105–120.

Botting, N., & Conti-Ramsden, G. (2008). The role of language, social cognition, and social skill in the functional social outcomes of young adolescents with and without a history of SLI. *British Journal of Developmental Psychology, 26*, 281–300.

Burleson, B. R. (1982). The development of comforting communication skills in childhood and adolescence. *Child Development, 53*, 1578–1588.

Burling, R. (1986). The selective advantage of complex language. *Ethology and Sociobiology, 7*, 1–16.

Castro-Caldas, A., Petersson, K. M., Reis, A., Stone-Elander, S., & Ingvar, M. (1998). The illiterate brain: Learning to read and write during a childhood influences the functional organization of the adult brain. *Brain, 121*, 1053–1063.

Chomsky, N. (1959). Review of *Verbal Behavior*, by B. F. Skinner. *Language, 35*, 26–58.

Chomsky, N. (1967). The formal nature of language. Appendix A, Lenneberg, E. *Biological foundations of language*. New York, NY: Wiley.

Chomsky, N. (1980). *Rules and representations*. Oxford, UK: Basil Blackwell.

Chomsky, N. (2002). *On nature and language*. Cambridge, UK: Cambridge University Press.

Collins, S. A. (2000). Men's voices and women's choices. *Animal Behaviour, 60*, 773–780.

Collins, S. A., & Missing, C. (2003). Vocal and visual attractiveness are related in women. *Animal Behaviour, 65*, 997–1004.

Conti-Ramsden, G., & Botting, N. (2004). Social difficulties and victimization in children with SLI at 11 years of age. *Journal of Speech, Language, and Hearing Research, 47*, 145–161.

Cook, C. D., & Hamann, J. F. (1961). Relation of lung volumes to height in healthy persons between the ages of 5 and 38 years. *Journal of Pediatrics, 59*, 710–714.

Dabbs, J. M., & Mallinger, A. (1999). Higher testosterone levels predict lower voice pitch among men. *Personality and Individual Differences, 27*, 801–804.

De Bellis, M. D., Keshavan, M. S., Beers, S. R., Hall, J., Frustaci, K., Masalehdan, A., … Boring, A. M. (2001). Sex differences in brain maturation during childhood and adolescence. *Cerebral Cortex, 11*, 552–557.

DeCasper, A., & Fifer, W. P. (1980). On human bonding: Newborns prefer their mothers' voices. *Science, 208*, 1174–1176.

de Laguna, G. A. (1927). *Speech: Its function and development*. New Haven, CT: Yale University Press.

Dorval, B., & Eckerman, C. O. (1984). Developmental trends in the quality of conversation achieved by small groups of acquainted peers. *Monographs of the Society for Research in Child Development* (Serial No. 206), *49*, 1–91.

Dunbar, R. I. M. (1993). Coevolution of neocortical size, group size and language in humans. *Behavioral and Brain Sciences, 16*, 681–694.

Dundes, A., Leach, J. W., & Özkök, B. (1970). The strategy of Turkish boys' verbal dueling rhymes. In J. J. Gumperz & D. Hymes (Eds.), *Directions in sociolinguistics: The ethnography of communication.* New York, NY: Holt, Rinehart and Winston.

Durkin, K., & Conti-Ramsden, G. M. (2007). Language, social behaviour, and the quality of friendships in adolescents with and without a history of specific language impairment. *Child Development, 78*, 1441–1457.

Eckert, P. (1988). Adolescent social structure and the spread of linguistic change. *Language and Society, 17*, 183–207.

Engström, I., Karlberg, P., & Kraepellen, S. (1956). Respiratory studies in children. *Acta Paediatrica, 46*, 277–294.

Feinberg, D. R., Jones, B. C., Law Smith, M. J., Moor, F. R., DeBruine, L. M., Cornwell, R. E., ... Perrett, D. I. (2006). Menstrual cycle, trait estrogen level, and masculinity preferences in the human voice. *Hormones and Behavior, 49*, 215–222.

Feinberg, D. R., Jones, B. C., Little, A. C., Burt, M. D., & Perrett, D. I. (2005). Manipulations of fundamental frequency and formant frequencies influence the attractiveness of human male voices. *Animal Behaviour, 69*, 561–568.

Fitch, W. T. (2004). Kin selection and "mother tongues": A neglected component in language evolution. In D. K. Oller & U. Griebel (Eds.), *The evolution of communication systems: A comparative approach.* Cambridge, MA: MIT Press.

Fitch, W. T., & Giedd, J. (1999). Morphology and development of the human vocal tract: A study using magnetic resonance imaging. *Journal of the Acoustical Society of America, 106*, 1511–1522.

Flege, J. E., & Fletcher, K. L. (1992). Talker and listener effects on the perception of degree of foreign accent. *Journal of the Acoustical Society of America, 91*, 370–389.

Garstang, W. (1922). The theory of recapitulation: A critical re-statement of the biogenetic law. *Journal of the Linnaean Society (Zoology), 35*, 81–101.

Giedd, J. N. (2005). Structural magnetic resonance imaging of the adolescent brain. *Annals of the New York Academy of Science, 1021*, 77–85.

Giedd, J. N., Blumenthal, J., Jeffries, N. O., Castellanos, F. X., Liu, H., Zijdenbos, A., ... Rapoport, J. L. (2001). Brain development during childhood and adolescence: A longitudinal MRI study. *Nature Neuroscience, 2*, 861–863.

Girolametto, L., Wiigs, M., Smyth, R., Weitzman, E., & Pearce, P. S. (2001). Children with a history of expressive vocabulary delay: Outcomes at 5 years of age. *American Journal of Speech-Language Pathology, 10*, 358–369.

Gleason, J. B., & Weintraub, S. (1976). The acquisition of routines in child language. *Language in Society, 5*, 129–136.

Goody, J. (1977). *The domestication of the savage mind.* Cambridge, UK: Cambridge University Press.

Gordon, R. G. (Ed.). (2005). *Ethnologue: Languages of the world* (15th ed.). Dallas, TX: SIL International.

Gossen, G. (1976a). Verbal dueling in Chamula. In B. Kirshenblatt-Gimblett (Ed.), *Speech play: Research and resources for the study of linguistic creativity.* Philadelphia, PA: University of Pennsylvania Press.

Gossen, G. H. (1976b). Chamula genres of verbal behavior. In A. Paredes & R. Bauman (Eds.), *Toward new perspectives in folklore.* Austin, TX: University of Texas Press.

Gottlieb, G. (2002). *Individual development and evolution: The genesis of novel behavior.* Mahwah, NJ: Erlbaum.

Gould, S. J. (1977). *Ontogeny and phylogeny.* Cambridge, MA: Harvard University Press.

Hall, B. K. (1999). *Evolutionary developmental biology.* London, UK: Chapman and Hall.

Hart, B., & Risley, T. (1995). *Meaningful differences in everyday parenting and intellectual development in young American children.* Baltimore, MD: Brookes.

Hauser, M. D., Chomsky, N., & Fitch, W. T. (2002). The faculty of language: What is it, who has it, and how did it evolve? *Science, 298,* 1569–1579.

Helliesen, P. J., Cook, C. D., Friedlander, L., & Agathon, S. (1958). Studies of respiratory physiology in children. I. Mechanics of respiration and lung volumes in 85 normal children 5 to 17 years of age. *Pediatrics, 22,* 80–93.

Hermann, J. (2008). The 'language' problem. *Language & Communication, 28,* 93–99.

Hibbert, M., Lannigan, A., Raven, J., Landau, L., & Phelan, P. (1995). Gender differences in lung growth. *Pediatric Pulmonology, 19,* 129–134.

Higgins, M. B., & Saxman, J. H. (1991). A comparison of selected phonatory behaviors of healthy aged and young adults. *Journal of Speech and Hearing Research, 34,* 1000–1010.

Hockett, C. F. (1960). The origin of speech. *Scientific American, 203,* 88–96.

Hogan, J. A. (1988). Cause and function in the development of behavior systems. In E. M. Blass (Ed.), *Handbook of behavioral neurobiology. Vol. IX. Developmental psychobiology and behavioral ecology.* New York, NY: Plenum.

Hoit, J. D., Hixon, T. J., Watson, P. J., & Morgan, W. J. (1990). Speech breathing in children and adolescents. *Journal of Speech and Hearing Research, 33,* 51–69.

Hrdy, S. B. (2006). Evolutionary context of human development. In C. S. Carter, L. Ahnert, K. E. Grossmann, S. B. Hrdy, M. E. Lamb, S. W. Porges, & N. Sachser (Eds.), *Attachment and bonding: A new synthesis.* Cambridge, MA: MIT Press.

Janson, C. H., & van Schaik, C. P. (1993). Ecological risk aversion in juvenile primates: Slow and steady wins the race. In M. E. Pereira & L. A. Fairbanks (Eds.), *Juvenile primates: Life history, development, and behavior.* Oxford, UK: Oxford University Press.

Jespersen, O. (1924/1963). *The philosophy of grammar.* London, UK: George Allen & Unwin.

Joffe, T. H. (1997). Social pressures have selected for an extended juvenile period in primates. *Journal of Human Evolution, 32,* 593–605.

Karmiloff-Smith, A. (1985). Some fundamental aspects of language development after age 5. In P. Fletcher & M. Garman (Eds.), *Language acquisition: Studies in first language development* (2nd ed.). Cambridge, UK: Cambridge University Press.

Kuiper, K. (1996). *Smooth talkers: The linguistic performance of auctioneers and sportscasters.* Mahwah, NJ: Lawrence Erlbaum.

Lakoff, G., & Johnson, M. (1980). *Metaphors we live by.* Chicago, IL: University of Chicago Press.

Lieberman, D. E., McCarthy, R. C., Hiiemae, K. M., & Palmer, J. B. (2001). Ontogeny of postnatal hyoid and larynx descent in humans. *Archives of Oral Biology, 46,* 117–128.

Linell, P. (2005). *The written language bias in linguistic: Its nature, origins and transformations.* London and New York: Routledge.

Locke, J. L. (1993a). *The child's path to spoken language.* Cambridge, MA: Harvard University Press.

Locke, J. L. (1993b). The role of the face in vocal learning and the development of spoken language. In B. de Boysson-Bardies, S. de Schonen, P. Jusczyk, P. MacNeilage, & J. Morton (Eds.), *Developmental neurocognition: Speech and face processing in the first year of life.* The Netherlands: Kluwer Academic Publishers.

Locke, J. L. (1994). Development of the capacity for spoken language. In P. Fletcher & B. MacWhinney (Ed.), *Handbook of child language*. Oxford, UK: Blackwell Publishers.

Locke, J. L. (1996). Why do infants begin to talk? Language as an unintended consequence. *Journal of Child Language, 23,* 251–268.

Locke, J. L. (1997). A theory of neurolinguistic development. *Brain and Language, 58,* 265–326.

Locke, J. L. (1998a). Social sound-making as a precursor to spoken language. In J. R. Hurford, M. Studdert-Kennedy, & C. Knight (Eds.), *Approaches to the evolution of language: Social and cognitive bases*. Cambridge, UK: Cambridge University Press.

Locke, J. L. (1998b). Are developmental language disorders primarily grammatical? Speculations from an evolutionary model. In R. Paul (Ed.), *Exploring the speech-language connection*. Baltimore, MD: Paul H. Brookes.

Locke, J. L. (1999). Towards a biological science of language development. In M. Barrett (Ed.), *The development of language*. Hove (East Sussex), UK: Psychology Press.

Locke, J. L. (2001a). Rank and relationships in the evolution of spoken language. *Journal of the Royal Anthropological Institute, 7,* 37–50.

Locke, J. L. (2001b). First communion: The emergence of vocal relationships. *Social Development, 10,* 294–308.

Locke, J. L. (2006). Parental selection of vocal behavior: Crying, cooing, babbling and the evolution of spoken language. *Human Nature, 17,* 155–168.

Locke, J. L. (2008a). The trait of human language: Lessons from the canal boat children of England. *Biology & Philosophy, 23,* 347–361.

Locke, J. L. (2008b). Cost and complexity: Selection for speech and language. *Journal of Theoretical Biology, 251,* 640–652.

Locke, J. L. (2009). Evolutionary developmental linguistics: Naturalization of the faculty of language. *Language Sciences, 31,* 33–59.

Locke, J. L., & Bogin, B. (2006). Language and life history: A new perspective on the evolution and development of linguistic communication. *Behavioral and Brain Science, 29,* 259–325.

Malinowski, B. (1923). The problem of meaning in primitive languages. In C. K. Ogden & I. A. Richards (Eds.), *The meaning of meaning*. London, UK: Routledge and Kegan Paul.

Marchman, V. A., & Bates, E. (1994). Continuity in lexical and morphological development: A test of the critical mass hypothesis. *Journal of Child Language, 21,* 339–366.

Mazur, A., & Booth, A. (1998). Testosterone and dominance in men. *Behavioral and Brain Sciences, 21,* 353–363.

McGhee, P. E. (1979). *Humor: Its origin and development*. San Francisco, CA: W. H. Freeman.

Meltzoff, A. N., & Moore, M. K. (1994). Imitation, memory, and the representation of persons. *Infant Behavior and Development, 17,* 83–99.

Miller, G. (2000). *The mating mind: How sexual choice shaped the evolution of human nature*. London, UK: William Heinemann.

Miller, G. A. (1965). Some preliminaries to psycholinguistics. *American Psychologist, 20,* 15–20.

Mivart, St. G. (1871). *On the genesis of species*. London, UK: Macmillan.

Moon, C., Cooper, R. P., & Fifer, W. P. (1993). Two-day olds prefer their native language. *Infant Behavior and Development, 16,* 495–500.

Morais, J. (2001). The literate mind and the universal human mind. In E. Dupoux (Ed.), *Language, brain, and cognitive development: Essays in honor of Jacques Mehler*. Cambridge, MA: MIT Press.

Navas, A. L. G. P. (2004). Implications of alphabetic instruction in the conscious and unconscious manipulations of phonological representations in Portuguese-Japanese bilinguals. *Written Language & Literacy, 7,* 119–131.

Nelson, K. (1996). Memory development from 4 to 7 years. In A. J. Sameroff & M. M. Haith (Eds.), *The five to seven year shift: The age of reason and responsibility.* Chicago, IL: University of Chicago Press.

Nelson, K. E., Carskaddon, G., & Bonvillian, J. D. (1973). Syntax acquisition: Impact of experimental variation in adult verbal interaction with the child. *Child Development, 44,* 497–504.

Newmeyer, F. J. (2003). What can the field of linguistics tell us about the origins of language? In M. H. Christiansen & S. Kirby (Eds.), *Language evolution.* Oxford, UK: Oxford University Press.

Nippold, M. A. (1998). *Later language development: The school-age and adolescent years.* Austin, TX: Pro-ED.

Northcutt, R. G. (1990). Ontogeny and phylogeny: A re-evaluation of conceptual relationships and some applications. *Brain, Behavior and Evolution, 36*(2–3), 116–140.

Ochs, E. (1982). Talking to children in Western Samoa. *Language and Society, 2,* 77–104.

Oguchi, T., & Kikuchi, H. (1997). Voice and interpersonal attraction. *Japanese Psychological Research, 39,* 56–61.

Oller, D. K. (2004). Underpinnings for a theory of communicative evolution. In D. K. Oller & U. Griebel (Eds.), *The evolution of communication systems: A comparative approach.* Cambridge, MA: MIT Press.

Oller, D. K., Eilers, R. E., Neal, A. R., & Schwartz, H. K. (1999). Precursors to speech in infancy: The prediction of speech and language disorders. *Journal of Communication Disorders, 32,* 223–245.

Olson, D. (1994). *The world on paper: The conceptual and cognitive implications of writing and reading.* Cambridge, UK: Cambridge University Press.

Ostrosky-Solís, F., Ramirez, M., & Ardila, A. (2004). Effects of culture and education on neuropsychological testing: A preliminary study with indigenous and nonindigenous population. *Applied Neuropsychology, 11,* 186–193.

Paul, R., & Jennings, P. (1992). Phonological behavior in toddlers with slow expressive language development. *Journal of Speech and Hearing Research, 35,* 99–107.

Paul, R., & Shiffer, M. E. (1991). Communicative initiations in normal and late-talking toddlers. *Applied Psycholinguistics, 12,* 419–431.

Pawlby, S. J. (1977). Imitative interaction. In H. R. Schaffer (Ed.), *Studies in mother-infant interaction.* New York, NY: Academic Press.

Pedersen, M. F., Moller, S., Krabbe, S., & Bennett, P. (1986). Fundamental voice frequency measured by electroglottography during continuous speech: A new exact secondary sex characteristic in boys in puberty. *International Journal of Pediatric Otorhinolaryngology, 11,* 21–27.

Pedersen, M. F., Møller, S., Krabbe, S., Bennett, P., & Svenstrup, B. (1990). Fundamental voice frequency in female puberty measured with electroglottography during continuous speech as a secondary sex characteristic: A comparison between voice, pubertal stages, oestrogens and androgens. *International Journal of Pediatric Otorhinolaryngology, 20,* 17–24.

Pinker, S. (1994). *The language instinct: The new science of language and mind.* London, UK: Penguin Press.

Pinker, S., & Bloom, P. (1990). Natural language and natural selection. *Behavioral and Brain Sciences, 13,* 707–784.

Plunkett, K., & Marchman, V. (1993). From rote learning to system building: Acquiring verb morphology in children and connectionist nets. *Cognition, 48,* 21–69.

Putallaz, M., & Gottman, J. M. (1981). Social skills and group acceptance. In S. R. Asher & J. M. Gottman (Eds.), *The development of children's friendships*. Cambridge, UK: Cambridge University Press.

Puts, D. A. (2005) Mating context and menstrual phase affect women's preferences for male voice pitch. *Evolution and Human Behavior, 26*, 388–397.

Puts, D. A., Gaulin, S. J. C., & Verdolini, K. (2006) Dominance and the evolution of sexual dimorphism in human voice pitch. *Evolution and Human Behavior, 27*, 283–296.

Rescorla, L., & Ratner, T. (1996). Phonetic profiles of toddlers with specific expressive language impairment (SLI-E). *Journal of Speech and Hearing Research, 39*, 153–165.

Sanches, M., & Kirshenblatt-Gimblett, B. (1976). Children's traditional speech play and child language. In B. Kirshenblatt-Gimblett (Ed.), *Speech play: Research and resources for studying linguistic creativity*. Philadelphia, PA: University of Pennsylvania Press.

Schleidt, W. M. (1973). Tonic communication: Continual effects of discrete signs in animal communication systems. *Journal of Theoretical Biology, 42*, 359–386.

Schrader, P. C., Quanjer, P. H., & Olievier, I. C. (1988). Respiratory muscle force and ventilatory function in adolescents. *European Respiratory Journal, 1*, 368–375.

Senghas, A., & Coppola, M. (2001). Children creating language: How Nicaraguan Sign Language acquired a spatial grammar. *Psychological Science, 12*, 323–328.

Senghas, A., Kita, S., & Ozyurek, A. (2004). Children creating core properties of language: Evidence from an emerging sign language in Nicaragua. *Science, 305*, 1779–1782.

Seyfarth, R. M., & Cheney, D. L. (2003). Signalers and receivers in animal communication. *Annual Reviews of Psychology, 54*, 145–173.

Shaw, P., Greenstein, D., Lerch, J., Clasen, L., Lenroot, R., Gogtay, N., … Giedd, J. (2006). Intellectual ability and cortical development in children and adolescents. *Nature, 440*, 676–679.

Sherzer, J. (2002). *Speech play and verbal art*. Austin, TX: University of Texas Press.

Shriberg, L. D., Tomblin, J. B., & McSweeny, J. L. (1999). Prevalence of speech delay in 6-year-old children and comorbidity with language impairment. *Journal of Speech, Language, and Hearing Research, 42*, 1461–1481.

Shultz, T. R., & Horibe, F. (1974). Development of the appreciation of verbal jokes. *Developmental Psychology, 10*, 13–20.

Simonton, D. K. (1999). Talent and its development: An emergenic and epigenetic model. *Psychological Review, 106*, 435–457.

Slomkowski, C. L., Nelson, K., Dunn, J., & Plomin, R. (1992). Temperament and language: Relations from toddlerhood to middle childhood. *Developmental Psychology, 28*, 1090–1095.

Smith, A. (2006). Speech motor development: Integrating muscles, movements, and linguistic units. *Journal of Communication Disorders, 39*, 331–349.

Stahl, W. R. (1967). Scaling of respiratory variables in mammals. *Journal of Applied Physiology, 22*, 453–460.

Starkweather, C. W. (1987). *Fluency and stuttering*. Englewood, NJ: Prentice-Hall.

Studdert-Kennedy, M. (1991). Language development from an evolutionary perspective. In N. Krasnegor, D. Rumbaugh, R. Schiefelbusch, & M. Studdert-Kennedy (Eds.), *Language acquisition: Biological and behavioral determinants*. Hillsdale, NJ: Erlbaum.

Studdert-Kennedy, M. (1998). The particulate origins of language generativity: From syllable to gesture. In J. R. Hurford, M. Studdert-Kennedy, & C. Knight (Eds.), *Approaches to the evolution of language: Social and cognitive biases.* Cambridge, UK: Cambridge University Press.

Studdert-Kennedy, M. (2005). How did language go discrete? In M. Tallerman (Ed.), *Language origins: Perspectives on evolution.* Oxford, UK: Oxford University Press.

Studdert-Kennedy, M., & Goldstein, L. (2003). Launching language: The gestural origin of discrete infinity. In M. Christiansen & S. Kirby (Eds.), *Language evolution.* Oxford, UK: Oxford University Press.

Tambiah, S. J. (1983). The magical power of words. *Man, 3,* 175–208.

Tenney, S. M., & Remmers, J. E. (1963). Comparative quantitative morphology of the mammalian lung: Diffusing area. *Nature, 197,* 54–56.

Thal, D., Oroz, M., & McCaw, V. (1995). Phonological and lexical development in normal and late-talking toddlers. *Applied Psycholinguistics, 16,* 407–424.

Thurlbeck, W. M. (1982). Postnatal human lung growth. *Thorax, 37,* 564–571.

Titze, I. (1989). Physiologic and acoustic differences between male and female voices. *Journal of the Acoustical Society of America, 85,* 1699–1707.

Tomblin, J. B., Records, N. L., Buckwalter, P., Zhang, X., Smith, E., & O'Brien, M. (1997). Prevalence of specific language impairment in kindergarten children. *Journal of Speech, Language, and Hearing Research, 40,* 1245–1260.

Tunmer, W. E., & Cole, P. G. (1991). Learning to read: A metalinguistic act. In C. S. Simon (Ed.), *Communication skills and classroom success: Assessment and therapy methodologies for language and learning disabled students.* Eau Claire, WI: Thinking Publishers.

van IJzendoorn, M. H., Kijkstra, J., & Bus, A. G. (1995). Attachment, intelligence, and language: A meta-analysis. *Social Development, 4,* 115–128.

Veneziano, E. (1988). Vocal-verbal interaction and the construction of early lexical knowledge. In M. D. Smith & J. L. Locke (Eds.), *The emergent lexicon: The child's development of a linguistic vocabulary.* New York, NY: Academic Press.

Vihman, M. M., Macken, M. A., Miller, R., Simmons, H., & Miller, J. (1985). From babbling to speech: A reassessment of the continuity issue. *Language, 61,* 397–446.

Vuorenkoski, V., Lenko, H. L., Tjernlund, P., Vuorenkoski, L., & Perheentupa, J. (1978). Fundamental voice frequency during normal and abnormal growth, and after androgen treatment. *Archives of Disease in Childhood, 53,* 201–209.

Waldstein, R. S. (1990). Effects of postlingual deafness on speech production: Implications for the role of auditory feedback. *Journal of the Acoustical Society of America, 88,* 2099–2114.

Walsh, B., & Smith, A. (2002). Articulatory movements in adolescents: Evidence for protracted development of speech motor control processes. *Journal of Speech, Language, and Hearing Research, 45,* 1119–1133.

West-Eberhard, M. J. (2003). *Developmental plasticity and evolution.* Oxford, UK: Oxford University Press.

Whitmire, K. A. (2000). Adolescence as a developmental phase: A tutorial. *Topics in Language Disorders, 20,* 1–14.

Wilson, G. D. (1984). The personality of opera singers. *Personality and Individual Differences, 5,* 195–201.

2 The Competition Model and Language Disorders

Nora Presson and Brian MacWhinney

INTRODUCTION

To understand language disorders, we need to contrast disordered language processing with normal language processing. In one sense, this is easy to do. We see that people with language disorders struggle with articulation, lexical access, syntactic structure, comprehension, and other language functions. But simply observing these behavioral differences is not enough. To understand the dynamics of communication disorders we need to articulate a processing model that explains in mechanistic terms how and why disordered processing differs from normal processing. Moreover, because communication abilities continue to develop throughout the life span, the model must also consider properties of language acquisition.

The Competition Model (MacWhinney, 2008a) addresses this challenge by providing a functionalist account of how languages are learned across the life span and how they are processed in real time. Three decades of research based on this model have shed light on aspects of first language learning, second language learning, bilingual processing, developmental language disorders, and language loss in aphasia.

The fundamental claim of the model is that alternative interpretations compete online during language processing. To probe these various competitions, researchers have used multifactorial experimental designs to measure the process of cue competition. As summarized in MacWhinney (2008a) and elsewhere, the predictions of the model have been uniformly supported across three decades of research involving 15 different languages (MacWhinney & Bates, 1989). In this chapter, we will focus on the ways in which this model can help explain behavioral and neural patterns of language disorders.

Readers of this volume are well aware of the many challenges involved in studying language disorders. Perhaps the biggest challenge is that these disorders come in so many alternative forms. Given the complexity of language, there are good reasons to expect that the patterns of language disorders should be at least as diagnostically complex as disorders of any other sophisticated biological system (such as the immune or the circulatory system). We know that the human brain is an extremely complex object (Buzsaki, 2006) and that no two human brains are totally alike. Rather, our brains differ substantially in terms of size, connectivity, and microstructure. Language is a complex and distributed process overlaid on this individually variable and complex system. Although language is a species-specific ability, the detailed shape of that ability involves many mutations across millions of years that have promoted a gradual and continual growth in communication skills (MacWhinney, 2008b). These changes have impacted dozens of traits relating to the size of the brain, patterns of neural connectivity, styles of neural processing, gestural expression, and the structure of the vocal apparatus.

Given this immense complexity, we might wonder how one could even begin to understand language disorders. Fortunately, language itself provides two powerful searchlights for our exploration. The first is that language use is grounded on social convention. This means that, no matter how variable our brains, we all learn to use the same socially shared system for communicating meaning. To illustrate this, Quine (1960) compared language use to the structure of hedges in a formal garden. Viewed from the inside, each hedge has its own idiosyncratic branching structure. Viewed from the outside, all of the hedges have the same straight edges. Social convention serves as the metaphorical gardener, making sure that each of us uses language in accordance with tightly specified patterns. No matter how individualistic our intentions or divergent our thought patterns, we all must end up conforming to the same grammatical rules. These core linguistic patterns are called "cues" in the Competition Model, and studies in that framework show that cues are acquired bit by bit during childhood. However, by adulthood, normal native speakers have acquired and coordinated all the relevant cues, weighing each cue by its normative strength. In this way, ensuring a common communicative system, normally developing speakers end up with nice, straight hedges.

There is also a second way in which language properties facilitate our exploration of language disorders. By its very nature, language rests on at least six separable data-processing systems: audition, articulation, lexicon, syntax, perspective switching, and mental model construction. A modular view of language (Fodor, 1983; Pinker, 1997) views these systems, and others, as executing in isolation and as represented in discrete local neuronal regions. This model suggests that we might expect to find easily distinguishable neural patterns in patients with language disorders.

In contrast, the Competition Model views these separable systems as interconnected and interactive (McClelland, 1989). From the viewpoint of the Competition Model, developmental language disorders should arise primarily from disturbances in the connections between these partially separable systems, rather than damage or malformation of particular areas. At the same time, we must recognize that some disorders, particularly in the aphasias, can arise from malformations, including lesions, within specific brain areas.

WHY USE A PROCESSING MODEL?

Some have argued that specific linguistic deficits are the basis for language disorders (Rice & Wexler, 1996). In some of these accounts, deficits are associated with specific brain areas that are damaged in aphasia (Caplan, 1992). In other accounts, the deficit is linked to some specific mutation that is thought to impact language functioning (van der Lely & Stollwerk, 1996). However, analyses have often over-simplified the actual patterns of disruptions in the linguistic system. Language is a complex process, consisting of many component skills. Semantic, lexical, phonological, and syntactic information must be processed online to produce or comprehend language. Viewing language as a dynamic interaction between many local brain areas is consistent with the available neuroanatomical and behavioral data (Bookheimer, 2002). One classic contrast emphasizes the role of Wernicke's area for lexical processing and the role of Broca's area for syntactic processing. Work in neuroimaging (Booth et al., 2001; Just, Carpenter, Keller, Eddy, & Thulborn, 1996) has supported aspects of this analysis. This work has shown that there is language task differentiation in neural tissue.

Why, then, would we suggest that research go beyond mapping particular competencies to specific disorders (such as SLI) or anatomical injuries (as in aphasia)? First, evidence suggests that even specific damage can exert broad and varying effects on language functioning (Bates, Wulfeck, & MacWhinney, 1991). The reverse is also true; similar symptoms in language production and comprehension can be elicited from different types of damage (Bates, Wulfeck, & MacWhinney, 1991). More fundamentally, it is a mistake to think that local areas operate in a simple and uniform way when involved with other areas online. Neuroimaging with fMRI can underestimate the dynamic real-time flexibility and complexity of the system. A processing approach, on the other hand, emphasizes the potential for systemwide deficits to stem from varying or multiple causes. Moreover, as Quine's analysis suggests, the specific symptoms of a language disorder will depend on how the linguistic processing network is configured. For example, because different languages are represented differently, we would expect noticeably different patterns of impairment in different languages. These observations underline the importance of a processing approach to communicative disorders.

AN INTRODUCTION TO THE COMPETITION MODEL

The Competition Model provides a processing account for both comprehension and production. In order to map form to meaning during comprehension, or meaning to form in production, a language user must use a set of cues specific to that language. Each of these cues has a certain *validity*, or general usefulness of a cue in the input. More specifically, we can think of cue validity in terms of the dimensions of *reliability* and *availability*. The availability of a cue is the degree to which it is accessible in the input. The reliability of a cue is the probability with which a cue leads to correct usage or understanding.

The original framing of the Competition Model (Bates & MacWhinney, 1982) relied exclusively on the concepts of reliability and availability. At that time, we viewed competition in terms of its final results, such as sentence role interpretation, often revealed in decisions made after subjects had finished hearing whole sentences. However, once experimenters began making online measurements of processing (Kempe & MacWhinney, 1998; MacWhinney & Pléh, 1988), it became clear that additional dimensions needed to be included in the model. This additional variance was described in terms of *cue cost*, a measure of the processing effort needed to make use of that cue during comprehension or production. Among the factors affecting cue cost, the most notable is *working memory load* (Gupta & MacWhinney, 1997; King & Just, 1991). Other factors include *detectability* and *systematicity*. For cues to compete, they must be maintained together for the short-term, necessitating some working memory or attentional focus mechanism. This integration is important because it plays a large role in predicting the effects of disorders in language.

Over the years, as the model has been extended to an increasingly wider range of phenomena in both first and second language learning, it has been necessary to add additional processing dimensions. The current version of the model, called the Unified Competition Model, provides a singular account of both first and second language learning. The Unified Model retains competition as the core mechanism by which form and meaning are mapped in comprehension and production. The model is described in terms of seven additional dimensions of cognitive processing that modulate this core process of competition, as illustrated in Figure 2.1.

In the Unified Model, competition arises between alternatives within specific cortical *maps*. The relevant maps represent cortical areas that encode patterns, across six areas language processing: audition, articulation, lexicon, syntax, perspective taking, and mental models. These maps are broadly tied to specific brain areas in the model: auditory cortex for audition, motor cortex for articulation, Wernicke's area for lexicon, Broca's area for syntax, dorsolateral prefrontal cortex for perspective taking, and more dorsal areas for mental models. In addition, morphological usage coordinates processing in posterior lexical areas and anterior syntactic areas. In lexical representation, there is a further distinction between localized phonological representations and distributed semantic representations. For details regarding the emergence and connectivity of lexical maps please consult Li, Zhao, and MacWhinney (2007).

The strength of a given competitor within a map is determined by its resting strength and the additional activation it receives from other items from *connectivity* both within and between brain areas. For example, the competition between

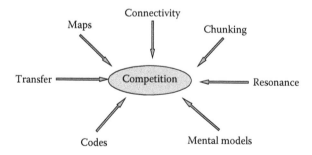

FIGURE 2.1 The Unified Competition Model. (For further details see MacWhinney, B., *Handbook of Cognitive Linguistics and Second Language Acquisition*. Mahwah, NJ: Lawrence Erlbaum Associates, 2008a. Reprinted with permission.)

the two readings of *port* in (1) and (2) can be resolved by connections to other lexical items (*captured* and *drank*). However, the competition between the two readings of *raced* in (3) and (4) is determined by syntactic patterns that extend beyond single lexical items.

1. The sailors captured the port at night.
2. The sailors drank the port at night.
3. The horse raced past the barn.
4. The horse raced past the barn fell.

The dimension of *connectivity* likewise influences the ways in which local areas communicate with each other. For example, the lexical cortex in Wernicke's area must be connected in some way to the motor cortex that produces articulatory output. The study of speech errors has shown that the lexicon maintains a function that assures that output forms are at least whole words. To do this, there must be some reciprocal connection between motor and lexical brain areas.

Within local maps, items that occur together frequently can become unified into *chunks*. For example, the phrase *as they say* functions as a single lexical item that is functionally equivalent to *reportedly*. Other chunks operate on the phonological level. For example, in Japanese, there are only 70 possible syllables and each of these, such as *na*, *ko*, or *ku* operate as single chunks. In syntax, chunks have a more flexible structure. For example, a phrase such as *what I really wanted to say was* can be processed as the same syntactic chunk that would produce *what I really meant to say was*.

The patterns of connection between local areas are further influenced by *resonance* in neural activation. During processing, attentional areas in the frontal cortex (Botvinick, Braver, Barch, Carter, & Cohen, 2001) maintain resonant activation in the local maps. This type of online resonance is particularly relevant to the study of language disorders, because it implements both the process of working memory and that of gating, which are necessary to language models. Working memory operates by maintaining a pattern of activation in an area or across areas. Gating operates in speech production to allow a candidate pattern in the output buffer to actually be produced (Levelt, 1989). Both of these aspects of resonance rely heavily on accurate timing of gating during production and preservation of material while it is still needed for sentence processing. If this connectivity is poorly wired or if resonance is inaccurate, errors in timing result, and the whole complex process of language production can fall apart.

Resonance also operates during language learning to consolidate new forms and chunks in memory. For example, when we read a new word, we represent that new word in terms of resonance between sound, meaning, and orthography. The hippocampus and other subcortical areas provide temporary support for these resonant connections (Wittenberg, Sullivan, & Tsien, 2002). The smooth functioning of resonance involves precise activation between corresponding linked areas. For example, a given lexical item in auditory cortex is linked to a corresponding representation in articulatory/motor cortex. This mapping between the two areas retains the fundamental property of resonance: auditory features must be mapped in a traceable way onto articulatory features. Another pathway of resonant connection links lexicon and syntax. Words that occupy a certain position in the lexical map also operate in similar ways in the syntactic map, and connectivity between the two areas is necessary. If these patterns of connection between areas are jumbled or disordered, it will be difficult to achieve smooth control of this type of resonance.

The Unified Model includes three additional dimensions. Two of these dimensions—transfer and code selection—are primarily important for the study of bilingualism and second language learning. The final dimension, mental model construction, is relevant primarily for those speakers with conceptual communication disorders (Craig & Evans, 1993). Mental model construction includes skills such as perspective shifting, theory of mind, imagery, and narrative construction. Problems with mental model construction have often been implicated in disorders such as autism (Pelphrey, Morris, & McCarthy, 2005), schizophrenia (Rochester & Martin, 1979), and Williams Syndrome (Karmiloff-Smith et al., 1997).

PREDICTIONS OF THE MODEL

Having reviewed the seven dimensions that control competitive processing in the Unified Model, we can now return to the original question. Specifically, how can a processing model add to the understanding of language disorders and treatment of patients diagnosed with those disorders? There are two main possibilities. First, understanding the greater systemwide features of these disorders can increase our ability to predict patient behavior. Second, this increased predictive power can influence how treatment can be designed and evaluated.

Research in communication disorders addresses three main theoretical questions: (1) To what degree can we characterize impairments as localized versus global? (2) Are the problems encountered by patients exclusively linguistic, or are domain-general cognitive processes also affected? (3) How much of language is "hard-wired"; that is, genetically specified and available independent of experience and learning? Let us examine how the Unified Model addresses each of these questions.

LOCALIZED VERSUS GLOBAL IMPAIRMENT

Reacting against his failure to locate the *engrams* of memory, Karl Lashley (1951) proposed that all cognitive functioning is global. However, given what we now know about the details of neural connectivity (Schmahmann et al., 2007; Van Essen, Felleman, DeYoe, Olavarria, & Knierim, 1990), it is difficult to deny that different neuronal areas have different functions. However, this functional differentiation does not invalidate the concept of global cognition. In the case of language impairments, we can think of language processing in terms of the performance of an acrobat who is simultaneously juggling across seven separate dimensions. At any given moment, there is a contribution from attentional areas, lexical processing, links from lexicon to syntax, and often elaboration of a mental model. If processing in any one of these coordinated areas suddenly crashes or breaks down, then the larger process is disrupted. In the case of normal speakers, the juggler is so skillful that this seldom happens, and when it does, there is a quick recovery. In a speaker with impairments, problems in any area can impact the whole system. Because of this, the Unified Model places an emphasis on overall patterns of cognitive *cost* or cognitive *load*. If stress to the system causes failure primarily in a highly vulnerable or costly area of language, then, within a language, there should be a common tendency *across disorders* for similar structures and processes to be harmed. That is, aphasics and SLI patients should be similar in *which* elements of language are impaired, either in comprehension or production. Moreover, a similar pattern of these impairments (albeit to a lesser degree) might be produced with normal language users under cognitive load. We will see that findings from Broca's and Wernicke's aphasics, as well as SLI patients, show support for this Competition Model prediction.

An important piece of evidence for the systemic properties of language disorders comes from nondisordered individuals under cognitive load. First, we know that marked increases in cognitive load can impair normal comprehension (Just & Carpenter, 1992). Moreover, varying the type and quality of cognitive load creates a performance profile in normal college students that closely resembles the one found in aphasics (Dick et al., 2001). Because we know there is no *systematic* physiological or genetic damage to the language system in these control participants, results like these support a model of language as a broad, complex, resource-intensive system that depends on smooth coordination between diverse local resources.

Moreover, aphasics and SLI patients have similar deficits in the specific elements of language that are impaired, both in comprehension or production. Most importantly, this prediction shifts the emphasis in language disorders from specific competency deficits (e.g., inflectional morphology in Broca's aphasics) and moves it to the *cause* of those deficits (i.e., less reliable, less frequent, more costly parts of the system, such as inflectional morphology are more vulnerable to deficits across the board). The resemblance between the areas of language affected under cognitive load and those affected in SLI is a good example of the ways in which processing models can illuminate the study of language disorders.

The Competition Model does not suggest there are no differences among different disorders. On the contrary, these dissociation help us understand the detailed functioning of chunking, connectivity, maps, and resonance within the framework of the Competition Model.

SPECIFIC LANGUAGE IMPAIRMENT

Specific language impairment is a disorder that is defined by normal cognitive function combined with markedly poor performance on language tasks. As such, the disorder is a logical testing ground for hypotheses about the domain-generality of language as well as possible genetic origins of grammatical competence.

Specific Language Impairment and *FOXP2*

Some researchers have argued that SLI is a genetic disorder resulting in a phenotypically unified competence deficit. For example, the Extended Optional Infinitive Model (Rice & Wexler, 1996) proposes that SLI is centrally a failure to develop verb agreement, delaying competent syntactic production. Similarly, the G-SLI model (van der Lely, 2005) proposes that there is at least some subgroup of SLI patients whose essential deficit is in grammatical processing; more specifically, there must be impairment in grammar but not in word learning, phonology, or working memory. However, we suggest that full application of these models depends on assumptions that lack strong biological evidence and general plausibility.

The strongest phrasing of these arguments includes each of three main tenets: (1) the cause of SLI is genetic in origin, (2) the deficits seen in SLI are fundamentally domain-specific, and (3) SLI has a common set of diagnostic criteria based on linguistic competence that mark the fundamental difference between SLI and comparison individuals. Let us examine each of these tenets.

Is the Cause of SLI Genetic in Origin?

In order to characterize SLI as a disorder with a single genetic cause, several inferences are needed. First, the argument requires an identifiable genetic source of the disorder. For example, in the KE family (Marcus, 2001), the disorder is linked to a dominant mutation on the *FOXP2 gene*.

What is known about *FOXP2*, however, does not lend itself to such an easy explanation. First, the fact that the gene exists in large concordance across species (Enard et al., 2002) makes it is necessary to differentiate what part of the *FOXP2 gene* is uniquely human. Second, a large-scale study of 270 four-year-old language-impaired children from a general population sample of 18,000 children (Meaburn, Dale, Craig, & Plomin, 2002) did not find the hypothesized *FOXP2* mutation in any participants. Therefore, there must be some alternative etiology that leads to language impairment, beyond a simple mutation in *FOXP2*.

Moreover, mutations of *FOXP2* in patients are also associated with small-scale orofacial motor control. Thus, behavioral deficits in these individuals extend beyond functional language processing to motor control (including motor control that is necessary for speech). Vargha-Khadem, Watkins, Alcock, Fletcher, and Passingham (1995) note that the disorder in affected members of the KE family "indicates that the inherited disorder does not affect morphosyntax exclusively, or even primarily; rather, it affects intellectual, linguistic, and orofacial praxic functions generally" (p. 930). Given the complex range of deficits, it is unclear how a mutation in this area could yield a phenotypically unified disorder such as that proposed by van der Lely, Rosen, and McClelland (1998).

This is not to say that such specific and mutation-based disorders are impossible; indeed, sickle cell anemia is a clear case of a disorder that is both phenotypically identifiable and genetic in origin. However, this example makes it clear that the level of specificity involved in describing such a disorder is much higher than that currently used in SLI. Genetic specification of the "one gene, one mutation" variety is unlikely. A more complex model, involving interactions between genetic factors, seems more probable. Recently, Vernes et al. (2008) traced the down-regulation of *FOXP2* on *CNTNAP2*, a gene that encodes a neurexin that influences cortical development. Looking at a British database of 847 individuals from families with at least one child with SLI, this group then focused on nine *CNTNAP2* polymorphisms. Each of these nine had a significant association with nonword repetition scores. The most powerful association was for a haplotype labeled ht1 linked to a lowering of nonword repetition scores by half a standard deviation. This same pattern is also heavily associated with autism. This new research illustrates the growing contribution of genetic analysis, as well as the complexity of genetic interactions involved and the ways in which they impact the formation of connections between areas in early brain development.

Van der Lely has emphasized the extent to which she can identify a highly specified subgroup of SLI language users. However, attempts to replicate this selection specificity (Bishop, Bright, James, Bishop, & van der Lely, 2000) have not succeeded. Moreover, even if such a distinct subtype were identified, and even if there were some statistical association between that disorder and some genetic mutation or set of mutations, we would still need a cognitive or neural model by which the mutations could be linked mechanistically to the disorder in question.

ARE SLI DEFICITS DOMAIN-SPECIFIC?

Claims of specific competence deficits in children with SLI have been used to support nativist views regarding the "faculty of language" (Hauser, Chomsky, & Fitch, 2002). The idea is that the specificity of this disorder implies that language learning and processing depend on a separate linguistic module, rather than on domain-general processes, and that damage to the module causes highly specified symptoms as hypothesized in SLI. However, the comorbidity of nonlinguistic task difficulties for children with SLI (Barry, Yasin, & Bishop, 2006) calls this interpretation into question.

Many studies have found deficits in nonlinguistic tasks in SLI patients, seemingly disputing the definition of SLI as an exclusively linguistic (or exclusively grammatical) disorder. The findings that SLI patients have impaired phonological short-term memory (Evans & MacWhinney, 1999), that the KE family and others have comorbid motor problems (Vargha-Khadem et al., 1995), and other trends toward cross-domain SLI symptoms are supportive of a richer understanding of SLI than that which restricts the impairment to one grammatical competency.

Finally, in a gating task of word identification from incomplete auditory data, an SLI group took longer to produce the correct response consistently (Mainela-Arnold, Evans, & Coady, 2008). These findings suggest a prolonged process of competition in SLI lexical processing. Such data help connect a potential perceptual deficit with the accompanying processing impairment.

Is SLI Exclusively a Deficit of Linguistic Competence?

Van der Lely and Christian (2000) describe the difference between processing models and competence deficit models as the difference between whether or not "impaired input processes and processing capacity cause SLI" (p. 35). That is, within a competence deficit model, any negative effects that stem from SLI should be restricted to the linguistic domain, and basic cognitive capacity (such as working memory) should remain within the normal range. More concretely, these competence models of SLI predict that genetic changes cause domain-specific effects, and that those effects consist of competence deficits such as the Extended Optional Infinitive stage. However, there is real variability in the symptoms and deficits showed by SLI children, and multiple cognitive limitations could be the source of these varied deficits.

First, as noted earlier, SLI is characterized by a variety of comorbid impairments (Norbury, Bishop, & Briscoe, 2002), such as phonological and oro-facial motor control disorders. The data from the KE family of language-impaired individuals are characterized by just such comorbidity (Bishop, 2002). Motor control problems, while clearly implicated in deficits in language production, do not fit the profile of a uniquely human mutation-based impairment in grammatical usage, as in a competence model. Van der Lely et al. (1998) differentiate between these comorbid impairments and the root cause of SLI by selecting participants who fall within normal range in these other language-related skills. This exclusion certainly increases the likelihood that there is a common etiology for the impairment in the grammatical SLI subgroup. However, there is no room in such a model to explain the nonlinguistic deficits of the many individuals excluded during this process. Unless there is some plausible explanation for the rest of these SLI subtypes, it is difficult to accept a model dependent on restricting any variance in the patient population.

Second, the competence impairments that serve as *cause* in models such as Rice and Wexler (1996) and van der Lely et al. (1998) could in fact be the *result* of impairments in processing, which need not be domain specific. For example, the Competition Model account would suggest that at least some children with SLI have problems with long-distance neural connectivity. Such problems could have a particularly strong impact on the coordination of information between posterior lexical areas and anterior syntactic areas. These problems would not impact linguistic competence, but rather the speed and accuracy of processing during interactive communication between these two separate areas. This emphasis on the vulnerability of between-area communication is in accord with the Competition Model emphasis on processing cost. According to the Competition Model, the SLI patient is performing a complex task with limited cognitive resources, and the limitation of those resources creates predictable and consistent negative effects for the most resource-intensive aspects of language processing.

Third, there is substantial evidence that the SLI diagnosis can be further subdivided based on whether the impairment in language competence extends to receptive as well as expressive language use (Evans & MacWhinney, 1999).

It is difficult to see how a competence account alone can explain this further dissociation. However, the Competition Model can account for this asymmetry as a result of differences in connectivity. Varieties of SLI that are exclusively expressive function much like Broca's aphasia. In typical speakers, Broca's area serves to gate the firing of lexical items during production. In expressive SLI, as in Broca's aphasia, disruption in the connectivity between Broca's and Wernicke's areas interrupt the smooth gating of lexical items for production. This gating is only important during production and is not involved in comprehension. In the case of receptive-expressive SLI, then we would expect to see a different, more general problem of information exchange between brain areas, affecting connections between Broca's area, DLPFC, Wernicke's area, and attentional areas generally.

APHASIA

These issues can be further explored by considering aphasic patients. Aphasia arises when a brain lesion from trauma or stroke produces a linguistic impairment. Traditionally, aphasia has been divided into three main categories: Broca's, or nonfluent aphasia; Wernicke's, or fluent aphasia; and anomia, or problems with word finding. Additional types include global and conduction aphasia. Because the etiology of aphasia is much clearer than that of SLI, and because the injuries are easier to map, aphasia provides a useful counterpoint to SLI. In SLI, the functional deficits are well-defined but etiology remains unclear. In aphasia, the opposite is true.

Although aphasia has a clear etiology, lesion site is not a strong predictor of symptom pattern. Two patients with lesions in very different areas will often have similar linguistic profiles. Similarly, patients with lesions in the same area often end up with very different profiles in language performance. Moreover, if a person with Wernicke's aphasia is impaired in grammaticality judgment in a way that resembles a person with Broca's aphasia, this does not necessarily mean that Broca's and Wernicke's areas perform the same processing tasks, or that they are neurally identical. Rather, it means that grammar is a complex computational task with certain high-risk components that can be impaired in similar ways through damage to various parts of the language network. In this way, aphasia often teaches us more about the nature of the language processing system than it does about the brain.

Crosslinguistic studies of aphasia (Bates et al., 1991) have illustrated and validated this approach. There is a rich literature demonstrating differences between Broca's aphasics who are native speakers of different languages. For example, the use of agreement in aphasic patients whose native language is Italian is relatively less impaired than in comparison patients whose native language is English. This result is predictable in a Competition Model framework, given the strength of agreement cues in Italian compared to English. In both Broca's and Wernicke's aphasics, obligatory structures such as SVO word order in German and Italian patients are preserved. These structures are also the most valid, least costly (as defaults in the language), and most highly frequent. Similarly, when Turkish speakers become aphasic, they still maintain the use of SOV word order, which is the standard in Turkish. As Elizabeth Bates would say, "You can take the Turks out of Turkey, but you can't take the Turkish out of the Turks." Overall, this research shows that the major determinant of cue survival in aphasia is the relative strength of the cue in the language of the aphasic.

The status of competence accounts in aphasia is similar to its status in SLI. In SLI, competence accounts look to a simple causal association between a damaged component (such as a specific mutation) and a language deficit. In aphasia, these accounts also require that a specific lesioned local area or module be the root cause of the aphasic disability. In both cases, the competence approach fails to consider the broader context of the language system, wherein levels of processing (semantics, syntax, lexicon, audition, comprehension) interact within a distributed functional neural network of brain areas (Bookheimer, 2002).

In the Competition Model analysis, the effects of lesions must be understood in terms of the damage inflicted on both grey matter and white matter. Damages to grey matter impact the content of the representational maps that are at the core of the system. In one view, these maps could be viewed as encoding specific linguistic competence. However, when grey matter is damaged, there is usually accompanying damage to the white matter that connects the local map with other processing regions. Thus, actual patterns of aphasia relate not just to the processing in local maps, but also disorders in connectivity and processing that occurs as two or more maps attempt to work in synchrony.

Gupta, MacWhinney, Feldman, and Sacco (2003) showed that, in children who had had early focal lesions, learning was quantitatively delayed in word learning, nonword repetition, and serial recall tasks. Although the level of performance was impaired overall, the relation between measures of verbal working memory and word learning was maintained, and those relations were similar to the control group. These data are consistent with the finding that children with focal lesions are able to achieve functional language use, although their overall reaction times are often slower than that of controls (MacWhinney, Feldman, Sacco, & Valdes-Perez, 2000).

A similar, and perhaps even more striking, finding comes from Wilson and Saygin (2004). They report evidence in direct contradiction to models that hypothesize that Broca's area is the unique site for comprehension of maximal trace projections (Grodzinsky, 2000). In Wilson and Saygin's study, *all patient groups*, including anomics, shared a general impairment pattern, although the quantitative performance of the patients varied, as expected. These results show that a number of injuries to the language network can create similar performance profiles. These data fit well with the analysis of the Competition Model.

Finally, data suggest that nonaphasic patients with left-hemisphere lesions have sentence comprehension and free word recall deficits compared to similar right-hemisphere lesion patients (Vallar, Papagno, & Cappa, 1988). The left hemisphere patients had lexical and syntactic deficits, as well as a decrement in verbal long-term memory. Consistent with the view of language as a complex and distributed system, the varied lesion sites all had some broad effect on linguistic *processing*, as demonstrated through varied behavioral measures.

SUMMARY AND CONCLUSION

This chapter has presented ways in which the Competition Model can be useful in understanding SLI and aphasia. The Competition Model framework suggests that there are multiple pathways that can produce SLI. As we have argued, impairment in processing capacity can result in symptoms that reflect weakened "vulnerable" linguistic structures. Such a processing deficit, however, could have multiple causes, consistent with accounts of decreased verbal working memory (Gathercole & Baddeley, 1993), phonological processing impairment (Tallal & Piercy, 1974), and orofacial motor impairment (Vargha-Khadem et al., 1995). In this sense, SLI can be viewed as linked to an *endophenotype* (Gottesman & Gould, 2003) in which a complex set of genetic variations produce a phenotypically consistent cognitive outcome. The current literature suggests that at the core of the SLI endophenotype is a set of individual variations that can influence the operation of verbal working memory. We must note that verbal working memory is not a single cognitive process. On the one hand, the six local cortical maps that support language each maintain some type of local memory through competitive activation patterns. However, this local activation is not enough to effectively control higher levels of language processing. Once an item is activated locally, it must receive additional support from other areas and it must also trigger activation in other areas.

For example, a word such as "more" may maintain activation in the posterior lexical area. This activation constitutes a certain level of local memory. However, this item must then activate Broca's area to trigger combination with a noun, as in "more campers." Once this phrase links up with a verb, as in "more campers visited the park," activation then spreads to frontal areas that encode perspective (MacWhinney, 2008c) and overall mental models. The distributed and interactive nature of this information flow requires smooth white matter connections between each of the areas involved in processing. This suggests that an SLI endophenotype involves disruptions that interrupt the timing or accuracy of this information flow.

This approach suggests that we should not imagine working memory as a discrete neural storage area. As Mainela-Arnold et al. (2008) write:

> Current developments in connectionist modeling and neuroscience suggest that what has been referred to as working memory capacity may be comprised of global competition of activation in large-scale neural networks with a top-down attentional bias from prefrontal cortex (PFC) circuits. (p. 390)

This is consistent with other domain-general models of working memory function (Schneider & Chien, 2003).

The Unified Competition Model is designed to interface with perceptual and memory processes and integrates working memory buffers at each level of processing. In this way, the model is aligned with cognitive models such as ACT-R (Anderson & Lebiere, 1998) that maintain local buffers. These accounts fit behavioral data that show competition and interference at multiple levels in online language processing. Because language depends on the integration of multiple inputs to produce either intelligible outputs or comprehension, describing the precise nature of this coordination is crucial for neurally grounded language models. By mapping connections between language areas with diffusion tensor imaging (DTI; Schmahmann et al., 2007), or by using functional connectivity analyses (MacDonald, Just, & Carpenter, 1992), we can provide further articulation of this account.

Although the Competition Model emphasizes the structural integrity of language, it also emphasizes the complexity of neurolinguistic processing. Although we expect a wide variety of lesions or endophenotypes to produce similar symptom patterns, we also expect that careful scientific work can eventually separate out the relative contributions of the six separate local processing regions and the complex patterns of white matter connections between them. We also expect that some symptom patterns will arise not from lesions, but from poor mappings between resonant areas and cellular-level problems with neuronal firing and consolidation. In this sense, we would agree with van der Lely (2005) when she notes "it is only by identifying pertinent ... phenotypes that we can illuminate functionally specialized cognitive systems" (p. 53). There are many contrasts that are illuminative in this way; for example, some aphasics are expressive (fluent), while others are nonfluent. Some subjects have affected prosody and labored articulation, whereas others do not. Similarly, in SLI, some subjects have reduced working memory and others are closer to normal. However, we do not want to use these dissociations to link impairments to modules. Rather, we need to look at the overall dimensions of cue strength and cue cost as the linguistic backdrop against which processing limitations should be measured. Only by collecting a rich set of measures of performance in both experimental and naturalistic contexts can we achieve clearer understandings of the various ways in which this integrated system can be impaired. Language, though unique in the types and complexity of the necessary calculations, is in the end a cognitive process, and this simple fact leads to a more complete understanding of language disorders.

REFERENCES

Anderson, J., & Lebiere, C. (1998). *The atomic components of thought.* Mahwah, NJ: Erlbaum.

Barry, J., Yasin, I., & Bishop, D. (2006). Heritable risk factors associated with language impairments. *Genes, Brain & Behavior, 6,* 66–76.

Bates, E., & MacWhinney, B. (1982). Functionalist approaches to grammar. In E. Wanner & L. Gleitman (Eds.), *Language acquisition: The state of the art* (pp. 173–218). New York, NY: Cambridge University Press.

Bates, E., Wulfeck, B., & MacWhinney, B. (1991). Crosslinguistic research in aphasia: An overview. *Brain and Language, 41,* 123–148.

Bishop, D. (2002). The role of genes in the etiology of specific language impairment. *Journal of Communication Disorders*, *35*, 311–328.

Bishop, D., Bright, P., James, C., Bishop, S. J., & van der Lely, H. (2000). Grammatical SLI: A distinct subtype of developmental language impairment. *Applied Psycholinguistics*, *21*, 159–181.

Bookheimer, S. (2002). Functional MRI of language: New approaches to understanding the cortical organization of semantic processing. *Annual Review of Neuroscience*, *25*, 151–188.

Booth, J. R., MacWhinney, B., Thulborn, K. R., Sacco, K., Voyvodic, J. T., & Feldman, H. M. (2001). Developmental and lesion effects during brain activation for sentence comprehension and mental rotation. *Developmental Neuropsychology*, *18*, 139–169.

Botvinick, M. M., Braver, T. S., Barch, D. M., Carter, C. S., & Cohen, J. D. (2001). Conflict monitoring and cognitive control. *Psychological Review*, *108*, 624–652.

Buzsaki, G. (2006). *Rhythms of the brain*. Oxford, UK: Oxford University Press.

Caplan, D. (1992). *Language: Structure, processing, and disorders*. Cambridge, MA: Bradford Books.

Craig, H., & Evans, J. (1993). Pragmatics and SLI: Within-group variations in discourse behaviors. *Journal of Speech and Hearing Research*, *36*, 777–789.

Dick, F., Bates, E., Wulfeck, B., Utman, J., Dronkers, N., & Gernsbacher, M. A. (2001). Language deficits, localization and grammar: Evidence for a distributive model of language breakdown in aphasics and normals. *Psychological Review*, *108*, 759–788.

Enard, W., Przeworski, M., Fisher, S. E., Lai, C. S. L., Wiebe, V., Kitano, T., … Pääbo, S. (2002). Molecular evolution of *FOXP2*, a gene involved in speech and language. *Nature*, *418*, 869–872.

Evans, J. L., & MacWhinney, B. (1999). Sentence processing strategies in children with expressive and expressive-receptive specific language impairments. *International Journal of Language and Communication Disorders*, *34*, 117–134.

Fodor, J. (1983). *The modularity of mind: An essay on faculty psychology*. Cambridge, MA: MIT Press.

Gathercole, V., & Baddeley, A. (1993). *Working memory and language*. Hillsdale, NJ: Lawrence Erlbaum Associates.

Gottesman, I. I., & Gould, T. D. (2003). The endophenotype concept in psychiatry: Etymology and strategic intentions. *American Journal of Psychiatry*, *160*, 636–645.

Grodzinsky, Y. (2000). The neurology of syntax: Language use without Broca's area. *Behavioral and Brain Sciences*, *23*, 1–21.

Gupta, P., & MacWhinney, B. (1997). Vocabulary acquisition and verbal short-term memory: Computational and neural bases. *Brain and Language*, *59*, 267–333.

Gupta, P., MacWhinney, B., Feldman, H., & Sacco, K. (2003). Phonological memory and vocabulary learning in children with focal lesions. *Brain and Language*, *87*, 241–252.

Hauser, M., Chomsky, N., & Fitch, T. (2002). The faculty of language: What is it, who has it, and how did it evolve? *Science*, *298*, 1569–1579.

Just, M., & Carpenter, P. (1992). A capacity theory of comprehension: Individual differences in working memory. *Psychological Review*, *99*, 122–149.

Just, M., Carpenter, P., Keller, T., Eddy, W., & Thulborn, K. (1996). Brain activation modulated by sentence comprehension. *Science*, *274*, 114–116.

Karmiloff-Smith, A., Grant, J., Berthoud, I., Davies, M., Howlin, P., & Udwin, O. (1997). Language and Williams syndrome: How intact is "intact"? *Child Development*, *68*, 246–262.

Kempe, V., & MacWhinney, B. (1998). The acquisition of case-marking by adult learners of Russian and German. *Studies in Second Language Acquisition*, *20*, 543–587.

King, J., & Just, M. (1991). Individual differences in syntactic processing: The role of working memory. *Journal of Memory and Language, 30*, 580–602.

Lashley, K. (1951). The problem of serial order in behavior. In L. A. Jeffress (Ed.), *Cerebral mechanisms in behavior*. New York, NY: Wiley.

Levelt, W. J. M. (1989). *Speaking: From intention to articulation*. Cambridge, MA: MIT Press.

Li, P., Zhao, X., & MacWhinney, B. (2007). Dynamic self-organization and early lexical development in children. *Cognitive Science, 31*, 581–612.

MacDonald, M., Just, M., & Carpenter, P. (1992). Working memory constraints on the processing of syntactic ambiguity. *Cognitive Psychology, 24*, 56–98.

MacWhinney, B. (2008a). A unified model. In P. Robinson & N. Ellis (Eds.), *Handbook of cognitive linguistics and second language acquisition*. Mahwah, NJ: Lawrence Erlbaum Associates.

MacWhinney, B. (2008b). Cognitive precursors to language. In K. Oller & U. Griebel (Eds.), *The evolution of communicative flexibility* (pp. 193–214). Cambridge, MA: MIT Press.

MacWhinney, B. (2008c). How mental models encode embodied linguistic perspectives. In R. Klatzky, B. MacWhinney, & M. Behrmann (Eds.) Embodiment, Ego-Space, and Action (pp. 369–410). Mahwah, NJ: Lawrence Erlbaum Associates.

MacWhinney, B., & Bates, E. (Eds.). (1989). *The crosslinguistic study of sentence processing*. New York, NY: Cambridge University Press.

MacWhinney, B., Feldman, H. M., Sacco, K., & Valdes-Perez, R. (2000). Online measures of basic language skills in children with early focal brain lesions. *Brain and Language, 71*, 400–431.

MacWhinney, B., & Pléh, C. (1988). The processing of restrictive relative clauses in Hungarian. *Cognition, 29*, 95–141.

Mainela-Arnold, E., Evans, J. L., & Coady, J. A. (2008). Lexical representations in children with SLI: Evidence from a frequency-manipulated gating task. *Journal of Speech, Language, and Hearing Research, 51*, 381–393.

Marcus, G. (2001). *The algebraic mind*. Cambridge, MA: MIT Press.

McClelland, J. L. (1989). Parallel distributed processing: Implications for cognition and development. In R. G. M. Morris (Ed.), *Parallel distributed processing: Implications for psychology and neurobiology*. Oxford, UK: Oxford University Press.

Meaburn, E., Dale, P. S., Craig, I., & Plomin, R. (2002). Language-impaired children: No sign of the FOXP2 mutation. *Neuroreport, 13*, 1075–1077.

Norbury, C., Bishop, D., & Briscoe, J. (2002). Does impaired grammatical comprehension provide evidence for an innate grammar module? *Applied Psycholinguistics, 23*, 247–268.

Pelphrey, K. A., Morris, J. P., & McCarthy, G. (2005). Neural basis of eye gaze processing deficits in autism. *Brain, 128*, 1038–1048.

Pinker, S. (1997). *How the mind works*. New York, NY: W. W. Norton & Company.

Quine, W. (1960). *Word and object*. Cambridge, MA: MIT Press.

Rice, M. L., & Wexler, K. (1996). Toward tense as a clinical marker of specific language impairment in English-speaking children. *Journal of Speech and Hearing Research, 39*(6), 1239–1257.

Rochester, S., & Martin, J. R. (1979). *Crazy talk: A study of the discourse of schizophrenic speakers*. New York, NY: Plenum.

Schmahmann, J. D., Pandya, D. N., Wang, R., Dai, G., D'Arceuil, H. E., de Crespigny, A. J., & Wedeen, V. J. (2007). Association fibre pathways of the brain: Parallel observations from diffusion spectrum imaging and autoradiography. *Brain, 130*, 630–653.

Schneider, W., & Chien, J. (2003). Controlled and automatic processing: Behavior, theory, and biological mechanisms. *Cognitive Science, 27*, 525–559.

Tallal, P., & Piercy, M. (1974). Developmental aphasia: Rate of auditory processing and selective impairment of consonant perception. *Neuropsychologia, 12*, 83–93.

Vallar, G., Papagno, C., & Cappa, S. F. (1988). Latent dysphasia after left hemisphere lesions: A lexical-semantic and verbal memory deficit. *Aphasiology, 2*, 463–478.

van der Lely, H. (2005). Domain-specific cognitive systems: Insight from grammatical-SLI. *Trends in Cognitive Sciences, 9*, 53–59.

van der Lely, H., & Christian, V. (2000). Lexical word formation in children with grammatical SLI: A grammar-specific versus an input-processing deficit? *Cognition, 75*, 33–63.

van der Lely, H., Rosen, S., & McClelland, A. (1998). Evidence for a grammar-specific deficit in children. *Current Biology, 8*, 1252–1258.

van der Lely, H., & Stollwerk, L. (1996). A grammatical specific language impairment in children: An autosomal dominant inheritance? *Brain and Language, 52*, 484–504.

Van Essen, D. C., Felleman, D. F., DeYoe, E. A., Olavarria, J. F., & Knierim, J. J. (1990). Modular and hierarchical organization of extrastriate visual cortex in the macaque monkey. *Cold Spring Harbor Symposium on Quantitative Biology, 55*, 679–696.

Vargha-Khadem, F., Watkins, K., Alcock, K., Fletcher, P., & Passingham, R. (1995). Praxic and nonverbal cognitive deficits in a large family with a genetically transmitted speech and language disorder. *Proceedings of the National Academy of Sciences of the United States of America, 92*, 930–933.

Vernes, S. C., Newbury, D. F., Abrahams, B. S., Winchester, L., Nicod, J., Groszer, M., ... Fisher, S. E. (2008). A functional genetic link between distinct develomental language disorders. *The New England Journal of Medicine, 359*(22), 2337–2345.

Wilson, S. M., & Saygin, A. P. (2004). Grammaticality judgments in aphasia: Deficits are not specific to syntactic structures, aphasic syndromes, or lesion sites. *Journal of Cognitive Neuroscience, 16*(2), 238–252.

Wittenberg, G., Sullivan, M., & Tsien, J. (2002). Synaptic reentry reinforcement based network model for long-term memory consolidation. *Hippocampus, 12*, 637–647.

Wittgenstein, L. (1953). *Philosophical investigations*. Oxford, UK: Blackwell.

3 Language Processing in Normal Aging

Lise Abrams and Meagan T. Farrell

INTRODUCTION

Older adults' ability to perceive, comprehend, and produce language has been an area of interest to researchers in recent years. One of the core questions under study has been whether aging affects the processing of language universally or only in specific ways. In general, an asymmetric pattern emerges, where older adults experience greater difficulties when producing language compared to comprehending it (e.g., Burke, MacKay, & James, 2000). In particular, word-retrieval problems are some of the most noticeable and frustrating language difficulties reported by older adults (e.g., Lovelace & Twohig, 1990). Although these difficulties are much less significant than the profound language impairments found in clinical disorders such as aphasia, they nonetheless have important consequences for older adults' ability to communicate. For example, difficulty retrieving someone's name during a conversation can result in negative perceptions of older adults' competence, both from the listener and the speaker (e.g., Cohen, 1994; Hummert, Garstka, Ryan, & Bonnesen, 2004; Kemper & Lacal, 2004; Ryan, See, Meneer, & Trovato, 1994). This negative perception of aging is misleading, as there are positive aspects of aging, such as consistent increases in vocabulary that occur across the life span (e.g., Verhaeghen, 2003).

The purpose of this chapter is to review the literature on language processing in healthy older adults, with a particular focus on the cognitive processes underlying language and the circumstances that lead to impairments in older adults' language comprehension and production. This chapter begins with a brief review of theories of cognitive aging, as they relate specifically to language processing. The remainder of the chapter discusses research-based findings regarding language processing in old age, covering comprehension and production of both oral and written language as well as language use in conversational settings. We conclude with some discussion about our own directions for future research and suggestions for enhancing the ability to communicate with older adults.

THEORIES OF COGNITIVE AGING

Salthouse (1988) suggested that there was a paucity of theories of cognitive aging in comparison to the number of empirical findings at that time. In the two subsequent decades, a number of theoretical explanations have been proposed to explain age-related changes in language processing. Generally, these theories can apply to other aspects of cognition besides language, but for the purposes of this chapter, we have highlighted their relevance to language processing specifically. Brief descriptions of each theory and some corresponding empirical evidence are given below.

WORKING MEMORY

Working memory is a limited-capacity memory system that temporarily holds and manipulates information as we perform cognitive tasks (e.g., Baddeley, 1986). Some theorists suggest that older adults suffer overall decreases in working memory capacity, the amount of information that can be held at a given time (e.g., Craik, 1983; Salthouse, 1991). An alternative viewpoint is that aging is accompanied by changes in processing efficiency in working memory, not necessarily capacity (e.g., MacDonald & Christiansen, 2002). In this view, older adults have less efficient processing, such as slower spreading of activation throughout the networks of the language system, which in turn constrains the amount of information that they are able to process concurrently. Regardless of the cause of working memory deficits in old age, older adults do have greater difficulty with language tasks that are dependent on working memory, such as the production and comprehension of complex grammar or semantically difficult content (e.g., Kemper, 1987, 1992; Kemper & Kemtes, 1999; Kemper & Sumner, 2001; Kemper, Thompson, & Marquis, 2001; Obler, Fein, Nicholas, & Albert, 1991; Zurif, Swinney, Prather, Wingfield, & Brownell, 1995). For example, Kemper and Sumner (2001) reported that several measures of grammatical complexity were positively correlated with traditional working memory span measures, including reading span and digit span.

INHIBITION DEFICITS

Another explanation for age-related changes in language processing comes from inhibition deficit theory (e.g., Hasher, Lustig, & Zacks, 2007; Hasher & Zacks, 1988). In this theory, aging weakens inhibitory processes, which are responsible for regulating the information that enters and leaves working memory. The main consequence of older adults' inefficient inhibitory processes is that irrelevant information gains entry into working memory, is not deleted, and thus creates interference. Inhibition deficits have been used to explain various impairments in older adults' perception and comprehension of language, such as older adults having greater difficulty understanding speech when background speech or noise is present (e.g., Pichora-Fuller, Schneider, & Daneman, 1995; Tun, O'Kane, & Wingfield, 2002) or when there is competition from similar-sounding words (e.g., Sommers, 1996; Sommers & Danielson, 1999). Older adults also have greater difficulty ignoring visually distracting information during reading (e.g., Connelly, Hasher, & Zacks, 1991; Li, Hasher, Jonas, May, & Rahhal, 1998). Difficulties with inhibition have also been used to explain some age-related deficits in language production, such as older adults producing more speech that is off-topic (e.g., Arbuckle, Nohara-LeClair, & Pushkar, 2000; Gold, Andres, Arbuckle, & Schwartzman, 1988).

GENERAL SLOWING

Theories of general slowing propose that age-related deficits in language processing are due to slowing of component processes (e.g., Birren, 1965; Cerella, 1985; Myerson, Hale, Wagstaff, Poon, & Smith, 1990; Salthouse, 2000). Specifically, processing speed, the speed at which older adults execute cognitive operations, may be too slow to accomplish a task in a given amount of time (e.g., Salthouse, 1996). Age-related declines in processing speed have been used to explain older adults' deficits in time-limited tasks, such as comprehension of speeded speech (e.g., Wingfield, 1996; Wingfield, Poon, Lombardi, & Lowe, 1985). Processing speed deficits have also been used to explain some of older adults' difficulties with sentence comprehension, such as a reduction in the use of contextual information to help resolve ambiguity (e.g., Dagerman, MacDonald, & Harm, 2006). Although general slowing theories have been applied to some language tasks, they generally are used to explain older adults' performance on a much broader range of cognitive tasks (e.g., Salthouse, 1985).

TRANSMISSION DEFICIT HYPOTHESIS

The Transmission Deficit Hypothesis offers the most specific mechanism to explain the asymmetric effect of aging on language processing, where certain aspects of language processing, namely semantic representations and retrieval, are actually well-preserved into late adulthood, relative to phonological and orthographic representations (e.g., Burke et al., 2000). In this framework, linguistic information is stored as nodes in a vastly interconnected network separated into multiple systems, including a semantic system for word meanings, a phonological system for sounds, and an orthographic system for spellings (MacKay, 1987; MacKay & Abrams, 1998). As people age, the strength of connections between these nodes becomes gradually degraded throughout the entire network (Burke & MacKay, 1997; MacKay & Abrams, 1996; MacKay & Burke, 1990), which influences the speed and amount of activation that is transmitted between nodes. The architecture of the network leaves the phonological and orthographic systems particularly vulnerable to age-related transmission deficits because it relies on single connections between the semantic representation of a word's meaning and the word's phonological/orthographic form. Evidence in support of the Transmission Deficit Hypothesis comes from an age-associated increase in tip-of-the-tongue (TOT) experiences, a temporary inability to produce a word despite knowing its meaning (e.g., Burke, MacKay, Worthley, & Wade, 1991; White & Abrams, 2002), more frequent slips of the tongue (e.g., MacKay & James, 2004), and increased spelling errors (e.g., Abrams & Stanley, 2004; MacKay & Abrams, 1998; Margolin & Abrams, 2007).

LANGUAGE COMPREHENSION

Current theories of cognitive aging need to account for the observation that while some language functions are maintained or even improved throughout most of late adulthood, other capacities are significantly corrupted by the cognitive aging process. This age-linked asymmetry in linguistic abilities is classically demonstrated by the comparison of input- to output-side language processes (Burke et al., 2000; James & MacKay, 2007). We focus first on input processes, which refer to the perception of speech sounds and letters and comprehension at the word, sentence, and discourse level. Aging appears to have a less deleterious effect on input-side processes, although some deficits do emerge.

SENSORY/PERCEPTUAL VERSUS COGNITIVE DEFICITS

A common cause of deficits in older adults' comprehension of language is sensory and perceptual deficits. With respect to vision, older adults experience declines in visual acuity, retinal blurring (e.g., Artal, Ferro, Miranda, & Navarro, 1993), a reduction in the accuracy of voluntary saccadic eye movements (e.g., Scialfa, Hamaluk, Pratt, & Skaloud, 1999), and reduced light transmitted to the retina (e.g., Scialfa, 2002). These changes in vision have consequences for visual language processing, such as a reduction in the speed and accuracy of recognizing words and reading text (e.g., Akutsu, Legge, Ross, & Schuebel, 1991; Scialfa, 2002; Steenbekkers, 1998). Similar sensory and perceptual declines occur in the auditory system, where aging is frequently accompanied by presbycusis, or pure-tone hearing loss characterized by the loss of higher frequencies (e.g., CHABA, 1988; Cheesman, 1997; Frisina & Frisina, 1997; Willott, 1991). These age-related auditory changes can lead to poorer identification of individual sounds and words, even in ideal listening situations (e.g., Humes, 1996).

However, when younger and older adults are equated on hearing ability, age differences sometimes still emerge, suggesting that higher-level cognitive deficits may also contribute to age-related impairments in spoken language processing (e.g., CHABA, 1988; Frisina & Frisina, 1997; Schneider & Pichora-Fuller, 2000; Wingfield & Tun, 2001). Specifically, reductions in processing resources described earlier, such as working memory capacity, processing speed, or inhibitory control, have been proposed to explain age differences in spoken language processing (see Sommers, 2008, for a review). Support for this view comes from studies showing that increasing or decreasing the cognitive demands on speech perception and comprehension determines the degree of impairment that older adults experience. For example, older adults show exacerbated declines under listening conditions that increase the amount of resources required for successful perception and comprehension, such as background noise (e.g., Frisina & Frisina, 1997; Pichora-Fuller et al., 1995; Tun, 1998; Tun & Wingfield, 1999), accelerated speaking rates (e.g., Gordon-Salant & Fitzgibbons, 1999; Stine, Wingfield, & Poon, 1986; Wingfield, Peelle, & Grossman, 2003), multiple people talking at once relative to a single talker (e.g., Sommers, 1997; Sommers & Danielson, 1999; Tun & Wingfield, 1999), or unfamiliar talkers (e.g., Yonan & Sommers, 2000). Conversely, circumstances that reduce the cognitive demands of spoken language processing facilitate older adults' performance, often more so than younger adults. For example, older adults' speech perception is improved by presenting words in highly predictive or semantic contexts (e.g., Frisina & Frisina, 1997; Pichora-Fuller et al., 1995; Sommers & Danielson, 1999; Wingfield, Aberdeen, & Stine, 1991; Yonan & Sommers, 2000), when speaking rates are slower (e.g., Wingfield & Ducharme, 1999; Wingfield, Tun, Koh, & Rosen, 1999), or when prosodic and syntactic information is provided (e.g., MacKay & Miller, 1996; Wingfield, Lindfield, & Goodglass, 2000).

WORD-LEVEL COMPREHENSION

Despite the additive effects of hearing loss and cognitive declines, the majority of healthy older adults maintain an ability to successfully communicate in a variety of settings (e.g., Wingfield & Grossman, 2006). One explanation is that older adults may be able to make use of environmental and contextual cues as a compensatory strategy to offset their sensory, perceptual, and cognitive changes (e.g., Craik, 1986; Humphrey & Kramer, 1999; Sommers, 2008). Alternatively, older adults may be able to employ effective top-down strategies that make use of preserved semantic knowledge, which appears to resist the age-related degradation observed in other domains of cognition (e.g., Burke et al., 2000; Burke & Shafto, 2008; Kemper, 1992; Thornton & Light, 2006). Since input-type lexical processes rely on the ability to link current linguistic information onto existing semantic knowledge, many aspects of language comprehension remain markedly intact among older adults, at least at the single-word level (e.g., Burke & MacKay, 1997; Thornton & Light, 2006).

Semantic priming studies, which examine how word meanings are processed and organized in the semantic network, have demonstrated that older adults experience the benefit of semantic priming at least to the same degree as younger adults (e.g., Balota, Watson, Duchek, & Ferraro, 1999; Burke, White, & Diaz, 1987; Faust, Balota, & Multhaup, 2004; Howard, McAndrews, & Lasaga, 1981; Lazzara, Yonelinas, & Ober, 2002; Tree & Hirsh, 2003; White & Abrams, 2004). Individuals are faster to identify a target word (e.g., DOCTOR) when it is preceded by a semantically related prime (e.g., NURSE), compared to an unrelated word (e.g., TABLE), and the degree of facilitation from the semantic prime is comparable for younger and older adults (see Laver & Burke, 1993 for a meta-analysis). Similarly, both age-groups benefit equivalently from exposure to contextually related sentences prior to single-word comprehension tasks (e.g., Burke & Yee, 1984; Stine & Wingfield, 1994). Furthermore, older adults are equally if not more accurate in making decisions about the lexical status of linguistic stimuli, such as decisions about whether visually presented items are actual words or not (e.g., James & MacKay, 2007).

In sum, although age-related sensory declines restrict the speed with which older adults are able to comprehend lexical items, there seems to be little or no change in their ability to process and organize the meanings of words. The findings that older adults perform consistently well on these comprehension tasks are likely the product of a superior vocabulary and a dense semantic network, which continues to grow throughout most of adulthood.

SENTENCE AND DISCOURSE COMPREHENSION

The picture is somewhat more complex when considering older adults' comprehension at the sentence and discourse level. Unlike the observed pattern in word-level comprehension, older adults do show impairment in comprehension and retention of sentences and longer texts (e.g., Johnson, 2003; Kemper & Sumner, 2001; see also reviews by Burke & Shafto, 2008 Kemper, 2006; Thornton & Light, 2006; Wingfield & Stine-Morrow, 2000). Age differences in comprehension have largely been attributed to declines in component cognitive processes like working memory (e.g., De Beni, Borella, & Carretti, 2007; Margolin & Abrams, 2009; Stine-Morrow, Soederberg Miller, Gagne, & Hertzog, 2008). Sentence and discourse comprehension requires processing current linguistic input and integrating it with previously read material in order to create a cohesive representation of the text. As a result, older adults are more vulnerable to syntactically complex or ambiguous sentences (e.g., Kemper, Crow, & Kemtes, 2004; Kemtes & Kemper, 1997; Zurif et al., 1995) and prefer segmenting text into smaller chunks in order to offset the demands on working memory (e.g., Wingfield et al., 1999). However, difficulties with processing negation during sentence comprehension do not seem to increase with age (Margolin & Abrams, 2009).

Most comprehension measures used in research rely on readers' memory for the text; as a result, older adults' impairments in comprehension may more accurately reflect age-related declines in episodic memory (e.g., Burke & Shafto, 2008) and not a decline in reading ability. Furthermore, older adults may be able use their superior vocabulary and semantic knowledge to counteract processing deficits during the comprehension of discourse. A reader's *situation model* refers to his/her global representation of the text. It is created and constantly updated while reading to include information about the shifts in time and space, character and theme development, as well as to incorporate the textual information with preexisting knowledge structures (e.g., van Dijk & Kintsch, 1983; Zwaan, Magliano, & Graesser, 1995; Zwaan & Radvansky, 1998). Situation models differ from *surface level* and *textbase* representations, which are data-driven and exist independent of the reader's knowledge (e.g., Stine-Morrow et al., 2008). Surface-level representations consist of the individual meaning of words and the syntactic structure of sentences. At the next level, the textbase captures the semantic meaning explicitly provided in the text and links multiple concepts. Older adults demonstrate an intact ability to construct mental representations of discourse and update situation models as necessary during reading (e.g., Morrow, Stine-Morrow, Leirer, Andrassy, & Kahn, 1997; Radvansky, Copeland, & Zwaan, 2003; Radvansky, Zwaan, Curiel, & Copeland, 2001), despite impaired memory and comprehension for surface and textbase information.

Older adults may actually depend more on self-constructed situation models during reading because they are able to utilize existing knowledge when forming representations. As a result, older adults may not remember specific details (likely to be asked on typical comprehension measures) but will have preserved under-standing of the global meaning or gist of the text. For example, older adults' mem-ory for situation model information was superior to younger adults for passages about history (e.g., Radvansky et al., 2001) as well as narratives (e.g., Radvansky et al., 2003). Recently, Stine-Morrow et al. (2008) compared the reading abilities and strategies of younger and older readers using individual sentences, scientific expository texts, and narratives. Resource allocation was measured as a function of the amount of time readers spent on text features thought to reflect surface-level, textbase-level, and discourse-level processing. Collapsed across genre type, they found that compared to younger adults, older adults allocated more resources to surface-level processes (increased reading times for low-frequency and multi-syllabic words) and textbase processes (increased time spent on the introduction of new concepts) when reading individual sentences. However, these differences were diminished by contextual facilitation, as age differences disappeared for narrative texts and were less pronounced for the expository texts. Stine-Morrow et al. (2008) proposed that older adults may compensate for obvious processing deficits, such as declines in working memory capacity, by relying on superior knowledge-based processing and preserved contextual understanding, as well as by allocating additional resources as needed.

SPOKEN LANGUAGE PRODUCTION

In contrast to the input side, the output side of language requires the activation and retrieval of phonological information (for spoken language production) and orthographic information (for written language production). Comparisons of input-and output-side processes demonstrate significantly greater age-related deficits on production tasks, relative to comprehension tasks (e.g., Burke et al., 2000; James & MacKay, 2007; MacKay & Abrams, 1998). Tasks of production typically involve lexical retrieval, in spoken or written form.

TIP-OF-THE-TONGUE (TOT) STATES

On some occasions, word production fails and results in a TOT state, a temporary and often frustrating inability to retrieve a known word (e.g., Brown & McNeill, 1966). TOT states increase with aging, both in the laboratory and in everyday life (e.g., Abrams, 2008; Brown & Nix, 1996; Burke et al., 1991; Burke, Locantore, Austin, & Chae, 2004; Cross & Burke, 2004; Evrard, 2002; Gollan & Brown, 2006; Heine, Ober, & Shenaut, 1999; Maylor, 1990), despite older adults having larger vocabularies (e.g., Verhaeghen, 2003). TOT states are thought to reflect phono-logical encoding failure after the selection of an appropriate word. The inability to retrieve phonology (and result in a TOT) increases with age, presumably because aging reduces transmission of excitation to phonological representations (MacKay & Burke, 1990), a difficulty that seems to derive from atrophy in the left insula (Shafto, Burke, Stamatakis, Tam, & Tyler, 2007). Consistent with this explanation, compared to younger adults, older adults can retrieve less phonological information about the TOT word, such as number of syllables or first and last letters (e.g., Burke et al., 1991; Brown & Nix, 1996; Heine et al., 1999; James & Burke, 2000), and they are less likely to have an alternate word during a TOT state, an incorrect word that involuntarily comes to mind and often overlaps phonologically with the TOT word (e.g., Burke et al., 1991; Heine et al., 1999; White & Abrams, 2002). TOT states are more likely to occur for low- than high-frequency words (e.g., Vitevitch & Sommers, 2003), and proper names have the greatest susceptibility to TOT states, especially in old age (e.g., Burke et al., 1991; Evrard, 2002; James, 2006; Rastle & Burke, 1996).

Research has shown that activation of phonological representations thought to cause TOT states can be achieved by prior production of words that share phonology with the TOT word (e.g., James & Burke, 2000; see Abrams, Trunk, & Margolin, 2007a for a review). For example, James and Burke (2000) showed that after pronouncing a list of words that included *abstract, indigent, truncate, tradition,* and *locate,* people were less likely to have a TOT for *abdicate.* Pronouncing phonologically related words during a TOT can also help to resolve the TOT, resulting in retrieval of the intended word (e.g., Abrams & Rodriguez, 2005; Abrams, Trunk, & Merrill, 2007b; Heine et al., 1999; James & Burke, 2000; Meyer & Bock, 1992), and the initial syllable is the key to TOT resolution in both age groups (Abrams, White, & Eitel, 2003; White & Abrams, 2002). There are some age-related changes in the ability to resolve TOT states following phonologically related words, but the deficits are specific to older adults in their late 70s and 80s. Adults in their 60s and early 70s show an increase in resolving their TOT states following phonologically related words to the same degree as younger adults (e.g., Heine et al., 1999; James & Burke, 2000; White & Abrams, 2002), whereas adults in their late 70s and 80s have significantly less or no TOT resolution following phonologically related words (e.g., Heine et al., 1999; White & Abrams, 2002).

Recent research has documented instances where phonologically related words do not facilitate TOT resolution. Abrams and Rodriguez (2005) discovered that phonologically related words only help to resolve TOT states when these words are from a different part of speech as the TOT word. For example, when in a TOT state for the noun *bandanna,* reading *banish* (a verb) helped to resolve the TOT state, but reading *banjo* (a noun) did not. Abrams et al. (2007b) found that adults aged 61–73 showed a similar pattern, while adults aged 75–89 not only did not benefit from reading *banish,* but their retrieval of *bandanna* was worse after reading *banjo* compared with an unrelated word. These findings suggest that similar sounding words in the same grammatical class as the TOT word may compete with the TOT word for production and that these potential alternative words become more competitive for retrieval as we age.

PICTURE NAMING

The suggestion that older adults have an increased difficulty in activating the connections between words and their phonology is also supported by research on picture naming. Studies requiring older adults to produce the names of visually presented pictures have shown that older adults name objects less accurately and more slowly than younger adults (e.g., Feyereisen, 1997). However, age deficits in picture naming are not always found in individual studies (e.g., Goulet, Ska, & Kahn, 1994). One possible explanation is that older adults' larger vocabularies give them greater familiarity with the rarer picture names than younger adults, which then masks the age-linked decline in picture naming that would have appeared if both age groups were equally familiar with the words (e.g., Schmitter-Edgecombe, Vesneski, & Jones, 2000). Furthermore, similar to research on TOT states, there are differences within the older adult group, namely that many of the age differences in picture naming are found only when older adults reach their 70s (e.g., Barresi, Nicholas, Connor, Obler, & Albert, 2000; Connor, Spiro, Obler, & Albert, 2004; MacKay, Connor, Albert, & Obler, 2002; Morrison, Hirsh, & Duggan, 2003; Nicholas, Obler, Albert, & Goodglass, 1985).

Another use of picture naming studies has been to measure the influence of distractors, but there are virtually no studies with older adults. The only published study of which we are aware is Taylor and Burke (2002), who examined picture–word interference effects in younger and older adults as a function of auditory semantic and phonological distractors presented either before or after the picture appeared. Relative to unrelated distractors, interference (slower latencies) emerged when semantic distractors preceded the pictures, and older adults showed greater interference than younger adults. In contrast, facilitation (faster latencies) occurred when phonologically related distractors were presented after the picture, and this facilitation was equivalent for both age groups. These findings are consistent with the idea that older adults have a more elaborate semantic network, which results in greater priming to related concepts and subsequently more interference. Conversely, the lack of an age difference in degree of phonological facilitation suggests that presentation of phonologically related words strengthens the transmission of excitation to all connected words and that this "priming" process remains stable with age, a claim supported by research in other production tasks (e.g., James & Burke, 2000; White & Abrams, 2004).

Speech Errors

Compared to TOT states and picture naming, there is considerably less research on aging and speech errors. Speech errors provide us with an understanding about how language production is planned and how this planning can sometimes go awry and lead to errors in articulation. The patterns of speech errors that emerge have given researchers insight into the mechanisms that underlie speech production more generally. Two classes of errors that have been studied in aging include slips-of-the-tongue and dysfluencies. A slip-of-the-tongue occurs when a speaker rearranges one or more sounds across words to be produced, such as *darn bore* instead of *barn door*, or swaps entire words, for example, *I'm writing a mother to my letter* instead of *I'm writing a letter to my mother*. Similar to other forms of speech production, a word's frequency appears to influence the likelihood of a speech error. Compared to high-frequency words, low-frequency words appear more often in natural speech error corpuses (e.g., Stemberger & MacWhinney, 1986) and result in more sound misorderings in experiments that induce speech errors (e.g., Dell, 1990).

The majority of research on speech errors initially emerged via observational methods, which examined the distribution of linguistic features in large samples of spontaneous speech (e.g., Fromkin, 1971; Garrett, 1975). Since speech errors occurred relatively infrequently in spontaneous speech, experimental methods of error elicitation were developed to create processing circumstances that lead to making speech errors. MacKay and James (2004) used the transform technique with younger and older adults, where they were asked to change /p/ to /b/, or /b/ to /p/, whenever there was a /p/ or /b/ in a visually presented word. Age differences in speech errors in their responses occurred for some error types but not others. For example, older adults were more likely than younger adults to make an omission error (e.g., *pans* misproduced as *pan*), whereas younger adults were more likely than older adults to make a nonsequential substitution error (e.g., *pug* misproduced as *puck*). This selective increase in certain types of speech errors with age conflicts with the findings of Vousden and Maylor (2006), who used the repetition of tongue twisters (e.g., *a bucket of blue bug's blood*) to induce speech errors in younger and older adults. They found no age-related increase in the number of errors, as younger and older adults had equivalent error rates, but they pointed out some methodological issues, such as older adults' inability to produce speech at the desired rate when the rate was relatively fast.

Another type of speech error is dysfluencies, which represent interruptions in otherwise fluent speech. Dysfluencies can be nonlexical (e.g., *uh, um*) or lexical (e.g., *you know*) and include pauses, stutters, word repetitions, and errors in stress and intonation. Older adults produce more dysfluencies than younger adults (see Mortensen, Meyer, & Humphreys, 2006 for a review), especially during difficult tasks and during tasks that place few constraints on the content of the utterance, such as picture description tasks (e.g., Cooper, 1990; Heller & Dobbs, 1993; Kemper, Rash, Kynette, & Norman, 1990; Le Dorze & Bédard, 1998; Schmitter-Edgecombe et al., 2000), sentence production tasks (e.g., Altmann, 2004; Kemper, Herman, & Lian, 2003), and conversational interactions (e.g., Bortfeld, Leon, Bloom, Schober, & Brennan, 2001). These age-related increases in dysfluencies are thought to result from older adults having more word retrieval problems (e.g., Bortfeld et al., 2001), as dysfluencies could serve the purpose of giving them more time to locate the intended word.

WRITTEN LANGUAGE PRODUCTION

Compared to speech, there is considerably less research on older adults' ability to produce language in written form. The main area of research has focused on older adults' orthographic production (i.e., spelling). Subjectively, older adults often report that they notice a decrease in their ability to spell (e.g., MacKay & Abrams, 1998; Margolin & Abrams, 2007), and this intuition has been supported empirically. Stuart-Hamilton and Rabbitt (1997) found that adults in their 70s produced written correct spellings less often than adults in their 60s, who were less accurate than adults in their 50s. MacKay and Abrams (1998) found that older adults (aged 60 and above) were more likely to produce misspellings when spelling auditorily presented words than college students. Furthermore, the oldest half of the older adult group (aged 73–88) made certain types of errors more often than the other adults, such as misspelling the "c" in *calendar* as "k," despite "c" being the more common spelling for that sound. Interestingly, these age-related declines in spelling occur even when older adults are able to accurately perceive that a word was correctly spelled (e.g., Abrams & Stanley, 2004; MacKay, Abrams, & Pedroza, 1999). Using visually presented words shown very briefly, these studies showed that older adults were as accurate as younger adults in detecting whether or not a word was correctly spelled, but made more errors in producing the spellings that they just saw. These findings are consistent with an age-linked asymmetry between input-side and output-side language processes mentioned earlier, where deficits in production are consistently larger than those in comprehension, and extend this asymmetry to the perception and retrieval of orthographic information.

While these results suggest a universal decline in spelling with increasing age, Margolin and Abrams (2007) showed that age-related declines in spelling only occurred for poor spellers. Older adults who were poor spellers were less accurate in recognizing and producing correct spelling than younger adults who were poor spellers. In contrast, no age differences occurred for good spellers. These results indicate that aging alone is not detrimental to the processes underlying recognition or production of spelling but instead compounds existing problems caused by poor spelling. In any case, access to orthographic representations seems to weaken with age, similar to phonological representations, consistent with the idea that lower-level language representations are particularly susceptible to age-related changes (e.g., MacKay & Abrams, 1998; MacKay et al., 1999).

Spelling rare words in isolation or under time pressure is a relatively limited context to explore older adults' written production. Recently, White and her colleagues (White, Abrams, McWhite, & Hagler, 2010; White, Protasi, & Abrams, 2010; White, Abrams, Zoller, & Gibson, 2008b) have developed an innovative method to study whether older adults are susceptible to written errors for more commonly used words embedded in context, specifically homophones presented in sentences. Homophones are words that are pronounced identically but have different spellings and meanings (e.g., *beech* and *beach*). In these studies, sentences are presented auditorily for people to write down, and homophone spelling errors occur when the contextually appropriate word (e.g., *beech*) is instead replaced with its homophone, for example, "The lawyer was most proud of the *beach* tree in his garden." Unlike traditional spelling errors, older adults produced fewer homophone errors than younger adults (White et al., 2008a). White et al. also explored the influence of a homophone's spelling probability, which is defined as the frequency with which a particular spelling is used for a given sound. For example, the spelling *ail* is a high-probability spelling because it is a more common spelling for those sounds than is *ale*. Although both younger and older adults made more errors on homophones with a low-probability spelling relative to those with a high-probability spelling, this increase in errors due to spelling probability was *greater* for younger adults than older adults.

These findings are consistent with Cortese, Balota, Sergent-Marshall, and Buckner (2003), who found that when spelling spoken homophones in isolation (so that either spelling is correct), older adults relied more on a homophone's meaning, producing the spelling corresponding to the most commonly used meaning even when the spelling was low probability. In contrast, younger adults relied more on spelling probability, producing the high-probability spelling even when it corresponded to a less frequently used meaning. These findings suggest a shift from reliance on orthography to semantics with normal aging. One explanation for this shift is that older adults might shift to a reliance on semantics as a way to compensate for deficits in lower-level language representations, such as phonology and orthography (MacKay & Burke, 1990).

LANGUAGE IN CONVERSATION

The magnitude of age differences in language processing seems to depend on a number of factors, such as the type of experimental task, type of linguistic material, or even the individual goals of the speaker (e.g., Wingfield & Stine-Morrow, 2000). Given this variability, it is important to consider the degree to which empirical evidence translates into the *practical* language abilities of older adults. How do these selective changes in language processing influence the everyday interactions of older adults? Likewise, how do perceptions about the aging process affect the quality of communication? Language samples procured in the laboratory are useful for modeling the changing architecture of language abilities throughout the life span. However, it is important to keep in mind the social and pragmatic function that language plays in the real world; it enables and enriches social interactions and allows for the communication of crucial information about health, finances, and family.

STORYTELLING

Older adults' difficulties with speech production, such as word-finding problems during TOT states, might lead to the assumption that older adults are less engaging in conversation and poorer communicators. However, research on older adults' competence at socially driven communication has suggested the opposite. Results from storytelling and collaborative communication studies have shown that older adults have a heightened understanding of the interpersonal dynamics of communication (e.g., Gould, Kurzman, & Dixon, 1994; Kemper et al., 1990; Mergler, Faust, & Goldstein, 1985). Overall, older adults are rated as better storytellers than younger adults, a preference that is not limited to their own cohort (James, Burke, Austin, & Hulme, 1998; Kemper, Kynette, Rash, O'Brien, & Sprott, 1989; Kemper et al., 1990; see also Wingfield & Stine-Morrow, 2000 for a review). Younger adult listeners preferred stories read by older adults compared to younger adult readers (e.g., Mergler et al., 1985), and listeners from a variety of ages rated personal narratives told by older adults as more interesting and enjoyable than those told by younger and middle-aged adults (e.g., Pratt & Robins, 1991). Some have argued that older adults' superior storytelling is due to structural choices made by older adults, like using more complex narrative structures (e.g., Kemper et al., 1990) or using an exciting climactic build-up that is resolved at the end (e.g., Pratt & Robins, 1991). On the other hand, older adults' stories could be preferred because of their reduced speech rate, more appealing prosody, or their ability to focus the story directly at their listener (e.g., Wingfield & Stine-Morrow, 2000).

OFF-TOPIC SPEECH

Off-topic speech (OTS), or off-topic verbosity, has been defined as speech that may start out on-topic, but quickly becomes prolonged, unconstrained, and irrelevant to the present topic at hand (e.g., Arbuckle & Pushkar Gold, 1993; Gold et al., 1988). Some researchers have suggested that older adults are more verbose in autobiographical contexts such as life-history interviews, in nonautobiographical contexts such as referential communication tasks, and in the ability to tell stories based on pictures (e.g., Arbuckle et al., 2000; Arbuckle & Pushkar Gold, 1993; Glosser & Deser, 1992; Juncos-Rabadan, 1996). However, other research has failed to demonstrate a uniform, age-linked increase in OTS (e.g., Gould & Dixon, 1993; Heller & Dobbs, 1993; James et al., 1998; Trunk & Abrams, 2009), possibly because of the heterogeneous measures used to assess OTS, some of which involve more subjective assessments than others. For example, many studies that observed an age-related increase in OTS focused on individual words as either on- or off-topic, which may overestimate OTS by not accounting for the entire context in which words are used.

One explanation for extraneous wordiness in old age has been linked to a processing deficit in inhibiting irrelevant material (e.g., Arbuckle & Pushkar Gold, 1993; Pushkar Gold & Arbuckle, 1995), but more recent claims suggest that this impairment only applies to a minority of older adults (e.g., Arbuckle et al., 2000; Pushkar et al., 2000). Another explanation is that because older adults typically have had more experience with telling stories throughout their life (e.g., Boden & Bielby, 1983; Kemper, 1992), they may simply possess different goals for communicating, some of which encourage elaborative speech, particularly in autobiographical situations (e.g., James et al., 1998). Recently, Trunk and Abrams (2009) quantified younger and older adults' communicative goals and showed that age-related changes in OTS emerged only when *younger* adults changed their goals (i.e., selecting goals designed to produce more succinct stories for certain types of topics). In contrast, older adults consistently reported the same communicative goals for various topics, possibly because these goals lead them to consistently produce higher quality stories as discussed above (e.g., James et al., 1998; Pratt & Robins, 1991).

ELDERSPEAK

Communication can be influenced by the style that people use when speaking with older adults. In particular, there is a type of speech style called "elderspeak" that represents a specific set of accommodations used to address older adults, often when difficulties in communication are expected (e.g., Hummert et al., 2004; Kemper, 2006; Kemper & Harden, 1999; Ryan, Giles, Bartlucci, & Henwood, 1986). These accommodations are intended to simplify speech for older adults by using shorter and less syntactically complex sentences, speaking more slowly, repeating and paraphrasing, altering pitch and intonation for emphasis, and using terms of endearment such as "honey." Research has addressed whether elderspeak is helpful or harmful to older adults (e.g., Kemper & Harden, 1999). Some studies have shown that some aspects of elderspeak increase older adults' comprehension, specifically repetitions and elaborations as well as less syntactically complex sentences (which minimize the demands on working memory). Other aspects of elderspeak, such as slower speech rates and exaggerated intonation, actually impair comprehension. In addition to comprehension, elderspeak has a significant influence on older adults' self-perceptions. Older adults generally perceive elderspeak as condescending, although it can also be associated with positive feelings, such as affection (e.g., Ryan et al., 1986). If older adults feel like they are being patronized, they are more likely to question their language competence (e.g., Kemper & Harden, 1999), which in turn can lead to negative social consequences, such as withdrawing from social interaction.

COGNITIVE DEMANDS AND COMMUNICATIVE STRATEGIES

Age differences in communication styles may also reflect pragmatic choices made by older adults during speech production. One measure thought to reflect these pragmatic choices is the syntactic complexity of spoken and written language, measured by counts of different types of embedded clauses and of clauses per utterance. Research has shown that when responding to questions (e.g., Kemper & Sumner, 2001), describing pictures (e.g., Mackenzie, 2000), or writing in diaries or essays (e.g., Kemper, 1987; Kemper, Greiner, Marquis, Prenovost, & Mitzner, 2001), older adults tend to use sentences with restricted grammatical complexity. Age-associated declines in working memory may leave older adults with insufficient capacity to produce complex syntactic structures. As a result, older adults may unconsciously shift their communicative strategies to reduce the cognitive burden (produce simpler sentences) while simultaneously preserving the integrity of the intended message.

If older adults are choosing to produce simpler sentences as a pragmatic choice, then dual-task situations should be especially likely to reveal age-related declines in grammatical complexity. However, not all studies support this claim (e.g., Kemper et al., 2003; Kemper, Herman, & Nartowicz, 2005). For example, Kemper et al. (2003) examined the fluency, complexity, and content of spoken language samples of younger and older adults who were simultaneously performing one of three motor activities: walking, simple finger tapping, and complex finger tapping. Younger adults experienced greater dual-task costs than older adults in some areas, evidenced by decreased sentence length, grammatical complexity, and content when doing concurrent tasks. Older adults also exhibited dual-task costs by decreasing their speech rate, but the level of grammatical complexity of their responses was unaffected. This result is difficult to interpret because older adults' baseline language (in absence of a concurrent task) was less grammatically complex and content-filled than the younger adults, making further reductions in grammatical complexity more difficult to obtain. More research is needed to better understanding the relationship between working memory processes and the complexity of discourse production as well as the interaction between resource limitations and strategy use.

CONCLUSIONS

This chapter highlights the complexity of the relationship between aging and language processes. Unlike other cognitive functions, late adulthood is not accompanied by pervasive deterioration of language abilities, but instead results in declines only for specific functions, with spared or even improved abilities in other areas. Despite our growing knowledge about the language processing capabilities of healthy older adults, there are many gaps left to be filled. The focus of our research is to fill some of those gaps, specifically those in our knowledge about aging and language production, a topic that can be methodologically challenging (see, e.g., Vousden & Maylor, 2006). By creating novel methods and measures that are appropriate for multiple age groups, older adults' language abilities can be assessed under conditions where their cognitive, sensory, and perceptual deficits are less critical to performance. For example, our laboratory is currently conducting an experiment using a visual picture–word interference task with younger adults and two groups of older adults. Given that phonological distractors generally facilitate picture naming, we are investigating whether the picture's word frequency and the distractor's grammatical class are relevant to these findings and how these factors interact with age. Through this work, we aim to better understand why age-related declines in production are more prevalent than those in comprehension, in hopes of refining current theories of cognitive aging, which ultimately will lead to discovering ways to reduce these declines.

A second focus of our research is the differences that are emerging *within* the older adult group, to which future research on aging and language processing needs to be sensitive. The oldest adults seem to exhibit greater declines in various language tasks, such as TOT resolution (e.g., Abrams et al., 2007b; Heine et al., 1999; White & Abrams, 2002), spelling production (e.g., MacKay & Abrams, 1998), and even vocabulary (e.g., Lindenberger & Baltes, 1997). Unfortunately, a large proportion of aging research still reports data from an "older adult group" that spans three or four decades, thereby neglecting the cognitive changes likely to occur throughout those years. Making generalizations about aging without acknowledging that declines may be due to the very oldest members presents an overly pessimistic picture about language processing that may not be illustrative of the population it intends to represent. More precisely specifying the age at which language declines begin to emerge may also lead to the development of methods for combating impairments as well as a greater understanding of the changes in language that should be viewed as normal.

Finally, it is important to use the findings of research to improve communication with older adults. For example, despite knowledge that some aspects of elderspeak can facilitate communication with older adults, there is no evidence that speakers are accommodating their speech to highlight the beneficial components (e.g., Kemper & Kemtes, 2000). Similarly, understanding the causes of increased word finding failures in old age (and that they are a normal part of the aging process) may improve the way older adults view themselves in communicative settings and identify better ways for listeners to respond in situations where an older adult speaker is struggling to recover a specific word. Findings of research need to be disseminated to the people who can most benefit from them: clinicians working with older adults, family members who interact with an aging parent, and most importantly, the older adults themselves.

REFERENCES

Abrams, L. (2008). Tip-of-the-tongue states yield language insights. *American Scientist, 96,* 234–239.

Abrams, L., & Rodriguez, E. L. (2005). Syntactic class influences phonological priming of tip-of-the-tongue resolution. *Psychonomic Bulletin and Review, 12,* 1018–1023.

Abrams, L., & Stanley, J. H. (2004). The detection and retrieval of spelling in older adults. In S. P. Shohov (Ed.), *Advances in psychology research* (Vol. 33, pp. 87–109). Hauppauge, NY: Nova Science Publishers, Inc.

Abrams, L., Trunk, D. L., & Margolin, S. J. (2007a). Resolving tip-of-the-tongue states in young and older adults: The role of phonology. In L. O. Randal (Ed.), *Aging and the elderly: Psychology, sociology, and health* (pp. 1–41). Hauppauge, NY: Nova Science Publishers, Inc.

Abrams, L., Trunk, D. L., & Merrill, L. A. (2007b). Why a superman cannot help a tsunami: Activation of grammatical class influences resolution of young and older adults' tip-of-the-tongue states. *Psychology and Aging, 22,* 835–845.

Abrams, L., White, K. K., & Eitel, S. L. (2003). Isolating phonological components that increase tip-of-the-tongue resolution. *Memory and Cognition, 31,* 1153–1162.

Akutsu, H., Legge, G. E., Ross, J. A., & Schuebel, K. J. (1991). Psychophysics of reading: X. Effects of age-related changes in vision. *Journal of Gerontology: Psychological Sciences, 46,* P325–P331.

Altmann, L. J. P. (2004). Constrained sentence production in probable Alzheimer disease. *Applied Psycholinguistics, 25,* 145–173.

Arbuckle, T. Y., Nohara-LeClair, M., & Pushkar, D. (2000). Effect of off-target verbosity on communication efficiency in a referential communication task. *Psychology and Aging, 15,* 65–77.

Arbuckle, T. Y., & Pushkar Gold, D. P. (1993). Aging, inhibition and verbosity. *Journal of Gerontology: Psychological Sciences, 48,* P225–P232.

Artal, P., Ferro, M., Miranda, I., & Navarro, R. (1993). Effects of aging in retinal image quality. *Journal of the Optical Society of America A, 10,* 1656–1662.

Baddeley, A. D. (1986). *Working memory.* New York, NY: Oxford University Press.

Balota, D. A., Watson, J. M., Duchek, J. M., & Ferraro, F. R. (1999). Cross-modal semantic and homograph priming in healthy young, healthy old, and in Alzheimer's disease individuals. *Journal of the International Neuropsychological Society, 5,* 626–640.

Barresi, B. A., Nicholas, M., Connor, L. T., Obler, L., & Albert, M. L. (2000). Semantic degradation and lexical access in age-related naming failures. *Aging, Neuropsychology, and Cognition, 7,* 169–178.

Birren, J. E. (1965). Age changes in speed of behavior: Its central nature and physiological correlates. In A. T. Welford & J. E. Birren (Eds.), *Behavior, aging, and the nervous system: Biological determinants of speed of behavior and its changes with age* (pp. 191–216). Springfield, IL: Charles C. Thomas.

Boden, D., & Bielby, D. (1983). The past as resource: A conversational analysis of elderly talk. *Human Development, 26,* 308–319.

Bortfeld, H., Leon, S. D., Bloom, J. E., Schober, M. F., & Brennan, S. E. (2001). Disfluency rates in conversation: Effects of age, relationship, topic, role, and gender. *Language and Speech, 44,* 123–147.

Brown, A. S., & Nix, L. A. (1996). Age-related changes in the tip-of-the-tongue experience. *American Journal of Psychology, 109,* 79–91.

Brown, R., & McNeill, D. (1966). The "tip of the tongue" phenomenon. *Journal of Verbal Learning and Verbal Behavior, 5,* 325–337.

Burke, D. M., Locantore, J., Austin, A., & Chae, B. (2004). Cherry pit primes Brad Pitt: Homophone priming effects on young and older adults' production of proper names. *Psychological Science, 15,* 164–170.

Burke, D. M., & MacKay, D. G. (1997). Memory, language and ageing. *Philosophical Transactions of the Royal Society: Biological Sciences, 352,* 1845–1856.

Burke, D. M., MacKay, D. G., & James, L. E. (2000). Theoretical approaches to language and aging. In T. Perfect & E. Maylor (Eds.), *Models of cognitive aging* (pp. 204–237). Oxford, UK: Oxford University Press.

Burke, D. M., MacKay, D. G., Worthley, J. S., & Wade, E. (1991). On the tip of the tongue: What causes word finding failures in younger and older adults. *Journal of Memory and Language, 30,* 542–579.

Burke, D. M., & Shafto, M. A. (2008). Language and aging. *The handbook of aging and cognition* (3rd ed., pp. 373–443). New York, NY: Psychology Press.

Burke, D. M., White, H., & Diaz, D. L. (1987). Semantic priming in young and older adults: Evidence for age constancy in automatic and attentional processes. *Journal of Experimental Psychology: Human Perception and Performance, 13,* 542–579.

Burke, D. M., & Yee, R. L. (1984). Semantic priming during sentence processing by young and older adults. *Developmental Psychology, 20,* 903–910.

Cerella, J. (1985). Information processing rates in the elderly. *Psychological Bulletin, 98,* 67–83.

CHABA (Committee on Hearing and Bioacoustics Working Group on Speech Understanding and Aging). (1988). Speech understanding and aging. *Journal of the Acoustical Society of America, 83,* 859–895.

Cheesman, M. F. (1997). Speech perception by elderly listeners: Basic knowledge and implications for audiology. *Journal of Speech-Language Pathology and Audiology, 21,* 104–110.

Cohen, G. (1994). Age-related problems in the use of proper names in communication. In M. L. Hummert, J. M. Wiemann, & J. N. Nussbaum (Eds.), *Interpersonal communication in older adulthood* (pp. 40–57). Thousand Oaks, CA: Sage Publications.

Connelly, S. L., Hasher, L., & Zacks, R. T. (1991). Age and reading: The impact of distraction. *Psychology and Aging, 6,* 533–541.

Connor, L. T., Spiro, A., Obler, L. K., & Albert, M. L. (2004). Change in object naming ability during adulthood. *Journal of Gerontology: Psychological Sciences, 59*, P203–P209.

Cooper, P. V. (1990). Discourse production and normal aging: Performance on oral picture description tasks. *Journal of Gerontology: Psychological Sciences, 45*, P210–P214.

Cortese, M. J., Balota, D. A., Sergent-Marshall, S. D., & Buckner, R. L. (2003). Spelling via semantics and phonology: Exploring the effects of age. Alzheimer's disease and primary semantic impairment. *Neuropsychologia, 41*, 952–967.

Craik, F. I. M. (1983). On the transfer of information from temporary to permanent memory. *Philosophical Transactions of the Royal Society of London, B302*, 341–359.

Craik, F. I. M. (1986). A functional account of age differences in memory. In F. Klix & H. Hagendorf (Eds.), *Human memory and cognitive capabilities: Mechanisms and performance* (pp. 409–422). North Holland, The Netherlands: Elsevier.

Cross, E. S., & Burke, D. M. (2004). Do alternative names block young and older adults' retrieval of proper names? *Brain and Language, 89*, 174–181.

Dagerman, K. S., MacDonald, M. C., & Harm, M. W. (2006). Aging and the use of context in ambiguity resolution: Complex changes from simple slowing. *Cognitive Science, 30*, 311–345.

De Beni, R., Borella, E., & Carretti, B. (2007). Reading comprehension in aging: The role of working memory and metacomprehension. *Aging, Neuropsychology, and Cognition, 14*, 189–212.

Dell, G. S. (1990). Effects of frequency and vocabulary type on phonological speech errors. *Language and Cognitive Processes, 5*, 313–349.

Evrard, M. (2002). Ageing and lexical access to common and proper names in picture naming. *Brain and Language, 81*, 174–179.

Faust, M. E., Balota, D. A., & Multhaup, K. S. (2004). Phonological blocking during picture naming in dementia of the Alzheimer type. *Neuropsychology, 18*, 526–536.

Feyereisen, P. (1997). A meta-analytic procedure shows an age-related decline in picture naming: Comments on Goulet, Ska, and Kahn. *Journal of Speech and Hearing Research, 40*, 1328–1333.

Frisina, D. R., & Frisina, R. D. (1997). Speech recognition in noise and presbycusis: Relations to possible neural mechanisms. *Hearing Research, 106*, 95–104.

Fromkin, V. A. (1971). The non-anomalous nature of anomalous utterances. *Language, 47*, 27–52.

Garrett, M. F. (1975). The analysis of sentence production. In G. Bower (Ed.). *Psychology of learning and motivation* (Vol. 9, pp. 133–177). New York, NY: Academic Press.

Glosser, G., & Deser, T. (1992). A comparison of changes in macrolinguistic and micro-linguistic aspects of discourse production in normal aging. *Journal of Gerontology: Psychological Sciences, 47*, P266–P272.

Gold, D., Andres, D., Arbuckle, T., & Schwartzman, A. (1988). Measurement and corre-lates of verbosity in elderly people. *Journal of Gerontology: Psychological Sciences, 43*, P27–P33.

Gollan, T. H., & Brown, A. S. (2006). From tip-of-the-tongue (TOT) data to theoretical impli-cations in two steps: When more TOTs means better retrieval. *Journal of Experimental Psychology: General, 135*, 462–483.

Gordon-Salant, S., & Fitzgibbons, P. (1999). Profile of auditory temporal processing in older listeners. *Journal of Speech, Language, and Hearing Research, 42*, 300–311.

Gould, O. N., & Dixon, R. A. (1993). How we spent our vacation: Collaborative storytell-ing by young and old adults. *Psychology and Aging, 8*, 10–17.

Gould, O. N., Kurzman, D., & Dixon, R. A. (1994). Communication during prose recall conversations by young and old dyads. *Discourse Processes, 17*, 149–165.

Goulet, P., Ska, B., & Kahn, H. J. (1994). Is there a decline in picture naming with advancing age? *Journal of Speech and Hearing Research, 37,* 629–644.

Hasher, L., Lustig, C., & Zacks, R. (2007). Inhibitory mechanisms and the control of attention. In A. Conway, C. Jarrold, M. Kane, A. Miyake, & J. Towse (Eds.), *Variation in working memory.* New York, NY: Oxford University Press.

Hasher, L., & Zacks, R. T. (1988). Working memory, comprehension, and aging: A review and a new view. In G. H. Bower (Ed.), *The psychology of learning and motivation* (Vol. 2, pp. 193–225). San Diego, CA: Academic Press.

Heine, M. K., Ober, B. A., & Shenaut, G. K. (1999). Naturally occurring and experimentally induced tip-of-the-tongue experiences in three adult age groups. *Psychology and Aging, 14,* 445–457.

Heller, R. B., & Dobbs, A. R. (1993). Age differences in word finding in discourse and nondiscourse situations. *Psychology and Aging, 8,* 443–450.

Howard, D. V., McAndrews, M. P., & Lasaga, M. I. (1981). Semantic priming of lexical decisions in young and old adults. *Journal of Gerontology, 36,* 707–714.

Humes, L. E. (1996). Speech understanding in the elderly. *Journal of the American Academy of Audiology, 7,* 161–167.

Hummert, M. L., Garstka, T. A., Ryan, E. B., & Bonnesen, J. L. (2004). The role of age stereotypes in interpersonal communication. In J. F. Nussbaum & J. Coupland (Eds.), *Handbook of communication and aging research* (2nd ed., pp. 91–114). Hillsdale, NJ: Lawrence Erlbaum Associates, Inc.

Humphrey, D. G., & Kramer, A. F. (1999). Age-related differences in perceptual organization and selective attention: Implications for display segmentation and recall performance. *Experimental Aging Research, 25,* 1–26.

James, L. E. (2006). Specific effects of aging on proper name retrieval: Now you see them, now you don't. *Journal of Gerontology: Psychological Sciences, 61,* P180–P183.

James, L. E., &, Burke, D. M. (2000). Phonological priming effects on word retrieval and tip-of-the-tongue experiences in young and older adults. *Journal of Experimental Psychology: Learning, Memory, and Cognition, 26,* 1378–1391.

James, L. E., Burke, D. M., Austin, A., & Hulme, E. (1998). Production and perception of "verbosity" in younger and older adults. *Psychology and Aging, 13,* 355–367.

James, L., & MacKay, D. G. (2007). New age-linked asymmetries: Aging and the processing of familiar versus novel language on the input versus output side. *Psychology and Aging, 22,* 94–103.

Johnson, R. E. (2003). Aging and the remembering of text. *Developmental Review, 23,* 261–346.

Juncos-Rabadan, O. (1996). Narrative speech in the elderly: Effects of age and education on telling stories. *International Journal of Behavioral Development, 19,* 669–685.

Kemper, S. (1987). Life-span changes in syntactic complexity. *Journal of Gerontology, 42,* 323–328.

Kemper, S. (1992). Language and aging. In F. I. M. Craik & T. A. Salthouse (Eds.), *The handbook of aging and cognition* (pp. 213–270). Hillsdale, NJ: Lawrence Erlbaum Associates, Inc.

Kemper, S. (2006). Language in adulthood. In E. Bialystok & F. I. M. Craik (Eds.) *Lifespan cognition: Mechanisms of change* (pp. 223–238). New York, NY: Oxford University Press.

Kemper, S., Crow, A., & Kemtes, K. (2004). Eye-fixation patterns of high- and low-span young and older adults: Down the garden path and back again. *Psychology and Aging, 19,* 157–170.

Kemper, S., Greiner, L. H., Marquis, J. G., Prenovost, K., & Mitzner, T. L. (2001). Language decline across the life span: Findings from the nun study. *Psychology and Aging, 16,* 227–239.

Kemper, S., & Harden, T. (1999). Experimentally disentangling what's beneficial about elderspeak from what's not. *Psychology and Aging, 14,* 656–670.

Kemper, S., Herman, R., & Lian, C. (2003). Age differences in sentence production. *Journal of Gerontology: Psychological Sciences, 58,* P260–P268.

Kemper, S., Herman, R. E., & Nartowicz, J. (2005). Different effects of dual task demands on the speech of young and older adults. *Aging, Neuropsychology, and Cognition, 12,* 340–358.

Kemper, S., & Kemtes, K. (1999). Limitations on syntactic processing. In S. Kemper & R. Kliegl (Eds.), *Constraints on language: Aging, grammar, and memory* (pp. 79–106). Boston, MA: Kluwer.

Kemper, S., & Kemtes, K. (2000). Aging and message production and comprehension. In D. C. Park & N. Schwarz (Eds.), *Cognitive aging: A primer* (pp. 197–213). New York, NY: Psychology Press.

Kemper, S., Kynette, D., Rash, S., O'Brien, K., & Sprott, R. (1989). Life-span changes to adults' language: Effects of memory and genre. *Applied Psycholinguistics, 10,* 49–66.

Kemper, S., & Lacal, J. C. (2004). Addressing the communication needs of an aging society. In R. W. Pew & S. B. Van Hemel (Eds.), *Technology for adaptive aging* (pp. 129–149). Washington, DC: The National Academies Press.

Kemper, S., Rash, S. R., Kynette, D., & Norman, S. (1990). Telling stories: The structure of adults' narratives. *European Journal of Cognitive Psychology, 2,* 205–228.

Kemper, S., & Sumner, A. (2001). The structure of verbal abilities in young and older adults. *Psychology and Aging, 16,* 312–322.

Kemper, S., Thompson, M., & Marquis, J. (2001). Longitudinal change in language production: Effects of aging and dementia on grammatical complexity and propositional content. *Psychology and Aging, 16,* 227–239.

Kemtes, K. A., & Kemper, S. (1997). Younger and older adults' on-line processing of syntactically ambiguous sentences. *Psychology and Aging, 12,* 362–371.

Laver, G. D., & Burke, D. M. (1993). Why do semantic priming effects increase in old age? A meta-analysis. *Psychology and Aging, 8,* 34–43.

Lazzara, M. M., Yonelinas, A. P., & Ober, B. A. (2002). Implicit memory in aging: Normal transfer across semantic decisions and stimulus format. *Aging, Neuropsychology, and Cognition, 9,* 145–156.

Le Dorze, G., & Bédard, C. (1998). Effects of age and education on the lexico-semantic content of connected speech in adults. *Journal of Communication Disorders, 31,* 53–71.

Li, K. Z. H., Hasher, L., Jonas, D., May, C. P., & Rahhal, T. A. (1998). Distractibility, circadian arousal, and aging: A boundary condition? *Psychology and Aging, 13,* 574–583.

Lindenberger, U., & Baltes, P. B. (1997). Intellectual functioning in old and very old age: Cross-sectional results from the Berlin Aging Study. *Psychology and Aging, 12,* 410–432.

Lovelace, E. A., & Twohig, P. T. (1990). Healthy older adults' perceptions of their memory functioning and use of mnemonics. *Bulletin of the Psychonomic Society, 28,* 115–118.

MacDonald, M. C., & Christiansen, M. H. (2002). Reassessing working memory: Comment on Just and Carpenter (1992) and Waters and Caplan (1996). *Psychological Review, 109,* 35–54.

MacKay, A. I., Connor, L. T., Albert, M. L., & Obler, L. K. (2002). Noun and verb retrieval in healthy aging. *Journal of the International Neuropsychological Society, 8,* 764–770.

MacKay, D. G. (1987). *The organization of perception and action: A theory for language and other cognitive skills.* New York, NY: Springer-Verlag.

MacKay, D. G., & Abrams, L. (1996). Language, memory, and aging: Distributed deficits and the structure of new-versus-old connections. In J. E. Birren & K. W. Schaie (Eds.), *Handbook of the psychology of aging* (4th ed., pp. 251–265). San Diego, CA: Academic Press.

MacKay, D. G., & Abrams, L. (1998). Age-linked declines in retrieving orthographic knowledge: Empirical, practical, and theoretical implications. *Psychology and Aging, 13,* 647–662.

MacKay, D. G., Abrams, L., & Pedroza, M. J. (1999). Aging on the input versus output side: Theoretical implications of age-linked asymmetries between detecting versus retrieving orthographic information. *Psychology and Aging, 14,* 3–17.

MacKay, D. G., & Burke, D. M. (1990). Cognition and aging: New learning and the use of old connections. In T. M. Hess (Ed.), *Aging and cognition: Knowledge organization and utilization* (pp. 213–263). Amsterdam, The Netherlands: North Holland.

MacKay, D. G., & James, L. E. (2004). Sequencing, speech production, and selective effects of aging on phonological and morphological speech errors. *Psychology and Aging, 19,* 93–107.

MacKay, D. G., & Miller, M. D. (1996). Can cognitive aging contribute to fundamental psychological theory? Repetition deafness as a test case. *Aging, Neuropsychology, and Cognition, 3,* 169–186.

Mackenzie, C. (2000). Adult spoken discourse: The influences of age and education. *International Journal of Language and Communication Disorders, 35,* 269–285.

Margolin, S. J., & Abrams, L. (2007). Individual differences in young and older adults spelling: Do good spellers age better than poor spellers? *Aging, Neuropsychology, and Cognition, 14,* 529–544.

Margolin, S. J., & Abrams, L. (2009). Not may not be too difficult: The effects of negation on older adults' sentence comprehension. *Educational Gerontology, 35,* 306–320.

Maylor, E. A. (1990). Recognizing and naming faces: Aging, memory retrieval and the tip of the tongue state. *Journal of Gerontology: Psychological Sciences, 45,* P215–P225.

Mergler, N. L., Faust, M., & Goldstein, M. D. (1985). Storytelling as an age-dependent skill: Oral recall of orally presented stories. *International Journal of Aging and Human Development, 20,* 205–228.

Meyer, A. S., & Bock, K. (1992). The tip-of-the-tongue phonemenon: Blocking or partial activation. *Memory and Cognition, 20,* 715–726.

Morrison, C. M., Hirsh, K. W., & Duggan, G. B. (2003). Age of acquisition, ageing, and verb production: Normative and experimental data. *Quarterly Journal of Experimental Psychology: Human Experimental Psychology, 56,* 705–730.

Morrow, D. G., Stine-Morrow, E. A. L., Leirer, V. O., Andrassy, J. M., & Kahn, J. (1997). The role of reader age and focus of attention in creating situation models from narratives. *Journal of Gerontology: Psychological Sciences, 52,* P73–P80.

Mortensen, L., Meyer, A. S., & Humphreys, G. W. (2006). Age-related effects on speech production: A review. *Language and Cognitive Processes, 21,* 238–290.

Myerson, J., Hale, S., Wagstaff, D., Poon, L. W., & Smith, G. A. (1990). The information-loss model: A mathematical theory of age-related cognitive slowing. *Psychological Review, 97,* 475–487.

Nicholas, M., Obler, L. K., Albert, M. L., & Goodglass, H. (1985). Lexical retrieval in healthy aging. *Cortex, 21,* 595–606.

Obler, L. K., Fein, D., Nicholas, M., & Albert, M. L. (1991). Auditory comprehension and aging: Decline in syntactic processing. *Applied Psycholinguistics, 12,* 433–452.

Pichora-Fuller, M. K., Schneider, B. A., & Daneman, M. (1995). How young and old adults listen to and remember speech in noise. *Journal of the Acoustical Society of America, 97,* 593–608.

Pratt, M. W., & Robins, S. L. (1991). That's the way it was: Age differences in the structure and quality of adults' narratives. *Discourse Processes, 14,* 73–85.

Pushkar, D., Basevitz, P., Arbuckle, T. Y., Nohara-LeClair, M., Lapidus, S., & Peled, M. (2000). Social behavior and off-target verbosity in elderly people. *Psychology and Aging, 15,* 361–374.

Pushkar Gold, D. P., & Arbuckle, T. Y. (1995). A longitudinal study of off-target verbosity. *Journal of Gerontology: Psychological Sciences, 50,* P307–P315.

Radvansky, G. A., Copeland, D. E., & Zwaan, R. A. (2003). Aging and functional spatial relations in comprehension and memory. *Psychology and Aging, 18,* 161–165.

Radvansky, G. A., Zwaan, R. A., Curiel, J. M., & Copeland, D. E. (2001). Situation models and aging. *Psychology and Aging, 16,* 145–160.

Rastle, K. G., & Burke, D. M. (1996). Priming the tip of the tongue: Effects of prior processing on word retrieval in young and older adults. *Journal of Memory and Language, 35,* 586–605.

Ryan, E. B., Giles, H., Bartlucci, G., & Henwood, K. (1986). Psycholinguistic and social psychological components of communication by and with the elderly. *Language and Communication, 6,* 1–24.

Ryan, E. B., See, S. K., Meneer, W. B., & Trovato, D. (1994). Age-based perceptions of conversational skills among younger and older adults. In M. L. Hummert, J. M. Wiemann, & J. N. Nussbaum (Eds.), *Interpersonal communication in older adulthood* (pp. 15–39). Thousand Oaks, CA: Sage Publications.

Salthouse, T. A. (1985). *A theory of cognitive aging.* Amsterdam, The Netherlands: North-Holland.

Salthouse, T. A. (1988). Resource-reduction interpretations of cognitive aging. *Developmental Review, 8,* 238–272.

Salthouse, T. A. (1991). *Theoretical perspectives on cognitive aging* (pp. 301–349). Hillsdale, NJ: Lawrence Erlbaum.

Salthouse, T. A. (1996). The processing-speed theory of adult age differences in cognition. *Psychological Review, 103,* 403–428.

Salthouse, T. A. (2000). Steps towards the explanation of adult age differences in cognition. In T. Perfect & E. Maylor (Eds.), *Models of cognitive aging* (pp. 19–49). Oxford, UK: Oxford University Press.

Schmitter-Edgecombe, M., Vesneski, M., & Jones, D. (2000). Aging and word finding: A comparison of discourse and nondiscourse tests. *Archives of Clinical Neuropsychology, 15,* 479–493.

Schneider, B. A., & Pichora-Fuller, M. K. (2000). Implications of perceptual deterioration for cognitive aging research. In F. I. M. Craik & T. A. Salthouse (Eds.), *Handbook of aging and cognition* (pp. 155–220). Mahwah, NJ: Lawrence Erlbaum Associates, Inc.

Scialfa, C. T. (2002). The role of sensory factors in cognitive aging research. *Canadian Journal of Experimental Psychology, 56,* 153–163.

Scialfa, C. T., Hamaluk, E., Pratt, J., & Skaloud, P. (1999). Age differences in saccadic averaging. *Psychology and Aging, 14,* 695–699.

Shafto, M. A, Burke, D. M., Stamatakis, E. A., Tam, P. P., & Tyler, L. K. (2007). On the tip-of-the-tongue: Neural correlates of increased word-finding failures in normal aging. *Journal of Cognitive Neuroscience, 19*, 2060–2070.

Sommers, M. S. (1996). The structural organization of the mental lexicon and its contribution to age-related declines in spoken-word recognition. *Psychology and Aging, 11*, 333–341.

Sommers, M. S. (1997). Stimulus variability and spoken word recognition. II: The effects of age and hearing impairment. *Journal of the Acoustical Society of America, 101*, 2278–2288.

Sommers, M. (2008). Age-related changes in spoken word recognition. *The handbook of speech perception* (pp. 469–493). Malden, MA: Blackwell Publishing.

Sommers, M. S., & Danielson, S. M. (1999). Inhibitory processes and spoken word recognition in young and older adults: The interaction of lexical competition and semantic context. *Psychology and Aging, 14*, 458–472.

Steenbekkers, L. P. A. (1998). Visual contrast sensitivity. In L. P. A. Steenbekkers & C. E. M. Beijsterveldt (Eds.), *Design-relevant characteristics of ageing users. Backgrounds and guidelines for product innovation* (pp. 131–136). Delft: Delft University Press.

Stemberger, J. P., & MacWhinney, B. (1986). Frequency and the lexical storage of regularly inflected forms. *Memory and Cognition, 14,* 17–26.

Stine, E. A. L., & Wingfield, A. (1994). Older adults can inhibit high-probability competitors in speech recognition. *Aging and Cognition, 1*, 152–157.

Stine, E. A. L., Wingfield, A., & Poon, L. W. (1986). How much and how fast: Rapid processing of spoken language in later adulthood. *Psychology and Aging, 1*, 303–311.

Stine-Morrow, E. A. L., Soederberg Miller, L. M., Gagne, D. D., & Hertzog, C. (2008). Self-regulated reading in adulthood. *Psychology and Aging, 23*, 131–153.

Stuart-Hamilton, I., & Rabbitt, P. (1997). Age-related decline in spelling ability: A link with fluid intelligence? *Educational Gerontology, 23,* 437–441.

Taylor, J. K., & Burke, D. M. (2002). Asymmetric aging effects on semantic and phonological processes: Naming in the picture-word interference task. *Psychology and Aging, 17,* 662–676.

Thornton, R., & Light, L. L. (2006). Language comprehension and production in normal aging. In J. E. Birren and K. Warner Schaie (Eds.), *Handbook of the psychology of aging* (6th ed., pp. 261–287). Burlington, MA: Elsevier.

Tree, J. J., & Hirsh, K. W. (2003). Sometimes faster, sometimes, slower: Associative and competitor priming in picture naming with young and elderly participants. *Journal of Neurolinguistics, 16*, 489–514.

Trunk, D. L., & Abrams, L. (2009). Do younger and older adults' communicative goals influence off-topic speech in autobiographical narratives? Psychology and Aging, *24*, 324–337.

Tun, P. A. (1998). Fast noisy speech: Age differences in processing rapid speech with background noise. *Psychology and Aging, 13*, 424–434.

Tun, P. A., O'Kane, G., & Wingfield, A. (2002). Distraction by competing speech in young and older adult listeners. *Psychology and Aging, 17*, 453–467.

Tun, P. A., & Wingfield, A. (1999). One voice too many: Adult age differences in language processing with different types of distracting sounds. *Journals of Gerontology: Psychological Sciences, 54*, P317–P327.

van Dijk, T. A., & Kintsch, W. (1983). *Strategies of discourse comprehension*. New York, NY: Academic Press.

Verhaeghen, P. (2003). Aging and vocabulary score: A meta-analysis. *Psychology and Aging, 18*, 332–339.

Vitevitch, M. S., & Sommers, M. S. (2003). The facilitative influence of phonological similarity and neighborhood frequency in speech production in younger and older adults. *Memory and Cognition, 31,* 491–504.

Vousden, J. I., & Maylor, E. A. (2006). Speech errors across the lifespan. *Language and Cognitive Processes, 21,* 48–77.

White, K. K., & Abrams, L. (2002). Does priming specific syllables during tip-of-the-tongue states facilitate word retrieval in older adults? *Psychology and Aging, 17,* 226–235.

White, K. K., & Abrams, L. (2004). Phonologically mediated priming of preexisting and new associations in young and older adults. *Journal of Experimental Psychology: Learning, Memory, and Cognition, 30,* 645–655.

White, K. K., Protasi, M. & Abrams, L., (2010). *Spelling homophones gets better with age: Influences from orthography and semantics.* Poster presented at the 13th biennial Cognitive Aging Conference, Atlanta, GA.

White, K. K., Abrams, L, McWhite, C. B., & Hagler, H. L. (2010). Syntactic constraints in the retrieval of homophone orthography. *Journal of Experimental Psychology: Learning, Memory, and Cognition, 36,* 160–169.

White, K. K., Abrams, L., Zoller, S. M., & Gibson, S. M. (2008b). Why did I right that? Factors that influence the production of homophone substitution errors. *The Quarterly Journal of Experimental Psychology, 61,* 977–985.

Willott, J. F. (1991). *Aging and the auditory system: Anatomy, physiology, and psychophysics.* San Diego, CA: Singular Press.

Wingfield, A. (1996). Cognitive factors in auditory performance: Context, speed of processing, and constraints of memory. *Journal of the American Academy of Audiology, 7,* 175–182.

Wingfield, A., Aberdeen, J. S., & Stine, E. A. (1991). Word onset gating and linguistic context in spoken word recognition by young and elderly adults. *Journal of Gerontology: Psychological Sciences, 46,* P127–P129.

Wingfield, A., & Ducharme, J. L. (1999). Effects of age and passage difficulty on listening rate preferences for time-altered speech. *Journal of Gerontology: Psychological Sciences, 54,* P199–P202.

Wingfield, A., & Grossman, M. (2006). Language and the aging brain: Patterns of neural compensation revealed by functional brain imaging. *Journal of Neurophysiology, 96,* 2830–2839.

Wingfield, A., Lindfield, K. C., & Goodglass, H. (2000). Effects of age and hearing sensitivity on the use of prosodic information in spoken word recognition. *Journal of Speech, Language, and Hearing Research, 43,* 915–925.

Wingfield, A., Peelle, J. E., & Grossman, M. (2003). Speech rate and syntactic complexity as multiplicative factors in speech comprehension by young and older adults. *Aging, Neuropsychology, and Cognition, 10,* 310–322.

Wingfield, A., Poon, L. W., Lombardi, L., & Lowe, D. (1985). Speed of processing in normal aging: Effects of speech rate, linguistic structure, and processing time. *Journal of Gerontology, 40,* 579–585.

Wingfield, A., & Stine-Morrow, E. A. L. (2000). Language and speech. In F. I. M. Craik & T. A. Salthouse (Eds.), *The handbook of aging and cognition* (2nd ed., pp. 359–416). Mahwah, NJ: Lawrence Erlbaum Associates, Inc.

Wingfield, A., & Tun, P. A. (2001). Spoken language comprehension in older adults: Interactions between sensory and cognitive change in normal aging. *Seminars in Hearing, 22,* 287–301.

Wingfield, A., Tun, P. A., Koh, C. K., & Rosen, M. J. (1999). Regaining lost time: Adult aging and the effect of time restoration on recall of time-compressed speech. *Psychology and Aging, 14,* 380–389.

Yonan, C. A., & Sommers, M. S. (2000). The effects of talker familiarity on spoken word identification in younger and older listeners. *Psychology and Aging, 15,* 88–99.

Zurif, E., Swinney, D., Prather, P., Wingfield, A., & Brownell, H. (1995). The allocation of memory resources during sentence comprehension: Evidence from the elderly. *Journal of Psycholinguistic Research, 24,* 165–182.

Zwaan, R., Magliano, J. P., & Graesser, A. C. (1995). Dimensions of situation model construction in narrative comprehension. *Journal of Experimental Psychology: Learning, Memory, and Cognition, 21,* 386–397.

Zwaan, R. A., & Radvansky, G. A. (1998). Situation models in language comprehension and memory. *Psychological Bulletin, 123,* 162–185.

4 Working Memory and Attention in Language Use

Nelson Cowan

INTRODUCTION

Working memory refers to a small amount of information held in the mind, readily accessible for a short time to help an individual comprehend language and solve problems. As such, it is not just any topic, but potentially the key mechanism that organizes and represents one's conscious experience as a human being; William James (1890) referred to it as primary memory, which he described as the trailing edge of consciousness. The purpose of this chapter is to alert you to the ways in which scientists in this field have been thinking about working memory and its implications for language, attention, and the mind. The discussion will be based on some important findings from various laboratories to illustrate our notions about working memory. It will come out in the discussion that there is a lot of debate in this field.

PLAN FOR THE CHAPTER

We will start with just a touch of history to give us our bearings about where the field came from. Then the discussion turns to the various ways in which working memory could be involved in language processing. This leads to an explanation of a couple of theoretical models that could help in understanding how working memory may operate. Finally, the chapter will focus on a single key issue. It is the issue of whether there is one central working memory function that uses attention and cuts across domains (such as verbal and nonverbal processing) or whether there are specific working memory modules for different types of materials. Research on individual differences and age differences will be woven into the fabric of this discussion about the key issue of the nature of working memory. The field of working memory is rich and diverse, but the aims of the chapter are more focused in order to keep our eye on the ball, which is gaining a useful perspective on what working memory means and what it is worth scientifically.

THE HISTORY OF WORKING MEMORY
RESEARCH IN A NUTSHELL

There is a difference between the vast information storehouse of the mind, known as *long-term memory*, and *working memory*, the small portion of that memory held in the mind for a brief time. George Miller kicked off the field in modern times with his famous article (1956) based on a long conference address he was cajoled into giving despite some reluctance as a young professor (see Miller, 1989). It helped establish this working memory concept and, in the process, helped launch the field of cognitive psychology that went beyond behavior to draw inferences about how ideas seem to be represented in the mind. His article relayed his entertaining observation that he was being persecuted by a number, the seven or so items that one could barely manage to recall from a just-encountered list. What was most important in Miller's observations was that anything meaningful to the individual—such as a letter, a word, an acronym, or an idiom—could serve as a meaningful unit or *chunk* among the seven or so apparently held in working memory. (Later the observation would be made that the seven or so items one might recall were themselves grouped into 3–5 chunks, which more fundamentally defines the working memory limit; see Broadbent, 1975; Cowan, 2001). Miller, Galanter, and Pribram (1960) coined the term working memory to refer to the use of this brief memory to keep track of one's current goals and subgoals while trying to accomplish them.

Soon afterward, George Miller turned his attention to other aspects of language but Alan Baddeley and Graham Hitch picked up the ball where Miller left off (Baddeley & Hitch, 1974), using a rich set of studies on list memory and reasoning to demarcate different aspects of working memory. According to their theory, working memory was a system that included a central and meaningful holding faculty related to consciousness and attention, echoing earlier contemplations by the extraordinary philosopher and armchair psychologist William James (1890). Working memory was also said to include some more automatic holding mechanisms supposedly specialized in speech sounds on the one hand, and visual and spatial patterns on the other hand. These faculties were all supposed to be coordinated in their functioning by mechanisms known to be dependent on the frontal lobes of the brain, termed central executive processes. Baddeley (1986) thought he could explain working memory data without the attention-related type of storage and dropped it, in contrast to others, including Cowan (1988), who resembled James (1890) in seeing that type storage and the focus of attention as a key basis of working memory. Baddeley (2000) later seemed to agree, adding an *episodic buffer* that was said to mediate similarly central, abstract types of storage. There are still vivid discussions about such theoretical topics as just what role attention plays in working memory and how general or specialized the working memory storage devices are in the brain. We will return to these questions after explaining how working memory may be involved in processing language.

WORKING MEMORY IN LANGUAGE PROCESSING

TYPES OF INFORMATION INCLUDED IN WORKING MEMORY FOR LANGUAGE

The theories of working memory were mostly developed to explain a rather focused body of knowledge in which certain variables were emphasized, such as the number of items in a list to be recalled, the semantic (meaning-based) or phonological (speech-sound-based) similarity between items in the list, or the presence or absence of a second task during the presentation of the list. Theoretically, though, we have to allow for the possibility that many levels of concepts in memory become active when a new stimulus is presented (or, for that matter, when one's mind wanders among the possibilities in long-term memory). Table 4.1 illustrates many of the levels of units that may become active in memory when one hears the sentence (from Alan Ginsburg's poem *Howl*, 1956, "I saw the best minds of my generation destroyed by madness"). Any of these active units could become part of working memory. One might, for example, remember a bit about the tone of voice in which the sentence was spoken. As a second or so elapses after the stimulus sentence, some of the acoustic and phonological information may drift out of working memory but it may be replaced by an increasing awareness of the meaning of the sentence, which also will leave working memory and awareness as time progresses.

MECHANISMS OF INFORMATION LOSS FROM WORKING MEMORY

There are several ways in which this temporary information could leave working memory, as shown in Table 4.2. The long history of considering these possibilities

TABLE 4.1
Possible Types of Verbal Working Memory and Examples of the Units for Each Type

STIMULUS: "I saw the best minds of my generation destroyed by madness..."
(Allen Ginsburg, *Howl*)

Possible Types of Verbal Working Memory	Example of Units
SENSORY	(speech sound frequency patterns as perceived)
PHONOLOGICAL	/... dəstrɔɪd baɪ madnəs.../
ARTICULATORY	(mouth movement plans to produce the phonemes)
LEXICAL	I, saw, the, best...
SEMANTIC	(self concept) (see + past) (def. article) (superlative)...
GRAMMATICAL	(subject – *I*) [verb phrase – (verb *saw*, object phrase *the best minds of my generation*)]...
CONSTRUCTED SCENE	(conception of intent and implications of the sentence)
PRIMING ACTIVATION	concepts related to *I, saw, best, minds*...
INTENDED SPEECH	plans for what one intends to say in response to stimulus

TABLE 4.2

Possible Mechanisms of Loss of Verbal Working Memory and Descriptions of the Mechanisms

Possible Mechanisms of Working Memory Loss	Description of Mechanism
DECAY	units are lost over time, in a matter of seconds
CAPACITY LIMITS	units are lost if there are more than a few to be retained at the same time
SPECIFIC INTERFERENCE	units are lost or contaminated if similar units occur afterward
ACID BATH	loss of units in which an interfering item has an effect that depends on the duration of its presentation
LOSS OF CONTEXT	as time elapses and conditions change, the retrieval cues present at encoding of the stimuli are no longer fully present

was reviewed by Cowan (2005). It is critical to realize that no matter how an item is lost from working memory, it presumably still might be retrieved from long-term memory if sufficient cues are presented, though there is no guarantee that the subject will remember that this particular unit from long-term memory was presented at a certain particular time or within a certain particular event.

In one possible mechanism of loss from working memory, called *decay*, information is simply lost as a function of time. This mechanism is analogous to radioactive decay, in which a particular element such as uranium has a known period of decay or half-life. This possibility is still a leading contender, for example, in the case of sensory memory, the memory of the way an event looked, sounded, felt, and so on. (Some researchers would not consider this part of working memory but it is according to the rather theory-neutral definition that I gave in the first sentence.) Decay also has been nominated as a mechanism for forgetting of phonological and visuospatial information by Baddeley (1986). People could recall as much as they could recite in about two seconds (Baddeley, Thomson, & Buchanan, 1975) and that can be explained on the basis that covert verbal rehearsal refreshes the information before it decays from working memory beyond the point at which retrieval becomes impossible, which presumably would happen in about two seconds. This feature of working memory has, however, been hotly contested over the years. As just one example, Lewandowsky, Duncan, and Brown (2004) had subjects recall letters in a list quickly (after saying "super" between each two letters recalled) or slowly (after saying "super, super, super" between each two letters). No difference in recall was observed despite the difference in the time course of recall.

Another way in which information could leave working memory is that there could be a limit in how many units can be retained at once. If too many items are presented, the subject may have to make a decision about which ones to retain, or perhaps this decision sometimes occurs automatically in the brain. This notion of capacity limits, too, has been controversial. Although Miller (1956) documented that people could recall lists of about seven items, he also provided enough information to provoke doubt as to whether each item was recalled as a separate chunk or whether subjects group together items to form larger chunks on the fly (for example, grouping 7-digit telephone numbers into a group of 3 digits followed by a group of 4 digits, which might be memorized separately). In that case, the important limit may be how many separate chunks are retained, and it may be fewer than seven. In situations in which it is difficult to group items together or rehearse them (because, for example, the items were not attended at the time they were presented or rehearsal was suppressed), normal adults most typically can recall only three to five items, not seven (Cowan, 2001). Nevertheless, as the commentaries at the end of the Cowan reference indicate, not everyone is convinced that there is a constant chunk capacity limit to working memory or some central part of it. Some researchers are just not convinced that the process of chunking has been controlled well enough to tell what the limit in chunks is, or whether that limit is truly constant across situations.

A third way in which information can be lost from working memory is through interference. This means that items replace other items in working memory. In this case, though, the replacement comes not because there is a fixed limit on how many items can be in working memory at once—a capacity limit—but because newly presented items that have features similar to items already in working memory replace or contaminate the representation of those pre-stored items in working memory.

Fourth, there can be a combination of interference and decay, degradation by an interfering stimulus over time, called an acid bath (Posner & Konick, 1966). In this mechanism, there is interference that depends not only on the similarity of the item in memory and the interfering item, but also the time during which an item is presented. In one good example of this type of forgetting, Massaro (1970) found that memory for the pitch of a tone was lost steadily over time during which another tone was presented; steadily but at a slower rate when a white noise was presented instead; and steadily at a very slow rate when there was no interfering sound.

It is very difficult to tell the difference between decay and an acid bath. Except possibly for sensory memory, it appears that people may prevent memory loss through rehearsal over time if there are no interfering stimuli. In order to prevent rehearsal, it is usually necessary to include stimuli to be recited. In that case, however, any memory loss over time can be attributed to an acid bath from the stimuli used to prevent rehearsal. Reitman (1971, 1974) tried to prevent rehearsal using a condition in which a subject listened carefully for a sound but, on particular trials, did not detect a sound. Some forgetting still seemed to occur. In our laboratory, Zwilling (2008) has replicated this type of experiment using a slightly different procedure, but did not find any forgetting. So it remains uncertain how it would be possible to detect decay.

One way that decay might be observed is by making the stimulus unattended at the time of its presentation. If an unattended stream of sounds is presented, one can present an occasional cue to switch attention to the sensory memory of that sound stream, which presumably will not have been rehearsed. Then it is possible to determine how the sensory memory is lost over time. Eriksen and Johnson

(1964) and Cowan, Lichty, and Grove (1990) did this, and did find some loss of memory as a function of the time between the sound and the retrieval cue.

There is, however, one additional mechanism of forgetting that can be confused with decay, loss of context. It is possible that the retrieval of information from working memory depends on retrieval cues that change rather rapidly over time. If one receives a stimulus and later is asked to retrieve it, loss of ability over time may not indicate decay. Instead, it may indicate that the retrieval cues have changed too much as the context has changed. A well-known result that indicates as much is one by Bjork and Whitten (1974). Ordinarily, there is especially good memory for the items at the end of a list to be recalled in a free recall task, in which the items can be recalled in any order. Subjects tend to recall the items at the end of the list first, and then go back and recall other list items. This list-final advantage or *recency effect* is lost if there is an interfering task lasting several seconds between the list and recall. Traditionally, this loss of the recency effect was attributed to decay of memory for items at the end of the list, with earlier items having been memorized and therefore unaffected by the delay (Glanzer & Cunitz, 1966). Bjork and Whitten, however, considered that it may be the relative rather than the absolute recency of the items at the end of the list that made them easy to recall. They placed an interfering task lasting 12 seconds between each pair of items to be recalled. When items were separated like this, it was found that the recency effect was not lost even after an interfering task between the list and recall. Apparently, the recency effect occurred at least partly because the most recent item was temporally distinct relative to the rest of the list (like a telephone pole that one is standing near compared to other poles down the line, which start to blend together in the distance), not because of decay. However, this "long-term recency effect" of Bjork and Whitten was not as large as the regular recency effect so it remains possible that decay plays a role, too.

COMPETING MODELS OF WORKING MEMORY

It is possible to proceed to consider working memory functioning without worrying overly much about which mechanisms of loss are at play. We will now examine a few simple theoretical models that can help you to conceptualize working memory, and these models assume particular mechanisms of loss or forgetting. It is instructive to think about what is similar between these models and what is different.

MODELS OF ALAN BADDELEY

Baddeley (1986) presented a model that included three components: the *phonological loop*, the *visuospatial sketchpad*, and the *central executive*. The model was designed to account for the results of various studies, including those of Baddeley and Hitch (1974) but actually beginning earlier, in which verbal or pictorial material was presented for immediate recall. The results suggested that verbal material interfered with other verbal material and that the source of interference was primarily in the sound system of language (as opposed to meaning, for example). This sound-based interference occurred even if the material was visually presented. For example, people have a great deal of difficulty recalling the order of the letters in the list *d, b, c, t, v, p, g* even if they are visually presented because, mentally, a speech-based code is formed and the rhyming letters cause speech-sound-based confusion (Conrad, 1964). In contrast, there is relatively little interference with working memory of a spatial layout from printed or spoken letters, and little interference with working memory of the letters from a spatial layout. This type of evidence was used to justify the separation of phonological and visuospatial *buffers*, which presumably each hold information of a particular type for a short time. The information is held automatically but a voluntary-attention-based system, the central executive, is responsible for helping to determine when and how the buffers are used. Certain processes are out of the control of the central executive nevertheless, such as the automatic entry of spoken language into the phonological buffer. A large corpus of evidence contributed to this sort of model.

This model was modified (Baddeley, 2000, 2001) on the grounds that people remember semantic information in working memory and bindings between different sorts of information, such as the association between a shape and a name that was assigned to it. On such grounds, an *episodic buffer* was added to account for information that is neither purely phonological nor purely visuospatial in nature. The resulting model is depicted in Figure 4.1. In this model, it was said that the phonological and visuospatial buffers contain information that is subject to decay, which is depicted by the subscript b in the diagram. (As an aside, I think we could substitute an acid bath here without doing terrible damage to the gist of the model.) The mechanism of loss characteristics of the episodic buffer were left for future research and might include both a capacity limit (Baddeley, 2001), a, and possibly decay, b.

Both Baddeley (1986; Baddeley & Hitch, 1974) and Cowan (1988) built their models largely in reaction to the standard information processing models of the early era of the field of cognitive psychology. The most influential of these models were the seminal model of Broadbent (1958) and the elaboration of that sort of model by Atkinson and Shiffrin (1968). The reactions of Baddeley and Cowan were for somewhat different reasons. In these early models, a single sensory memory fed information into a short-term store, which in turn fed information into long-term storage. Processes like the central executive processes governed the transfer of information from one store to the next, at least in the Atkinson and Shiffrin model in which details of processing were explored mathematically. Baddeley and Hitch (1974) reacted to the inclusion of only a single short-term store, regardless of the type of information stored. They found evidence that different types of information seem to be stored separately.

MODEL OF NELSON COWAN

Cowan (1988) was not so concerned with that point and was less inclined to like separate modules for the storage of phonological and visuospatial information. The differential interference results cannot be denied but they could be accounted for with the general principle that stimuli sharing features of various sorts are

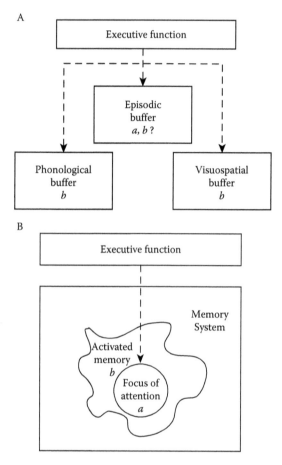

FIGURE 4.1   Two simple models of working memory. A. The model of Baddeley (2000). B. The model of Cowan (1988, 1999). In both models, a = stores assumed to be capacity-limited; b = stores assumed to be time-limited; a, b ? = store with limits open to debate.

more likely to interfere with one another (cf. Nairne, 1990). Baddeley's postulation of phonological and visuospatial stores seemed to rule out the untested possibility that storage differs in other, perhaps equally important ways: say, in the sensory modality of input, or in the speech versus nonspeech quality of sounds. There was also evidence that semantic information was saved in working memory, even though it was not so important in retaining the serial order of items in a list. In response to these considerations, Cowan (1988, p. 171) suggested that instead of separate buffers, various stimuli activated elements of long-term memory, which served a short-term retention function:

> The spectral, temporal, and spatial properties of sensation would be present as coded features in memory that behave in a way comparable to non-sensory features such as meaning and object categories. At least, this is the simplest hypothesis until

evidence to the contrary is obtained. One might hypothesize that premotor and prespeech plans ... also consist of activated memory elements.

What Cowan (1988) was reacting to in the early information processing models was not so much the problem of a single storage mechanism, but problem of the relation between memory and selective attention. In the early models, information from an all-encompassing but short-lived sensory memory was selectively forwarded for further processing and storage in short-term (or working) memory. This arrangement seemed to overlook the point that some features of memory were activated automatically by incoming stimuli. It also overlooked the point that not all information that was readily accessible had the same status. Some information was in the focus of attention and awareness, and this information could be readily integrated and deeply processed (as in the levels-of-processing conception of Craik and Lockhart, 1972). In contrast, other accessible information persisted for a short time in an unintegrated form. Examples might include the stream of sounds or phonemes from someone who just spoke when you were not paying attention, and a sentence to which you attended a few seconds ago but have now stopped attending.

The outcome of these concerns was a model like that developed by Cowan (1988), illustrated in Figure 4.2. Here it was suggested that there are two different working memory mechanisms that lose information in different ways. The temporarily activated elements of long-term memory lose activation through decay, denoted with subscript b (or, again, one could substitute an acid bath). In contrast, the subset of these activated elements that are in the focus of attention are resistant to decay but are limited to a handful of chunks at any one time, denoted with subscript a; about four chunks in normal adults, according to Cowan (2001).

In subsequent writing a further, important detail was discussed. Working memory should not be thought of as only the collection of activated features from long-term memory inasmuch as working memory must also include new links between features. One might have seen many blue objects and many different apples in one's life, but never a blue apple. If one is presented, this new binding between object identity and color must be retained in working memory as well as being stored in long-term memory. Cowan (1995, 1999, 2005) suggested that one function of the focus of attention is to store the bindings between features found in stimuli (or, for that matter, the results of creative thought), some of which may not already exist in long-term memory. It would retain, for example, information about what shape is in what location and what color goes with each shape in each location. At least, it would do so until a capacity limit is reached.

There is a new puzzle for this suggestion that the focus of attention retains binding information. When visual arrays are retained in working memory, retention of the binding between features (e.g., which shape goes with which color) does not differentially depend on attention. If you are distracted while retaining an array of objects, it will hurt your retention of the binding between features such as color and shape, or color and location, but it apparently will not do so more than it hurts your retention of the features themselves (Allen, Baddeley, & Hitch, 2006; Cowan, Naveh-Benjamin, Kilb, & Saults, 2006). This puzzle can be explained, though, under the premise that attention perceives and retains objects. Attention is needed to put the features together to perceive and retain the object but retaining the bindings between features may be part of that process of retaining the object, at no extra charge to working memory capacity (see Luck & Vogel, 1997). This process of binding between features and its cost to attention has not been examined as carefully in the domain of language.

MATHEMATICAL MODELS OF WORKING MEMORY

It is important not to leave the impression that the Baddeley (1986, 2001) and Cowan (1988, 2001) models are the only ones that treat working memory, or even the models that predict the results in the most detail. These two models were proposed in a spirit of a general framework for further research, with many details left unsettled. In contrast, many others have devised models with a different aim. These other models have aimed to generate numerical predictions of performance in working memory tasks. To do so, they have had to rely on some assumptions that cannot be verified, so there is a tradeoff in strengths and weaknesses of the methods. Some such models have been constructed to explain results in a certain domain, such as the recall of verbal lists (e.g., Burgess & Hitch, 1999). Some rely on principles different from the ones stressed by Baddeley or Cowan, such as retrieval cues and context changes over time (e.g., Brown, Neath, & Chater, 2007) or effects of interference between items on capacity (e.g., Davelaar, Goshen-Gottstein, Ashkenazi, Haarman, & Usher, 2005). Some were designed to account for memory and information processing as a whole, including working memory processes (e.g., Anderson & Lebiere, 1998; Grossberg, 1978; Newell, 1990). Continuing to refine and test such mathematical models is an important avenue for further research, though it is outside the scope of the present chapter.

A KEY ISSUE: THE DOMAIN GENERALITY VERSUS SPECIFICITY OF WORKING MEMORY

The models of Baddeley and Cowan seem to differ in a key prediction. (The difference may not hold when the episodic buffer is added to the model, as it may act in a way similar to the focus of attention.) The greater modularity of the Baddeley (1986) model means that there should be little interference between phonological and visuospatial information. In contrast, Cowan (1988) predicts that there can be interference between very different types of information provided that the information has to occupy the focus of attention. Which is it? Is working memory for language a separate faculty or set of faculties of the mind that can be used to comprehend and produce speech without taking into account other ongoing tasks that demand working memory such as, perhaps, keeping in mind what way you are driving? Or do all types of working memory tax a single, central resource such as attention? These are two very different conceptions of the mind.

In the remainder of the chapter we will discuss the contributions of several types of methods to resolve this basic question. To anticipate, the answer appears to be that there is some working memory mechanism related to attention that cuts across stimulus encoding domains, in addition to some domain-specific mechanisms. The issue can be investigated either by manipulating memory loads and examining the average effect of this, which is an experimental approach; or by determining how much individual difference variance is shared by different types of working memory task, which is a psychometric approach. I will discuss these methods in the abstract and then discuss some research using each method, within the following sections of the chapter. In the final sections, the application of these concepts to working memory for language will be examined in more detail.

THE POTENTIAL CONTRIBUTION OF EXPERIMENTAL METHODS

Experimental methods operate by manipulating variables in groups of normal subjects and examining the effects on the means. If two tasks share the same working memory resource, then it should be possible to show that requiring retention in both tasks at once is harmful to the recall in at least one of the tasks. For example, it should be possible to ask whether memory for a word or digit list shares a resource along with memory for an array of visual objects. One way to examine this question is to embed one task within another one on some trials, as shown in Figure 4.2A. This figure illustrates what I will call an *embedded task* procedure. Suppose, for example, that Set 1 is an array of visual objects and Set 2 is a list of spoken words. On dual-task trials, Set 1 (a visual array) will be

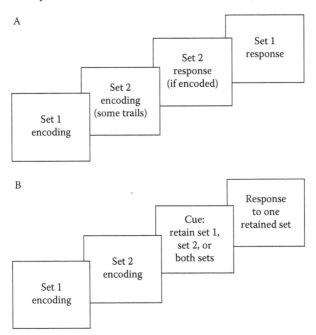

FIGURE 4.2　Two procedures to examine attention-sharing between tasks. A. Embedded-task procedure. B. Postcue procedure.

presented for perceptual encoding into working memory first, and then Set 2 (a word list) will be presented. After Set 2 is tested, Set 1 can be tested. For example, subjects might be asked to recognize one visual object and/or its location in the array, and then one word and/or its serial position in the list. During the entire task of encoding, retaining, and responding to Set 2, there is a visual memory load from retaining the items in Set 1. Also, during Set 1 retention, there is a memory load from doing all of the Set 2 activities. To measure these tasks, one can compare performance in those dual-task trials with performance in other, single-task trials that include only Set 1 or only Set 2.

If one cannot find interference between two tasks in an embedded task procedure, it seems likely that there is no common working memory resource between the tasks. However, if interference is found, the embedded task procedure is not able to indicate with certainty that it is working memory retention in the two tasks that conflict with one another. An alternative source of interference is that Set 1 retention could be hurt by Set 2 encoding or responding. Conversely, the effect of Set 1 on Set 2 performance could occur because retention of the Set 1 materials interfere with Set 2 encoding or responding.

One way to deal with this problem was developed by Cowan and Morey (2007), who used what we can call a *postcue* procedure, illustrated in Figure 4.2B. Both sets are presented for encoding. Then there is a cue to retain only the first set, only the second set, or both sets. The test is always on an item from one of the sets that the subject was supposed to retain according to the cue. Encoding of the sets is identical in all trial types because the subject does not know in advance what type of cue will be presented. If retention of either set is hurt by the cue to retain both sets at once, that dual-task interference can only be attributed to interference in working memory maintenance.

There are limitations of the postcue procedure as well. Set 2 encoding might be confined by the fact that Set 1 was already encoded. Therefore, the postcue procedure does not necessarily pick up the entire conflict between maintenance in the two sets. If the two sets are encoded into distinctly different modules with no resource overlap, however, encoding of Set 2 should not be impeded by maintenance of Set 1. At any rate, if an effect of a dual-set postcue is in fact obtained, that effect cannot be attributed to effects taking place at encoding. We will return to these methods with results after explaining a very different, psychometric method of looking at the issue of a common resource between different types of working memory tasks.

THE POTENTIAL CONTRIBUTION OF PSYCHOMETRIC METHODS AND INDIVIDUAL VARIATION

The psychometric method involves careful testing of individual differences in performance, making use of the pattern of correlations (and regressions) between tasks. Fundamentally, if performance on verbal and spatial working memory tasks correlate highly, it is possible that they stem from a common working memory mechanism. If they do not correlate at all, it is highly improbable that they stem from a common mechanism. This logic can also be taken to another level. Many have suggested that working memory is critical for intelligence (e.g., Engle, Tuholski, Laughlin, & Conway, 1999). If two different measures of working memory account for a common pool of variance in intelligence tests, they may be measuring the same working memory mechanism.

I have stated these conclusions about mechanisms based on correlations in a guarded way because one must be careful about the inferences that are drawn. To see this, it helps to go into a little detail about hypothetical research scenarios. Imagine a situation in which there are four task types: verbal memory, verbal perception, nonverbal memory, and nonverbal perception. Imagine further that the perception tasks require the same skills as the memory tasks, except for holding the information in working memory. For example, a verbal memory task could be to hear a series of seven digits and recall the digits from memory; the equivalent perception task could be to hear a series of seven digits and write them down while listening. Suppose there is a common memory faculty, *CM*, shared between the two memory tasks; a separate verbal memory faculty, *VM*; a common perceptual faculty shared between the two verbal tasks, *VP*; a separate nonverbal memory faculty, *NM*; and a common perceptual faculty shared between the two nonverbal tasks, *NP*. (For the sake of the argument let us present the items quickly so that perception is not trivial.) Then according to a linear model, each individual *i* would have performance levels on the four tasks as follows:

$$\text{Verbal memory}_i = CM_i + VM_i + VP_i + error_1 \tag{4.1}$$

$$\text{Verbal perception}_i = VP_i + error_2 \tag{4.2}$$

$$\text{Nonverbal memory}_i = CM_i + NM_i + NP_i + error_3 \tag{4.3}$$

$$\text{Nonverbal perception}_i = NP_i + error_4 \tag{4.4}$$

In these formulas, *error* in each case refers to measurement error. If there is a correlation between the types of memory task, it could be either because they both include CM_i or because some other terms are correlated. Assuming that the errors are uncorrelated, it could still be that there is a correlation between VM_i and NM_i even though they are different mechanisms. By analogy, the hands and feet are very different body parts but there is a correlation between the size of one's hands and of one's feet.

It could also be that there is a correlation between VP_i and NP_i. If we find, however, that verbal and nonverbal perception tasks are uncorrelated, we can be assured that the correlation between memory tasks does not occur for perceptual reasons.

The central question under examination is whether CM_i is too large to be neglected, which would indicate that there is a common memory resource across types of task. Even if the memory tasks are correlated it is hard to be sure of that because there is no independent estimate of VM_i and NM_i and they could correlate with one another. In terms of classifying people, this issue may not be important. By analogy, one might want to classify people into those with large hands and feet, versus those with small hands and feet. Still, one would not want to claim that hands and feet are the same things.

A combination of experimental and correlational findings is most powerful. One can find out whether there is a common working memory mechanism according to a dual-task experimental design, and also whether a common mechanism is possible according to a correlational design. Let us now put these methods to use.

WITHIN-DOMAIN AND GENERAL, CROSS-DOMAIN MECHANISMS OF WORKING MEMORY

Within-Domain Mechanisms

Baddeley (1986) very clearly described a large body of evidence suggesting that the coding of word lists relies heavily on a specialized, phonological storage mechanism. Semantic similarities between items in a list (e.g., rat, mouse, squirrel, etc.) are of very little consequence when the items must be recalled in order, which is serially; whereas phonological similarities (e.g., rat, mat, hat, etc.) are of great consequence, resulting in poor serial recall. Other phonological factors also play a special role in the serial recall of lists, including the length of words and the presence of irrelevant speech. A person is able to recall about as many items of a certain type as he or she can repeat in about two seconds. These findings were said to point toward a phonological storage mechanism from which information can decay, unless the phonological information is refreshed by the use of covert verbal rehearsal before the 2-second period is over.

According to Cowan (1999, 2005), the phonological store is only one type of activated information from long-term memory, which may include newly formed links between items such as the serial order of items in the list. These newly formed links become newly added information in long-term memory. Both theorists agree that covert verbal rehearsal is a very powerful and efficient way to retain phonological information, as one finds in verbal lists.

Unlike Baddeley (1986), Cowan (1988, 1995) emphasized that there are other sorts of activated information contributing to working memory performance as well. This point is underscored, for example, by the work on memory for quickly presented sentences described by Potter and Lombardi (1990). This work indicates that semantic information is constructed and used in working memory tasks. On each trial in the experiments described, a sentence was followed by a list of words presented very rapidly and then a probe, which was to be judged present or absent from the list. One of the unprobed words in the list was a lure item that was semantically related to a word in the sentence. Recall of the sentence turned out to be tainted by intrusion of the lure item on a large number of trials (compared to a small number of substitutions when there was no lure word in the list). For example, the sentence, *The knight rode around the palace searching for a place to enter* could be mis-remembered with the word *castle* replacing *palace*, a type of substitution that was much more likely when *castle* was among the list items in the probe task (even though this semantically related item was never used as the probe item). These results support the inference that a semantic representation of the sentence was held in working memory, in a vulnerable form. Providing related evidence, Romani and Martin (1999) found neurological patients with a specific deficit in working memory for semantic and lexical information. Potter (1993) summarized additional evidence that people ordinarily construct semantic representations in short-term (or working) memory.

It is not yet clear whether this sort of evidence can be accounted for best by the revised model of Baddeley (2000, 2001) or Cowan (1988, 1999). Baddeley's episodic buffer can hold semantic or lexical information but, in the 2001 paper, it was said to be subject to a capacity limit. In contrast, Cowan envisions semantic information as possibly present in the activated region of long-term memory with no capacity limit, just a time limit. (The focus of attention may be needed to make the semantic information active but that activated information was supposed to stay active for some time after it leaves the focus of attention). Until we know how much semantic information can be active outside of the focus of attention, we cannot tell the model that works better in this regard.

General, Cross-Domain Mechanisms

Some recent research seems to suggest that there is a common working memory mechanism across modalities or domains that might be based on the focus of attention as proposed, for example, by Cowan (1988, 1999, 2001, 2005). Much of it has relied on the embedded task procedure as described in Figure 4.2. Cocchini, Logie, Della Sala, MacPherson, and Baddeley (2002) carried out such a procedure using either verbal or spatial tasks as the first and second tasks and reported little interference between tasks. Morey and Cowan (2004, 2005) found somewhat different results in a study based on the visual array comparison procedure of Luck and Vogel (1997). In this procedure, an array of differently colored squares at haphazard locations is presented. In the version we used, a second array is presented but one item in the array is circled. Either the second array is identical to the first (except for the presence of the circle cue in the second array) or else the circled item has changed color. The task is to indicate whether that color has changed. This task becomes increasingly difficult when more than four items are in the array. Morey and Cowan sometimes required that a random list of six or seven spoken digits be retained in memory during the same period when the first array also had to be retained. The visual and verbal memory tasks interfered with one another substantially, provided that the digit list was recited aloud during this retention period. It was not simply verbal coding that interfered with the visual array memory, inasmuch as a simple recitation of the subject's known 7-digit telephone number had little effect on that memory. Stevanovski and Jolicoeur (2007) carried out a study with the visual array comparison task in which a tone identification task was presented between the arrays, and they included repetition of a single word ("banana") to prevent rehearsal. The finding was that the tone identification task impaired memory of the visual array; more so when the identification task included four tones rather than two and therefore was more difficult. These results suggest that there is a common capacity shared between verbal and visual materials.

Saults and Cowan (2007) took this conclusion further by suggesting that with sensory memory out of the way, all of the remaining capacity seemed to be central rather than modular in nature. Along with visual arrays they presented an array of spoken digits from four loudspeakers arranged around the subject. Each of the four digits was in a different voice (male or female adult or child). There was only one test, either a repetition of the visual array that might contain a change in one color or a repetition of the spoken array that might contain a change in one digit. In the best experiment, the auditory test involved digits that had been rearranged, so that the only potential cue that the subject could use was the link between the voice and the digit produced in that voice. Therefore, it did not allow the use of spatial information as in the visual stimuli. In other trial blocks, the subject knew they should attend only to the visual arrays or only to the spoken digits.

Saults and Cowan (2007) found that the results depended on whether there was a mask, a combination of complex squares and combined speech sounds to eliminate the sensory afterimage of the stimuli to be remembered. The mask was placed long enough after the arrays to allow good encoding of the abstract information. When there was no such mask, the two sets of stimuli interfered with one another but, still, subjects could remember more items when two modalities were to be remembered than when only one modality was to be remembered. However, when there was a mask, the amount that could be remembered if only visual items had to be remembered (about three and a half visual items) was almost exactly the same as the amount that could be remembered if both modalities had to be remembered (about three and a half items in all, some visual and some auditory). This suggests that any separate visual or verbal storage mechanism (possibly sensory in nature) can be masked out and that what remains when it is masked out is a substantial, remaining component that applies across modalities and holds three to four items in an abstract manner.

One nagging problem with these embedded task studies is that it is difficult to tell whether the conflict between tasks occurs in the process of retaining items from both modalities in working memory, or from the conflict between retention in one modality and encoding or, responding in the other modality. Cowan and Morey (2007) addressed this question using a postcue procedure as illustrated in Figure 4.2. On some trials, a visual array and a spoken list of digits or letters were presented, in either order. On other trials, two different visual arrays were presented (one with colored circles and one with colored squares) and, on still other trials, two different spoken lists were presented (one with digits and one with letters). After the presentation, there was a cue to keep remembering only the first set (array or list), only the second set (array or list), or both sets. The test was on one array item or one list item. In both cases, the item was shown in the correct location or in the wrong location; it was the correct or wrong spatial location for the visual item, or the correct or wrong serial position in the list for the spoken item. Overall, the cost of retaining a second visual set along with the visual set that was then tested (.61 item) was about the same as the cost of retaining a verbal set along with the visual set that was then tested (.58 item). Visual memory storage seems to occur in a form abstract enough that it can be interrupted equally by another set of visual items or a set of verbal items. For tests of verbal items, the cost of retaining a second verbal set along with the verbal set that was then tested was .65 items, versus .36 items for retention of a visual set along with the verbal set that was then tested. Although this difference did not reach significance, perhaps verbal working memory storage does include a modality-specific component, as we will discuss in a following section. Overall, though, these results tend to reinforce the notion from embedded task studies that there is a central, attention-demanding component of working memory retention.

Confirmation of this notion of a central, attention-demanding component of working memory retention comes also from a psychometric type of study conducted by Kane et al. (2004). They administered a variety of working memory tasks in which processing and storage were combined, including some verbally based and some spatially based tasks. It also included some simple span tasks that required storage and repetition of multiple items (e.g., a list of words or a series of spatial locations) but no separate processing component. The method of evaluation was structural equation modeling, a type of confirmatory factor analysis that produces a model of the various sources of variance that could contribute to the results. The best-fitting model did not need separate verbal and spatial working memory tasks of the complex, storage-and-processing sort. A single component fit the data across modalities and correlated well with both verbal and nonverbal intelligence measures. In contrast, the simple span tasks divided into more separate components for verbal versus spatial storage, with verbal span tasks accounting for some variance in intelligence tests using verbal materials and spatial span tasks accounting for some variance in intelligence tests using spatial materials.

The general factor for working memory tasks that include both storage and processing could reflect the contribution of an attention-demanding aspect of working memory storage, such as the focus of attention of Cowan (1999) or the episodic buffer of Baddeley (2000). Attention can be used to save information and to process it, and the attention-based mechanism deals with information in the abstract rather than tying it closely to the modality or code in which the information arrived. In contrast, the separation between simple verbal versus spatial span tasks could reflect skill in dealing with verbal versus spatial information. Although there is some correlation between an individual's ability to handle information in one modality and another, these specific skills are probably automatic and the profile of skills across modalities and codes can differ from one individual to the next; some people may be more interested in, experienced with, and/or naturally capable with verbal materials, and others with spatial materials.

WORKING MEMORY STRUCTURE AND THE LEVELS OF LANGUAGE

What we have discussed to this point could be consistent with either of the models shown in Table 4.1. Many or all of the levels of language shown in Table 4.1 are activated by the incoming speech or printed stimuli. If one has to remember a string of phonological information, an advantage is that the human mind is well-suited to rehearse the material. According to the model of Baddeley (2000), other forms of language information must be held in the episodic buffer and therefore would be limited to a few items (Baddeley, 2001).

According to the model of Cowan (1999, 2005), there is a slightly different analysis. Activated elements of long-term memory could include all sorts of language codes; but the focus of attention would be able to provide more integrated, analyzed information of up to a few items. As mentioned above, we do not yet know what model is correct. They differ in the mechanisms whereby nonphonological language information can be held in working memory.

Another hypothesis, beyond both of these theories, is that there is a specialized module that holds one type of grammatical information, namely the way in which words are combined to form sentences, or syntax (Caplan, Waters, & DeDe, 2007). That type of theory is in line with the theoretical work of Noam Chomsky, in which he suggests that the language acquisition device in children includes some innate syntactical information that can cut down on the possible grammars that have to be considered (Piattelli-Palmarini, 1980). Caplan et al. summarized a great deal of research looking at whether memory for syntax is affected by a memory load. That research included both dual task and psychometric factors. The conclusion was that syntactical working memory is separate, in that people with poor working memory are not impaired in syntactic analysis compared to people with good working memory, and that syntactic memory load and other types of memory load result in different patterns of activation in brain imaging studies.

A recent study by Fedorenko, Gibson, and Rohde (2007) may warrant a revision in all of these approaches. They compared easier, subject-extracted sentences (e.g., *The janitor who frustrated the plumber lost the key on the street*) to more difficult, object-extracted sentences (e.g., *The janitor who the plumber frustrated lost the key on the street*). The greater difficulty of the latter sentence type was attributed to the need to retrieve the subject of the sentence (*janitor*) as the object of the verb within the dependent clause (*frustrated*). Reading a sentence was combined with a math problem. For example, the subject might see the words *The janitor* with *12* above it, *who frustrated the plumber* with *+ 4* above it, and *lost the key* with *+ 5* above it, and *on the street* with *+ 4* above it. The math problem was either relatively easy or relatively hard; the one shown here is easy, involving small numbers. Subjects reported the sum and then answered questions about the sentence.

The most important dependent variable in the study of Fedorenko et al. (2007) was the speed with which subjects advanced through the parts of the problem. These reaction times were slower for object- than for subject-extracted sentences, mainly in the part of the sentence in which the interpretation of the relative clause was involved (*who frustrated the plumber* versus *who the plumber frustrated*). Moreover, this sentence type effect interacted with the difficulty of the math problem in that the added effect of difficult problems was larger for object-extracted sentences than for subject-extracted sentences. The result was replicated in two experiments.

So far, this result could be explained in at least two different ways. It could be that verbal information processing for the harder math problems interfered with difficult syntactic processing, or it could be that the drain on attention from the harder math problems interfered with difficult syntactic processing. A second pair of experiments, however, distinguished between these hypotheses by using spatial tasks instead of math. For example, one of them involved adding pie chart sections together visually. This visual task affected reaction times related to syntactic processing but there was no interaction between the difficulty of syntactic processing and the difficulty of the secondary task problem. The secondary task difficulty effect was the same for subject- and object-extracted sentences.

From these data, it seems possible to conclude that one part of the difficulty of working memory for syntax is specific to verbal materials. This is the part that causes the syntactic difficulty by math difficulty interaction. Additionally, the main effect of secondary task difficulty even with a spatial secondary task suggests that syntactic processing may require attention, to a comparable extent for each sentence type. Perhaps attention is needed in this procedure to discriminate whether the sentence is a subject- or object-extracted one, whereas subject-extracted sentence processing in ordinary life might not require as much attention as it does in this experimental setting with mixed sentence types.

The results of Fedorenko et al. (2007) seem to confirm that there is a specific verbal working memory component that depends on verbal processing. In contrast to the theoretical assertion of Caplan et al. (2007), though, it is not syntax-specific. It may well be a covert articulation component that is involved in both syntax processing and math. The finding, discussed by Caplan et al., that individual differences in working memory capacity tend not to affect syntactic processing may have a simple explanation. This may be found because most normal adults can use covert articulatory processes sufficiently well to process syntax. In fact, span tasks that allow articulation do not correlate very well with intelligence in adults (Cowan et al., 2005). One could predict, though, that individuals with impairment in articulatory processes may well display impaired syntax, as well as some impairment on working memory. Clearly, this question of whether there is a separate working memory for syntax is heating up and there is no agreement on it yet.

TRADEOFF BETWEEN STORAGE AND PROCESSING OF LANGUAGE

Last, it is important to acknowledge that the amount that can be retrieved in a working memory task depends on what other storage and processing is taking place (e.g., Bunting, Cowan, & Colflesh, 2008). Within an attention-based model, attention devoted to processing is used at the expense of some storage. A number of authors have suggested that the individuals who can store the most information and do the best processing are those who can inhibit the processing or storage of irrelevant information so that working memory can be devoted to the relevant information (e.g., Gernsbacher, 1993; Hasher, Stolzfus, Zacks, & Rypma, 1991; Kane, Bleckley, Conway, & Engle, 2001). On the other hand, at least one study suggests that the ability to control attention and the capacity of working memory are partly independent of one another among adults (Cowan, Fristoe, Elliott, Brunner, & Saults, 2006).

CONCLUSION

Working memory is a surprisingly encompassing concept that is involved in most information processing, including most language comprehension and production. This makes it important but also difficult to analyze. I have suggested that working memory for language depends on an ensemble of attention-dependent and automatic activation processes. The exact best model is not yet known but I have indicated several types of evidence that would help to clarify it. The goal was to sketch a model or set of models (see Figure 4.1) simple enough to be helpful in thinking about language processing, yet accurate enough to make useful predictions.

REFERENCES

Allen, R. J., Baddeley, A. D., & Hitch, G. J. (2006). Is the binding of visual features in working memory resource-demanding? *Journal of Experimental Psychology: General, 135*, 298–313.

Anderson, J. R., & Lebiere, C. (1998). *Atomic components of thought.* Hillsdale, NJ: Erlbaum.

Atkinson, R. C., & Shiffrin, R. M. (1968). Human memory: A proposed system and its control processes. In K. W. Spence & J. T. Spence (Eds.), *The psychology of learning and motivation: Advances in research and theory* (Vol. 2, pp. 89–195). New York, NY: Academic Press.

Baddeley, A. (2000). The episodic buffer: A new component of working memory? *Trends in Cognitive Sciences, 4*, 417–423.

Baddeley, A. (2001). The magic number and the episodic buffer. *Behavioral and Brain Sciences, 24*, 117–118.

Baddeley, A. D. (1986). *Working memory.* Oxford, UK: Clarendon Press.

Baddeley, A. D., & Hitch, G. (1974). Working memory. In G. H. Bower (Ed.), *The psychology of learning and motivation* (Vol. 8, pp. 47–89). New York, NY: Academic Press.

Baddeley, A. D., Thomson, N., & Buchanan, M. (1975). Word length and the structure of short-term memory. *Journal of Verbal Learning and Verbal Behavior, 14*, 575–589.

Bjork, R. A., & Whitten, W. B. (1974). Recency-sensitive retrieval processes in long-term free recall. *Cognitive Psychology, 6*, 173–189.

Broadbent, D. E. (1958). *Perception and communication.* New York, NY: Pergamon Press.

Broadbent, D. E. (1975). The magic number seven after fifteen years. In A. Kennedy & A. Wilkes (Eds.), *Studies in long-term memory* (pp. 3–18). Oxford, UK: John Wiley & Sons.

Brown, G. D. A., Neath, I., & Chater, N. (2007). A temporal ratio model of memory. *Psychological Review, 114*, 539–576.

Bunting, M. F., Cowan, N., & Colflesh, G. H. (2008). The deployment of attention in short-term memory tasks: Tradeoffs between immediate and delayed deployment. *Memory & Cognition, 36*, 799–812.

Burgess, N., & Hitch, G. J. (1999). Memory for serial order: A network model of the pho-nological loop and its timing. *Psychological Review, 106,* 551–581.

Caplan, D., Waters, G., & DeDe, G. (2007). Specialized verbal working memory for lan-guage comprehension. In A. R. A. Conway, C. Jarrold, M. J. Kane, A. Miyake, & J. N. Towse (Eds.), *Variation in working memory* (pp. 272–302). New York, NY: Oxford University Press.

Cocchini, G., Logie, R. H., Della Sala, S., MacPherson, S. E., & Baddeley, A. D. (2002). Concurrent performance of two memory tasks: Evidence for domain-specific work-ing memory systems. *Memory & Cognition, 30,* 1086–1095.

Conrad, R. (1964). Acoustic confusion in immediate memory. *British Journal of Psychology, 55,* 75–84.

Cowan, N. (1988). Evolving conceptions of memory storage, selective attention, and their mutual constraints within the human information processing system. *Psychological Bulletin, 104,* 163–191.

Cowan, N. (1995). Attention and memory: An integrated framework. Oxford Psychology Series, No. 26. New York: Oxford University Press. (Paperback edition: 1997).

Cowan, N. (1999). An embedded-processes model of working memory. In A. Miyake & P. Shah (Eds.), *Models of working memory: Mechanisms of active maintenance and executive control* (pp. 62–101). Cambridge, UK: Cambridge University Press.

Cowan, N. (2001). The magical number 4 in short-term memory: A reconsideration of mental storage capacity. *Behavioral and Brain Sciences, 24,* 87–185.

Cowan, N. (2005). *Working memory capacity.* Hove, East Sussex, UK: Psychology Press.

Cowan, N., Elliott, E. M., Saults, J. S., Morey, C. C., Mattox, S., Hismjatullina, A., & Conway, A. R. A. (2005). On the capacity of attention: Its estimation and its role in working memory and cognitive aptitudes. *Cognitive Psychology, 51,* 42–100.

Cowan, N., Fristoe, N. M., Elliott, E. M., Brunner, R. P., & Saults, J. S. (2006). Scope of attention, control of attention, and intelligence in children and adults. *Memory & Cognition, 34,* 1754–1768.

Cowan, N., Lichty, W., & Grove, T.R. (1990). Properties of memory for unattended spoken syllables. *Journal of Experimental Psychology: Learning, Memory, & Cognition, 16,* 258–269.

Cowan, N., & Morey, C. C. (2007). How can dual-task working memory retention limits be investigated? *Psychological Science, 18,* 686–688.

Cowan, N., Naveh-Benjamin, M., Kilb, A., & Saults, J. S. (2006). Life-span develop-ment of visual working memory: When is feature binding difficult? *Developmental Psychology, 42,* 1089–1102.

Craik, F. I. M., & Lockhart, R. S. (1972). Levels of processing: A framework for memory research. *Journal of Verbal Learning and Verbal Behavior, 11,* 671–684.

Davelaar, E. J., Goshen-Gottstein, Y., Ashkenazi, A., Haarman, H. J., & Usher, M. (2005). The demise of short-term memory revisited: Empirical and computational investiga-tions of recency effects. *Psychological Review, 112,* 3–42.

Engle, R. W., Tuholski, S. W., Laughlin, J. E., & Conway, A. R. A. (1999). Working mem-ory, short-term memory, and general fluid intelligence: A latent-variable approach. *Journal of Experimental Psychology: General, 128,* 309–331.

Eriksen, C. W., & Johnson, H. J. (1964). Storage and decay characteristics of nonattended auditory stimuli. *Journal of Experimental Psychology, 68,* 28–36.

Fedorenko, E., Gibson, E., & Rohde, D. (2007). The nature of working memory in linguis-tic, arithmetic and spatial integration processes. *Journal of Memory and Language, 56,* 246–269.

Gernsbacher, M. A. (1993). Less skilled readers have less efficient suppression mecha-nisms. *Psychological Science, 4,* 294–298.

Glanzer, M., & Cunitz, A. R. (1966). Two storage mechanisms in free recall. *Journal of Verbal Learning & Verbal Behavior, 5*, 351–360.

Grossberg, S. (1978). A theory of human memory: Self-organization and performance of sensory-motor codes, maps, and plans. In R. Rosen & F. Snell (Eds.), *Progress in theoretical biology* (Vol. 5, pp. 500–639) New York, NY: Academic Press.

Hasher, L., Stolzfus, E. R., Zacks, R. T., & Rypma, B. (1991). Age and inhibition. *Journal of Experimental Psychology: Learning, Memory, & Cognition, 17*, 163–169.

James, W. (1890). *The principles of psychology*. New York, NY: Henry Holt.

Kane, M. J., Bleckley, M. K., Conway, A. R. A., & Engle, R. W. (2001). A controlled-attention view of working-memory capacity. *Journal of Experimental Psychology: General, 130*, 169–183.

Kane, M. J., Hambrick, D. Z., Tuholski, S. W., Wilhelm, O., Payne, T. W., & Engle, R. E. (2004). The generality of working-memory capacity: A latent-variable approach to verbal and visuo-spatial memory span and reasoning. *Journal of Experimental Psychology: General, 133*, 189–217.

Lewandowsky, S., Duncan, M., & Brown, G. D. A. (2004). Time does not cause forgetting in short-term serial recall. *Psychonomic Bulletin & Review, 11*, 771–790.

Luck, S. J., & Vogel, E. K. (1997). The capacity of visual working memory for features and conjunctions. *Nature, 390*, 279–281.

Massaro, D. W. (1970). Retroactive interference in short-term recognition memory for pitch. *Journal of Experimental Psychology, 83*, 32–39.

Miller, G. A. (1956). The magical number seven, plus or minus two: Some limits on our capacity for processing information. *Psychological Review, 63*, 81–97.

Miller, G. A. (1989). George A. Miller. In Lindzey Gardner (Ed.), *A history of psychology in autobiography* (Vol. VIII, pp. 391–418). Stanford, CA: Stanford University Press.

Miller, G. A., Galanter, E., and Pribram, K. H. (1960). *Plans and the structure of behavior*. New York, NY: Holt, Rinehart and Winston, Inc.

Morey, C. C., & Cowan, N. (2004). When visual and verbal memories compete: Evidence of cross-domain limits in working memory. *Psychonomic Bulletin & Review, 11*, 296–301.

Morey, C. C., & Cowan, N. (2005). When do visual and verbal memories conflict? The importance of working-memory load and retrieval. *Journal of Experimental Psychology: Learning, Memory, and Cognition, 31*, 703–713.

Nairne, J. S. (1990). A feature model of immediate memory. *Memory & Cognition, 18*, 251–269.

Newell, A. (1990). *Unified theories of cognition*. Cambridge, MA: Harvard University Press.

Piattelli-Palmarini, M. (1980). *Language and learning: The debate between Jean Piaget and Noam Chomsky*. London, UK: Routledge and Kegan Paul.

Posner, M. I., & Konick, A. F. (1966). On the role of interference in short-term retention. *Journal of Experimental Psychology, 72*, 221–231.

Potter, M. C. (1993). Very short-term conceptual memory. *Memory & Cognition, 21*, 156–161.

Potter, M. C., & Lombardi, L. (1990). Regeneration in the short-term recall of sentences. *Journal of Memory & Language, 29*, 633–654.

Reitman, J. S. (1971). Mechanisms of forgetting in short term memory. *Cognitive Psychology, 2*, 185–195.

Reitman, J. S. (1974). Without surreptitious rehearsal, information in short-term memory decays. *Journal of Verbal Learning & Verbal Behavior, 13*, 365–377.

Romani, C., & Martin, R. (1999). A deficit in the short-term retention of lexical-semantic information: Forgetting words but remembering a story. *Journal of Experimental Psychology: General, 128*, 56–77.

Saults, J. S., & Cowan, N. (2007). A central capacity limit to the simultaneous storage of visual and auditory arrays in working memory. *Journal of Experimental Psychology: General, 136*, 663–684.

Stevanovski, B., & Jolicoeur, P. (2007) Visual short-term memory: Central capacity limitations in short-term consolidation. *Visual Cognition, 15*, 532–563.

Zwilling, C. E. (2008). *Forgetting in short-term memory: The effect of time.* Unpublished master's thesis, University of Missouri, Columbia, MO.

5 Neurobiological Bases of the Semantic Processing of Words

Karima Kahlaoui, Bernadette Ska,
Clotilde Degroot, and Yves Joanette

INTRODUCTION

Language is defined as a brain-based system allowing for interpersonal communication using sounds, symbols, and words to express a meaning, idea, or abstract thought. Human beings' ability to understand and produce language involves a considerable amount of brain resources. For over a century, our understanding of brain mechanisms for language came mainly from lesion studies; essentially, lesion studies pointed to the existence of some association between a damaged brain region and a given set of language deficits (e.g., Broca, 1865; Wernicke, 1874). In recent decades, imaging methods—which permit one to measure various indirect indices of ongoing neural activities arising from the brain "in action"—have revolutionized cognitive neuropsychology and neurolinguistics, providing a new way of mapping language abilities and, in particular, much better evidence about both the anatomical and temporal aspects of brain processes. Currently, a fundamental question in cognitive neuroscience concerns where and how the normal brain constructs meaning, and how this process takes place in real time (Kutas & Federmeier, 2000). Imaging methods have been highly successful in investigating semantic information processing, revealing cortical area networks that are certainly plausible, given our previous knowledge of cerebral anatomy and lesion studies. Several imaging methods allow one to explore different aspects of the brain: spatial distribution (using hemodynamic methods), temporal deployment (using electrophysiological methods) or both (using emerging imaging methods). This chapter focuses on the convergent contribution of different imaging methods to our understanding of the neural bases of the semantic processing of words. First, an overview of imaging methods will be presented. Then, the converging results concerning the neurobiological bases of semantic processes will be reported for each method mentioned above. Since the number of publications on language processing and, more specifically, on the neurobiological bases of the semantic processing of words exceeds what can be reviewed here, this chapter focuses on the most representative papers in each area.

AN OVERVIEW OF IMAGING METHODS

Notwithstanding the existence of specific imaging approaches using Positron Emission Tomography (PET) along with specific neurochemical markers, the non-invasive methods currently available for human brain research are most frequently divided into two general approaches: hemodynamic and electrophysiological.

*   The most important of the methods based on hemodynamic principles are PET and functional magnetic resonance imaging (fMRI). Although both PET and fMRI present an approximation of neural activation by detecting the locally specific changes in blood composition and flow that accompany brain activity, there are some subtle differences between them. PET detects blood flow changes relatively directly using labeled oxygen as a marker, while fMRI, which is based on the principle of blood oxygenation level dependent (BOLD) measures blood flow via changes in the magnetization properties linked with the relative concentration of deoxyhemoglobin (HHb) on the venous side of the capillary bed. Overall, these methods have a very good spatial resolution and, in the case of fMRI, have the advantage of being able to provide a functional map that can be plotted on the anatomical image collected during the same session. The main limitation of these methods is their poor temporal resolution (>1 second). This is because of the intrinsic nature of the hemodynamic signal, which lags behind the corresponding neuronal signal by several seconds (for a thorough review, see Shibasaki, 2008).
*   Methods based on electrophysiological principles include event-related potentials (ERPs) and magnetoencephalography (MEG). These methods measure the neuronal activity of the brain, in particular postsynaptic discharges that can be recorded at the scalp in response to specific stimuli or events (e.g., a sound). The most important advantage of ERPs and MEG is their excellent temporal resolution (milliseconds) of brain neural activity, which makes it possible to investigate the whole sequence of cognitive processes occurring from sensory signal arrival to meaning comprehension. However, their major limitation is their poor spatial resolution.
*   Since the pioneering work of Jöbsis (1977), a third class of noninvasive brain imaging techniques has begun to emerge: optical imaging methods. These methods—which provide spatial and/or time course resolution—are based on the absorption and scattering properties of near-infrared light, which allow users to measure the functional activity occurring in the brain tissue (Gratton, Fabiani, Elbert, & Rockstroh, 2003). The principle is simple: the near-infrared light penetrates the head and permits one to measure some of the optical properties of the cortical tissue. The two main optical imaging methods are near-infrared spectroscopy (NIRS, estimating hemodynamic signals) and event-related optical signal (EROS, estimating neuronal signals). With the NIRS technique, one

can assess changes in both oxyhemoglobin (O_2Hb) and deoxyhemoglobin (HHb), in contrast to fMRI, which makes use of only the relative changes in HHb and cerebral blood volume. Oxygen consumption during brain activation results in a decrease in HHb and an increase in O_2Hb and total hemoglobin (Hb-tot; i.e., the sum of O_2Hb and HHb). In contrast, the EROS technique allows identifying fast optical signals in cortical tissue. The advantages of optical methods include good portability, low cost, and the possibility of executing acquisitions in a natural setting. Since these methods are light, low-cost, and do not require strict motion restriction, they are particularly suitable for research and applications in newborns, children, and healthy or sick adults.

NEUROBIOLOGICAL BASES OF WORD SEMANTIC PROCESSING

Since the advent of the various imaging methods, the exploration of the neural substrates of semantic memory and semantic processes has become a frequent focus of investigation, in both neurologically healthy individuals and patients. Semantic memory is usually described as our organized general world knowledge, which includes meanings of words, properties of objects and other knowledge that is not dependent on particular time and space contexts (Tulving, 1972). An important cognitive tool for investigating the structure of semantic memory, and particularly the mental representations of word meanings and their interrelationships in the brain, is the semantic priming paradigm. In behavioral studies, a semantic priming effect occurs when participants are faster at recognizing a target word, as indicated by lexical decision or semantic categorization, for example (e.g., nurse), when it is preceded by a related word (e.g., doctor) than when it is preceded by an unrelated word (e.g., bread; Meyer & Schvaneveldt, 1971). Such priming effects reflect the fact that lexical concepts in semantic memory are clustered according to a network of semantic similarity (Collins & Loftus, 1975). According to the spreading activation model, the activity in semantic networks spreads quickly between strongly connected nodes (as in the case of related words) and decays exponentially as the distance between nodes increases (as in the case of unrelated words). By modulating the time period between prime and target presentation (i.e., stimulus onset asynchrony; SOA), it is possible to distinguish at least two different types of mechanisms underlying semantic priming effects: automatic spreading activation and controlled semantic processing (Neely, 1991). When the SOA is short, automatic processing is generally believed to take place because not enough time is available to develop a strategy. In contrast, a longer SOA gives participants enough time to consciously process the relationship between prime and target, including both facilitation and inhibition components, and thus leads to attentional or strategic processing. Priming effects can also be influenced by the relatedness of prime–target pairs and by the instructions given to participants; a lower proportion of relatedness pairs and instructions that avoid any allusion to related pairs in a stimulus set influence automatic processes (Neely, 1991).

HEMODYNAMIC-BASED NEUROIMAGING OF THE
SEMANTIC PROCESSING OF WORDS

Historically, the retrieval of semantic information has been associated with the left temporal lobe, based mainly on the evidence of clinical data from patients with aphasia, Alzheimer's disease, or semantic dementia (Hodges & Gurd, 1994; Hodges, Salmon, & Butters, 1990, 1992). This pattern has been supported by neuroimaging PET and fMRI studies showing that semantic knowledge is represented in a distributed manner and its storage and retrieval depend primarily on the inferior and lateral temporal cortical regions (Damasio, Tranel, Grabowski, Adolphs, & Damasio, 2004; Démonet, Thierry, & Cardebat, 2005). Usually, semantic priming effects are reflected by a decrease in the amount of brain activation ("response suppression") for related compared to unrelated pairs of stimuli (Mummery, Shallice, & Price, 1999). It has been suggested that this phenomenon reflects the decrease in neural activity required to recognize targets, given that these words are easier to process because they have lower recognition thresholds as a result of spreading activation (Copland et al., 2003). However, a so-called *inverse pattern* (i.e., an increase in brain activity for related compared to unrelated prime–target pairs) has also been observed in some imaging studies. Using PET, Mummery et al. (1999) investigated the neural substrates of semantic priming by manipulating the proportion of related prime–target word pairs from 0% to 100%. The results showed a decrease in activity in the left anterior temporal lobe with increasing relatedness, except for the highest proportion of pairs, where an increase in activity was observed. This complex pattern was explained as the result of two processes: automatic (reflected in the decrease in activity) and strategic (reflected in the increase in activity) priming. More recently, Copland et al. (2003; Copland, de Zubicaray, McMahon, & Eastburn, 2007) also observed a decrease in brain activity for related compared to unrelated prime–target pairs of words using a short SOA (150 ms) but an increase in brain activity in the same condition using a long SOA (1000 ms). One suggested explanation is that the increased brain activity may reflect either postlexical semantic integration (Kotz, Cappa, von Cramon, & Friederici, 2002) or the detection of the semantic relationships between words (Copland et al., 2007; Rossell, Price, & Nobre, 2003).

Other brain regions are activated during semantic processing, such as the left inferior prefrontal gyrus (LIPG). Evidence for the involvement of the LIPG during semantic processing came from an fMRI study that demonstrated that repeated access to semantic knowledge is associated with a decrease of LIPG activity. Demb et al. (1995) investigated repetition priming effects in both semantic (abstract/concrete judgment) and perceptual (uppercase/lowercase) decision tasks. Activation of the LIPG decreased as a function of item repetition but only in the semantic task, suggesting that the LIPG is a part of a semantic executive system that participates in the retrieval of semantic information. This reduced activation during repetition priming has been interpreted as indicating more efficient or faster word processing because lower thresholds activate existing representations (Henson, Shallice, & Dolan, 2000). In line with these data, several fMRI and

PET studies have shown an activation of the LIPG in different semantic process-ing tasks, including the generation of semantically similar words, word classifi-cation (Gabrieli et al., 1996), and semantic monitoring (Démonet et al., 1992). The manipulation of the number of semantic items has also been reported to influence LIPG activation (Gabrieli, Poldrack, & Desmond, 1998; Wagner, Pare-Blagoev, Clark, & Poldrack, 2001). In addition, clinical data showed that patients with lesions to the LIPG, although impaired on some semantic tasks, do not typi-cally present semantic deficits such as those seen following a temporal lobe lesion (Swick & Knight, 1996). Based on these observations, it has been argued that the LIPG mediates either central executive retrieval of semantic knowledge (Wagner et al., 2001) or semantic working memory processes (Gabrieli et al., 1998).

Challenging these hypotheses, a different interpretation of the contribution of the LIPG to the semantic processing of words emerges from a series of fMRI and neuropsychological studies. According to Thompson-Schill, Aguirre, D'Esposito, and Farah (1999) and Thompson-Schill, D'Esposito, Aguirre, and Farah (1997), the LIPG is involved in the selection of semantic knowledge from among compet-ing alternative responses. To test their hypothesis, Thompson-Schill et al. (1997) compared high- and low-selection conditions in three different semantic tasks (generation vs. classification vs. comparison tasks) using fMRI. For example, in the classification task, participants classified line drawings of common objects. In the high-selection condition, the classification of items was based on a specific attribute of the object's representation (e.g., a line drawing of a car was associ-ated with the word "expensive"). In the low-selection condition, the classification was based on the object's name (e.g., a line drawing of a fork was associated with the corresponding word: "fork"). Overall, the results showed that activation occurs in a similar region of the LIPG for high- and low-selection conditions, suggesting that it is the selection process, not retrieval of semantic knowledge that triggered activity in the LIPG. Similarly, Thompson-Schill et al. (1999) investi-gated the effects of repeated word generation under different conditions during whole-brain echoplanar fMRI. Participants performed a word generation task. During the second presentation of a word stimulus, participants were asked to generate either the same response as with the first presentation ("same" condition) or a different response than with the first presentation ("different" condition). At the behavioral level, priming effects were found for both relevant ("same") and irrelevant ("different") information. At the brain activation level, relevant primes produced a decrease in LIPG activation, while irrelevant primes produced an increase in LIPG activation. The authors attributed the LIPG decrease to a reduc-tion in competition and, hence, in selection demands. The LIPG increase has been interpreted as an increase in the selection of competing responses because the word has already been retrieved once. In other words, the selection of a semantic representation is more demanding in the irrelevant than the relevant condition, because the generation of a target word in the latter condition was facilitated by relevant priming. The pattern of activation is different in the left temporal lobe: item repetition produced a decrease in activation in the left temporal cortex for both relevant and irrelevant conditions, suggesting a decrease in retrieval of the semantic information. According to Thompson-Schill et al. (1999), this disso-ciation suggests that selection of competing responses and retrieval are separate processes subserved by different regions, namely the LIPG and the left temporal cortex, respectively. Nevertheless, studies have recently shown that the temporal cortex may also be sensitive to the presence of semantic competitors in some con-ditions (Noppeney, Phillips, & Price, 2004; Spalek & Thompson-Schill, 2008), restarting the debate.

The LIPG has also been reported to be involved in the phonological process-ing of words (e.g., Fiez, 1997). Indeed, the LIPG, and in particular the posterior part, has been associated with speech production for a long time (Broca, 1865). Individuals with lesions in this area are characterized by motor and phonological deficits affecting language production (Damasio & Damasio, 1992). Thus, some researchers have suggested that there is a functional dissociation between the anterior and posterior parts of the LIPG, which play a specific role in semantic and phonological processing, respectively. This dissociation between anatomi-cal regions in the LIPG for phonological and semantic processes is supported by numerous clinical and functional neuroimaging studies (Bookheimer, 2002; Costafreda et al., 2006; Démonet et al., 2005). These observations, however, are not unanimously accepted. In some studies, similar activations have been reported for both phonological and semantic processes in the anterior and posterior LIPG (Devlin, Matthews, & Rushworth, 2003; Gold & Buckner, 2002), suggesting that some common underling cognitive processing is involved.

While a number of variables appear to influence semantic processes, one impor-tant factor is the categorization of objects. Semantic categorization is a basic prop-erty of the semantic information organization process that permits the recognition of semantic items and relates them to other familiar entities, but also needs to clas-sify new objects into the existing knowledge structure. Classically, most models of semantic knowledge organization are based on hierarchical or taxonomic catego-ries (e.g., natural categories, such as animals or fruits; and artifact categories, such as furniture or tools). Studies of category-specific effects have become increas-ingly important in revealing the organization of semantic memory. This field of research originated in neuropsychological studies with brain-damaged patients (e.g., Warrington & McCarthy, 1994). Most reports of category-specific deficits describe patients with impaired recognition of natural objects (e.g., animals, fruits) rather than artifacts (e.g., furniture, tools); the opposite pattern is reported much less frequently (for reviews, see Capitani, Laiacona, Mahon, & Caramazza, 2003; Laws, 2005). Three main explanations have been advanced to account for these dissociations: the *sensory-functional* (Humphreys & Forde, 2001; Warrington & Shallice, 1984), *domain-specific* (Caramazza & Shelton, 1998), and *correlated feature* hypotheses (Tyler & Moss, 2001).

- The sensory-functional hypothesis suggests that conceptual knowledge is organized according to semantic object features. Sensory features are claimed to be more relevant for distinguishing natural items, while functional features are critical for recognizing artifacts. Hence, the loss of sensory or functional knowledge impairs natural or artifact categories.

- The domain-specific hypothesis assumes that evolutionary pressure has segregated the neural systems dedicated to natural and artifact objects.
- Finally, the correlated feature account suggests that category effects need not always reflect segregation within the semantic system because the conceptual features are stored in a single semantic system in which natural objects share more features than artifacts.

Each of these hypotheses makes different assumptions about the underlying neuroanatomy, which can be evaluated by different functional neuroimaging methods.

Several reports using PET and fMRI have provided anatomical confirmation of the natural object/artifact dissociation in the brain. Brain activations related to semantic categories have been observed during different semantic tasks (e.g., picture naming, semantic decisions; Chao & Martin, 2000; Mummery, Patterson, Hodges, & Price, 1998; Perani et al., 1999). Classically, natural objects (e.g., animals) produced stronger activation in visual association areas of the occipito-temporal cortex, while artifacts (e.g., tools) elicited relatively stronger activation in brain areas involved in action representation, namely the pre-motor areas, left middle temporal cortex, and parietal cortex. A meta-analysis based on seven PET studies reported on the influence of an experimental task in probing the stored semantic knowledge (Devlin et al., 2002). This review demonstrated specific activations for each category: while natural objects activated the bilateral anterior temporal cortex, artifacts activated the left posterior middle temporal region. Most of these neuroanatomical dissociations are in agreement with the sensory-functional hypothesis. Importantly, Devlin et al. (2002) showed that category-specific effects were found for semantic decision (i.e., location, color, action, real-life size) and word retrieval (i.e., category fluency, picture naming, and word reading) tasks but not for perceptual tasks (e.g., screen size judgment). Consequently, category effects seem to be specific to semantic context.

Other models proposed that the organization of semantic knowledge is based on thematic representation. These models propose that categories are held together by a context (scene or event) in which certain objects are encountered (e.g., dog and leash). Sachs, Weis, Krings, Huber, & Kircher (2008a) recently compared categorical and thematic representation using fMRI. Their results showed that both kinds of representations activated similar neural substrates: the left inferior frontal, middle temporal, and occipital regions, suggesting that comparable mechanisms may be involved in the processing of taxonomic and thematic conceptual relations. Interestingly, the same authors (Sachs et al., 2008b) again investigated the neural substrates of these categories but this time under automatic processing conditions (i.e., with SOA of 200 ms), in order to minimize the effect of strategic processes on categorical processing. Participants performed a lexical decision task with four different experimental conditions: thematically related prime-target pairs (e.g., jacket: button), taxonomically related pairs (e.g., jacket: vest), unrelated pairs (e.g., jacket: bottle), and pairs with pseudoword targets (e.g., jacket: neuz). The behavioral data show that the size of a priming effect is greater for thematic than taxonomic categories, arguing that members of thematic categories share a *stronger and more salient conceptual relationship.* The neuroimaging data show activations mainly located in the right hemisphere: while taxonomic priming effects involve activation in the right precuneus, posterior cingulate, right middle frontal, superior frontal, and postcentral gyrus, thematic priming effects are observed in the right middle frontal gyrus and anterior cingulate. Strangely, no activation is reported in the LIPG or the middle temporal gyrus. Another important result reported by the authors is the involvement of the right precuneus, which was only observed for taxonomic categories, suggesting that these categories require increased effort to resolve semantic ambiguity because they are considered to be less salient. Considering both behavioral and neuroimaging data, and data from other neuroimaging studies (e.g., Cavanna & Trimble, 2006), the authors argue that episodic memory—which has previously been found to be associated with the precuneus—is likely to be more involved in taxonomic categories. According to Sachs et al. (2008b), "it seems much more likely to have an episodic memory of a car in a garage or a button in a coat, than a dog and a goat or a cup and a glass" (p. 201).

Another way to investigate semantic networks is by analyzing the pattern of activation while the individual is engaged in word production. The verbal fluency task (also referred to as *oral naming*) is a classical language production paradigm in which participants are asked to generate as many words as possible. The most common measures of verbal fluency are orthographic (letter-based, such as "F" or "L") and semantic (category-based, such as "animals" or "sports"). To successfully perform this task, participants need to have intact lexical and semantic knowledge, efficient word access and retrieval, and well-organized semantic networks (Posner & DiGirolamo, 1998). Most neuroimaging studies of verbal fluency have shown that orthographic and semantic fluency tasks activate different brain regions. For example, using PET, Mummery, Patterson, Hodges, and Wise (1996) demonstrated that letter fluency activated left frontal regions, while semantic fluency yielded activation in left temporal regions (including the anteromedial region and inferior temporal gyrus). These early data were replicated by other studies using fMRI, PET and, more recently, voxel-based lesion symptom mapping (e.g., Baldo, Schwartz, Wilkins, & Dronkers, 2006). Similar clinical data were also reported (e.g., Troyer, Moscovitch, Winocur, Alexander, & Stuss, 1998). These dissociations can be explained by the use of different retrieval strategies for words associated with different criteria in the fluency tasks. For example, for letter-based fluency, the retrieval of words on the basis of their initial letter is not a natural component of language processing; consequently, unlike semantic retrieval, participants have to use an unfamiliar access route to the lexicon (Wood, Saling, Abbott, & Jackson, 2001) and a strategic search across graphophonemic or lexical memory. Thus, letter fluency can be harder because lexical stores are broader and less well defined than semantic stores. In contrast, semantic verbal fluency is more dependent on semantic memory because participants have to search for semantic associations within a given category; thus, this task depends mainly on the integrity of the semantic memory. For this reason, deficits in the semantic fluency task reflect semantic memory impairments and not executive dysfunctions.

These findings are not uncontroversial. Indeed, Gourovitch et al. (2000) investigated the neural substrates of both letter and semantic fluency in healthy participants using PET. A relatively greater activation of the inferior frontal cortex and temporo-parietal cortex was observed during letter fluency tasks, while greater activation of the left temporal cortex was observed during semantic fluency tasks. However, relative to the control task (i.e., participants had to generate days of the week and months of the year), this study showed that similar brain regions were activated during both fluency tasks, including the anterior cingulate and left prefrontal regions. It is also relevant that a meta-analysis by Henri and Crawford (2004) has demonstrated that focal frontal lesions are associated with equivalent letter and semantic impairments, suggesting that the frontal lobes are involved in executive control processes and effortful retrieval of semantic knowledge. However, temporal damage was found to be associated with more deficits on semantic than letter fluency. The involvement of the LIPG has also been reported during verbal fluency tasks. Recently, a meta-analysis of fMRI studies demonstrated that the two kinds of verbal fluency tasks activate different parts of the LIPG. While semantic fluency tasks tend to activate a more ventral-anterior portion of the IFG, orthographic fluency appeared to involve a more dorsal posterior part (Costafreda et al., 2006), in line with previous neuroimaging studies (e.g., Fiez, 1997). Given that verbal fluency tasks involve the monitoring of several items in working memory, it has been suggested that these activations reflect working memory rather than semantic processes (Cabeza & Nyberg, 2000). To explain these contradictory data, some authors suggest that semantic and graphophonemic processes might be closely related. It may be the case that some graphophonemic processes are involved in semantic fluency and, similarly, some semantic processes might be involved in orthographic fluency. According to Costafreda et al. (2006), this "noise" would fail to detect spatial differences in brain activations. Although this meta-analysis is significant, none of the fMRI studies included by the authors was conducted with the same participants. The comparison of experimental tasks in a single group of participants is a powerful tool allowing the precise assessment of activation differences. A recent study by Heim, Eickhoff, & Amunts (2008) compared three different types of verbal fluency (orthographic vs. semantic vs. syntactic, i.e., generating nouns in the masculine gender) in the same participants using fMRI. Activations were found in both anterior and posterior parts of the LIPG for all verbal fluency tasks, suggesting that certain unspecific aspects—and not condition-specific demands—of verbal fluency are similar for three tasks. These data, which are in line with Gold and Buckner's (2002) results, may reflect the controlled retrieval of lexical information. In addition, these results are in accordance with the hypothesis whereby the LIPG mediates lexical selection processes (Snyder, Feigenson, & Thompson-Schill, 2007).

Troyer et al. (1998) and, more recently, Hirshorn and Thompson-Schill (2006) proposed that letter/semantic fluency dissociation can be described in terms of clustering (i.e., words produced inside the same subcategory) and switching (i.e., ability to change subcategory). When participants have to produce as many words as possible as a function of a given category or letter, they spontaneously tend to produce more clusters of semantically or phonetically related items. This approach can provide information on the structure of semantic memory, but also on the dynamic interaction between different semantic links. Such spontaneous clusters of words are consistent with the spreading activation model (Collins & Loftus, 1975), according to which a prime word can automatically activate a local network of related concepts. A series of clinical studies demonstrated that the switching is sustained by the frontal lobes whereas clustering is sustained by temporal regions (Troyer et al., 1998). In a recent fMRI study, Hirshorn and Thompson-Schill (2006) demonstrated that the LIPG is involved in the switching of subcategories during semantic fluency. The involvement of the LIPG in switching is due to the high semantic selection demands underlying this process. The switching/clustering dissociation echoes the selection/retrieval dissociation (Hirshorn &Thompson-Schill, 2006).

ELECTROPHYSIOLOGICAL NEUROIMAGING OF THE SEMANTIC PROCESSING OF WORDS

Functional neuroimaging studies provide crucial insights into the neurobiological bases of the semantic processing of words. However, given that neural activity occurs very fast, electrophysiological measures are essential to gain a better understanding of the time course of language processing. In ERP studies, the N400 component, which is a negative deflection that emerges at about 250 ms and peaks approximately 400 ms after word onset, is highly sensitive to semantic processing and, in particular, to semantic priming. The N400 component was first reported to be sensitive to the integration of words in a sentence context (Kutas & Hillyard, 1980). The amplitude of the N400 response to the sentence's final word is reduced if that word is semantically expected in the sentence context (e.g., "The pizza was too hot to *eat*") compared to an unexpected word (e.g., "The pizza was too hot to *cry*"). Consequently, it is inversely proportional to the ease with which the stimulus may be integrated into the current semantic context. An N400 component has also been reported during semantic priming paradigms with words (in both visual and auditory modalities: Federmeier & Kutas, 2001; Holcomb, 1993) and pictures of objects (McPherson & Holcomb, 1999), as well as for the processing of other meaningful or potentially meaningful stimuli, such as faces, odors, environmental sounds, and pronounceable pseudowords (Gunter & Bach, 2004; Koelsch et al., 2004). The N400 amplitude has been found to decrease with repetition priming and high word frequency (Kutas & Federmeier, 2000). It has been argued that the N400 component reflects the access and integration of a semantic representation into a current context (Holcomb, 1993).

Similarly to fMRI and PET studies, electrophysiological data have confirmed the importance of the involvement of the temporal cortex in semantic memory and semantic processing in general. Field potentials from intracranial electrodes in patients have demonstrated that the N400 is generated in the temporal cortex (in the area of the collateral sulcus and the anterior fusiform gyrus), confirming the crucial role this area plays in the storage and/or retrieval of semantic knowledge (Nobre, Allison, & McCarthy, 1994). Similar areas have been identified in MEG studies showing that the N400 generators are localized in bilateral fronto-temporal areas (left more than right hemisphere), as well as in the hippocampus, the parahippocampal gyri, the amygdala, and the superior and middle temporal gyri (e.g., Halgren et al., 2002; Marinkovic et al., 2003). Such convergences were explored simultaneously in combined fMRI/ERP studies. For example, Matsumoto, Iidaka, Haneda, Okada, and Sadato (2005) found a significant correlation between BOLD signal and N400 semantic priming effect in the left superior temporal gyrus but not in the LIPG. Interestingly, clinical data show that lesions in the left temporal lobe and temporo-parietal junction produce both decreased amplitudes and delayed latencies for N400 component, whereas LIPG lesions have little or no impact on the N400 (see Van Petten & Luka, 2006). Overall, these data confirm that the left temporal cortex is involved in the retrieval of semantic knowledge and suggest that, although the frontal lobe is required for some aspects of language processing, it does not appear to be involved in the semantic context effects. Matsumoto et al. (2005) proposed that the processes linked to the LIPG (i.e., selection or working memory) could be associated with another ERP component, possibly the Late Positive Component (LPC), which seems to underlie many aspects of language processing such as working memory, episodic memory retrieval, response selection, and reallocation of cognitive resources.

At the same time, the mechanisms underlying the N400 priming effect are still a matter of debate. Comparing short and long SOAs (200 vs. 1000 ms) during lexical decision tasks, Rossell et al. (2003) found an N400 semantic priming effect for both conditions. Surprisingly, though, this effect starts significantly earlier in the long-SOA condition (300–320 ms) than in the short-SOA condition (360–380 ms). The authors interpret that result as indicating a facilitation effect of semantic processing by controlled expectancies. In contrast, other ERP studies suggest that the difference in N400 reflects either automatic processes (Kellenbach, Wijers, & Mulder, 2000) or both automatic and controlled processes (Kutas & Federmeier, 2000).

Among the word semantic properties that modulate ERP components, one that is often reported is the object category. A series of ERP studies conducted by Kiefer (2001, 2005) generated some important insights into the temporal aspects of category-specific effects. Kiefer (2001) investigated the time course of both perceptual and semantic aspects of natural and artifact objects during superordinate object categorization (e.g., animal: cat) with pictures and words. At the early—perceptual—level (around 160–200 ms), the ERP data show greater perceptual processing for pictures of natural objects than artifacts. In contrast, at the later—semantic—level (around 300–500 ms), category-specific effects were observed in both modalities and associated with a reduction of N400 amplitude in specific electrodes (i.e., occipito-temporal areas for natural and fronto-central areas for artifact objects). In particular, the second study by Kiefer (2005) demonstrates that category-specific effects are obtained in lexical tasks and not only on semantic tasks, as was previously reported in the fMRI literature (e.g., Devlin et al., 2002). More specifically, the aim of his study was to track the time course of brain activation associated with category-specific effects during a lexical decision task. In order to test the relevance of these effects for semantic memory, a repetition priming paradigm was used. In line with Kiefer (2001), the ERP data showed a greater positive component over occipito-parietal areas in the N400 (about 350–450 ms) and LPC (about 500–600 ms) time windows for natural objects, and a greater positive component over fronto-central regions for artifact objects in the N400 time window for a lexical decision task. Overall, these scalp distribution data are in line with previous PET and fMRI studies, which demonstrate that the occipito-temporal regions subserve visual semantic knowledge, which is more specific to natural objects. Conversely, the frontal cortex, and especially the motor areas, is involved in action-related knowledge, which is more specific to artifacts (Chao & Martin, 2000; Perani et al., 1999). Another important result reported by Kiefer (2005) concerns repetition effects. Consistent with the ERP literature, repetition produces less category-related activity than the initial presentation of words; this reduction occurs over the occipito-parietal and frontal areas for both natural and artifact objects in the N400 and LPC time windows. In addition, an earlier onset of repetition effects is observed for natural than for artifact categories, suggesting that there is a specific temporal dynamic for different types of knowledge and supporting the hypothesis that there are multiple cortical semantic systems. This finding is particularly interesting because it highlights some of the weaknesses related to hemodynamic methods, and in particular concerning the temporal aspects of information processing. Indeed, if the neural signal decays rapidly, hemodynamic methods, due to the relatively slow changes in blood flow, can fail to detect reliable brain activations for specific processes (e.g., Devlin et al., 2002).

In addition, the high temporal resolution of electrophysiological methods is crucial for understanding the interhemispheric dynamics underlying various aspects of language processing. For example, using the ERP method, Bouaffre and Faïta-Ainseba (2007) have recently demonstrated that semantically associated word pairs are activated with delay in the right compared to the left hemisphere, highlighting the left hemisphere's primacy for this kind of processing. Similarly, by using MEG, some researchers (Dhond, Witzel, Dale, & Halgren, 2007; Liu et al., 2008) showed that there are spatio-temporal differences in concrete versus abstract word processing. Combining MEG and synthetic aperture magnetometry (i.e., analysis that volumetrically localizes language processing), Liu et al. (2008) found no neuromagnetic differences between abstract and concrete words in the primary visual and auditory cortices. However, significant differences were observed over the frontal regions: more neurons were activated in the left frontal areas for abstract words, while more neurons were activated in the right frontal areas for concrete words. Neuromagnetic changes were also observed in the left posterior temporal areas and LIPG for all words but as a function of specific frequency band. The authors suggest that processing of abstract words is lateralized in the left hemisphere, whereas processing of concrete words is bilateral (with the right hemisphere sustaining imagistic processing). Dhond et al. (2007) observed differences between processing of abstract and concrete words in the fronto-temporal regions from 300 to 400 ms, arguing that, although the encoding of both concrete and abstract words seems similar, different parts of the network are more specialized for concrete versus abstract words.

Data From Emerging Imaging Methods

The new imaging methods now emerging are likely to complement current approaches exploring the physiological substrates of cognitive processes and the time course of their involvement. In addition, analysis methods are becoming increasingly well developed, allowing us to address such fundamental issues as the connectivity (i.e., functional or effective) and the interaction (how and in which direction) between different neural networks. For example, fMRI or functional neuroimaging data can now be analyzed in such a way as to allow for the description of putative networks associated with a given ability or task. Those networks are said to be *functional* or *effective* depending on whether or not they include causality indications. The nature of the information they provide is complementary to those of traditional activation pattern data. They can even offer converging evidence such as the results from Walter, Jbabdi, Marrelec, Benali, and Joanette (2006) showing that the functional connectivity associated with the semantic processing of words (semantic categorization decision task) includes a neural network involving both right- and left-hemisphere-based loci, whereas the network associated with grapho-phonological processing (rhyme decision task) is limited to the left hemisphere.

Regarding emerging imaging techniques, NIRS has been successfully used to detect brain activation related to a number of language tasks. Among cognitive tasks known to activate the prefrontal cortex, the verbal fluency task is often reported on in the literature about NIRS use. During semantic and orthographic fluency tasks, activations (i.e., increased O_2Hb and decreased HHb) are reported in inferior and dorsolateral prefrontal areas in healthy individuals (Herrmann, Ehlis, & Fallgatter, 2003; Quaresima et al., 2005), as well as patients with neurological (Hermann, Langer, Jacob, Ehlis, & Fallgatter, 2008) or psychiatric diseases (Ehlis, Herrmann, Plichta, & Fallgatter, 2007; Quaresima, Giosuè, Roncone, Casacchia, & Ferrari, 2009). The data concerning lateralization effects are contradictory. Activation in the bilateral prefrontal cortex is observed in most NIRS studies (Hermann et al., 2003; Herrmann, Walter, Ehlis, & Fallgatter, 2006; Kameyama, Fukuda, Uehara, & Mikuni, 2004; Kameyama et al., 2006; Matsuo, Watanabe, Onodera, Kato, & Kato, 2004; Watanabe, Matsuo, Kato, & Kato, 2003). This bilateral activation has been interpreted as underlying executive processes related to verbal fluency and not to specific language processes. However, other NIRS studies have reported a clear lateral effect, with higher oxygenation in the left hemisphere, according to most fMRI studies on verbal fluency (Fallgatter et al., 1997; Hermann et al., 2005, 2006). Why are there such discrepancies between studies? Several possible explanations can be put forward, such as number of NIRS channels (very limited in many studies), position of NIRS optodes on scalp, number of participants, and data analysis method. Recently, Quaresima et al. (2009) found high variability between participants performing verbal fluency and visuospatial working memory tasks. In particular, single-subject analysis demonstrated bilateral prefrontal activation for only a few participants. In addition, significant interindividual variations in O_2Hb and HHb were reported in response to both tasks. The authors proposed some explanations of these phenomena and emphasized the importance of single-subject analysis, which provides more anatomical information about the changes in brain activity. In addition, to improve the poor spatial resolution related to single- or two-channel studies, multichannel NIRS systems have been introduced (e.g., Schecklmann, Ehlis, Plichta, & Fallgatter, 2008).

Using high spatial and temporal sampling, the EROS approach allows users to obtain brain images with very good spatial and temporal resolution: on the order of a few millimeters and a few milliseconds, respectively (Tse et al., 2007). The first EROS study of language processing has recently been carried out by Tse et al. (2007), who reported on the spatial and temporal dynamics in processing semantic and syntactic anomalies in sentences. A rapid interaction between left superior/middle temporal cortices and the IFC was obtained during semantically and syntactically anomalous sentence processing using both EROS and ERP. Remembering that semantic and syntactic anomalies induce typical ERP patterns at the N400 and P600 components, respectively, it is interesting to note that EROS data show an increase in activation first in the left superior/middle temporal cortices then in the inferior frontal cortices, suggesting that activation moves from posterior (temporal) to anterior (frontal) regions in the course of sentence processing.

CONCLUSION

The emergence of imaging methods has had a tremendous impact for the development of cognitive neurosciences over the last decades. In particular, they have allowed a unique understanding of the spatial and/or temporal aspects of the neurobiological bases of the semantic processing of words. However, because of the large number of intrinsic (e.g., nature of semantic features) and extrinsic (e.g., characteristics/limitations of a given neuroimaging acquisition and/or data analysis technique) factors that can influence the results, one should not be surprised to find nonconverging—and sometimes contradictory—results in the literature. Thus, direct comparisons between studies is difficult because of differences in the kind of method used but also because of the nature of stimuli, experimental tasks that reflect different levels of semantic processing, the way the data were analyzed, and the methodology used. In fact, we are only starting to unveil the neurobiological bases of the semantic processing of words. The present review shows that this question is very complex since the semantic processing of words appears to result from a large and distributed neural network of which components are modulated by a myriad of semantic features, characteristics, and representations. The addition of new emerging imaging methods, along with the quest for converging evidence across the different neuroimaging approaches, will reveal new and important insights regarding language processing in general and the semantic processing of words in particular.

REFERENCES

Baldo, J. V., Schwartz, S., Wilkins, D., & Dronkers, N. F. (2006). Role of frontal versus temporal cortex in verbal fluency as revealed by voxel-based lesion symptom mapping. *Journal of the International Neuropsychological Society, 12*, 896–900.

Bookheimer, S. (2002). Functional MRI of language: New approaches to understanding the cortical organization of semantic processing. *Annual Review of Neuroscience, 25*, 151–188.

Bouaffre, S., & Faïta-Ainseba, F. (2007). Hemispheric differences in the time-course of semantic priming processes: Evidence from event-related potentials (ERPs). *Brain and Cognition, 63*, 123–135.

Broca, P. 1865. Du siège de la faculté du langage articulé. *Bulletin de la Société d'Anthropologie, 6*, 337–393.

Cabeza, R., & Nyberg, L. (2000). Imaging cognition II: An empirical review of 275 PET and fMRI studies. *Journal of Cognitive Neuroscience, 12*, 1–47.

Capitani, E., Laiacona, M., Mahon, B., & Caramazza, A. (2003). What are the facts of semantic category-specific deficits? A critical review of the clinical evidence. *Cognitive Neuropsychology, 20*, 213–261.

Caramazza, A., & Shelton, J. R. (1998). Domain-specific knowledge systems in the brain the animate-inanimate distinction. *Journal of Cognitive Neuroscience, 10*, 1–34.

Cavanna, A. E., & Trimble, M. R. (2006). The precuneus: A review of its functional anatomy and behavioural correlates. *Brain, 129*, 564–583.

Chao, L. L., & Martin, A. (2000). Representation of manipulable man-made objects in the dorsal stream. *Neuroimage, 12*, 478–484.

Collins, A. M., & Loftus, E. F. (1975). A spreading-activation theory of semantic processing. *Psychological Review, 82*, 407–428.

Copland, D. A., de Zubicaray, G. I., McMahon, K., & Eastburn, M. (2007). Neural correlates of semantic priming for ambiguous words: An event-related fMRI study. *Brain Research, 1131*, 163–172.

Copland, D. A., de Zubicaray, G. I., McMahon, K., Wilson, S. J., Eastburn, M., & Chenery, H. J. (2003). Brain activity during automatic semantic priming revealed by event-related functional magnetic resonance imaging. *Neuroimage, 20*, 302–310.

Costafreda, S. G., Fu, C. H., Lee, L., Everitt, B., Brammer, M. J., & David, A. S. (2006). A systematic review and quantitative appraisal of fMRI studies of verbal fluency: Role of the left inferior frontal gyrus. *Human Brain Mapping, 27*, 799–810.

Damasio, A. R., & Damasio, H. (1992). Brain and language. *Scientific American, 267*, 88–95.

Damasio, H., Tranel, D., Grabowski, T., Adolphs, R., & Damasio, A. R. (2004). Neural systems behind word and concept retrieval. *Cognition, 92*, 179–229.

Demb, J. B., Desmond, J. E., Wagner, A. D., Vaidya, C. J., Glover, G. H., & Gabrieli, J. D. (1995). Semantic encoding and retrieval in the left inferior prefrontal cortex: A functional MRI study of task difficulty and process specificity. *Journal of Neuroscience, 15*, 5870–5878.

Démonet, J. F., Chollet, F., Ramsay, S., Cardebat, D., Nespoulous, J. L., Wise, R., ... Frackowiak, R. (1992). The anatomy of phonological and semantic processing in normal subjects. *Brain, 115*, 1753–1768.

Démonet, J. F., Thierry, G., & Cardebat, D. (2005). Renewal of the neurophysiology of language: Functional neuroimaging. *Physiological Reviews, 85*, 49–95.

Devlin, J. T., Matthews, P. M., & Rushworth, M. F. (2003). Semantic processing in the left inferior prefrontal cortex: A combined functional magnetic resonance imaging and transcranial magnetic stimulation study. *Journal of Cognitive Neuroscience, 15*, 71–84.

Devlin, J. T., Moore, C. J., Mummery, C. J., Gorno-Tempini, M. L., Phillips, J. A., Noppeney, U., . . . Price, C. J. (2002). Anatomic constraints on cognitive theories of category specificity. *Neuroimage, 15*, 675–685.

Dhond, R. P., Witzel, T., Dale, A. M., & Halgren, E. (2007). Spatiotemporal cortical dynamics underlying abstract and concrete word reading. *Human Brain Mapping, 28*, 355–362.

Ehlis, A. C., Herrmann, M. J., Plichta, M. M., & Fallgatter, A. J. (2007). Cortical activation during two verbal fluency tasks in schizophrenic patients and healthy controls as assessed by multi-channel near-infrared spectroscopy. *Psychiatry Research, 156*, 1–13.

Fallgatter, A. J., Roesler, M., Sitzmann, L., Heidrich, A., Mueller, T. J., & Strik, W. K. (1997). Loss of functional hemispheric asymmetry in Alzheimer's dementia assessed with near-infrared spectroscopy. *Cognitive Brain Research, 6*, 67–72.

Federmeier, K. D., & Kutas, M. (2001). Meaning and modality: Influences of context, semantic memory organization, and perceptual predictability on picture processing. *Journal of Experimental Psychology: Learning Memory and Cognition, 27*, 202–224.

Fiez, J. A. (1997). Phonology, semantics, and the role of the left inferior prefrontal cortex. *Human Brain Mapping, 5*, 79–83.

Gabrieli, J. D. E., Desmond, J. E., Demb, J. B., Wagner, A. D., Stone, M. V., Vaidya, C. J., & Glover, G. H. (1996). Functional magnetic resonance imaging of semantic memory processes in the frontal lobes. *Psychological Science, 7*, 278–283.

Gabrieli, J. D. E., Poldrack, R. A., & Desmond, J. E. (1998). The role of left prefrontal cortex in language and memory. *Proceedings of the National Academy of Sciences of the USA, 95*, 906–913.

Gold, B. T., & Buckner, R. L. (2002). Common prefrontal regions coactivate with dissociable posterior regions during controlled semantic and phonological tasks. *Neuron, 35*, 803–812.

Gourovitch, M. L., Kirkby, B. S., Goldberg, T. E., Weinberger, D. R., Gold, J. M., Esposito, G., ... Berman, K. F. (2000). A comparison of rCBF patterns during letter and semantic fluency. *Neuropsychology, 14*, 353–360.

Gratton, G., Fabiani, M., Elbert, T., & Rockstroh, B. (2003). Seeing right through you: Applications of optical imaging to the study of the human brain. *Psychophysiology, 40*, 487–491.

Gunter, T. C., & Bach, P. (2004). Communicating hands: ERPs elicited by meaningful symbolic hand postures. *Neuroscience Letters, 372*, 52–56.

Halgren, E., Dhond, R. P., Christensen, N., Van Petten, C., Marinkovic, K., Lewine, J. D., & Dale, A. M. (2002). N400-like magnetoencephalography responses modulated by semantic context, word frequency, and lexical class in sentences. *Neuroimage, 17*, 1101–1116.

Heim, S., Eickhoff, S. B., & Amunts, K. (2008). Specialisation in Broca's region for semantic, phonological, and syntactic fluency? *Neuroimage, 40*, 1362–1368.

Henri, J. D., & Crawford, J. R. (2004). A meta-analytic review of verbal fluency performance following focal cortical lesions. *Neuropsychology, 18*, 284–295.

Henson, R., Shallice, T., & Dolan, R. (2000). Neuroimaging evidence for dissociable forms of repetition priming. *Science, 287,* 1269–1272.

Herrmann, M. J., Ehlis, A. C., & Fallgatter, A. J. (2003). Frontal activation during a verbal-fluency task as measured by near-infrared spectroscopy. *Brain Research Bulletin, 61,* 51–56.

Herrmann, M. J., Langer, J. B., Jacob, C., Ehlis, A. C., & Fallgatter, A. J. (2008). Reduced prefrontal oxygenation in Alzheimer disease during verbal fluency tasks. *The American Journal of Geriatric Psychiatry, 16,* 125–135.

Herrmann, M. J., Walter, A., Ehlis, A. C., & Fallgatter, A. J. (2006). Cerebral oxygenation changes in the prefrontal cortex: Effects of age and gender. *Neurobiology of Aging, 27,* 888–894.

Hirshorn, E. A., & Thompson-Schill, S. L. (2006). Role of the left inferior frontal gyrus in covert word retrieval: Neural correlates of switching during verbal fluency. *Neuropsychologia, 44,* 2547–2557.

Hodges, J. R., & Gurd, J. M. (1994). Remote memory and lexical retrieval in a case of frontal Pick's disease. *Archives of Neurology, 51,* 821–827.

Hodges, J. R., Salmon, D. P., & Butters, N. (1990). Differential impairment of semantic and episodic memory in Alzheimer's and Huntington's diseases: A controlled prospective study. *Journal of Neurology, Neurosurgery, and Psychiatry, 53,* 1089–1095.

Hodges, J. R., Salmon, D. P., & Butters, N. (1992). Semantic memory impairment in Alzheimer's disease: Failure of access or degraded knowledge? *Neuropsychologia, 30,* 301–314.

Holcomb, P. J. (1993). Semantic priming and stimulus degradation: Implications for the role of the N400 in language processing. *Psychophysiology, 30,* 47–61.

Humphreys, G. W., & Forde, E. M. (2001). Hierarchies, similarity, and interactivity in object recognition: "Category-specific" neuropsychological deficits. *The Behavioral and Brain Sciences, 24,* 453–476.

Jöbsis, F. F. (1977). Noninvasive, infrared monitoring of cerebral and myocardial oxygen sufficiency and circulatory parameters. *Science, 198,* 1264–1267.

Kameyama, M., Fukuda, M., Uehara, T., & Mikuni, M. (2004). Sex and age dependencies of cerebral blood volume changes during cognitive activations: A multichannel near-infrared spectroscopy study. *Neuroimage, 22,* 1715–1721.

Kameyama, M., Fukuda, M., Yamagishi, Y., Sato, T., Uehara, T., Ito, M., … Mikuni, M. (2006). Frontal lobe function in bipolar disorder: A multichannel near-infrared spectroscopy study. *Neuroimage, 29,* 172–184.

Kellenbach, M. L., Wijers, A. A., & Mulder, G. (2000). Visual semantic features are activated during the processing of concrete words: Event-related potential evidence for perceptual semantic priming. *Cognitive Brain Research, 10,* 67–75.

Kiefer, M. (2001). Perceptual and semantic sources of category-specific effects: Event-related potentials during picture and word categorization. *Memory and Cognition, 29,* 100–116.

Kiefer, M. (2005). Repetition-priming modulates category-related effects on event-related potentials: Further evidence for multiple cortical semantic systems. *Journal of Cognitive Neuroscience, 17,* 199–211.

Koelsch, S., Kasper, E., Sammler, D., Schulze, K., Gunter, T., & Friederici, A. D. (2004). Music, language and meaning: Brain signatures of semantic processing. *Nature Neuroscience, 7,* 302–307.

Kotz, S. A., Cappa, S. F., von Cramon, D. Y., & Friederici, A. D. (2002). Modulation of the lexical-semantic network by auditory semantic priming: An event-related functional MRI study. *Neuroimage, 17,* 1761–1772.

Kutas, M., & Federmeier, K. D. (2000). Electrophysiology reveals semantic memory use in language comprehension. *Trends in Cognitive Sciences, 4*, 463–470.

Kutas, M., & Hillyard, S. A. (1980). Reading senseless sentences: Brain potentials reflect semantic incongruity. *Science, 207*, 203–205.

Laws, K. R. (2005). "Illusions of normality": A methodological critique of category-specific naming. *Cortex, 6*, 842–851.

Liu, Y., Xiang, J., Wang, Y., Vannest, J. J., Byars, A. W., & Rose, D. F. (2008). Spatial and frequency differences of neuromagnetic activities in processing concrete and abstract words. *Brain Topography, 20*, 123–129.

Marinkovic, K., Dhond, R. P., Dale, A. M., Glessner, M., Carr, V., & Halgren, E. (2003). Spatio-temporal dynamics of modality-specific and supramodal word processing. *Neuron, 38*, 487–497.

Matsumoto, A., Iidaka, T., Haneda, K., Okada, T., & Sadato, N. (2005). Linking semantic priming effect in functional MRI and event-related potentials. *Neuroimage, 24*, 624–634.

Matsuo, K., Watanabe, A., Onodera, Y., Kato, N., & Kato, T. (2004). Prefrontal hemodynamic response to verbal-fluency task and hyperventilation in bipolar disorder measured by multi-channel near-infrared spectroscopy. *Journal Affective Disorders, 82*, 85–92.

McPherson, W. B., & Holcomb, P. J. (1999). An electophysiological investigation of semantic priming with pictures of real objects. *Psychophysiology, 36*, 53–65.

Meyer, D. E., & Schvaneveldt, R. W. (1971). Facilitation in recognizing pairs of words: Evidence of a dependence between retrieval operations. *Journal of Experimental Psychology, 90*, 227–234.

Mummery, C. J., Patterson, K., Hodges, J. R., & Price, C. J. (1998). Functional neuroanatomy of the semantic system: Divisible by what? *Journal of Cognitive Neuroscience, 10*, 766–777.

Mummery, C. J., Patterson, K., Hodges, J. R., & Wise, R. J. S. (1996). Generating 'tiger' as an animal name or a word beginning with T: Differences in brain activation. *Proceedings Biological Sciences, 263*, 989–995.

Mummery, C. J., Shallice, T., & Price, C. J. (1999). Dual-process model in semantic priming: A functional imaging perspective. *Neuroimage, 9*, 516–525.

Neely, J. H. (1991). Semantic priming effects in visual word recognition: A selective review of current findings and theory. In D. Besner & G. W. Humphreys (Eds.), *Basic processes in reading. Visual word recognition* (pp. 264–336). Hillsdale, NJ: Erlbaum.

Nobre, A. C., Allison, T., & McCarthy, G. (1994). Word recognition in the human inferior temporal lobe. *Nature, 37*, 260–263.

Noppeney, U., Phillips, J., & Price, C. (2004). The neural areas that control the retrieval and selection of semantics. *Neuropsychologia, 42*, 1269–1280.

Perani, D., Schnur, T., Tettamanti, M., Gorno-Tempini, M., Cappa, S. F., & Fazio, F. (1999). Word and picture matching: A PET study of semantic category effects. *Neuropsychologia, 37*, 293–306.

Posner, M. I., & DiGirolamo, G. J. (1998). Executive attention: Conflict, target detection, and cognitive control. In R. Parasuraman (Ed.), *The attentive brain*. Cambridge, MA: MIT Press.

Quaresima, V., Ferrari, M., Torricelli, A., Spinelli, L., Pifferi, A., & Cubeddu, R. (2005). Bilateral prefrontal cortex oxygenation responses to a verbal fluency task: A multichannel time-resolved near-infrared topography study. *Journal of Biomedical Optics, 10*, 11012.

Quaresima, V., Giosuè, P., Roncone, R., Casacchia, M., & Ferrari, M. (2009). Prefrontal cortex dysfunction during cognitive tests evidenced by functional near-infrared spectroscopy. *Psychiatry Research: Neuroimaging, 171*(3), 252–257.

Rossel, S. L., Price, C. J., & Nobre, A. C. (2003). The anatomy and time course of semantic priming investigated by fMRI and ERPs. *Neuropsychologia*, *41*, 550–564.

Sachs, O., Weis, S., Krings, T., Huber, W., & Kircher, T. (2008a). Categorical and thematic knowledge representation in the brain: Neural correlates of taxonomic and thematic conceptual relations. *Neuropsychologia*, *46*, 409–418.

Sachs, O., Weis, S., Zellagui, N., Hubert, W., Zvyagintsev, M., Mathiak, K., & Kircher, T. (2008b). Automatic processing of semantic relations in fMRI: Neural activation during semantic priming of taxonomic and thematic categories. *Brain Research*, *1218*, 194–205.

Schecklmann, M., Ehlis, A. C., Plichta, M. M., & Fallgatter, A. J. (2008). Functional near-infrared spectroscopy: A long-term reliable tool for measuring brain activity during verbal fluency. *Neuroimage*, *43*, 147–155.

Shibasaki, H. (2008). Human brain mapping: Hemodynamic response and electrophysiology. *Clinical Neurophysiology*, *119*, 731–743.

Snyder, H. R., Feigenson, K., & Thompson-Schill, S. L. (2007). Prefrontal cortical response to conflict during semantic and phonological tasks. *Journal of Cognitive Neuroscience*, *19*, 761–775.

Spalek, K., & Thompson-Schill, S. L. (2008). Task-dependent semantic interference in language production: An fMRI study. *Brain and Language*, *107*, 220–228.

Swick, D., & Knight, R. T. (1996). Is prefrontal cortex involved in cued recall? A neuropsychological test of PET findings. *Neuropsychologia*, *34*, 1019–1028.

Thompson-Schill, S. L., Aguirre, G. K., D'Esposito, M., & Farah, M. J. (1999). A neural basis for category and modality specific of semantic knowledge. *Neuropsychologia*, *37*, 671–676.

Thompson-Schill, S. L., D'Esposito, M., Aguirre, G. K., & Farah, M. J. (1997). Role of left inferior prefrontal cortex in retrieval of semantic knowledge: A reevaluation. *Proceedings of the National Academy of Sciences of the USA*, *94*, 14792–14797.

Troyer, A. K., Moscovitch, M., Winocur, G., Alexander, M. P., & Stuss, D. (1998). Clustering and switching on verbal fluency: The effects of focal frontal- and temporal-lobe lesions. *Neuropsychologia*, *36*, 499–504.

Tse, C. Y., Lee, C. L., Sullivan, J., Garnsey, S. M., Dell, G. S., Fabiani, M., & Gratton, G. (2007). Imaging cortical dynamics of language processing with the event-related optical signal. *Proceedings of the National Academy of Sciences of the USA*, *104*, 17157–17162.

Tulving, E. (1972). Episodic and semantic memory. In E. Tulving & W. Donaldson (Eds.), *Organization of memory*. New York, NY: Academic Press.

Tyler, L. K., & Moss, H. E. (2001). Towards a distributed account of conceptual knowledge. *Trends in Cognitive Sciences*, *5*, 244–252.

Van Petten, C., & Luka, B. J. (2006). Neural localization of semantic context effects in electromagnetic and hemodynamic studies. *Brain and Language*, *97*, 279–293.

Wagner, A. D., Pare-Blagoev, E. J., Clark, J., & Poldrack, R. A. (2001). Recovering meaning: Left prefrontal cortex guides controlled semantic retrieval. *Neuron*, *31*, 329–338.

Walter, N., Jbabdi, S., Marrelec, G., Benali, H., & Joanette, Y. (2006, March 1–4). Carl Wernicke was essentially right: FMRI brain interactivity analysis of phonological and semantic processing of isolated word. Communication presented at the *World Federation of Neurology: Aphasia and Cognitive Disorders Research Group*, Buenos Aires (Argentina).

Warrington, E. K., & McCarthy, R. A. (1994). Multiple meaning systems in the brain: A case of visual semantics. *Neuropsychologia*, *32*, 1465–1473.

Warrington, E. K., & Shallice, T. (1984). Category specific semantic impairments. *Brain, 107*, 829–854.

Watanabe, A., Matsuo, K., Kato, N., & Kato, T. (2003). Cerebrovascular responses to cognitive tasks and hyperventilation measured by multi-channel near-infrared spectroscopy. *The Journal of Neuropsychiatry and Clinical Neurosciences, 15*, 442–449.

Wernicke, C. 1874. Der aphasische Symptomenkomplex. Eine psychologische Studie auf anatomischer Basis. Breslau, Poland: Max Cohn & Weigert.

Wood, A. G., Saling, M. M., Abbott, D. F., & Jackson, G. D. (2001). A neurocognitive account of frontal lobe involvement in orthographic lexical retrieval: An fMRI study. *Neuroimage, 14*, 162–169.

6 From Phonemes to Discourse: Event-Related Brain Potential (ERP) Componentry and Paradigms for Investigating Normal and Abnormal Language Processing

Marta Kutas, Katherine DeLong, and Michael Kiang

INTRODUCTION

Remarkably, over the past few decades technological advances have made it possible and relatively economical (compared to other neuroimaging methodologies) to investigate normal and abnormal language processing and communication by "reading" patterns of voltage differences between pairs of electrodes on the human scalp. Indeed, electrical brain activity triggered by written, spoken, signed, gestured, or depicted events in the physical world can serve as "potential" windows on the brain's language-related sensitivities and processing operations. Critically, such electrical potentials can be recorded at all stages of development (from neonates to elderly adults), at various levels of consciousness (from alert or sleeping healthy individuals to comatose or vegetative state patients), and in populations diverse in their abilities to produce motor outputs (as with individuals with apraxia, or who stutter, or Parkinson's disease patients). These electrical "snapshots" of mental operations do not provide an exhaustive view of all neural processes engaged in, or even essential for, language and thus are not by themselves optimal for localization purposes. They do, however, offer a relatively sensitive index of qualitatively different aspects of neural activity in the neocortex before, during, and after various linguistic and communicative acts, even in individuals who cannot otherwise effectively relay their messages, desires, or level of understanding.

In this review we examine normal linguistic and communicative processes by means of scalp-recorded brainwave studies of reading, listening, signing, and gesture. The scope of topics will range from how the brain responds to small linguistic units (e.g., phonemes) to higher levels of linguistic analysis (e.g., pragmatic aspects of discourse comprehension). We aim to provide a backdrop of paradigms, findings, and interpretations against which electrophysiological investigations within the field of language and communicative disorders can be crafted. Space limitations prohibit us from detailed coverage of even the past 30-some years of ERP language research, much less the longer history of cognitive ERP research. If language processes were special and encapsulated, not overlapping with other cognitive domains, this would not be worth mentioning. However, we believe that language processing cannot be properly investigated in isolation: sensory coding, attention, working memory, implicit memory, semantic memory, episodic memory, source memory, response preparation, inhibitory processes, novelty detection, task switching, assessing feedback, and error monitoring are but a subset of the processes that play a role in language as they do in other cognitive domains. And, although not all of these have been thoroughly investigated within the realm of language, clever and thoughtful research on these processes offers useful insights to psycholinguists and neurolinguists working with all sorts of individuals.

ELECTROPHYSIOLOGICAL MEASURES OF BRAIN ACTIVITY

The electroencephalogram (EEG) reflects ongoing, so-called background electrical activity of the brain, which is typically decomposed into different frequency bands (delta, theta, alpha, beta, and gamma), and analyzed as power in each of these frequency bands as a function of recording site and task conditions. Of critical importance for ERP researchers—even if background EEG is presumably averaged out in the calculation of an average ERP—are changes in resting EEG as a function of both age (albeit in different rates in different cortical areas) and clinical condition. Clinical groups, for example, often show less power in the higher (relative to lower) frequency bands, perhaps implicating a maturational lag, given that normal maturation is accompanied by a decreased power in the lower frequencies and increased power in the higher frequencies (Clarke, Barry, McCarthy, & Selikowitz, 2001; Somsen, van't Klooster, van der Molen, van Leeuwen, & Licht, 1997). EEG measures clearly can be used to assess cognitive functions across the age span (taking maturational course into account). In the past few decades, electrophysiologists also have looked at spectral changes of both power and phase in different frequency bands that occur in response to various stimuli or events (known as event-related synchronization, ERS, or desynchronization, ERD; Pfurtscheller & Lopes da Silva, 1999), as well as the systematic relationships between these evoked and induced rhythms and various cognitive processes. A smaller group of researchers also have scrutinized the coherence between the power and phase dynamics in the EEG activity at two or more sites, as a proxy for information exchange and coordination between brain areas (Varela, Lachaux, Rodriguez, & Martinerie, 2001). These, too, are likely to be reliably affected by various clinical conditions. Although these techniques comprise a promising new area within cognitive (and language) EEG research, in this chapter we will limit ourselves to cognitive ERP language-related research, as that is where the lion's share of investigations have been conducted over the past 30-odd years.

Event-related brain potential (ERPs) are the electrical brain activity synchronized in time to a stimulus, response, event, or even an event's absence. ERPs can be recorded intracranially with depth electrodes (typically in individuals with intractable epilepsy) or at the scalp with surface electrodes embedded in an electrode cap or net. ERPs are presumed to be the brain's (or at least the cortical regions') response to eliciting events, comprised of millisecond-by-millisecond time series of voltages at individual recording sites, affording inferences about brain sensitivities and computations. Because the time-locked response to an event coincides with electrical brain activity *not* time-locked to the eliciting event (either at all or in phase), ERPs are typically extracted via averaging across multiple repetitions of the eliciting event. These repetitions need not be exactly the same stimulus or event (though they may be) as long as they are conceptually similar with respect to the experimental manipulations: for instance, averaging the ERPs within a condition comprised of 40 different, but similarly anomalous, sentences. The ERP waveform is used to track the course of information processing as "sensory inputs" travel from the eye or ear to mind for comprehension, or in reverse, as "outputs" travel from mind to tongue or hand, for production. The scalp ERP, at each recording site, is an instantaneous reflection of the sum of all the brain activity that meets the criteria for being recordable at the scalp surface (see Kutas & Dale, 1997). Measuring how such signals change over normal or abnormal development, as a function of healthy or pathological aging, or due to various sorts of brain damage, are just a few excellent applications for which the ERP may be especially advantageous, as they are elicited without need for any overt motor response.

ERPs offer an image of cortical brain activity across time at multiple timescales, from milliseconds to seconds in a continuous, and relatively noninvasive manner. Of the studies to be reviewed herein, all rely on the ERP technique, using paradigms in which various stimulus types are presented (or omitted), at a rate under the experimenter's control or occasionally self-paced. The moment of stimulus onset—or for missing items, the point at which the item would have occurred—is considered "zero" on the time axis, and in this way the ERP is temporally synchronized to the eliciting event. With respect to this zero time point, however, what exactly the event-related potential voltage waveforms represent is a matter of some theoretical debate. On one view, it is assumed that the electrical brain activity synchronized to stimulus onset is a reflection of the brain processing of that item at that particular point in time. On another view, the presentation of the stimulus item acts to perturb (and realign) the ongoing EEG rhythms. In either case, such recordings provide a time series of dependent measures generated by the brain's processing of the events that can be meaningfully interpreted in the context of any experimental design to reveal something about how the brain construes or produces language inputs.

While the methodology has many attributes to recommend it for the study of cognitive—and in the present case particularly language—phenomena, the "reading" of the actual ERP waveforms is neither straightforward nor intuitive. Although electrical brain activity is sensitive to and reflects a wide variety of factors (including how recently one ate, how tired one is, or one's general mood at the time of the experiment), the elicited potentials do not come with a road map. At any given point, the ERP waveform is negative, positive, or unchanged relative to some baseline, but these negativities and positivities per se have no intrinsic meaning relative to their neural generators. Nonetheless, cognitive ERPers have been developing a glossary of ERP components and effects by discovering manipulations that *usually* lead to them. These in turn are defined in terms of their polarity, shape, topography across the scalp, and latency relative to zero. The labeled patterns—which by convention get their names either from a combination of their polarity and/or approximate latency (e.g., N400, P600, left anterior negativity or LAN) or by their theorized functional significance (e.g., lateralized readiness potential or LRP, Mismatch Negativity or MMN, NoGo N200, error related negativity or ERN)—then serve as proxies for particular constructs or information processing operations (e.g., response preparation, sensory discrimination, focused selective attention, error processing, semantic processing, working memory updating, grammatical processing, etc.) and can sometimes be used to adjudicate between alternative theoretical accounts of some psychological phenomenon.

We hedge in noting that certain manipulations *usually* lead to particular brainwave patterns because sometimes they do not, contrary to well-conceived hypotheses (a case in point being the N400, discovered in a study designed to elicit a P300). ERPs are a sharp tool that can leave a messy trail if not handled with care. The ERP literature is a testament to the view that there are few, if any, linguistic/cognitive processes under the purview of the neocortex that cannot benefit from ERP analyses. That said, the language ERP literature across the life span, even in healthy individuals, is vast, and a single chapter could in no way do it justice. We thus offer an overview of the methodology's flexibility and utility in investigating language-related processing, beginning with production and progressing through multiple levels of language comprehension.

INVESTIGATING PRODUCTION VIA RESPONSE PREPARATION AND MONITORING

Until recently, ERP investigations of language "production" have been few and far between, mostly due to the fact that ERPs, like most neuroimaging methods, are not particularly tolerant of facial, head, or body movements. Over the past 25 years or so, however, two major advances have led to an upswing in such studies: first, the development of analytic procedures such as independent components analysis (ICA) and the like (e.g., Second Order Blind Identification or SOBI) for decomposing scalp-recorded signals and extracting relevant/discarding irrelevant (artifactual) subcomponents (Delorme, Sejnowski, & Makeig, 2007; Romero, Mananas, & Barbanoj, 2008), and second, the development of clever experimental paradigms for monitoring production preparation (even if the ultimate decision is not to generate any response) as well as response outcome, including errors. The following ERP components have been especially useful in delineating stages of information processing, in general, and language production, in particular: the LRP, our primary focus here, the NoGo-N200 (a fronto-central negative stimulus-locked ERP peaking around 200 ms or later depending on information availability, reflecting response inhibition) and the error-related negativity or ERN (also known as Ne), an ERP often linked to errors or conflict processing, that occurs within 100 ms after an incorrect response or feedback stimulus.

The readiness potential (RP), or Bereitschaftspotential, from which the LRP is derived, is a gradually increasing ERP negativity beginning about 500 ms to one second prior to a prepared movement (onset defined by switch closure or muscle activity). The prepared movement may be either self-paced (Kornhuber & Deecke, 1964) or in response to an "imperative" stimulus (Kutas & Donchin, 1980; Rohrbaugh, Syndulko, & Lindsley, 1976), and can be initiated by the wrist, arm, knee, foot, or toe, as well as movements associated with swallowing, speaking, and writing, among others. The initial portion of the RP is bilaterally symmetric and is contingent on intact functioning of the supplementary motor cortex; its latter asymmetric portion is generated in the primary motor cortex but is contingent on normal functioning of the cerebello-thalamo-cortical loop. The RP has been examined in a host of clinical populations with motor problems but also has been used to investigate "free will," as it has been found to begin before the time when individuals indicate awareness of their intent to move (Libet, Gleason, Wright, & Pearl, 1983; Sirigu et al., 2004). Critically, the RP is not seen before speeded responses to stimuli occurring at unpredictable intervals without prior warning for which individuals cannot prepare (Kutas & Donchin, 1980; Papa, Artieda, & Obeso, 1991). Thus, the RP appears to reflect some aspect of movement preparation, rather than a necessary component for overt movement per se. This correlation in combination with two other of its characteristics: (a) the somatotopic and contralateral distribution of the latter half of the RP—more negative over right central sites preceding left finger, hand, or arm movements, and vice versa, and (b) the ability to monitor this asymmetry even in stimulus-locked (not just response-locked) ERP waveforms, have made the RP an especially useful ERP index in investigations of the timing of mental events (mental chronometry).

The lateralized readiness potential, derived from the RPs elicited in paradigms in which the response-related asymmetry over central sites serves as a proxy for response activation (De Jong, Wierda, Mulder, & Mulder, 1988; Gratton, Coles, Sirevaag, Eriksen, & Donchin, 1988) in particular, has been of great utility in analyzing the stimulus versus response aspects of information processing. The LRP can be derived in a number of different ways (e.g., double subtraction method or subtraction averaging method), which are equivalent as long as the design is such that within a given condition, a right hand response is correct for half the trials and the left hand is correct for the remaining half. In the subtraction averaging procedure, the ERP from the central site ipsilateral to the responding hand is subtracted from that on the contralateral site, separately for each hand, and the two are averaged. The resultant LRP, if any, reflects lateralization due to motor preparation with direction (polarity) indicating the response that has been preferentially activated, magnitude indicating the degree of the preferential activation, and latency indicating when the response was preferentially activated.

Accordingly, cognitive electrophysiologists have generally used the LRP to address questions about the dynamics of information processing (e.g., partial information transmission), the order in which information about a stimulus is extracted, the processing locus of particular experimental effects, and individual differences. Whenever the question of interest can be phrased in terms of the relative activation of the two responses (right and left hands), an LRP analysis can provide an answer. The most common ways of eliciting an RP for LRP derivation are the conflict and Go-NoGo paradigms. In both, it is essential that the experimental stimuli have multiple attributes which can be mapped onto the different responses (hands) in the conflict paradigm, or to different aspects of response (which hand, whether or not to respond) in the Go-NoGo paradigm. In the conflict paradigm, these different attributes are mapped onto the same hand in some conditions and onto different hands in other conditions, with critical inferences drawn from the direction of the LRP on conflict trials. In the Go-NoGo paradigm one attribute determines the hand that is to respond and the other attribute determines whether or not to respond at all, with critical inferences drawn from the presence and timing of the LRP on NoGo trials. This Go-NoGo paradigm is also the experimental milieu for eliciting an N2 NoGo response (an index of response inhibition), whose timing likewise affords inferences about the time point by which information needed for halting a (prepared) response must have been available. The Go-NoGo paradigm has proven especially fruitful for testing alternative views of language production.

Schmitt, Münte, and Kutas (2000), for instance, used the LRP and NoGo N200 to determine the relative timing of access to semantic and phonological information during tacit picture naming. Participants viewed pictures of animals or inanimate objects (the semantic attribute) whose names began with a vowel or a consonant (the phonological attribute). In one condition (*go/no-go = semantics; dual-choice = phonology*), the Go-NoGo decision was contingent on the semantic attribute, and the response hand was contingent on a phonological attribute while in the other (*go/no-go = phonology; dual-choice = semantics*), the mapping was reversed; namely, the Go-NoGo decision was contingent on the phonological attribute, and the response hand on the semantic attribute. Regardless of condition, Go trials should be associated with large indistinguishable LRPs (as long as the isolated semantic and phonological decisions are of equal difficulty, as reflected in a similar time course). Of critical interest for the question at hand, however, is the ERP pattern on the NoGo trials in these two conditions. The presence of an LRP—even a short-lived one—on a NoGo trial implies that the information indicating what hand to prepare is available before the information indicating whether or not any response is to be given. Its duration provides an upper limit on the time by when the information not to respond has become available. By contrast, the absence of an LRP on a NoGo trial implies that the information on which the response hand hinges is available either coincident with or sometime after the information on which the Go-NoGo response hinges. Schmitt et al. found a reliable LRP on NoGo trials in the (*go/no-go = phonology; dual-choice = semantics*) condition, but not in the (*go/no-go = semantics; dual-choice = phonology*) condition, suggesting that access to semantic information preceded that to phonological information (see Figure 6.1a).

In these types of experiments, participants are not asked to name the pictures aloud so as to minimize potentially contaminating muscle artifacts associated with the act of speaking. Rather it is assumed that participants engage the same semantic and phonological processes in tacit naming as in overt naming. LRP analyses in dual-choice Go-NoGo tasks of this type have indicated that semantic information (animal vs. object) is available before phonological information (van Turennout, Hagoort, & Brown, 1997) and that semantic information (an object's weight) is available before syntactic gender in German or Dutch (Schmitt, Schiltz, Zaake, Kutas, & Münte, 2001). Using a slightly different LRP design, Abdel Rahman, van Turennout and Levelt (2003) showed that phonological retrieval is not contingent on retrieval of semantic information—as proposed by serial models of language production (e.g., Levelt, Roelofs, & Meyer, 1999); but, rather, can occur before semantic access, consistent with parallel processing of semantic and phonological information (e.g., Dell & O'Seaghdha, 1992).

To date, the obvious potential of the LRP (and NoGo N200, which is larger and more robust than the LRP) to examine whether, and if so how, clinical (cognitive or motor) disorders might affect the timing of various language processes has remained largely untapped. By identifying the time points at which semantic and phonological information are accessed, for example, LRPs in a Go-NoGo paradigm could provide evidence on the contribution, if any, of the diminished availability of semantic information in Alzheimer's dementia patients to their documented naming deficits (Garrard, Lambon Ralph, Patterson, Pratt, & Hodges, 2005; Salmon, Butters, & Chan, 1999).

LANGUAGE COMPREHENSION

While a few well-crafted experiments have examined language production in preparation for, but in the absence of, speaking, the bulk of the ERP language literature has focused on language comprehension. ERPs have proven especially useful for studying speech processing because their exquisite temporal sensitivity spans the analysis of speech signals from phonemes to discourse.

LANGUAGE OR NOT? EARLY SENSORY COMPONENTS

Event-related brain potential components that occur within the first 200 ms following stimulus onset are obligatory responses presumed to reflect sensory processing and occasionally attentional modulation of the input. These so-called sensory evoked potentials (EPs) are modality specific and sensitive in their amplitude and/or latency to the physical parameters of the stimulus. In fact, abnormalities in these early sensory potentials are routinely used to assess the integrity of the sensory system. For instance, the auditory brainstem response (ABR), an EP occurring within the first 10 ms after an auditory click, is used to screen hearing in newborns, determine hearing loss in children, or neurophysiologically assess hearing in brainstem lesion patients. In an ideal world in which time and money were not practical constraints, every ERP investigation of language and nonlanguage auditory processing would begin with an ABR assessment, along with audiometric tests. This would seem especially critical for ruling out peripheral abnormalities in patient populations with auditory language deficits.

Early EP componentry such as the N1-P2 complex, thought to reflect preattentive processing of sound in the auditory cortex, has been utilized to monitor speech segmentation and detection processes. Using an experimental design that contrasted EPs recorded before and after training on multisyllabic nonsense words (e.g., *babupu* or *bupada*), Sanders, Newport, and Neville (2002) found that the N1 component could serve as a marker of word onsets in continuous speech (see also Tremblay & Kraus, 2002 for similar use of the N1-P2 to track speech-sound training). We believe that such ERP markers of speech segmentation and detection can prove unquestionably useful for monitoring learning in individuals for whom behavioral testing is not a viable option (e.g., infants or some patient populations), and also may be instrumental for studying dyslexic or autistic individuals, delayed talkers, and second language learners, among others. In this regard, however, it is important to note that the N1 is comprised of three functionally distinct subcomponents: the N1a generated in the supratemporal plane of auditory cortex, and the N1b and N1c, both generated from the lateral surface of superior temporal gyri, but with different maturational curves. This suggests caution when generalizing across studies (whether within or across individuals) employing different electrode montages. Among the clear benefits of many ERP components is that as reflections of postsynaptic activity they are good indices of synaptic plasticity (due to experience and learning) and can be reliably recorded with about equal sensitivity in different clinical groups and across the age span, starting with infants.

PHONEMIC DISCRIMINATION AND CATEGORICAL PERCEPTION: MISMATCH NEGATIVITIES

A case in point is the so-called mismatch negativity (MMN) that not only can be recorded in neonates (as early as preterm infants born 30–35 weeks after conception), but in a sleeping, inattentive babies at that (Cheour-Luhtanen, Alho, Sainio, Rinne, & Reinikainen, 1996; Cheour, Alho, Sainio, & Reinikainen, 1997)! The MMN is a fronto-central negativity generated near primary auditory cortex (with a contentious frontal lobe contribution), which in the earliest studies was recorded between 100 and 300 ms poststimulus onset to infrequent tones that deviated in pitch, intensity, or duration from those of the more frequent, standard tone stream in which they were embedded (Näätänen, Gaillard, & Mantysalo, 1978). The greater the deviance, the earlier the MMN onset and the larger its amplitude (Tiitinen, May, Reinikainen, & Näätänen, 1994). Critically, the MMN can be elicited in the absence of attention, even when participants are actively engaged in a cognitively demanding distractor task (playing a video game or watching a silent movie), although the component is not impervious to attentional manipulations. As a sensitive index of auditory sensory (echoic) memory, the MMN has been the ERP tool of choice for analyzing early auditory processing and short-term memory. The MMN, however, has proven especially useful for investigating issues in speech perception (e.g., categorical perception of speech) because it is not restricted to tone stimuli or to simple physical deviations thereof. Once a representation has been formed, an MMN can be elicited by phonemes, syllables, words, and other abstract patterns including complex regularities where the commonality of the "standard" lies more in a "rule-like" association (e.g., to a descending tone pair deviant in a stream of ascending tone pair standards; Paavilainen, Jaramillo, Näätänen, & Winkler, 1999). MMN findings reveal what sorts of auditory perceptual patterns are stored in the auditory cortex, and since the late 1990s have demonstrated how these patterns (e.g., speech) are modulated by experience (for recent trends in MMN research, see Näätänen, Paavilainen, Rinne, & Alho, 2007).

The MMN has been broadly used to monitor the acquisition of both native and nonnative, real and artificial, speech contrasts in infants, children, and adults. Cheour et al. (1998), for example, adopted an MMN paradigm in a cross-linguistic analysis with Finnish and Estonian infants to demonstrate that language-specific memory traces develop during the latter half of the first year of life (6–12 months). These languages were chosen due to their similar vowel structures. The standard stimulus was a vowel prototype found in both languages (/e/), as was one of the deviants (/ö/); the other deviant was found only in Estonian (/õ/). Both infant groups showed larger amplitude MMNs to the Finnish–Estonian /ö/ deviant at 1 year than at 6 months of age. However, only the Estonian infants showed a similar age-related increase to the Estonian /õ/ deviant; Finnish infants showed only a small acoustic-based MMN to the Estonian deviant, regardless of age. Thus within the first year there is a diminution in the ability of humans to discriminate nonnative speech sounds and a noticeable improvement in their ability to discriminate native vowel sounds. Winkler et al. (1999) used a similar MMN paradigm with adult monolingual and bilingual speakers to demonstrate preattentive categorization of second language phonemes with language experience. Finns and "Finnish fluent" Hungarians, but not "Finnish naïve" Hungarians, showed increased MMNs to vowel categories perceptually distinctive in Finnish, but not Hungarian. Such results argue for long-term changes in the adult brain areas involved in phonetic analysis (see Figure 1b).

The MMN also has been used to assess auditory discrimination accuracy in clinical groups with various types of language impairments, including but not limited to dyslexia (e.g., Baldeweg, Richardson, Watkins, Foale, & Gruzelier, 1999), specific language impairment for speech sounds (e.g., Kraus et al., 1996), aphasia (e.g., Ilvonen et al., 2004), developmental stuttering (e.g., Corbera, Corral, Escera, & Idiazabal, 2005), and Asperger's syndrome (Kujala, Lepisto, Nieminen-von Wendt, Näätänen, & Näätänen, 2005). For example, Baldeweg et al. (1999) used the MMN in conjunction with Näätänen's (1992) model of auditory atten-tion to explore the hypothesis that specific low-level auditory perceptual deficits are implicated in dyslexia. Specifically, they predicted that the N1 (indexing the neural coding of auditory stimulus onset and offset) would be normal in dyslexics as would the MMNs in response to duration-based deviants, whereas the MMNs to pitch-based deviants would be abnormal. By choosing a(n electro)physiological measure that does not rely on attentional resources, potential confounds in those with dyslexia comorbid with attention-deficit hyperactivity disorder could be cir-cumvented. The MMN results were as predicted, thereby substantiating parallel deficits in a tone frequency discrimination task, as well as correlating with pho-nological impairments inferred from off-line reading errors. Two aspects of this study are worth noting. This study underscores the fact that as a multidimensional dependent measure, the ERP waveform allows a simultaneous scrutiny of mul-tiple processing operations—early and late—which may prove especially useful for confirming or ruling out impairments in one level as the cause for difficulties at another. This study also highlights an important design decision to show speci-ficity; namely, including a condition that is expected to be normal in addition to one which is expected to be problematic (also see MMNs to different tones versus speech sounds in aphasic patients, Ilvonen et al., 2004; and individuals with per-sistent developmental stuttering, Corbera et al., 2005).

In sum, the MMN offers an index of the functioning of the auditory sensory memory system that is sensitive to long-term perceptual learning. Critically for diagnostic purposes, the MMN is easy to record, and does not require active engage-ment of the participant. As a consequence, the MMN has proven especially useful in auditory research with infants and others with temporary or permanent limitations in their communicative abilities. As noted, the MMN paradigm has found numer-ous clinical applications, for example, in the study of developmental language and literacy impairments (see Bishop, 2007 for a review), the evaluation of auditory per-ceptual deficits in aphasia (Aaltonen, Tuomainen, Laine, & Niemi, 1993), the assess-ment of auditory sensory memory in Alzheimer's (Pekkonen, Jousmäki, Könönen, & Reinikainen, 1994) and Parkinson's (Pekkonen, Jousmaki, Reinikainen, & Partanen, 1995) patients, among others. Given the MMN's sensitivity to long-term experi-ence with the perceptual properties of language, its utility as an analytic tool is limited only by the cleverness of the experimenter in choosing what to deviate from what background—this despite the fact that the MMN is unquestionably not a language-specific response.

A final note related to the MMN—based on the data to date, there is no sub-stantive, if any, relationship between the MMN and the so-called phonological mismatch negativity (PMMN). Indeed, whether or not a PMMN exists at all (Connolly & Phillips, 1994) or is merely the initial phase of an N400 congruity effect (Van Petten, Coulson, Rubin, Plante, & Parks, 1999) or a type of N200 (van den Brink, Brown, & Hagoort, 2001; van den Brink & Hagoort, 2004) remains highly controversial. In some sense, the label is inconsequential because whatever its name, the data from each of these laboratories are similar in showing that context affects spoken word processing and contextual integration even before a word is fully identified.

WORD, SENTENCE, AND DISCOURSE LEVEL COMPREHENSION

Although ERPs can be used to explore language comprehension at multiple levels of granularity, the great majority of the work to date has focused on words in isolation, in word pairs, within sentences, and more recently in short discourses. Although there are some differences as a function of input modality, the most robust ERP comprehension-sensitive effects—in particular, the N400 and P600 effects—are observed whether the eliciting stimuli are in written, spoken, signed, or even pictorial formats (i.e., not language specific). The most likely ERP effect to be language-specific (although that too is controversial) is the so-called left anterior negativity or LAN often seen in response to violations of word class (to a word from one lexical class when another was expected, e.g., to a verb when a preposition was contextually expected).

Measures of Meaning: From Words to Pragmatics

ERP research with words, pseudowords, pictures, gestures, acronyms, environmental sounds, and indeed other potentially meaningful items has revealed that the interval between 200 and 500 or so ms poststimulus (i.e., the N400 region) is especially sensitive to many of the factors that influence ease of lexical access such as frequency of occurrence, repetition, semantic relationships, context, among others (see Table 6.1).

The averaged electrical brain activity during this window to such items occurring in isolation is typically negative (relative to a prestimulus baseline and mastoid reference) or negative-going, and peaks around 400 ms. This is what it means when

---

TABLE 6.1
Some Linguistic Factors That Influence N400 Amplitude

Linguistic Factor	Influence on N400 Amplitude
Lexical association	Semantically related primes reduce N400 amplitude to target words
Repetition	Reduced negativity to repeated words
Frequency	Smaller negativity to more frequent than rare words
Word class (open/closed)	Larger negativity to open-class words over posterior sites
Concreteness	Larger negativity to isolated concrete compared to abstract words over frontal sites
Off-line expectancy (cloze probability)	Reduced negativity to more versus less expected words within a sentence/discourse context
Sentence position	Reduced negativity for open-class words across sentence position: larger for initial than approaching sentence end

we say that an N400 is the default response to any potentially meaningful item; ERPs to true nonwords or nonenvironmental sounds, for instance, do not exhibit an N400 in this time window even in isolation. The presence of surrounding context of many sorts (including representations in semantic memory) modulates the activity in the N400 region, generally reducing its amplitude with increasing contextual fit (with its actual polarity depending on the nature and strength of the relationship between the context and the item). For instance, the N400 to the second of a pair of words is smaller if the two words are semantically related (e.g., cat–dog) than if they are not (table–dog). Likewise, the N400 to a sentence medial or sentence final word is smaller if the word is semantically congruent with the prior sentence fragment (*I take coffee with cream and sugar.*) than if it is not (*I take coffee with cream and dog.*). These examples illustrate two classic N400-eliciting paradigms: the word pair paradigm and the anomalous sentence paradigm. Word pair studies have been used with a variety of tasks including lexical decision, and have revealed that the N400 region is also sensitive to phonological and morphological priming, not just semantic, associative, and conceptual priming (see Kutas & Hillyard, 1989 for discussion of task choice in the word pair paradigm). The anomalous sentence paradigm similarly has been employed with a variety of tasks, even though the best thing about the sentence paradigm is that participants need have no other task than to read or to listen—comprehension being the only (and unquestionably most natural) task. This is all the more awesome as a psycholinguistic tool for all subject populations, including various clinical groups, because numerous studies have unequivocally demonstrated that the whereas semantic anomalies may lead to very large N400s, readily measurable and manipulable N400s also can be seen in garden variety sentences—with no complex structure, no anomaly, and no ambiguities of any sort (e.g., *He was soothed by the gentle wind*). Moreover, the amplitude of the N400 in such sentences is inversely correlated ($r = -.90$) with the eliciting word's off-line cloze probability (see DeLong, Urbach, & Kutas, 2005; Kutas & Hillyard, 1984; see Figure 6.1c).

In young adults, the N400 has a 400 ms peak latency that is relatively stable across experimental paradigms, with a centro-posterior scalp distribution varying slightly depending on the modality (visual or auditory) and nature (visual, pictorial, linguistic, or nonlinguistic) of the eliciting stimuli. The N400's amplitude decreases and its latency increases with normal aging (e.g., Kutas & Iragui, 1998) and are impacted even more by dementia.

It is worth noting that it is primarily N400 amplitude rather than N400 latency that varies with most manipulations, although latency shifts have been observed with flash presentation rates of 10 words/s eliciting an N480 (Kutas, 1987), with bilinguals who show longer latency N400s in their weaker language (Kutas, Moreno, & Wicha, 2009), and in clever experimental designs where processing leading to auditory N400s can be delayed (Van Petten et al., 1999). With every potentially meaningful item exhibiting an N400, its true utility comes from being able to capitalize on the N400 effect, the amplitude difference between conditions attributable to differential contextual analysis. More generally, the benefit of any "bump" in the ERP waveform lies not necessarily in identifying and labeling

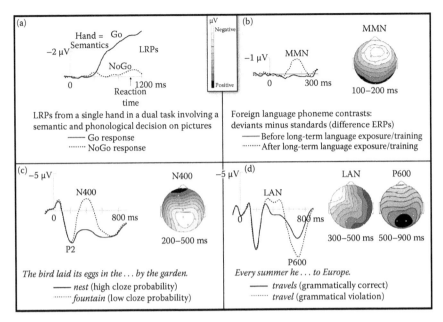

FIGURE 6.1 Idealized versions of five ERP effects (waveforms and scalp topography) used for investigating language. By convention, negative voltage is plotted upward. (a) LRPs (see text for derivation) in a dual task Go-NoGo paradigm, with responding hand determined by the outcome of a semantic decision and whether to respond (go) or not (nogo) determined by the outcome of a phonological decision. There is a large LRP on go trials, but also a reliable nogo response (~400 ms), indicating response activation, on nogo trials. (b) The mismatch negativity (MMN) created by subtracting the ERP to standards from ERPs to deviants; compared are MMNs to the same phoneme contrasts salient in a second—but not native—language, prior to and following long-term language exposure/training. The large, fronto-central MMN indicates perceptual sensitivity to the phoneme distinction as a result of language training. (c) A centro-parietal N400 effect for more versus less contextually expected continuations within a written sentence. (d) The left anterior negativity (LAN) and P600 elicited to subject–verb agreement errors in written sentences. The LAN (as shown here) has a frontal and left-lateralized focus and the P600 has a centro-parietal focus, though the scalp distributions of both effects vary across studies.

it as a distinct component (though this too could be informative), but rather in determining those factors that it is sensitive to and utilizing that knowledge to investigate well-specified research questions.

McLaughlin, Osterhout, and Kim (2004), for example, used an N400 word pair paradigm to determine how many hours of second language (L2) exposure were needed before a second language learner's brain processing of L2 words resembled that of a native speaker. French learners were tested three times—toward the beginning, middle, and end of an introductory course—as they performed a lexical decision task on the second of a pair of written items including semantically related word pairs, semantically unrelated word pairs, and word–pseudoword pairs. Compared to a control group receiving no French instruction, L2 learners showed differences in N400 amplitude to nonwords versus words after only 14 hours of instruction, indicating a sensitivity to lexicality within the second language (prior to any reliable sensitivity in overt behavior). Additionally, after only 63 hours of instruction, L2 learners exhibited smaller N400s to related than unrelated words, paralleling the native language response typically observed to such stimuli, and indicative of comprehension.

Both the word pair and sentence paradigms have been crossed with the visual half field paradigm (presenting stimuli approximately two degrees to the right or left of fixation), so as to expose only the contralateral hemisphere to that stimulus for 10 ms or so. Remarkably, the consequence of such a short head start in processing reveals reliable differences in the pattern of ERPs elicited and, by inference, differences in the ways that the two hemispheres deal with semantic relationships and sentential constraint, joke processing, and so on. One testable hypothesis that has come from such work is that the left hemisphere is predictive (using context to preactivate word meaning, among other features), while the right hemisphere is more integrative in its approach to meaning construction, waiting until it receives the input to link up word meaning with the accrued contextual representation (Federmeier & Kutas, 1999).

Intuitively it seems that sentence processing and discourse level processing should be similar (same mechanisms and same brain areas), though as with many such questions the answer might depend on what is meant by the same. Psycholinguists, however, have long distinguished the two, and at least on some serial accounts, not only do word level effects precede sentence level effects but sentence level effects precede discourse level effects. Likewise, the neuropsychological literature has implicated a greater contribution of the right hemisphere in discourse than sentence or word processing. From the moment that ERP (especially N400) analyses were routinely applied to language processing, it became clear that language processing is not strictly serial: lexical, sentential, and discourse factors all impact a word's processing as reflected in N400 activity at essentially the same time and in essentially the same way. Word (lexical) level, sentence level, and discourse level effects on word processing each systematically modulate the electrical brain activity triggered by a word between approximately 200–500 ms post-target word onset. As already stated, a semantically, categorically, or associatively related word reduces N400 amplitude, a congruent sentence context also reduces N400 amplitude, and a congruent and constraining discourse likewise reduces N400 amplitude; indeed all these "contexts" lead to a similar, graded reduction in N400 amplitude. In fact, the brain activity during the N400 time window is also sensitive to world knowledge stored in semantic memory, co-occurring information in the visual environment, and different sorts of information about a speaker (e.g., mismatch between content of a message and stereotype of the person delivering the message). N400 amplitudes, for example, to *married* in a spoken sentence such as *"Last year I got married in a beautiful castle"* are found to be smaller if spoken by an adult female voice than that of a little girl (Van Berkum, van den

Brink, Tesink, Kos, & Hagoort, 2008). Nieuwland and Van Berkum (2006) further demonstrated that global context can overrule local (sentential) pragmatic anomalies. They contrasted animacy violations (e.g., *"The peanut was in love"*) legitimized by discourse context, to discourse anomalous but pragmatically congruent completions (e.g., *"The peanut was salted"*) in the same context, and found larger N400s to the discourse-incongruent completion (*salted*). Such findings are rock solid evidence negating Gricean semantics-before-pragmatics models.

A recent trend in electrophysiological language research has been to investigate the more nonliteral aspects of language including humor, sarcasm, and gesture. Wu and Coulson (2005), for instance, investigated the role of gesture in comprehension, assessing perspectives ranging from the view that gesture is inconsequential in comprehension to the view that it is part and parcel of the comprehension process, routinely contributing to semantic analysis and meaning construction when co-present. In their study, participants viewed excerpts from television cartoons, each followed by a video of a person whose gesture was either congruent or incongruent with the particular cartoon. In one version, participants judged the congruency of the cartoon-gesture pairing, and in another, they judged the relatedness of a probe word that followed each cartoon-gesture pair. In both cases, measurements within the N400 time widow, time-locked to gesture onsets, indicated greater negativities to the incongruent relative to congruent ones. The results are noteworthy first because they show that interpretable ERP effects can be recorded to nonstatic gestures (as for nonstatic signs within sign language) and second because the nature of the effects—modulations in the amplitude of the potential in the N400 time window—indicate that the gestures are processed and integrated into a semantic/conceptual representation much like words and pictures. They also open the door to questions about the relation between gesture and language processing in various types of aphasias, no aspect of communication and language being immune to ERP monitoring and probing.

Eliciting a robust N400 response is not difficult. Even the average 4-year-old shows a greater negativity (N400) to a spoken noun that is semantically anomalous within a sentence context, although as with any brain response, a small percentage of the (presumably healthy) population does not elicit an N400 to canonical lexico-semantic violations. While this is not a problem on average, it can be problematic for case studies. Likewise, we also know many of the factors that will reliably modulate N400 amplitude within word pairs and sentences with these sorts of canonical semantic anomalies (nouns or verbs). Less is known however about lexico-semantic violations of adjectives, verbs, and other lexical classes.

Indeed, even a well-established component like the N400 is not completely clear from controversy. One debate centers on the degree to which N400 can be modulated by information occurring outside the focus of attention or outside of conscious awareness, operationally defined as verbal report (e.g., during masked priming, the attentional blink, sleep, or coma). The exact nature of the neural and/or mental operation(s) that the N400 (brain activity between 200–500 ms following a potentially meaningful item) indexes is also still a matter of considerable discussion. In fact, one might question whether it makes sense to talk about the N400 as if it is "a thing" given its sensitivity to a very broad range of factors and concomitant activity in a significant part of the cortex. In a scholarly review of the neuropsychological, intracranial, and magnetoencephalography literature, Van Petten and Luka (2006) conclude that large portions of the temporal lobes—especially in the left hemisphere—are responsible for the scalp-recorded N400 component, at least the canonical N400 elicited by visual words alone, in word pairs or anomalous sentences. However, as they aptly note, very little is known about generators of the N400 in other modalities or by other types of stimulus conditions, because researchers have yet to look; there is no reason to assume that N400s to jokes and N400s to gestures and N400 modulations by speaker identity will all be generated in the exact same brain areas. These are empirical questions! Likewise, despite the general consensus on what is needed to modulate N400 amplitude, there is as of yet no consensus on what "computation" it (assuming an it) reflects. Many different types of information are coming together—whether literally onto some common representation or in space or in temporal coincidence—during the region of the N400 to influence what information is "active" in the comprehender's mind/brain and to influence what they understand. Some refer to this process as contextual integration, others like Hagoort and colleagues (Hagoort, Baggio, & Willems, in press) refer to it as semantic unification (see van Berkum, 2009 and Chwilla & Kolk for their specific takes on the N400). Hot off the presses, an interesting set of questions about just what aspect of semantic analysis the N400 reflects have been raised by the results of a handful of studies that have reported N400 effects in response to seemingly grammatical violations (e.g., Hopf, Bayer, Bader, & Meng, 1998). These studies are particularly intriguing because they raise some fundamental questions not just about the N400 component itself, but also about the juxtaposition between how we as researchers draw clear distinctions between semantics and syntax, for example, versus how the brain appreciates this human divide.

Because so much is known about the factors that influence N400 parameters, its potential for researching special language populations is great. Researchers have exploited N400 sensitivity to word class to examine potential differences in processing for open versus closed class words in aphasic patients (ter Keurs, Brown, Hagoort, & Stegeman, 1999), to assess semantic categorization in normal aged as well as dementia populations (Iragui, Kutas, & Salmon, 1996), and to track longitudinal N400 patterns in children at risk for developmental language disorders such as specific language impairment (Friedrich & Friederici, 2006), to name but a few. The N400 is an excellent diagnostic tool for assessing semantic analysis and meaning construction in humans of all ages, in all languages—written, spoken, and signed. Whatever the experimental conditions, one can always include a safety net of sorts by including 25 or so sentences (and an equal number of controls, though not the exact same sentences within participants) including a semantically anomalous noun known to elicit a canonical N400. The properties of this N400 can provide a basis for comparing all other ERP or N400-like effects within the same individual and group.

As already noted, it is relatively easy to elicit a large N400 in most young adults—all it takes is five or so semantically anomalous sentences. Of course, for many reasons one needs to record many more trials—25 minimum (and preferably 35–40). However, just because one can, it does not mean one (e.g., one interested in language and/or communicative disorders) should. Seeing "what if" is not generally a recommended approach to rigorous scientific inquiry (although it could have a place in testing the waters). On the other hand, if there is a specific hypothesis about how or how quickly one group versus another makes sense of conceptual input then by all means adopt or adapt one of the N400-eliciting paradigms and have a go at it! Keep in mind that the N400 takes a huge hit with normal aging, and that variance can often be so great that it may not make much sense merely to compare the size of one group's N400 to that of another, rather compare N400 effects. And, never forget that there is no direct path from physiological (or behavioral) measures to psychological constructs (e.g., semantic analysis).

Effects of Structure and Syntax

Of course, lexico-semantic violations (especially of nouns) are not the only linguistic violations that elicit some systematic brain response. In fact, with history as our guide, we know that almost every violation—be it physical, orthographic, phonological, syntactic, pragmatic, and so on—elicits some sort of ERP effect compared to its nondeviant counterpart. In fact, many researchers seem to place a lot of stock in the identities of the ERPs elicited and what these say about whether or not two representations/processes are the same or different and about the psychological reality of the level under investigation. The issue of psychological reality notwithstanding, there is no question that language has hierarchical structure with regularities occurring at multiple levels—phonemes, letters, morphemes, words, phrases, clauses, and sentences, among others. Linguists have documented many of these regularities in remarkably nuanced and formal ways. Nonetheless, there is no single consensus view on how best to partition language representations and processes, much less syntax and syntactic processes. Thus it is not surprising that there is no single electrical brain manifestation of syntactic violation, even with syntax defined loosely as a system of "rules governing sentence structure." The ways, degrees, and timing with which the brain is sensitive to such rules during online comprehension are matters for empirical testing, and we believe they need to be investigated giving due consideration to working memory, sequencing, inhibition, attention, and monitoring operations, to name a few. These involve critical brain operations that may be effectively experimentally targeted within various patient populations and are unarguably important in many others. ERP investigations of syntax are on the rise, and indeed, there is no simple story to be told; for instance, not only the types of violation but individual differences have proven to be important for the ERP patterns seen, sometimes including, as already noted, N400s. Most grammatical/syntactic violations, however, do not elicit N400 activity.

In 1983, Kutas and Hillyard demonstrated that morphosyntactic violations do not elicit posterior N400 activity, being associated instead with more frontally distributed negativities and/or later positivities. More linguistically sophisticated studies have since highlighted three main effects (in order of reliability): the P600 (for a brief period also referred to as syntactic positive shift or SPS), the left anterior negativity or LAN, and an early left anterior negativity or ELAN. The P600 is a positivity beginning approximately 450–500 ms after the onset of a syntactically anomalous, ambiguous, or complex word, with a waveform shape alternating between peaked and broad. Its relative amplitude distribution across the scalp also varies considerably, though clear P600 identification is often tied to a centro-parietal maximum, with several researchers proposing specific links between the scalp distribution of the P600 and the grammatical process that elicited it (Friederici, Hahne, & Saddy, 2002; Kaan & Swaab, 2003; see Figure 6.1d). The range of conditions under which auditory and/or visual P600s have been observed includes violations of:

1. Subject–verb number agreement (Coulson, King, & Kutas, 1998; Münte, Szentkuti, Wieringa, Matzke, & Johannes, 1997) *Every Monday he *mow the lawn.*
2. Pronoun case (Coulson et al., 1998) *The plane took *we to paradise and back.*
3. Noun case (Münte, Heinze, Matzke, Wieringa, & Johannes, 1998) *The witch used her *broom's to fly to the forest.*
4. Pronoun gender agreement (Osterhout & Mobley, 1995) *The hungry waitress ordered *himself a burger.*
5. Pronoun number agreement (Osterhout & Mobley, 1995) *The bitter employees prepared *herself for the confrontation.*
6. Verb inflection (Friederici, Pfeifer, & Hahne, 1993) *The parquet was *polish.*
7. Phrase structure (Friederici, Pfeifer, & Hahne, 1993; Friederici, Steinhauer, & Frisch, 1999; Hagoort & Brown, 2000; Neville, Nicol, Barss, Forster, & Garrett, 1991) *The scientist criticized Max's *of proof the theorem.*

P600s in response to violations of phrase structure or word order/lexical class are also preceded by a negativity largest over left frontal sites and known as the early LAN or ELAN (see Figure 6.1d). Some would argue that ELANs are only seen in response to this type of violation, in which they are hypothesized to reflect automatic, first-pass parsing processes as the later parietal P600 reflects more strategically controlled, second-pass parsing processes (e.g., Friederici & Mecklinger, 1996).

P600s have been seen even in response to grammatical errors in senseless prose composed of real words (e.g., *Two mellow graves *sinks by the litany* compared to *Two mellow graves sink by the litany*), but not by apparent grammatical errors in prose comprising pseudowords (e.g., *The slithy toves *gimbles in the wabe* versus *The slithy toves gimble in the wabe*; Münte, Matzke, & Johannes, 1997). Like the N400, the P600 is not merely a response to a patent grammatical/

syntactic violation. P600s, for instance, were observed in response to the word *to* in "*The woman persuaded to...*" versus "*The woman struggled to...*" (Osterhout & Holcomb, 1992). In the first instance, *to* is not grammatically incorrect, as it could be part of a sentence in which *persuaded* introduces a passivized reduced relative clause, as in "*The woman persuaded to make a donation opened her checkbook*," although it is presumably less expected than one in which *persuaded* is followed by its direct object, as in "'*The woman persuaded her husband to make a donation.*"

An intriguing recent trend in P600 sentence comprehension literature reports P600s (aka late positivities) in response to manipulations that would typically not fall under the rubric of "syntactic." In some cases, a P600 is observed to what the authors considered an N400-eliciting semantic violation (e.g., Kuperberg, Sitnikova, Caplan, & Holcomb, 2003, in response to thematic role animacy violations, "*Every morning at breakfast the eggs would eat...*"; Kim & Osterhout, 2005, to anomalous verb forms, "*The hearty meal was devouring...*"; Kolk, Chwilla, van Herten, & Oor, 2003 and Hoeks, Stowe, & Doedens, 2004, to semantically associated verb and arguments, "*The cat that fled from the mice...*" and "*The javelin has thrown the athletes...*", respectively). In other cases, the P600s more clearly occur in conjunction with N400s or N400-like components (e.g., Federmeier, Wlotko, De Ochoa-Dewald, & Kutas, 2007, in response to unexpected sentence completions to highly constraining contexts; Vissers, Kolk, van de Meerendonk, & Chwilla, 2008, in response to violations of sentence truth-values in relation to picture stimuli; van de Meerendonk, Kolk, Vissers, & Chwilla, 2010, to highly but not mildly implausible sentence continuations). While it is not uncommon to observe multiple ERP effects (e.g., LAN, N400, P600) within a given condition, component co-occurrence is a finding that begs closer examination. Currently, we do not know why some of these studies give rise to an N400–P600 pattern while others exhibit only P600s, but the choice of control or baseline conditions must matter. Clearly, these studies do bring into question the "syntactic" nature of the P600 component: what exactly is being reflected in modulations of the P600?

The viable answers run the gamut from language-specific to domain general. Some researchers have proposed that the P600 reflects some form of syntactic reanalysis, based on data suggesting the following: (a) that the P600 is decomposable (using principal-components analysis) into subcomponents that distinguish it from a late posterior positivity variously known as the P3, P3b, or P300 in the literature on general information processing, categorization, or decision making (Friederici, Mecklinger, Spencer, Steinhauer, & Donchin, 2001), and (b) that P600 amplitude is proportional to the difficulty of syntactic reanalysis (Munte et al., 1997). Other researchers have argued, on the basis of experimental results suggesting that P600 and P3 amplitudes are sensitive to the same probabilistic parameters, that the P600 is a P3 in language contexts—a response to unexpected, infrequent syntactic anomalies or irregularities (Coulson et al., 1998; Gunter, Stowe, & Mulder, 1997). Depending on the question under investigation, whether or not the P600 is a member of the P3 family, or even if the two components are the same thing, may not matter.

With regard to P600 studies of patient populations, it has been found that for Broca's aphasia patients, who are characterized by difficulties producing and comprehending grammatical structures, P600s are reduced or absent in response to subject–verb number agreement violations (Wassenaar, Brown, & Hagoort, 2004) and word-class (noun vs. verb) violations (Wassenaar & Hagoort, 2005). Moreover, across patients, poorer performance on neuropsychological tests of syntactic comprehension correlates with smaller P600s. These results imply that Broca's aphasia patients' deficits in syntactic comprehension stem from disruption of processes that must be intact to elicit normal P600s—this could be any process prior to and including those manifest in the P600. It remains to be investigated whether P600 testing could have diagnostic or research utility in profiling aphasic patients' impairment in comprehending different types of grammatical structures, or in predicting such patients' prognosis for improvement. Again, it is not obvious the extent to which it matters whether or not the P600 is syntax-specific.

The same can be said for the left anterior negativity (LAN) that sometimes—but not always, for reasons unknown—precedes the P600 in response to various grammatical/syntactic violations. (Note that despite its moniker there are a substantial number of instances where the LAN is not left-lateralized, nor anterior, being more broadly distributed along the anterior-posterior axis.) The LAN, too, is currently the object of much debate regarding its special relation to syntax. In contrast to the proposal that the LAN is a specific response to syntactic violations (Münte, Heinze, & Mangun, 1993; Osterhout & Holcomb, 1992) is the proposal that it reflects the use of more general-purpose, working-memory resources during syntactic reanalysis, with an amplitude sensitive to working-memory load (Kluender & Kutas, 1993; Vos, Gunter, Kolk, & Mulder, 2001).

A final note on the use of ERPs to study language processing. If the electro-physiological study of language processing were contingent on the presence of violations and anomalies, ERP researchers would be hard pressed to argue that the results and inferences generalize to normal language comprehension. Whether this is a reasonable conclusion depends on exactly what is meant by a violation, whether violations are considered all-or-none or can be graded, the extent to which comprehenders must be "aware" that a violation has occurred, and so on. We believe a good argument can be made that as a (predictive) neural machine, the brain is continually generating (mostly unconscious) expectancies and thus experiencing violations of these expectancies to varying degrees. However, the beauty of ERP research is that overt violation manipulations are not necessary. Just ask participants to read, listen, gesture, and make sense of the world around them, and then monitor the electrical reflections of these activities at the scalp surface!

CONCLUDING REMARKS

The background and examples detailed herein paint a diverse picture of the types of language processing questions that ERPs can be used to answer. Some of the paradigms described are tried-and-true (e.g., the N400 semantic anomaly, the LRP in a Go-NoGo or conflict paradigm, and the MMN oddball). This means that we can be fairly certain that if we follow the "paradigm recipe," we know what ERP effects we are likely to observe, and thus that we can interpret systematic deviations in overall amplitude, relative amplitudes across the scalp or latency in meaningful ways. Of course, now and then, we may obtain findings somehow other than expected even in a "normal" population, presumably because we changed some aspect of the paradigm that was not considered crucial to the canonical effect that in fact may be. In that case, the cognitive electrophysiology field learns more about the factors leading to a particular ERP effect in a particular paradigm, and the design-inference cycle starts again. Moreover, it is not always possible to use or even to adapt an extant paradigm to the question at hand. That, however, need not be a cause for dismay, although it probably does mean more work ahead—the slow process of finding out first if this new paradigm generates any reliable ERP effects, then discovering what are the factors that manipulate the ERP effects, parameters, and so on. This process is the bread and butter of cognitive ERPers' existence. For others, it may be more rewarding to understand the ins and outs of each paradigm and the sorts of questions that each is especially suited to answer, and then to choose the right one to investigate a problem of interest, ever mindful that most cognitive ERP paradigms are not language specific, but can nonetheless serve psycholinguists and neurolinguists (in particular, researchers interested in communicative disorders) well.

ACKNOWLEDGMENT

Marta Kutas (and some of the work reported herein) is supported by grants AG08313 and HD22614.

REFERENCES

Aaltonen, O., Tuomainen, J., Laine, M., & Niemi, P. (1993). Cortical differences in tonal versus vowel processing as revealed by an ERP component called mismatch negativity (MMN). *Brain and Language, 44*(2), 139–152.

Abdel Rahman, R., van Turennout, M., & Levelt, W. J. M. (2003). Phonological encoding is not contingent on semantic feature retrieval: An electrophysiological study on object naming. *Journal of Experimental Psychology: Learning, Memory, and Cognition, 29*, 850–860.

Baldeweg, T., Richardson, A., Watkins, S., Foale, C., & Gruzelier, J. (1999). Impaired auditory frequency discrimination in dyslexia detected with mismatch evoked potentials. *Annals of Neurology, 45*(4), 495–503.

Bishop, D. (2007). Using mismatch negativity to study central auditory processing in developmental language and literacy impairments: Where are we, and where should we be going? *Psychological Bulletin, 133*(4), 651–672.

Cheour, M., Alho, K., Sainio, K., & Reinikainen, K. (1997). The mismatch negativity to changes in speech sounds at the age of three months. *Developmental Neuropsychology. Special Issue: Psychological Correlates of Infant Cognition, 13*(2), 167–174.

Cheour, M., Ceponiene, R., Lehtokoski, A., Luuk, A., Allik, J., Alho, K., & Näätänen, R. (1998). Development of language-specific phoneme representations in the infant brain. *Nature Neuroscience, 1*(5), 351–353.

Cheour-Luhtanen, M., Alho, K., Sainio, K., Rinne, T., & Reinikainen, K. (1996). The onto-genetically earliest discriminative response of the human brain. *Psychophysiology, 33*(4), 478–481.

Chwilla, D. J., & Kolk, H. H. J. (2005). Accessing world knowledge: Evidence from N400 and reaction time priming. *Cognitive Brain Research*, 25(3), 589–606.

Clarke, A. R., Barry, R. J., McCarthy, R., & Selikowitz, M. (2001). Age and sex effects in the EEG: Development of the normal child. *Clinical Neurophysiology, 112*(5), 806–814.

Connolly, J. F., & Phillips, N. A. (1994). Event-related potential components reflect phono-logical and semantic processing of the terminal word of spoken sentences. *Journal of Cognitive Neuroscience, 6*(3), 256–266.

Corbera, S., Corral, M. J., Escera, C., & Idiazabal, M. A. (2005). Abnormal speech sound representation in persistent developmental stuttering. *Neurology, 65*(8), 1246–1252.

Coulson, S., King, J. W., & Kutas, M. (1998). Expect the unexpected: Event-related brain response to morphosyntactic violations. *Language and Cognitive Processes, 13*(1), 21–58.

De Jong, R., Wierda, M., Mulder, G., & Mulder, L. J. M. (1988). Use of partial information in responding. *Journal of Experimental Psychology: Human Perception and Performance, 14*, 682–692.

Dell, G. S., & O'Seaghdha, P. G. (1992). Stages of lexical access in language production. *Cognition, 42*(1–3), 287–314.

DeLong, K. A., Urbach, T. P., & Kutas, M. (2005). Probabilistic word pre-activation during language comprehension inferred from electrical brain activity. *Nature Neuroscience, 8*(8), 1117–1121.

Delorme, A., Sejnowski, T., & Makeig, S. (2007). Enhanced detection of artifacts in EEG data using higher-order statistics and independent component analysis. *Neuroimage, 34*(4), 1443–1449.

Federmeier, K. D., & Kutas, M. (1999). A rose by any other name: Long-term memory structure and sentence processing. *Journal of Memory and Language, 41*(4), 469–495.

Federmeier, K. D., Wlotko, E. W., De Ochoa-Dewald, E., & Kutas, M. (2007). Multiple effects of sentential constraint on word processing. *Brain Research. Special Issue: Mysteries of Meaning, 1146*, 75–84.

Friederici, A. D., Hahne, A., & Saddy, D. (2002). Distinct neurophysiological pat-terns reflecting aspects of syntactic complexity and syntactic repair. *Journal of Psycholinguistic Research, 31*(1), 45–63.

Friederici, A. D., & Mecklinger, A. (1996). Syntactic parsing as revealed by brain responses: First-pass and second-pass parsing processes. *Journal of Psycholinguistic Research, 25*(1), 157–176.

Friederici, A. D., Mecklinger, A., Spencer, K. M., Steinhauer, K., & Donchin, E. (2001). Syntactic parsing preferences and their on-line revisions: A spatio-temporal analysis of event-related brain potentials. *Brain Research: Cognitive Brain Research, 11*(2), 305–323.

Friederici, A. D., Pfeifer, E., & Hahne, A. (1993). Event-related brain potentials during nat-ural speech processing: Effects of semantic, morphological and syntactic violations. *Brain Research: Cognitive Brain Research, 1*(3), 183–192.

Friederici, A. D., Steinhauer, K., & Frisch, S. (1999). Lexical integration: Sequential effects of syntactic and semantic information. *Memory and Cognition, 27*(3), 438–453.

Friedrich, M., & Friederici, A. D. (2006). Early N400 development and later language acquisition. *Psychophysiology, 43*(1), 1–12.

Garrard, P., Lambon Ralph, M. A., Patterson, K., Pratt, K. H., & Hodges, J. R. (2005). Semantic feature knowledge and picture naming in dementia of Alzheimer's type: A new approach. *Brain and Language, 93*(1), 79–94.

Gratton, G., Coles, M. G. H., Sirevaag, E., Eriksen, C. W., & Donchin, E. (1988). Pre- and post-stimulus activation of response channels: A psychophysiological analysis. *Journal of Experimental Psychology: Human Perception and Performance, 14*, 331–344.

Gunter, T. C., Stowe, L. A., & Mulder, G. (1997). When syntax meets semantics. *Psychophysiology, 34*(6), 660–676.

Hagoort, P., Baggio, G., & Willems, R. M. (In press). Semantic unification. To appear in M. S. Gazzaniga (Ed.), *The new cognitive neurosciences*. Cambridge, MA: The MIT Press.

Hagoort, P., & Brown, C. M. (2000). ERP effects of listening to speech compared to reading: The P600/SPS to syntactic violations in spoken sentences and rapid serial visual presentation. *Neuropsychologia, 38*(11), 1531–1549.

Hoeks, J. C. J., Stowe, L. A., & Doedens, G. (2004). Seeing words in context: The interaction of lexical and sentence level information during reading. *Cognitive Brain Research, 19*(1), 59–73.

Hopf, J., Bayer, J., Bader, M., & Meng, M. (1998). Event-related brain potentials and case information in syntactic ambiguities. *Journal of Cognitive Neuroscience, 10*(2), 264–280.

Ilvonen, T., Kujala, T., Kozou, H., Kiesiläinen, A., Salonen, O., Alku, P., & Näätänen, R. (2004). The processing of speech and non-speech sounds in aphasic patients as reflected by the mismatch negativity (MMN). *Neuroscience Letters, 366*(3), 235–240.

Iragui, V., Kutas, M., & Salmon, D. P. (1996). Event-related brain potentials during semantic categorization in normal aging and senile dementia of the Alzheimer's type. *Electroencephalography & Clinical Neurophysiology: Evoked Potentials, 100*(5), 392–406.

Kaan, E., & Swaab, T. Y. (2003). Repair, revision, and complexity in syntactic analysis: An electrophysiological differentiation. *Journal of Cognitive Neuroscience, 15*(1), 98–110.

Kim, A., & Osterhout, L. (2005). The independence of combinatory semantic processing: Evidence from event-related potentials. *Journal of Memory and Language, 52*(2), 205–225.

Kolk, H. H., Chwilla, D. J., van Herten, M., & Oor, P. J. (2003). Structure and limited capacity in verbal working memory: A study with event-related potentials. *Brain and Language, 85*(1), 1–36.

Kornhuber, H. and Deecke, L. (1964). Hirnpotentialänderungen beim Menschen vor und nach Willkürbewegungen, dargestellt mit Magnetbandspeicherung und Rückwärtsanalyse. *Pflügers Arch. ges. Physiol.* 281, p. 52.

Kraus, N., McGee, T. J., Carrell, T. D., Zecker, S. G., Nicol, T. G., & Koch, D. B. (1996). Auditory neurophysiologic responses and discrimination deficits in children with learning problems. *Science, 273*(5277), 971–973.

Kujala, T., Lepisto, T., Nieminen-von Wendt, T., Näätänen, P., & Näätänen, R. (2005). Neurophysiological evidence for cortical discrimination impairment of prosody in Asperger syndrome. *Neuroscience Letters, 383*(3), 260–265.

Kuperberg, G. R., Sitnikova, T., Caplan, D., & Holcomb, P. J. (2003). Electrophysiological distinctions in processing conceptual relationships within simple sentences. *Brain Research: Cognitive Brain Research, 17*(1), 117–129.

Kutas, M. (1987). Event-related brain potentials (ERPs) elicited during rapid serial visual presentation of congruous and incongruous sentences. *Electroencephalography and Clinical Neurophysiology. Supplement, 40*, 406–411.

Kutas, M., & Dale, A. (1997). Electrical and magnetic readings of mental functions. In M. D. Rugg (Ed.), *Cognitive neuroscience* (pp. 197–242). Cambridge, MA: MIT Press.

Kutas, M., & Donchin, E. (1980). Preparation to respond as manifested by movement-related brain potentials. *Brain Research, 202*(1), 95–115.

Kutas, M., & Hillyard, S. A. (1983). Event-related brain potentials to grammatical errors and semantic anomalies. *Memory and Cognition, 11*(5), 539–550.

Kutas, M., & Hillyard, S. A. (1984). Brain potentials during reading reflect word expectancy and semantic association. *Nature, 307*(5947), 161–163.

Kutas, M., & Hillyard, S. A. (1989). An electrophysiological probe of incidental semantic association. *Journal of Cognitive Neuroscience, 1*(1), 38–49.

Kutas, M., & Iragui, V. (1998). The N400 in a semantic categorization task across 6 decades. *Electroencephalography & Clinical Neurophysiology: Evoked Potentials, 108*(5), 456–471.

Kutas, M., Moreno, E. M., & Wicha, Y. Y. (2009). Code-switching and the brain. In B. E. Bullock & A. J. Toribio (Eds.), *The Cambridge handbook on linguistic code-switching.* Cambridge, UK: Cambridge University Press.

Levelt, W. J. M., Roelofs, A., & Meyer, A. S. (1999). A theory of lexical access in speech production. *Behavioral and Brain Sciences, 22*(1), 1–75.

Libet, B., Gleason, C. A., Wright, E. W., & Pearl, D. K. (1983). Time of conscious intention to act in relation to onset of cerebral activity (readiness-potential). The unconscious initiation of a freely voluntary act. *Brain, 106*(3), 623–642.

McLaughlin, J., Osterhout, L., & Kim, A. (2004). Neural correlates of second-language word learning: Minimal instruction produces rapid change. *Nature Neuroscience, 7*(7), 703–704.

Münte, T. F., Heinze, H. J., & Mangun, G. R. (1993). Dissociation of brain activity related to syntactic and semantic aspects of language. *Journal of Cognitive Neuroscience, 5*(3), 335–344.

Münte, T. F., Heinze, H. J., Matzke, M., Wieringa, B. M., & Johannes, S. (1998). Brain potentials and syntactic violations revisited: No evidence for specificity of the syntactic positive shift. *Neuropsychologia, 36*(3), 217–226.

Münte, T. F., Matzke, M., & Johannes, S. (1997). Brain activity associated with syntactic incongruencies in words and pseudo-words. *Journal of Cognitive Neuroscience, 9*(3), 318–329.

Münte, T. F., Szentkuti, A., Wieringa, B. M., Matzke, M., & Johannes, S. (1997). Human brain potentials to reading syntactic errors in sentences of different complexity. *Neuroscience Letters, 235*(3), 105–108.

Näätänen, R. (1992). *Attention and brain function.* Hillsdale, NJ, England: Lawrence Erlbaum Associates, Inc.

Näätänen, R., Gaillard, A. W., & Mantysalo, S. (1978). Early selective-attention effect on evoked potential reinterpreted. *Acta Psychologica, 42*(4), 313–329.

Näätänen, R., Paavilainen, P., Rinne, T., & Alho, K. (2007). The mismatch negativity (MMN) in basic research of central auditory processing: A review. *Clinical Neurophysiology, 118*(12), 2544–2590.

Neville, H., Nicol, J. L., Barss, A., Forster, K. I., & Garrett, M. F. (1991). Syntactically based sentence processing classes: Evidence from event-related brain potentials. *Journal of Cognitive Neuroscience, 3*(2), 151–165.

Nieuwland, M. S., & Van Berkum, J. J. A. (2006). When peanuts fall in love: N400 evidence for the power of discourse. *Journal of Cognitive Neuroscience, 18*(7), 1098–1111.

Osterhout, L., & Holcomb, P. J. (1992). Event-related potentials elicited by syntactic anomaly. *Journal of Memory and Language, 31*(6), 785–806.

Osterhout, L., & Mobley, L. A. (1995). Event-related potentials elicited by failure to agree. *Journal of Memory and Language, 34*(6), 739–773.

Paavilainen, P., Jaramillo, M., Näätänen, R., & Winkler, I. (1999). Neuronal populations in the human brain extracting invariant relationships from acoustic variance. *Neuroscience Letters, 265*(3), 179–182.

Papa, S. M., Artieda, J., & Obeso, J. A. (1991). Cortical activity preceding self-initiated and externally triggered voluntary movement. *Movement Disorders, 6*(3), 217–224.

Pekkonen, E., Jousmäki, V., Könönen, M., & Reinikainen, K. (1994). Auditory sensory memory impairment in Alzheimer's disease: An event-related potential study. *Neuroreport: An International Journal for the Rapid Communication of Research in Neuroscience, 5*(18), 2537–2540.

Pekkonen, E., Jousmaki, V., Reinikainen, K., & Partanen, J. (1995). Automatic auditory discrimination is impaired in Parkinson's disease. *Electroencephalography and Clinical Neurophysiology, 95*(1), 47–52.

Pfurtscheller, G., & Lopes da Silva, F. H. (1999). Event-related EEG/MEG synchronization and desynchronization: Basic principles. *Clinical Neurophysiology, 110*(11), 1842–1857.

Rohrbaugh, J. W., Syndulko, K., & Lindsley, D. B. (1976). Brain wave components of the contingent negative variation in humans. *Science, 191*(4231), 1055–1057.

Romero, S., Mananas, M. A., & Barbanoj, M. J. (2008). A comparative study of automatic techniques for ocular artifact reduction in spontaneous EEG signals based on clinical target variables: A simulation case. *Computers in Biology and Medicine, 38*(3), 348–360.

Salmon, D. P., Butters, N., & Chan, A. S. (1999). The deterioration of semantic memory in Alzheimer's disease. *Canadian Journal of Experimental Psychology/Revue Canadienne De Psychologie Expérimentale, 53*(1), 108–117.

Sanders, L. D., Newport, E. L., & Neville, H. J. (2002). Segmenting nonsense: An event-related potential index of perceived onsets in continuous speech. *Nature Neuroscience, 5*(7), 700–703.

Schmitt, B. M., Münte, T. F., & Kutas, M. (2000). Electrophysiological estimates of the time course of semantic and phonological encoding during implicit picture naming. *Psychophysiology, 37*(4), 473–484.

Schmitt, B. M., Schiltz, K., Zaake, W., Kutas, M., & Münte, T. F. (2001). An electrophysiological analysis of the time course of conceptual and syntactic encoding during tacit picture naming. *Journal of Cognitive Neuroscience, 13*(4), 510–522.

Sirigu, A., Daprati, E., Ciancia, S., Giraux, P., Nighoghossian, N., Posada, A., & Haggard, P. (2004). Altered awareness of voluntary action after damage to the parietal cortex. *Nature Neuroscience, 7*(1), 80–84.

Somsen, R. J., van't Klooster, B. J., van der Molen, M. W., van Leeuwen, H. M., & Licht, R. (1997). Growth spurts in brain maturation during middle childhood as indexed by EEG power spectra. *Biological Psychology, 44*(3), 187–209.

ter Keurs, M., Brown, C. M., Hagoort, P., & Stegeman, D. F. (1999). Electrophysiological manifestation of open- and closed-class words in patients with Broca's aphasia with agrammatic comprehension. An event-related brain-potential study. *Brain: A Journal of Neurology, 122*(5), 839–854.

Tiitinen, H., May, P., Reinikainen, K., & Näätänen, R. (1994). Attentive novelty detection in humans is governed by pre-attentive sensory memory. *Nature, 372*(6501), 90–92.

Tremblay, K. L., & Kraus, N. (2002). Auditory training induces asymmetrical changes in cortical neural activity. *Journal of Speech, Language, and Hearing Research, 45*(3), 564–572.

Van Berkum, J. J. A., van den Brink, D., Tesink, C. M. J. Y., Kos, M., & Hagoort, P. (2008). The neural integration of speaker and message. *Journal of Cognitive Neuroscience, 20*(4), 580–591.

van Berkum, J. J. A. (2009). Does the N400 directly reflect compositional sense-making? *Psychophysiology*, Special Issue: Society for Psychophysiological Research Abstracts for the Forty-Ninth Annual Meeting, *46*(Suppl. 1), s2.

van de Meerendonk, N., Kolk, H. H. J., Vissers, C. T. W. M., & Chwilla, D. J. (2010). Monitoring in language perception: Mild and strong conflicts elicit different ERP patterns. *Journal of Cognitive Neuroscience, 22* (1), 67–82.

van den Brink, D., Brown, C. M., & Hagoort, P. (2001). Electrophysiological evidence for early contextual influences during spoken-word recognition: N200 versus N400 effects. *Journal of Cognitive Neuroscience, 13*(7), 967–985.

van den Brink, D., & Hagoort, P. (2004). The influence of semantic and syntactic context constraints on lexical selection and integration in spoken-word comprehension as revealed by ERPs. *Journal of Cognitive Neuroscience, 16*(6), 1068–1084.

Van Petten, C., Coulson, S., Rubin, S., Plante, E., & Parks, M. (1999). Time course of word identification and semantic integration in spoken language. *Journal of Experimental Psychology: Learning, Memory, and Cognition, 25*(2), 394–417.

Van Petten, C., & Luka, B. J. (2006). Neural localization of semantic context effects in electromagnetic and hemodynamic studies. *Brain and Language, 97*(3), 279–293.

van Turennout, M., Hagoort, P., & Brown, C. M. (1997). Electrophysiological evidence on the time course of semantic and phonological processes in speech production. *Journal of Experimental Psychology: Learning, Memory, and Cognition, 23*(4), 787–806.

Varela, F., Lachaux, J. P., Rodriguez, E., & Martinerie, J. (2001). The brainweb: Phase synchronization and large-scale integration. *Nature Reviews Neuroscience, 2*(4), 229–239.

Vissers, C. T. W. M., Kolk, H. H. J., van de Meerendonk, N., & Chwilla, D. J. (2008). Monitoring in language perception: Evidence from ERPs in a picture-sentence matching task. *Neuropsychologia, 46*(4), 967–982.

Vos, S. H., Gunter, T. C., Kolk, H. H., & Mulder, G. (2001). Working memory constraints on syntactic processing: An electrophysiological investigation. *Psychophysiology, 38*(1), 41–63.

Wassenaar, M., & Hagoort, P. (2005). Word-category violations in patients with Broca's aphasia: An ERP study. *Brain and Language*, 92(2), 117–137.

Winkler, I., Kujala, T., Tiitinen, H., Sivonen, P., Alku, P., Lehtokoski, A., … Näätänen, R. (1999). Brain responses reveal the learning of foreign language phonemes. *Psychophysiology, 36*(5), 638–642.

Wu, Y. C., & Coulson, S. (2005). Meaningful gestures: Electrophysiological indices of iconic gesture comprehension. *Psychophysiology, 42*(6), 654–667.

7 Early Word Learning: Reflections on Behavior, Connectionist Models, and Brain Mechanisms Indexed by ERP Components

Manuela Friedrich

INTRODUCTION

From the neurobiological perspective, learning consists in pre- and postsynaptic molecular changes and in structural modifications of synaptic connectivity within specific brain areas, which are triggered by the previous processing of external signals, and in turn affect future signal transmission between neurons. At the behavioral level, learning allows an organism to modify and fine-tune its behavior to the requirements of the environment. It is however, largely unknown, how the molecular and structural changes at the neural level alter the systemic behavior at the psychological level.

Mathematical models, in principle, have the potential to bridge the gap between learning at the neural level and learning at the behavioral level, and to comprise the complex interplay of neuronal, systemic, and environmental effects. Massively parallel architectures, called artificial neural networks or connectionist models, provide an idea of how the complex interactions of a great many individual neuronal units result in systemic behavior. In these systems learning is studied by simulations, by which the "behavior" of a net; that is, its output under certain internal and environmental learning conditions is compared with the behavior in animals or humans observed experimentally. But even though the simulation results are often compatible with behavioral data and the basic principles of neural network dynamics are copied from biological neuronal signal transmission, most connectionist models are arbitrary designed architectures and their specific mechanisms described mathematically may not necessarily have a neurobiological basis.

On the other hand, brain imaging techniques and electrophysiological methods such as event-related brain potentials (ERPs) allow observation of the activity within certain brain structures or the related spatio-temporal voltage fluctuations at the scalp surface during perception, cognition, attention, and learning. The ERP, especially, has a high temporal resolution and is therefore particularly suitable for separating successive stages of stimulus processing. It consists of so-called components that systematically vary with certain experimental manipulations and that are assumed to reflect specific neural processes. ERP components mark the presence or absence of certain perceptual, cognitive, or linguistic processing stages; they indicate processing speed, the amount of resources allocated, or the effort necessary to realize the processing. ERP components also reflect learning-related changes of stimulus processing and are therefore used as brain signatures of a certain ability or a specific developmental stage. However, we do not know the brain mechanisms that cause the responses and what kind of neural interaction involved in the perceptual, cognitive, or linguistic processing stages is responsible for the activity patterns observed.

The present chapter is an attempt to bridge the levels of description in the case of early word learning by bringing together findings on behavioral development, ERP research, and neural network dynamics. In particular, the mechanism responsible for the elicitation of the N400 component of the ERP, interpreted as an index of context-dependent semantic memory use (Kutas & Hillyard, 1980), is proposed to be functionally similar to an artificial mechanism that has been developed to stabilize learning within a flexible connectionist memory system (Carpenter & Grossberg, 1987). The implications of the assumed real existence of such a mechanism will be discussed with respect to the development of categorization and word learning abilities in young children.

The structure of the chapter is the following: First, behavioral aspects of early word acquisition are described particularly with regard to the flexibility of the human lexical–semantic system. This part comprises the reformulating of basic questions of early word learning with respect to neural functioning. In a second step, ERP findings on lexical–semantic processing in infants and toddlers are reviewed. The course of N400 development observed in these studies and its interrelation with the children's language outcome raise questions about the nature of the N400 component and its direct involvement in the process of word learning. In connection with the nature of the N400, the term *semantic focus* is introduced as concept to refer to the flexible use of the representations established within the human lexical–semantic system and to the adjustment of these representations to internal needs and environmental requirements. The next paragraph describes the neural network model ART 1 (Carpenter & Grossberg, 1987) that provides a mathematical description of how the setting and the change of the semantic focus could be realized by neural dynamics. Finally, such a mechanism involved in changing the semantic focus is proposed to be reflected in the N400 component of the ERP. This assumption is further used to explain both the developmental course of the N400 and behavioral findings of early word acquisition.

Generally, the chapter is intended to encourage multidisciplinary work in developmental research, and in particular, the relation proposed here might lead to a deeper understanding of how words and their meanings are acquired by the infant brain.

BEHAVIORAL FINDINGS OF EARLY WORD LEARNING

Word learning includes the acquisition of phonological word forms, the extraction of relevant meanings, and the mapping between word form and word meaning memory representations. In order to learn words and their meanings the infant has to handle the variability of the environment in a response-appropriate manner. Basically, the infant brain must learn to differentiate what kind of variability is relevant for word learning and needs to be included into lexical–semantic memory representations and what is irrelevant and can be ignored.

WORD FORM AND WORD MEANING ACQUISITION

It has been found that infants early tune to the acoustic properties relevant in their native language; they acquire native language phoneme categories, prosodic features like typical word stress patterns, and the statistic distributions of phoneme combinations occurring in their target language (e.g., Friederici, Friedrich, & Christophe, 2007; Friederici & Wessels, 1993; Jusczyk, Cutler, & Redanz, 1993; Jusczyk, Friederici, Wessels, & Svenkerud, 1993; Kuhl, Williams, Lacerda, Stevens, & Lindblom, 1992; Werker & Lalonde, 1988; Werker & Tees, 2002). These skills facilitate the segmentation of the speech stream into single words, and they provide a basis for word form acquisition. Those variations of acoustic properties that are lexically relevant are included as features into the word form representations, whereas changes in the phonetic realization caused by the talker's age, gender, speech rate, or emotional state do not signal linguistic distinction and should therefore not be stored within lexical representations though they contain information relevant for social communication.

The acquisition of concepts and the mapping of words and concepts render word learning much more complex than word form acquisition alone. The infant brain must figure out what kind of meaningful information is relevant and what is not. In general concept formation occurs spontaneously without supervision by naming. This spontaneous structuring is influenced by words and behavioral relevant information, both guiding the formation and modification of concepts. For example, cats and dogs are initially seen as four-legged mammals, but naming cats as *cat* and dogs as *dog* facilitate the acquisition of separate concepts for cats and dogs. Similarly, the unexpected acerbity of a green apple may trigger the finer differentiation of different types of apples by the formation of representations that include color as distinctive feature. Thus, information that first appeared to be nonmeaningful may become meaningful in new situations, and different weightings of certain features are relevant in different contexts. During the course of development the human semantic system learns to semantically view a certain object or event in very different ways. The system becomes able to task-dependently switch between different points of view (i.e., between several semantic memory representations), and almost at each moment it must be able to create a new representation if the already acquired representations are not sufficiently appropriate. This enormous capacity enables the semantic system to handle very different objects or events as if they were the same, thereby broadly generalizing and transferring associated knowledge and expected outcomes, as well as discriminating between very similar objects or events if this is behaviorally relevant. The potential availability of the various memory representations with different weighting of semantic features makes the semantic system flexible and powerful allowing effective and optimal responses to the requirements of the environment. The knowledge about the neural basis of the ability to task-dependently adjust the threshold determining equality and dissimilarity in the external or internal environment would mainly contribute to our understanding of how the human lexical–semantic system can be stable, flexible, and constructive in parallel.

CATEGORIZATION AND THE DEGREE OF GENERALIZATION

In general, categorization realizes the balance between dissimilarity and equality by considering relevant features and abstracting from irrelevant information. Relevant features of a category are not represented in an all-or-none manner. Rather, the feature representation within a category depends on statistic properties such as the frequency of feature occurrence within exemplars that are considered as instances of the category. This leads to a graded prototypical structure of naturally acquired categories, including the effect that the prototype of a category is rated as a better exemplar than other category members and, even if never seen before, the prototype appears to be more familiar than previously observed exemplars that have constituted the category (e.g., Posner & Keele, 1968; Rosch, 1973). Such a prototypical structure of categories develops very early, it has been observed even in 3–4-month-old infants (Bomba & Siqueland, 1983; Quinn, 1987).

Categories extremely differ in their level of inclusiveness; that is, their degree of generalization. The degree of generalization is often described by three levels of abstraction, by global categories such as animals, basic level categories like dogs, and subordinate categories like poodles. However, there are a lot of categories at various intermediate levels of generality, such as, for example, mammals, four-legged mammals, fur-bearing animals, or several subspecies of poodles. The developmental course of categorization abilities appears to undergo a shift from global to basic level to subordinate categories (e.g., Younger & Fearing, 2000). However, results on categorization in infancy strongly depend on the behavioral method used (for a review, see Mareschal & Quinn, 2001). In studies that do not require a familiarization phase, infants categorize into broad global categories from about seven months on, and they show first signs of basic level knowledge at the end of their first year of life, although not consistently within the first 2 years. These broad categories cause overgeneralizations (e.g., a cat is referred to as a *dog*) that are massively observed in 1–2-year-olds, both in comprehension and production (e.g., McDonough, 2002). In contrast, in studies that require a familiarization phase, when infants have the possibility to form the categories during familiarization within the experiment, infants tune their category width in response to the requirements of the task, they form either global or basic level categories depending on the material used. In visual preference studies, even 3–4-month-old infants are able to form narrow, basic-level categories. The categorization results of these young infants sometimes display asymmetries (i.e., dogs are discriminated from the cat category, but cats are not discriminated from the dog category), which has been shown to depend on the overlap of the feature value distributions of the categories (French, Mareschal, Mermillod, & Quinn, 2004).

The results of behavioral studies clearly indicate that short lasting basic level categories can be acquired at a very early age, but the representations in long-term memory are much broader, and they are broader for a relatively long time. Although, in principle, the different results obtained with different behavioral methods can be attributed to the amount of information that is acquired by short-term learning during the experiment, the interaction of short- and long-term memory mechanisms involved in the formation of categories at varying levels of abstraction is completely unknown. Generally, little is known about how information is transferred from short-term memory into long-term memory and, even less, we know how a certain part of that information resulting in short-term basic level category formation is selected for consolidation and how this consolidation process leads to the establishment of more general categories in long-term memory.

MAPPING OF WORDS AND MEANINGS: TWO MODES OF EARLY WORD LEARNING

Full word learning requires the mapping of word form and word meaning memory representations and their reciprocal activation. Already at 6 months, infants associate the words *mama* and *papa* with the faces of their mother and father (Tincoff & Jusczyk, 1999). Around 8–10 months infants comprehend their first words (Bates, Thal, & Janowsky, 1992; Benedict, 1979). Thus, infants are able to establish associative links between phonological and semantic representations well before their first birthday. During this early stage, word learning appears to be a slow and time-consuming process that requires very frequent exposure to the word form within the appropriate context. Some weeks after the children's first birthday, however, infants become able to quickly learn a novel word for a novel meaning on the basis of only a few exposures (Schafer & Plunkett, 1998; Werker, Cohen, Lloyd, Casasola, & Stager, 1998; Woodward, Markman, & Fitzsimmons, 1994).

This *fast mapping ability* that develops between 12 and 14 months is assumed to be the basis of the rapid increase in vocabulary, the so-called *vocabulary spurt* that sets in at around 18 months. A main question and an ongoing debate in developmental research are related to the causes that underlie the qualitative change in infants' word learning ability. Several cognitive and sociocommunicative factors are discussed to affect the infant word learning rate (for an overview, see Nazzi & Bertoncini, 2003; Woodward et al., 1994). The assumption that before the vocabulary spurt children are not able to use the principle of linguistic reference is seen as the primary causation of the initial word learning restrictions in infants. According to this account, young children are able to slowly associate objects and words, but they learn a word as an associative context for an object instead of learning a word as symbolic reference that stands for an object even if this object is actually not present. Independent of whether the behaviorally observed qualitative change in the infant's word learning capacity is caused by the development of cognitive, linguistic, or social abilities, the decoding and consolidation of words and concepts appears to be radically changed when children become able to perform fast mapping. It is, however, completely unknown, what kind of changes in the neural mechanisms of perceptual, lexical–semantic, and memory processes are associated with the development of the fast mapping ability, and whether these changes are indeed qualitative or still quantitative in their nature. If assuming that the main developmental step is the ability to acquire and use referential knowledge, then the question will be, in which way the neural coding of referential connections and their involvement in specific stages of perceptual and cognitive stimulus processing differ from those of associative connections.

HIERARCHICAL KNOWLEDGE AND CONSTRAINTS IN EARLY WORD LEARNING

Once children have learned an initial meaning for a word, they must reach the appropriate level of generalization that the word refers to, they expand and refine their lexicon by learning other words with similar meanings, and they begin to reorganize the acquired concepts and to integrate them into hierarchically interpretable (but not necessarily hierarchically stored) knowledge structures.

Behavioral researchers have proposed several constraints that guide the acquisition of new word meanings. Some of these constraints are developed to explain the finding that 1–3-year-old children consistently map a novel word to a novel object when presented with two objects, one familiar and one unfamiliar, and asked for the referent of the novel word (*disambiguation effect*). It has been proposed that young children assume that an object can have only one name (*Mutual Exclusivity Constraint,* Markman & Wachtel, 1988), that they are motivated to label an unnamed category (*Novel Name-Nameless Category Principle,* Golinkoff, Mervis, & Hirsh-Pasek, 1994), or that they assume the meaning of a new word differs from the meaning of previously known words (*Contrast Principle,* Clark, 1987). However, the early age at which the disambiguation effect is observed suggests that it is not triggered by meta-cognitive abilities (e.g., pragmatic strategies), and therefore, it is not realized by intentional top-down guided neurocognitive processes. For this reason, the primary question is what neural mechanisms generate the behavior that results in the disambiguation effect and that can be described by constraints at the psycholinguistic level. More generally, one could ask what constraints in the maturing and developing brain cause the constraint behavior observed in young children.

Behavioral research has moreover shown that young children have particular difficulties in acquiring conceptual hierarchies. When 2–4-year-old children are trained with a new word for a subset of objects belonging to a known concept and having a known name (i.e., a word for a flower-subcategory like *rose*), after successful learning, many children do not anymore consider the objects of the subcategory to be members of the known concept. That is, for these children, roses are not flowers anymore, even though, before learning, children considered all target objects to be flowers. Goede and Friedrich (1995) showed that this *temporary exclusion of category members* that follows the acquisition of a subcategory depends on exemplar typicality and is not caused by one of the above mentioned constraints of early word learning. Rather, the exclusion of objects from a known, more general concept after learning a specific concept suggests that competition or inhibition processes are involved in the acquisition of new words and new concepts for already known objects. However, the neural processes of semantic specification and reorganization, which allow flexibly considering an object as belonging to several different concepts within a conceptual hierarchy, are largely unknown.

ERP COMPONENTS RELATED TO LEXICAL–
SEMANTIC PROCESSING

Besides advancements in behavioral methods, during the last decade, electrophysiological and brain imaging methods have been established in developmental research. By early pioneering studies, the electrophysiological responses on acoustic and visual stimuli were explored in infants. Here, researchers have observed several infant-specific ERP components that have no clear adult equivalent (e.g., the P100-N250 complex on acoustic stimulation instead of the obligatory N1 and P2 components in adults), the positive mismatch response instead of the adult mismatch negativity, and the Nc as an infant attentional response (e.g., Courchesne, Ganz, & Norcia, 1981; Dehaene-Lambertz & Dehaene, 1994; Kushnerenko et al., 2002). Recent research has moreover focused on the development of adult-like ERP components, particularly on those that are related to the development of certain language abilities, such as components reflecting semantic or syntactic processing stages (for an overview, see Friederici, 2005).

THE N400 COMPONENT IN ADULTS

Semantic processing in adults is reflected in the N400 component of the ERP. The N400 is a centro-parietally distributed negative wave with peak latency at around 400 ms, which was first observed in response to semantically incorrect sentence endings, for example in response to the word socks in the sentence *He spread the warm bread with socks* (Kutas & Hillyard, 1980). Initially the N400 was assumed to reflect lexical search and access, but a number of studies have shown that the N400 is not only elicited by words but also in response to other potentially meaningful stimuli, such as pictures, pseudowords, and natural sounds when they do not match an expectation established by a word, a sentence, a picture story, or even by an odor prime (Barrett & Rugg, 1990; Federmeier & Kutas, 2001; Ganis, Kutas & Sereno, 1996; Holcomb & McPherson, 1994; Nigam, Hoffman, & Simons, 1992; Sarfarazi, Cave, Richardson, Behan, & Sedgwick, 1999; Van Petten & Rheinfelder, 1995; West & Holcomb, 2002). Today the common view is that the N400 amplitude reflects the cognitive effort involved in integrating a non-expected or inappropriate meaningful stimulus into a given semantic context held in working memory (Holcomb, 1993). A relative reduction in the N400 amplitude indicates that a semantic expectation triggered by a prime, a sentence, or any other context, is matched and has facilitated subsequent semantic processing of a target stimulus.

The matching of incoming semantic information with a semantic expectation is not the only factor that affects N400 amplitude. It moreover depends on the general frequency of item usage (e.g., word frequency), on the specific frequency of an item within the experiment (the number of repetitions), on the overlap of physical, functional, and situational features of meaningful items (semantic similarity), and on the overlap of these features with those coded within semantic representations (typicality; for a review see Kutas & Federmeier, 2000). Therefore, the N400 has been proposed to reflect the recognition of meaningful stimuli and the structure and organization of semantic long-term memory, even though it is not known how the mechanisms that underlie N400 generation operate on semantic long-term memory.

THE N200-500 COMPONENT IN INFANTS AND TODDLERS

In infants and toddlers, two ERP components have been found to vary in response to lexical–semantic processing, the adult-like N400 and the infant-specific N200-500.

The N200-500 is a fronto-laterally distributed negativity in the 200–500 ms range, which reflects a processing stage involved in *word form* recognition, such as acoustic-phonological or lexical processing. In 11–20-month-olds it is enhanced to known or familiar words as compared to unknown or unfamiliar words, and it is more negative to unknown words than to backward presented words (Mills, Coffey-Corina, & Neville, 1993, 1997; Thierry, Vihman, & Roberts, 2003). A study with 10-month-olds moreover demonstrated that, within an experimental session, the N200-500 emerges during online familiarization with repeatedly presented, initially unfamiliar words (Kooijman, Hagoort, & Cutler, 2005).

The N200-500 is not only affected by word familiarity depending on the current number of repetitions or on previous word frequency. It is moreover sensitive to the expectation of a word form, which can be induced by priming within a picture–word priming paradigm (Friedrich & Friederici, 2004, 2005a, 2005b, 2006; for a review see Friedrich, 2008). This cross-modal experimental design was particularly developed to explore the neural correlates of lexical–semantic processing in 1-year-olds, their developmental course during early word learning, and the role that semantic priming and semantic integration mechanisms play in the progression of word learning in infants and toddlers. In this priming paradigm, pictures of known objects represent a simple, early acquired and easily accessible context for words. During the experimental session, children sat in front of a monitor, they looked at sequentially presented objects (e.g., a sheep) and listened to words or nonsense words presented acoustically 1900 ms post picture onset, when primary visual processing was finished but the object was still visible on the screen. Words were either congruous (i.e., named the objects correctly, *sheep*), or incongruous (i.e., named a semantically unrelated concept, *ball*). Nonsense words were either pseudowords that are legal according to the rules of German, and thus sound like a real German word (e.g., *Fless*), or nonwords that had a phonotactically illegal word-onset; that is, a phoneme combination that never occurs at the onset of a German word (e.g., *Rlink*). Each word and each nonsense word was preceded by the German indefinite article *ein* that represented an attentional cue and prepared the infant perception for noun onset (i.e., it temporally triggered word form processing).

In all age groups investigated with this cross-modal design so far, the N200-500 was increased in response to congruous words as compared to either incongruous words (Figure 7.1) or nonsense words (Friedrich & Friederici, 2004, 2005a, 2005b). Since congruous and incongruous words, and thus the infants' familiarity with them, were the same in this design (they were physically identical, only the picture–word pairings varied between conditions), prior experience or acoustic variations could not have caused the N200-500 amplitude differences between the word conditions. Therefore, the N200-500 effect is attributed to the matching or nonmatching of the expectation that has been set by the pictured object. This ERP result shows that even in 12-month-olds, the first lexical–semantic knowledge established in memory affects the processing of word forms by cross-modal priming.

In 19-month-olds, moreover, the N200-500 amplitude displayed a gradual differentiation (Friedrich, 2008; Friedrich & Friederici, 2005b). In this age group congruous words elicited the most negative responses, relative to the other words. Incongruous words and phonotactically legal pseudowords, which both consisted of familiar phoneme combinations but were not primed by the pictured objects, elicited moderately positive responses, while nonsense words, which contain

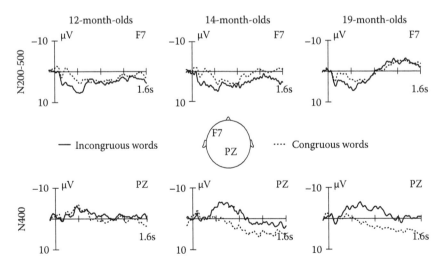

FIGURE 7.1 The N200-500 word form priming effect and the N400 semantic priming effect in different age groups.

phonotactically illegal phoneme combinations that were unfamiliar to the children, elicited the most positive responses. Thus, in these older children, the N200-500 was affected by priming and familiarity in parallel. This result indicates that the children's early experience with the legal phoneme combinations of their native language differentially affects their processing of novel word forms.

THE N400 COMPONENT IN INFANTS AND TODDLERS

In the same picture–word priming paradigm, an N400 semantic priming effect was observed in 14- and 19-month-olds (7.1), but this effect failed to appear in 12-month-olds (Friedrich & Friederici, 2004, 2005a, 2005b; for a review see Friedrich, 2008). In children of the two older age groups incongruous words elicited more negative responses than congruous words, which indicate that the processing of picture meanings primed the processing of word meanings. Moreover, the initiation of N400 semantic integration mechanisms was found to depend on the regularity of the phonotactic properties of nonsense words. Whereas semantic mechanisms indexed by the N400 are triggered by both words and legal pseudowords, these mechanisms were not triggered by phonotactically illegal nonwords. This result indicates that 19-month-old children consider phonotactically legal but not phonotactically illegal nonsense words as potential words of their native language (Friedrich & Friederici, 2005b).

By use of a longitudinal design, we further investigated how the N400 development is related to the children's language development later on. For this purpose, ERP data of the 19-month-old children were retrospectively analyzed according to the children's verbal language skills at 2 years 6 months as measured by a German language development test SETK-2 (Grimm, 2000). Children with age-adequate expressive language skills later on displayed an N400 priming effect at 19 months, whereas children with later, poorer language skills who are at risk for a developmental language disorder did not show it at that age (Friedrich & Friederici, 2006). This finding of a relation between the early functioning of the mechanisms underlying N400 generation and children's subsequent success in behavioral language development suits to the result of a study with 20-month-olds. Torkildsen and colleagues found that picture–word matches elicited an N400 priming effect in typically developing 20-month-olds, but not in 20-month-olds at familial risk for dyslexia, who also had lower productive vocabularies than the typically developing children (Torkildsen, Syversen, Simonsen, Moen, & Lindgren, 2007). Recently these findings were extended to the acquisition of new object-word associations. After training with novel pairs of pictures and words, 20-month-olds with high productive vocabularies displayed an N400 priming effect for trained picture–word associations, whereas 20-month-olds with low productive vocabularies did not (Torkildsen et al., 2008).

In both 12-month-olds and 19–20-month-olds with delayed language development, the mechanisms of semantic integration that cause N400 generation appears to be either not yet developed or not yet affected by semantic priming, even though the N200-500 effect indicates that, in the same children, objects do prime word forms (Friedrich & Friederici, 2005b, 2006). The presence of an N400 priming effect in normally developing children from 14 months upward suggests that the full functionality of these mechanisms develops between 12 and 14 months of age (Friedrich & Friederici, 2005a, 2005b). Thus, the first appearance of the N400 semantic word priming effect during development is temporally closely related to the first appearance of the fast mapping ability (i.e., the capacity of children to rapidly learn new words for new objects after only a few presentations). This temporal co-occurrence points to a possibly causal relationship between the brain mechanisms responsible for N400 elicitation and the qualitative shift from the slow to the fast word learning mode at the behavioral level.

The role that the N400 mechanisms plays in early word acquisition was further explored by analyzing the ERPs of 12-month-olds according to their word production at this age, which was rated by parents in a standardized questionnaire ELFRA-1 (Grimm & Doil, 2000). In infants with particularly early word production, an N400 priming effect was already present indicating that semantic integration mechanisms are functional in these infants. In normally and slowly developing children at that age, an N400 priming effect could not be observed, not even when only words that parents rated to be comprehended by their child were included in the analyses (Friedrich & Friederici, 2009).

In order to find out whether the missing N400 in slowly and normally developing 12-month-olds is caused by the general immatureness of the brain structures mediating the N400 response or by the fact that these mechanisms are not yet triggered by word stimuli, a picture–sound paradigm was developed as analog of the picture–word priming paradigm. Here, 12-month-old infants were presented with pictures of objects (e.g., a dog) and congruous or incongruous natural sounds (e.g., a barking or a ringing). In this study, we found an N400 priming effect on incongruous sounds, indicating that the mechanisms of semantic integration are already functional at 12 months. This result leads to the interpretation that the missing N400 priming effect on words is not caused by immature brain structures or immature N400 neural mechanisms at that age (Babocsai, Friedrich, & Pauen, 2007).

Overall, the studies reviewed here provide evidence that the early functioning of the N400 neural mechanisms interact with children's language development, but we do not know what kind of interaction this is. Although it might be the case that the N400 elicitation and the fast mapping ability are independent but require a similar state of brain development, the result of the picture–sound study argues against this hypothesis and provides evidence for a more direct interrelation. It rather appears that those brain structures realizing semantic integration are mature from early infancy on, but that the N400 neural mechanisms cannot operate on weakly established memory representations acquired in the slow word learning mode. It might even be possible that fast mapping requires the functioning of the mechanisms underlying N400 generation, and that these mechanisms are involved in the process of word learning. However, in order to understand the relation between the mechanisms responsible for N400 elicitation and the infant's word learning capacity, we would have to know what the N400 actually reflect and how semantic integration is realized at a neural level.

SEMANTIC FOCUS: THE CURRENT VIEW
OF THE SEMANTIC SYSTEM

The mechanisms reflected in the N400 component are involved in primary or secondary semantic processing stages, most likely in setting or changing the semantic focus. Here the term *semantic focus* means the selective activation of certain aspects of semantic knowledge, which are coded as assemblies of semantic features and stored in (one or more) semantic representations. The semantic focus is the current choice of the semantic system in a certain situation and it represents the context-dependent view of an object or event.* That means, from the possible representations available by the semantic system, only a subset is selected within a certain situation. But how does the neural system select the semantic knowledge that is appropriate in a situation?

In principle, selection can be realized by different mechanisms. One is the preactivation of memory structures either by long-lasting motivations and intentions, or by short-lasting representations currently active in working memory. This short-lasting priming of certain semantic aspects is caused by the activation of memory structures that are semantically related to the ongoing context. Priming is well known to affect response time by realizing faster stimulus processing, but it also modifies the quality of stimulus processing by preventing the unaffected, spontaneous focus of the corresponding neural system. Thus, priming as a semantic selection mechanism sets the focus according to the current semantic context and the organization of this semantic information in long-term memory. Although the N400 is extremely sensitive to semantic priming and it also depends on the organization of semantic memory, it does not reflect the priming process itself (i.e., the semantic preactivation) but rather the effect of semantic preactivation on the semantic processing of a subsequent stimulus.

Another way of selection that more directly depends on memory, is the differentiated modification of activity during neuronal signal transmission. An object that is perceived (or generally, any incoming meaningful information) always activates several possible semantic representations with which the object shares common features. One (or some) of these representations sets the semantic focus, which means it is activated strongest and remains temporally stable in short-term memory. In addition to semantic priming, this focus mainly depends on the overlap of features activated by the object with features coded within potentially relevant representations and on the selective strengths of features (i.e., the weighting of features within these representations). Thus, this kind of selection mainly sets the current semantic focus according to previously acquired knowledge that has been affected by the frequency of activations and the quality of consolidation. N400 amplitude has been shown to depend on semantic similarity and on the typicality of an exemplar as member of a category, both reflected

---

* The term semantic focus mainly follows the concept of the attentional focus as internal state of selection; it is not necessarily triggered externally by linguistic input as it is the case in the linguistic notion of focus.

in the overlap of semantic features, as well as on item frequency and previous exposure to items (Kutas & Federmeier, 2000). Therefore it might be involved in the primary activation of semantic representations and in a potential competition between relevant representations. Since these basic mechanisms of neuronal signal transmission are essential for any further semantic processing, one would expect that they are mature very early and that they are present even in infants. The missing N400 in 12-month-olds suggest that the N400 does not represent a mechanism that is involved in such an obligatory semantic processing stage.

With respect to behavioral relevance a third mechanism of knowledge selection would be necessary in the case of an inappropriate semantic focus. If the current focus does not match the expectation of the ongoing semantic context, or if the consequences associated with this focus (such as the predicted lexical-semantic context or the expected emotional impact) are not matched by the actual consequences, then the current semantic focus caused by priming and previous knowledge should be inhibited. This inhibition should trigger the memory search for a more appropriate semantic focus, and in doing so would realize semantic integration. If existing representations cannot be successfully integrated, this should lead to the acquisition of a new semantic representation that better fits the current contextual situation, and refines, corrects, or complements the representations available within the lexical–semantic system. Such a mechanism would moreover automatically be applied to pseudowords as potential references of meaning; therefore pseudowords would also "reset" the current state of activity of the semantic system. This supposed selection mechanism would set a new focus according to the evaluation of the previous focus with respect to behavioral consequences, emotional relevance, and both the previous and the forthcoming semantic context. A mismatch of a semantic focus with the semantic context is exactly what the N400 triggers. Like the N400, such an evaluation mechanism would moreover be affected by the organization of semantic memory, and its functioning might depend on a certain developmental state of the representations established within the semantic system.

THE STABILITY–PLASTICITY DILEMMA

But how is the semantic system able to evaluate its own current focus? How does it overcome inappropriate activations? Moreover, how does it know whether the knowledge it already has acquired is appropriate or whether it should rather form a new semantic representation? An even more general question is, how is the human neural system able to learn new semantic representations for objects or events while holding in memory old representations acquired for similar objects or events. With respect to artificial learning systems, this question is called *stability–plasticity dilemma* (Grossberg, 1987). It refers to the fact that during training artificial neural networks adjust their weight patterns to the environmental statistics, and a changing environment (i.e., changing probabilities of feature occurrence) can erase previously learned knowledge. Moreover, if neural networks are trained with a new output for an input pattern that has already been trained in another learning environment, then most systems either do not learn the new classification or they "forget" the first learned mapping. This means that these systems are unable to learn new classifications for the same input set while preserving already established knowledge; they are either stable or flexible, but they are not both stable and flexible in parallel. Thus, they cannot acquire hierarchical semantic knowledge without having an explicitly designed hierarchical structure. A predefined hierarchical architecture, however, would strongly limit the flexibility of abstraction. For example, if there are predefined levels to categorize a certain rose as rose, as flower, and as plant, additional levels would be necessary to code it as cut flower, as ornamental plant, as cultivated plant, or as any other category exemplar. The human semantic system does not appear to rely on such hard-wired hierarchies, since it can create and store an unlimited number of partly overlapping representations that, moreover, do not erase each other.

ADAPTIVE RESONANCE THEORY

Adaptive Resonance Theory (ART) was particularly developed to resolve the stability–plasticity dilemma (e.g., Grossberg, 1976a, 1976b, 1980, 1987). This advanced theory provides sophisticated artificial neural mechanisms for stable prototype formation and self-adjusted attention switching, which are mathematically formalized and incorporated into powerful neural network models (e.g., Carpenter & Grossberg, 1987; Carpenter, Grossberg, & Reynolds, 1991; Carpenter, Martens, & Ogas, 2005). The network dynamic fully relies on neurobiologically plausible local and real-time computations, and it incorporates attentional mechanisms, such as attentional gain control, attentional priming, vigilance regulation, and orienting, which realize self-evaluation, self-adjusted memory search, and the stable formation of memory representations, even of those with strongly overlapping features.

The basic model of the ART family, the ART 1 (Carpenter & Grossberg, 1987), is an unsupervised neural network, which means that the net is not given explicit information of the categorical membership of an input exemplar or of the mapping of an input to a certain output. Rather, the net creates its own category structures depending on the feature frequency distributions and the feature correlation structure within the learning environment. This unsupervised learning produces prototypes based on similarity. In contrast, supervised learning models enable arbitrary mappings and the formation of categories that are sensitive to other distinctions such as culturally mediated or linguistically triggered categorizations. In the supervised ARTMAP (Carpenter et al., 1991), the output of an unsupervised ART 1 module is used to determine the categorization of a second ART 1 module. Thus, one ART 1 supervises the other ART 1, which represents a kind of self-supervising as is the case in natural learning systems. This supervised ARTMAP can particularly be used to study the interaction of spontaneous and word guided concept formation and its developmental course.

ART 1 ARCHITECTURE AND THE CONCEPT OF ADAPTIVE RESONANCE

The ART 1 (7. 2) consists of an input layer (I) and two representational layers: one coding features (F1) and the other coding categories (F2). Categories are represented by their bidirectional weighted connections from and to the feature representations. Gain control and orienting subsystem are additional components complementing the basic network design. As common in neural networks, the artificial neurons within the layers are called *nodes* or *populations*. ART 1 short- and long-term dynamics (i.e., activation and learning), are described by differential equations that allow to simulate real-time processing. A specific characteristic of ART systems is that short- and long-term dynamics operate on different time scales. This main feature is inspired by the fact that the electro-chemical communication between real neurons is relatively fast as compared to the molecular and structural modifications of synaptic connections, which correspond to learning. With other words, learning needs time, and sufficiently stable learning can only take place in a temporally stable internal state. In ART systems this relative stability is given by the resonant state, in which short-term processing results and which is called *adaptive resonance*. The resonant state is characterized by the matching and the sustained reciprocal activation of bottom-up input and top-down learned expectations.

ART 1 SHORT-TERM DYNAMICS

The short-term dynamics of the ART 1 determines how the activation of the system changes in response to input activity that arises from a certain preprocessing stage. Figure 7.2 provides a slightly simplified illustration of the ART 1 short-term dynamics (for a detailed mathematical description, see Carpenter & Grossberg, 1987). *A:* An input pattern activates gain control (G), orienting subsystem (O), and specific feature detection nodes in F1. Gain control nonspecifically activates all nodes in F1. Those F1 nodes that receive activation of both input layer and gain control exceed a threshold and generate an output. Activity in F1 inhibits the orienting subsystem and prevents the activity of this subsystem by balancing the activation by the input pattern. The bottom-up signals from F1 to F2 are filtered by adaptive long-term weights, and the input that an F2 node receives is the sum of all weighted signals from F1 to the F2 node. Mathematically this is the scalar product between the F1 output vector and the weight vector to the F2 node, which can be interpreted as similarity of the input exemplar with the prototype of the category coded in F2. *B:* Competition between F2 nodes results in suprathreshold activity of that F2 node (or of several nodes) that has received the highest signal, whereas the activity of all other F2 nodes is suppressed. Note that strong weights of a few features may lead to the highest signal even though the whole feature pattern of the input might not be matched by the winning F2 node. Output of F2 inhibits gain control, such that F1 is no longer activated nonspecifically. Instead, F1 receives a specific signal from F2; namely, the output of the winning F2 node multiplied with the top-down weight vector from F2 to F1, which represents the feature pattern *expectation* read out by the category momentarily active

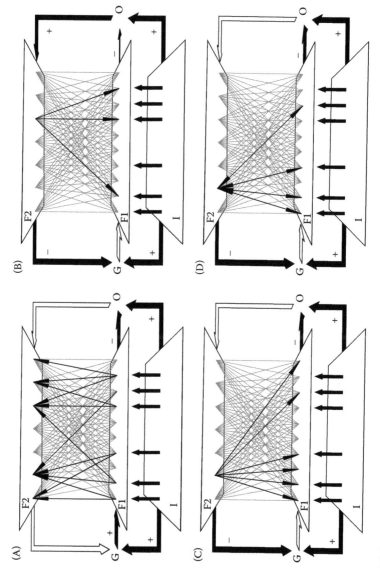

FIGURE 7.2   ART 1 short-term dynamics.

in F2. Suprathreshold activity in F1 is now possible if a node receives specific signals from both input and F2. Since normally the category expectation differs from the input pattern, total F1 activity is attenuated and likewise the inhibition of the orienting subsystem decreases. If this decrease is too strong with respect to the criterion set by the value of the *vigilance parameter* (p), mathematically, if the ratio of the inhibition by the total activity in F1 and the activation by the total input activity is smaller than p, then the orienting system becomes active and resets short-term activity by nonspecific activation of F2. This *reset* temporary inhibits the category node currently active in F2 and, as a consequence, inhibition of the gain control is removed.* *C:* Thus, (if the input is still present) the system returns into state A, except that the first-pass attracting category is temporary not sensitive to signals from F1 and therefore it does not win competition again. This enables another F2 category to win competition and to release an expectation in F1. Again, the associated activity decrease in F1 and the attenuated inhibition of the orienting subsystem is evaluated according to the current vigilant state of the system, which possibly leads to further memory search. *D:* If a category expectation sufficiently matches the input pattern, then the inhibition of the orienting subsystem remains strong enough, and a reset is prevented. Sustained reciprocal activation between F1 and F2 now constitutes the resonant state in which learning takes place.

ART 1 LONG-TERM DYNAMICS

The long-term dynamics of the ART 1 determines how the weights of connections change, that is, how the system learns. In ART systems, learning is only possible in the resonant state, in which bottom-up and top-down information is matched. In adaptive resonance the F1 activity of those features that are both present in the input and expected by the category is sustained by reciprocal activation between F1 and F2. Therefore, the connections between these feature nodes and the active category node, are strengthened during learning. Moreover, the weights to those features that are expected by the category but not present in the input are reduced.

Learning in ART 1 is time-dependent, and the differential equations can be used to simulate learning for several temporal conditions (Friedrich, 1994, 1997). In the case of *fast learning* sufficient time is available for weight changing such that the state of dynamic equilibrium is reached and no further weight change occurs. In this case, weights are fully adapted to the information in resonance; therefore categories contain only features that are present in each exemplar. In contrast, if there is not enough time for learning (i.e., if the resonant state is interrupted or the rate of leaning is low), then only a certain amount of information is transferred into weights. In this case of *slow learning*, categories represent features according

---

* F2 is designed according to the neurophysiological model of a gated dipole field, whose nodes respond to nonspecific arousal in a state-dependent fashion. In particular, those nodes that are active during arousal are selectively inhibited for a certain period (Grossberg, 1976b, 1980).

to their frequency distribution within the category exemplars. Thus, slow learning within ART 1 leads to the formation of prototypical categories with a pronounced graded structure.

VIGILANCE AND THE LEVEL OF GENERALIZATION

In ART systems, category inclusiveness (i.e., the level of generalization) depends on the value of the vigilance parameter that models the internal evaluation criterion involved in the sensitivity control mechanism of the orienting sub-system. Low vigilance represents a relaxed state, in which the system tolerates high variability between category exemplars. This state leads to the formation of broad, general categories. In contrast, if vigilance is high, then the system is in a state of low tolerance, which enables the fine discrimination between similar exemplars and the formation of narrow, specific categories. As a result of varying vigilance, categories at different levels of inclusiveness, which range from a very global level of abstraction up to representations of individual exemplars, coexist in ART systems.

The effect of vigilance, however, depends on the present learning state of the system, or more specifically, on the learning state of a certain category. The ART reset is only triggered by a mismatch between bottom-up input and the top-down expectations of the currently winning category, and thus, it requires sufficiently specified memory structures coded in that category. When learning is slow due to time or processing limitations, initially the system forms broad global categories that code a lot of features. These very fuzzy categories act as attractors, and they match lots of input patterns, thus, even in the case of maximal vigilance, reset is prevented and specific categories are not acquired. During the course of further learning categories become sharper and more specified. Now if vigilance is sufficiently high then reset will initiate memory search and specific categories can be formed (Friedrich, 1995, 1997).

IMPLICATIONS FOR EARLY WORD LEARNING AND N400 DEVELOPMENT

The ART neural networks are the first artificial neural memory system that can be stable, flexible, and constructive in parallel. They achieve these properties by incorporating a neural mechanism that enables the systems to evaluate their own categorization behavior, to suppress a current focus chosen by priming and first-pass competition of memory representations, and to adjust their category inclusiveness according to internal and external requirements. Since the human memory system is stable, flexible, and constructive in reality, the question can be posed, whether a functionally similar mechanism is actually working in the human brain. Here it is shown what the basic assumptions of ART and the real presence of an ART-like evaluation mechanism would imply with respect to early word learning. It is moreover suggested that if such a mechanism would actually exist, then it would have been reflected in the N400 component of the ERP.

THE SLOW LEARNING MODE

If following the assumption that a temporally stable state is required for natural learning too, one could further assume that this temporal stability is limited during early development, since the input from preprocessing stages might temporally not be stable, some activity loss during resonance might not be compensated by weak synaptic connections, and molecular and structural synaptic changes might require more time during early than later developmental states. Similar as in ART simulations (Friedrich, 1994, 1997), such temporal constraint in the maturing brain would result in behavioral constraints for category formation and word learning. According to ART, first naturally acquired categories would be very global with a fuzzy and pronounced prototypical structure that would cause massive overgeneralizations. The formation of specific categories would depend on the amount of previous learning of more global categories and it would involve the inhibition of global categories. A frequent successive presentation of exemplars of a certain subcategory (as in behavioral tests that include a familiarization phase) would shift the global category toward the specific features of the subcategory, such that exemplars of another subcategory could initiate reset and constitute its own category. This categorization behavior predicted by simulations is exactly what has been found for natural and experimentally induced categorizations in infants and toddlers (e.g., Bomba & Siqueland, 1983; Goede & Friedrich, 1995; Mareschal & Quinn, 2001; McDonough, 2002; Quinn, 1987; Younger & Fearing, 2000).

Moreover, temporally limited learning would not only result in constraint categorizations but also in weak associations between words and concepts, such as it is the case in the slow word learning mode before children acquire the fast mapping ability. At the neural level, the shift from the slow to the fast word learning mode would then be associated with quantitative rather than qualitative changes, such as longer temporal stability and therefore more time for synaptic modifications, or with a higher rate of learning-related changes.

OVERCOMING ERRORS BY ART RESET

The advantage of slow learning is that it is relatively robust with respect to the effect of errors. A few errors will be automatically erased by the representation of features according to their frequency distribution. Even false mappings between words and concepts are of no consequence for the whole learning process if the most frequent mappings are correct. Thus, an explicit mechanism for error correction is not required in the slow learning mode.

However, as infants become able to rapidly associate new words with newly built concepts, they may establish inappropriate conceptual representations or wrong associations between words and concepts, such that mechanisms for correcting them would need to develop. Without an explicit error correction mechanism, wrong associations could only be resolved by unspecific forgetting, that is some kind of synaptic weight decrease that is not specific to the invalid memory representation. The ART reset, however, represents an error correction mechanism that specifically detects wrong associations and enables the formation of new semantic concepts and the correct mappings between words and concepts. According to ART, the functioning of this mechanism actually sets in at the point in development at which it is necessary; that is, when learning becomes faster and therefore error correction becomes crucial.

N400 as the Reflection of a Semantic Short-Term Reset

It is proposed here that the mechanisms underlying the elicitation of the N400 component of the ERP are involved in a memory search process that is triggered to reinterpret a meaningful stimulus in a way that matches the whole contextual situation, whereby semantic integration of that stimulus into the meaningful context takes place. ART is the first theory that provides a model for real-time memory search in a massively parallel neural architecture. According to this model, memory search is realized by successive nonspecific arousal waves that reset short-term activity. This neural reset mechanism temporally inhibits the activity pattern of the first preferred representations and therefore it enables the system to focus on those aspects of the stimulus that are relevant in the present context.

In the unsupervised basic ART 1 model memory search is triggered by a nonmatching expectation read out from the currently active category representation. In the supervised ARTMAP model (Carpenter et al., 1991), reset is triggered in the same way, but vigilance regulation and therefore reset is moreover mediated by nonmatching outputs of the two ART 1 modules, such as a word active in one module, which does not match a concept active in the other module, as is the case in the picture–word ERP study with infants and young children.

Dissociation of N200-500 and N400
Priming During Early Development

In both ART 1 and ARTMAP, reset and therefore the memory search for an appropriate semantic focus does not only depend on the sensitivity parameter vigilance but also on the expectation read out by the currently active category, which must be sufficiently specified in order to cause a mismatch. If assuming that an ART-like reset mechanism (i.e., the inhibition of the current semantic focus) is reflected in the N400 component of the ERP, this behavior of the model can be used to explain the dissociation of N400 semantic priming and N200-500 word priming observed in the ERP of 12-month-old infants.

Suppose, for instance, an infant has not yet established specific cat or dog categories, but it has an unspecific global mammal representation that is (possibly weakly) associated with the word *dog* perceived most often in this context. If now, the infant sees a dog (or a cat), then, according to ART, the global mammal category would win first-pass competition and would release an expectation. If vigilance is low, this category is chosen for resonance and would prime the word *dog* such that the subsequent perceptual processing of the word *dog* is facilitated. In the infant ERP, this would be reflected as an N200-500 word priming effect; that is, an increased N200-500 amplitude in response to the word *dog*. If, in contrast, the infant either hears the unexpected word *cat* or a semantically unrelated word like *car*, vigilance increases. If the expectation of the mammal representation is sufficiently specified, then this vigilance increase leads to ART reset, which would be reflected as N400 in the ERP. However, ART reset will be prevented and activation will not be removed from the initially winning mammal representation, as long as the expectation of this global category is too unspecific to cause a clear mismatch. Consequently, memory search would not be initiated and the N400 would be missing in the ERP. According to this interpretation the N400 could however be elicited very early in development, if a sufficiently specified memory representation has first been established during a familiarization phase and is then violated in a subsequent test phase.

CONCLUSIONS

The ART neural networks provide an idea of how the developmental constraints at the neural level, such as the strength of synaptic connections, the global vigilant state of the system, and the time available for the learning of individual items may cause the systemic constraints observed in the categorization and word learning behavior of infants and toddlers. Most of the neural constraints that are crucial for the systemic behavior are related to ART reset, a mechanism that enables both the formation of new semantic memory representations and the task-dependent switch between several representations already available for an object or event. Here, ART reset is supposed to have a real natural equivalent that is reflected in the N400 component of the ERP. This identification theoretically relates the elicitation of the N400 to the learning state of semantic representations. Moreover, it interprets the developmental course of the N400 as depending on the frequency and the amount of learning. The identification of ART reset and N400 as proposed in the present chapter offers a general explanation for how the mechanisms that underlie N400 generation operate on semantic long-term memory, and how their functioning is related to the categorization and word learning capacities in infants and toddlers.

REFERENCES

Babocsai, L., Friedrich, M., & Pauen, S. (2007, March 29–April 1). Neural evidence for 12-month-olds' ability to integrate sight and sound in object categories. *Biennial Meeting of the Society for Research in Child Development (SRCD)*, Boston, Massachusetts.

Barrett, S. E., & Rugg, M. D. (1990). Event-related potentials and the semantic matching of pictures. *Brain and Cognition, 14,* 201–212.

Bates, E., Thal, D., & Janowsky, J. S. (1992). Early language development and its neural correlates. In I. Rapin & S. Segalowitz (Eds.), *Handbook of neuropsychology, child neurology* (Vol. 6, pp. 69–110). Amsterdam, The Netherlands: Elsevier.

Benedict, H. (1979). Early lexical development: Comprehension and production. *Journal of Child Language, 6,* 183–200.

Bomba, P. C., & Siqueland, E. R. (1983). The nature and structure of infant form categories. *Journal of Experimental Child Psychology, 35,* 294–328.

Carpenter, G. A., & Grossberg, S. (1987). A massively parallel architecture for a self-organizing neural pattern recognition machine. *Computer Vision, Graphics, and Image Processing, 37,* 54–115.

Carpenter, G. A., Grossberg, S., & Reynolds, J. H. (1991). ARTMAP: Supervised real-time learning and classification of nonstationary data by a self-organizing neural network. *Neural Networks, 4,* 565–588.

Carpenter, G. A., Martens, S., & Ogas, O. J. (2005). Self-organizing information fusion and hierarchical knowledge discovery: A new framework using ARTMAP neural networks. *Neural Networks, 18,* 287–295.

Clark, E. V. (1987). The principle of contrast: A constraint on language acquisition. In B. MacWhinney (Ed.), *Mechanisms of language acquisition* (pp. 1–33). Hillsdale, NJ: Erlbaum.

Courchesne, E., Ganz, L., & Norcia, A. M. (1981). Event-related brain potentials to human faces in infants. *Child Development, 52*(3), 804–811.

Dehaene-Lambertz, G., & Dehaene, S. (1994). Speed and cerebral correlates of syllable discrimination in infants. *Nature, 370,* 292–294.

Federmeier, K. D., & Kutas, M. (2001). Meaning and modality: Influence of context, semantic memory organization, and perceptual predictability on picture processing. *Journal of Experimental Psychology: Learning, Memory, and Cognition, 27*(1), 202–224.

French, R. M., Mareschal, D., Mermillod, M., & Quinn, P. C. (2004). The role of bottom-up processing in perceptual categorization by 3- to 4-month-old infants: Simulations and data. *Journal of Experimental Psychology: General, 133*(3), 382–397.

Friederici, A. D. (2005). Neurophysiological markers of early language acquisition: From syllables to sentences. *Trends in Cognitive Sciences, 9*(10), 481–488.

Friederici, A. D., Friedrich, M., & Christophe, A. (2007). Brain responses in 4-month-old infants are already language specific. *Current Biology, 17,* 1208–1211.

Friederici, A. D., & Wessels, J. M. I. (1993) Phonotactic knowledge of word boundaries and its use in infant speech-perception. *Perception & Psychophysics, 54,* 287–295.

Friedrich, M. (1994). Modellierung und Simulation kategorialer Strukturbildung: Eine Anwendung der Adaptiven Resonanztheorie auf die Begriffsbildung. Unpublished doctoral thesis.

Friedrich, M. (1997). Der Erwerb hierarchisch ordenbarer Kategorien in einem neuronalen Netz der Adaptiven Resonanztheorie. *ZASPIL, 8,* 57–80.

Friedrich, M. (2008). Neurophysiological correlates of picture-word priming in one-year-olds. In A. D. Friederici & G. Thierry (Eds.), *Early language development: Bridging brain and behaviour. Series "Trends in language acquisition research" (TiLAR),* (Vol. 5, 137–160). Amsterdam, The Netherlands: John Benjamins.

Friedrich, M., & Friederici, A. D. (2004). N400-like semantic incongruity effect in 19-month-olds: Processing known words in picture contexts. *Journal of Cognitive Neuroscience, 16,* 1465–1477.

Friedrich, M., & Friederici, A. D. (2005a). Lexical priming and semantic integration reflected in the ERP of 14-month-olds. *NeuroReport, 16*(6), 653–656.

Friedrich, M., & Friederici, A. D. (2005b). Phonotactic knowledge and lexical-semantic processing in one-year-olds: Brain responses to words and nonsense words in picture contexts. *Journal of Cognitive Neuroscience, 17*(11), 1785–1802.

Friedrich, M., & Friederici, A. D. (2006). Early N400 development and later language acquisition. *Psychophysiology, 43,* 1–12.

Friedrich, M., & Friederici, A. D. (2009). Maturing brain mechanisms and developing behavioral language skills. *Developmental Science* HYPERLINK "http://dx.doi.org/10.1016/j.bandl.2009.07.004" \t "doilink"doi:10.1016/j.bandl.2009.07.004.

Ganis, G., Kutas, M., & Sereno, M. (1996). The search for "Common Sense": An electrophysiological study of the comprehension of words and pictures in reading. *Journal of Cognitive Neuroscience, 8,* 89–106.

Goede, K., & Friedrich, M. (1995). Roses but not flowers: Phenomena of the development and the naming of concepts. In Maaike Verrips & Frank Wijnen (Hrsg.), *Papers from the Dutch-German colloquium on language acquisition* (Vol. 66, pp. 41–63). Amsterdam, The Netherlands: University of Amsterdam.

Golinkoff, R. M., Mervis, C. B., & Hirsh-Pasek, K. (1994). Early object labels: The case for lexical principles. *Journal of Child Language, 21,* 125–155.

Grimm, H. (2000). *SETK-2: Sprachentwicklungstest für zweijährige Kinder (2.0–2.11).* Diagnose rezeptiver und produktiver Sprachverarbeitungsfähigkeiten. Göttingen, Germany: Hogrefe.

Grimm, H., & Doil, H. (2000). *ELFRA: Elternfragebögen für die Früherkennung von Risikokindern (ELFRA-1, ELFRA-2).* Göttingen, Germany: Hogrefe.

Grossberg, S. (1976a). Adaptive pattern classification and universal recoding, I: Parallel development and coding of neural feature detectors. *Biological Cybernetics, 23,* 121–134.

Grossberg, S. (1976b). Adaptive pattern classification and universal recoding: II. Feedback, expectation, olfaction, illusions. *Biological Cybernetics, 23,* 187–202.

Grossberg, S. (1980). How does a brain build a cognitive code? *Psychological Review, 87,* 1–51.

Grossberg, S. (1987). Competitive learning: From interactive activation to adaptive resonance. *Cognitive Science, 11,* 1, 23–63.

Holcomb, P. J. (1993). Semantic priming and stimulus degradation: Implications for the role of the N400 in language processing. *Psychophysiology, 30,* 47–61.

Holcomb, P. J., & McPherson, W. B. (1994). Event-related brain potentials reflect semantic priming in an object decision task. *Brain and Cognition, 24,* 259–276.

Jusczyk, P. W., Cutler, A., & Redanz, N. J. (1993). Infant's sensitivity to the predominant stress pattern of English words. *Child Development, 64,* 675–687.

Jusczyk, P. W., Friederici, A. D., Wessels, J. M. I., Svenkerud, V. Y., & Jusczyk, A. M. (1993). Infant's sensitivity to the sound patterns of native language words. *Journal of Memory and Language, 32,* 402–420.

Kooijman, V., Hagoort, P., & Cutler, A. (2005). Electrophysiological evidence for prelinguistic infants' word recognition in continuous speech. *Cognitive Brain Research, 24*(1), 109–116.

Kuhl, P. K., Williams, K. A., Lacerda, F., Stevens, K. N., & Lindblom, B. (1992). Linguistic experience alters phonetic perception in infants by 6 months of age. *Science, 255,* 606–608.

Kushnerenko, E., Ceponiene, R., Balan, P., Fellman, V., Huotilainen, M., & Näätänen, R. (2002). Maturation of the auditory event-related potentials during the first year of life. *NeuroReport, 13,* 47–51.

Kutas, M., & Federmeier, K. D. (2000). Electrophysiology reveals semantic memory use in language comprehension. *Trends in Cognitive Sciences, 4,* 463–470.

Kutas, M., & Hillyard, S. A. (1980). Reading senseless sentences: Brain potentials reflect semantic incongruity. *Science, 207,* 203–205.

Mareschal, D., & Quinn, P. (2001). Categorization in infancy. *Trends in Cognitive Sciences, 5*(10), 443–450.

Markman, E. V., & Wachtel, G. F. (1988), Children's use of mutual exclusivity to constrain the meaning of words. *Cognitive Psychology, 20,* 121–157.

McDonough, L. (2002). Basic-level nouns: First learned but misunderstood. *Journal of Child Language, 29*(2), 357–377.

Mills, D. L., Coffey-Corina, S. A., & Neville, H. J. (1993). Language acquisition and cerebral specialization in 20-month-old infants. *Journal of Cognitive Neuroscience, 5,* 317–334.

Mills, D. L., Coffey-Corina, S. A., & Neville, H. J. (1997). Language comprehension and cerebral specialization from 13 to 20 months. *Developmental Neuropsychology, 13,* 397–445.

Nazzi, T., & Bertoncini, J. (2003). Before and after the vocabulary spurt: Two modes of word acquisition? *Developmental Science, 6*(2),136–142.

Nigam, A., Hoffman, J. E., & Simons, R. F. (1992). N400 to semantically anomalous pictures and words. *Journal of Cognitive Neuroscience, 4,* 15–27.

Posner, M. I., & Keele, S. W. (1968). On the genesis of abstract ideas. *Journal of Experimental Psychology, 77,* 353–363.

Quinn, P. C. (1987). The categorical representation of visual pattern information by young infants. *Cognition, 27,* 145–179.

Rosch, E. H. (1973). Natural categories. *Cognitive Psychology, 4,* 328–350.

Sarfarazi, M., Cave, B., Richardson, A., Behan, J., & Sedgwick, E. M. (1999). Visual event related potentials modulated by contextually relevant and irrelevant olfactory primes. *Chemical Senses, 24,* 145–154.

Schafer, G., & Plunkett, K. (1998). Rapid word learning by fifteen-month-olds under tightly controlled conditions. *Child Development, 69,* 309–320.

Thierry, G., Vihman, M., & Roberts, M. (2003). Familiar words capture the attention of 11-month-olds in less than 250 ms. *NeuroReport, 14,* 2307–2310.

Tincoff, R., & Jusczyk, P. W. (1999). Some beginnings of word comprehension in 6-month-olds. *Psychological Science, 10,* 172–175.

Torkildsen, J. V. K., Svangstu, J. M., Friis Hansen, H., Smith, L., Simonsen, H. G., Moen, I., & Lindgren, M. (2008). Productive vocabulary size predicts ERP correlates of fast mapping in 20-month-olds. *Journal of Cognitive Neuroscience, 20,* 1266–1282.

Torkildsen, J. V. K., Syversen, G., Simonsen, H. G., Moen, I., & Lindgren, M. (2007). Brain responses to lexical–semantic priming in children at-risk for dyslexia. *Brain and Language, 102,* 243–261.

Van Petten, C., & Rheinfelder, H. (1995). Conceptual relationships between spoken words and environmental sounds: Event-related brain potential measures. *Neuropsychologia, 33*(4), 485–508.

Werker, J. F., Cohen, L. B., Lloyd, V. L., Casasola, M., & Stager, C. L. (1998). Acquisition of word-object associations by 14-month-old infants. *Developmental Psychology, 34,* 1289–1309.

Werker, J. F., & Lalonde, C. E. (1988). Cross-language speech perception: Initial capabilities and developmental change. *Developmental Psychology, 24,* 1–12.

Werker, J. F., & Tees, R. C. (2002). Cross-language speech perception: Evidence for perceptual reorganization during the first year of life. *Infant Behavioral Development, 25,* 121.

West, W. C., & Holcomb, P. J. (2002). Event-related potentials during discourse-level semantic integration of complex pictures. *Cognitive Brain Research, 13,* 363–375.

Woodward, A. L., Markman, E., & Fitzsimmons, C. M. (1994). Rapid word learning in 13- and 18-month-olds. *Developmental Psychology, 30,* 553–566.

Younger, B. A., & Fearing, D. D. (2000). A global-to-basic trend in early categorization: Evidence from a dual-category habituation task. *Infancy, 1*(1), 47–58.

8 Connectionist Models of Aphasia and Other Language Impairments

Gary Dell and Audrey Kittredge

INTRODUCTION

Aphasia presents a bewildering variety of symptoms, both within and across individuals. In order to make sense of this variety, theorists have used models. For example, over 100 years ago, the hypothesized relation between aphasic syndromes and brain regions was elegantly expressed by Lichtheim (1885) in a diagram of a small network, with nodes for mental content and their associated brain loci (e.g., Broca's area containing motor patterns) and directional arrows between the nodes indicating the flow of processing (see Graves, 1997 for review). A syndrome could correspond to the loss of a node, such as Wernicke's aphasia resulting from damage to the node for auditory images, or the loss of an arrow, as in conduction aphasia where the transmission of auditory images in Wernicke's area to the motor patterns in Broca's area is compromised (see Figure 8.1).

Lichtheim's diagram well exemplifies the function of a model. A model mediates between scientific observations and a theory that explains those observations. It teaches us about the theory and helps us understand why particular findings follow from the theory. In fact, it is hard to imagine any characterization of aphasic language processing without diagrammatic models such as flow charts, "boxes-and-arrows," or other pictures of the hypothesized pathways that are traversed during the performance of linguistic tasks.

A computational model is a model expressed as a computer program. When a model's diagram is very complex or includes probabilistic notions, a theorist needs an automated way to determine the consequences of damage to components of the model. The program does this. It represents the hypothesized components and subcomponents of the model and the detailed processing operations that work within these to create behavior. Running the program is like following the arrows in the diagram. The program's output corresponds to simulated behavior (e.g., errors in the performance of some linguistic task), and hence the theory that inspired the model can be tested by comparing the output to human behavior. For a computational model of aphasia, brain damage can be simulated by removing or otherwise preventing the access of model components (e.g., blocking the retrieval

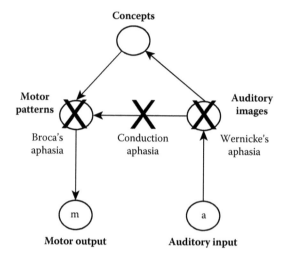

FIGURE 8.1 The Lichtheim model of aphasic syndromes. Xs indicate three of the possible damage loci.

of function morphemes) or changing the components' processing parameters so that they work less efficiently (e.g., reducing the capacity of working memory).

In this chapter we focus on *connectionist models*. Connectionist models, like all models, allow us to understand and work with theory, and they are computational in the sense that they are implemented as computer programs. It is important to note that although connectionist researchers use computers as tools, they often reject the computational metaphor for cognition—the idea that the brain is much like a standard computer, and cognition is the product of its programming. Instead, connectionist models are inspired by what is known about neural systems. For example, connectionist models mimic the assumption that the brain processes information in parallel, whereas the architecture that is the basis for most computers—the Von Neumann architecture—carries out instructions sequentially. Despite the affinity between connectionist models and neural systems, though, connectionist modelers rarely do what Lichtheim did; that is, link model parts with brain regions. Rather, as we will see, connectionist modelers aim to correctly characterize the cognitive mechanisms of language processing, with the hopes that eventually these mechanisms can be identified with brain areas.

The term *connectionist* actually means different things to different researchers and so we begin with some definitions. A connectionist model is a network of units that connect to one another through links (connections) that can vary in strength. The units or "nodes" possess an activation value (usually a real number, often between 0 and 1, or between −1 and 1), and this activation changes over time as activation passes through these links from unit to unit. If the strength or weight of a link is positive, the connection is excitatory and, if negative, it is inhibitory. Processing, that is, mapping from an input to an output, is carried out by *spreading activation*. The model is given an input by setting the activation levels of some of its units, called *input units*, to particular values. The input to a model of word retrieval during production, for example, might consist in setting the activations of units representing semantic features of the sought after word to positive values. Then the activation spreads, in parallel, throughout the network via the weighted connections. This spread is governed by the *activation rule*, an equation that specifies how each unit's activation changes when it receives activation from its neighboring units. Finally, the output of the model is determined by examining the activation levels of a set of *output units*. In a model of word production, the output units might represent the phonemes or phonetic features of the retrieved word.

Some connectionist models also include a learning component that determines the connection weights. Thus, a model with learning has to be trained before it can correctly map from its inputs to its outputs. The model is trained by giving it many trials, each of which consists of an input activation pattern and (typically) a desired output activation pattern. After the activation has spread on a particular trial, the connection weights are changed by the *learning rule*, an equation that determines how each weight is increased or decreased as a consequence of the activation of the network units. For example, a model of word retrieval might receive an input for the semantic features of, say, DOG, on a particular trial. But if the model has not yet been well trained, the activation might spread to the phonological units for HOG instead of DOG, resulting in an error. The learning rule might then change the connection weights so that the retrieval of /d/ is favored over the retrieval of /h/, when the semantic features of DOG are input, thus decreasing the chance of this error in the future. Eventually, the network's weights will become well adapted to its task, and its words will be accurately retrieved.

Connectionist models have been applied to language disorders for more than 20 years (e.g., for early applications see Cottrell, 1985; Harley, 1993; Hinton & Shallice, 1991). Models have been used to understand differences among aphasic syndromes (e.g., McNellis & Blumstein, 2001; Weems & Reggia, 2006), to characterize recovery (e.g., Harley, 1996; Martin, Saffran, & Dell, 1996), and even to suggest therapeutic interventions (e.g., Plaut, 1996). They have been applied to phenomena at both the sentence level (e.g., Chang, 2002) and the lexical level (e.g., Laine, Tikkala, & Juhola, 1998; Wright & Ahmad, 1997). Moreover, the kinds of connectionist models that have been applied to aphasia exhibit considerable variety. To illustrate this variety, we have chosen three models, which we will describe in sufficient detail to give a feel for how they explain language impairments. The first, the *interactive two-step model* of word production (Dell, Schwartz, Martin, Saffran, & Gagnon, 1997; Schwartz, Dell, Martin, Gahl, & Sobel, 2006) is a good place to start because it is conceptually simple and lacks a learning component.

THE INTERACTIVE TWO-STEP MODEL OF LEXICAL RETRIEVAL IN APHASIC SPEAKERS

The interactive two-step model is a model of single-word production derived from a general theory of production in which linguistic units are retrieved by spreading activation in a layered network. Figure 8.2 illustrates the three layers

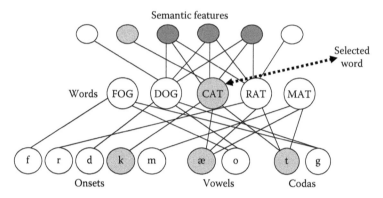

FIGURE 8.2   The interactive two-step model.

that were implemented in the model: a semantic input layer, a word layer, and a phonological output layer. The units in the network create *localist representations*; that is, units correspond directly to particular linguistic units: semantic features, words, and position-specific phonemes, respectively. Later, we will see an example of a model whose units form *distributed* rather than localist representations. In models with distributed representations, linguistic units correspond to a pattern of activation across many network units rather than to a single unit.

The connections in the interactive two-step model are all excitatory and run between adjacent layers. So, the semantic features of, say, CAT, have positive weights to the CAT word unit, which in turn is positively connected to its phonemes, /k/-onset, /ae/-vowel, and /t/-coda. The connections do not just run in a top-down or meaning-to-sound direction. There are also excitatory bottom-up connections from each word's phonemes to that word and from the word to its semantic features. The existence of both top-down and bottom-up connections makes the retrieval process *interactive*.

Lexical retrieval involves two steps, *word retrieval* and *phonological retrieval*. Word retrieval begins with a jolt of activation to the semantic features of the target word, for example, CAT. This activation then spreads throughout the network, down to word and phoneme units and upward as well. After a period of time, the most active word unit is selected, thus completing the word retrieval step. Hopefully, this is the target word CAT. Semantic errors such as DOG can occur, though, because some activation spreads to words that share semantic features with the target, and because the activation of all units is subject to random variation. Hence, there is some chance that DOG's activation will exceed CAT's. Words related to the target in phonological form also gain activation during the word retrieval step. When the target word CAT is active, this activation spreads down to its phonemes, which in turn send activation upward to formally similar words such as MAT. If a form-related word is sufficiently active, it could be selected, creating what is called a formal error. Moreover, lexical units that represent words that are related to the target both semantically and formally (e.g., RAT for the target CAT) gain activation both from shared semantic features and shared phonemes, and are especially likely to be erroneously selected, resulting in what is called a mixed error. Finally, if the word retrieval process is very noisy, there is a chance that an unrelated word (e.g., LOG for CAT) may be selected.

The phonological retrieval step begins with a jolt of activation to the selected word's lexical unit. Again, activation spreads through the network, both upward to semantics and downward to the phonemes. The phonological retrieval step is concluded by the selection of the most active phoneme units. This selection of phonemes is analogous to the prior selection of the most active word unit that concluded the word retrieval step. If the selected phoneme units do not correspond to that selected word unit, the result is a phonological error. Phonological errors can be nonwords (e.g., CAG for CAT), or they could be words, thus creating formal errors (e.g., MAT for CAT). Notice that formal errors can occur at either the word-retrieval step or the phonological-retrieval step. Notice, as well, that a phonological error can be made on top of a lexical error. If DOG was selected instead of CAT at the word retrieval step, poor phonological encoding of DOG may compound the error into something like MOG. These kinds of errors are extremely rare in normal speakers, but are not uncommon in aphasic speech (e.g., Martin, Dell, Saffran, & Schwartz, 1994). The model explains such errors through its assumption of two retrieval steps.

According to Schwartz et al. (2006), the central assumption of the model's account of aphasia is that aphasic errors are generated from the same mechanisms that create speech errors in unimpaired people. They called this the *continuity thesis*. To implement the continuity thesis, Schwartz and colleagues did four things. First, they set up the model so that it simulated the pattern of picture-naming errors made by control subjects. Next, they developed a theory of what might be damaged in aphasia, in effect, specifying the manner by which the model can be lesioned. After that, they compared the lesioned model's lexical access errors to those made by aphasic subjects who were doing the same picture-naming task that the control subjects did. As a result of this comparison, each subject was determined to have a specific lesion. And finally, they tested the model's characterization of each patient by seeing if the model could predict other features of the patient's production errors. Below, we expand on each of these aspects of the modeling process.

SIMULATING NAMING IN CONTROL SUBJECTS

The model's processing parameters were set up so that the model's probability of making a correct response (e.g., CAT), semantic error (e.g., DOG), formal error (e.g., MAT), mixed error (e.g., RAT), unrelated word error (e.g., LOG), and a nonword error (e.g., CAG) matched those of a group of 60 non-brain-injured control subjects who had taken a 175-item picture-naming test. The controls named 97% of the pictures correctly, with 2% semantic errors, 1% mixed errors, and very few errors in the other categories, and the model accurately simulated these probabilities (Dell et al., 1997).

SPECIFYING THE NATURE OF LESIONS IN THE MODEL

In principle, there are many properties of the model that could be "lesioned"; that is, altered in some way so that the model performs less accurately. The account of aphasia that seems to work best in this model is one in which brain damage is assumed to diminish the strengths of connections in the network. Specifically, the model has two lesionable parameters, the strength of the bidirectional connections between the semantic and lexical units (parameter s) and the strength of those between the phonological and lexical units (parameter p). Setting s and p to values of around .04 (e.g., during a small interval of time, a unit with activation a sends $.04 \times a$ to other units through these connections) makes the model behave like the normal controls. If s and/or p is reduced, less activation is transmitted and, because of inherent noise in the activations, the network becomes less accurate. Reducing s and reducing p have different effects on error patterns, though. Reducing s (a lexical-semantic lesion) creates more difficulty in word retrieval, leading to semantic and unrelated errors, while reducing p (a lexical-phonological lesion) impacts phonological retrieval more than word retrieval and especially promotes nonword errors.

FITTING THE MODEL TO NAMING DATA

We illustrate with an example patient from Schwartz et al. (2006). The NAC's naming response proportions were .74 correct, .07 semantic errors, .08 formal errors, .05 mixed errors, .06 unrelated word errors, and .01 nonwords. Schwartz and colleagues then fit the model to the data by looking for values of s and p that made the model's response pattern as close as possible to that of the patient. With $s = .0165$ and $p = .0382$, the model mimicked the pattern well: .73 correct, .10 semantic, .08 formal, .03 mixed, .06 unrelated, and .00 nonwords. Notice that the model's diagnosis is that NAC has a substantial lexical-semantic lesion (low s), but a close to normal value of the phonological parameter. Schwartz et al. quantified the difference between the model and the patient's pattern as the root mean squared deviation (*rmsd*) between the two sets of the six response proportions. For NAC, the *rmsd* was .018, which roughly means that, on average, the proportions differed between the patient and the model by .018. For 94 aphasic patients tested in Schwartz et al., the mean *rmsd* was .024.

The low mean *rmsd* tells us that, for most patients, the model did well. However, there were a few cases that the model could not simulate. Often, these were when a patient had a central semantic deficit. Notice that the model assumes that the semantic input to the model is intact; that is, the jolt of activation to the semantic features of the intended word is set at its normal value even when the model is lesioned. Hence, all the semantic errors in the model arise in the mapping between semantic and lexical representations (e.g., postsemantic semantic errors; e.g., Rapp & Goldrick, 2000) rather than from a poor semantic representation. So, if an aphasic individual has central semantic damage in addition to their language difficulties, the model will underpredict that person's semantic errors.

In Schwartz and colleague's sample, this underprediction happened for nine of their 94 patients.

TESTING PREDICTIONS FROM THE MODEL

The fact that the model can accurately simulate the naming errors of NAC and most other aphasic speakers is desirable, but the true test of a model is whether it can generate predictions that are verified. For example, the model's account of picture naming can be used to predict performance on another lexical task, word repetition (Dell, Martin, & Schwartz, 2007). In a repetition task, the patient hears a word and simply repeats it. The model's view of the relation between naming and repetition is that naming involves both word and phonological retrieval, but repetition only includes the phonological retrieval step. Specifically, the model assumes that, in repetition, the patient recognizes the word correctly, and then attempts to produce that word using exactly the same phonological retrieval mechanisms that are employed during naming. Consequently, all errors in repetition are assigned by the model to phonological retrieval during output. Repetition is just like naming, except that access to lexical representations from semantics is skipped.

The model's prediction of repetition from naming works like this: Consider patient HN, whose naming (35% correct, with many word-level errors) could be mimicked by the model with $s = .009$, and $p = .021$. If we then use these parameters and run the model on just the phonological retrieval step, we have HN's predicted repetition. Because HN has a larger phonological than semantic parameter, the model predicts repetition to be much better than naming, specifically .77 correct, .00 semantic, .06 formal, .01 mixed, .00 unrelated, and .16 nonwords. HN's actual repetition was .79 correct, .01 semantic, .07 formal, .01 mixed, .00 unrelated, and .13 nonwords. Thus, the model accurately predicted HN's correct repetition and error pattern (mostly nonword and formal errors).

Dell et al. (2007) concluded that most patients' word repetition could be predicted from naming (like HN), but that there were some whose repetition was unexpectedly good. This suggests that an additional source of information that is not available for naming may be used by some patients when they repeat words. This additional information likely comes from the phonology of the stimulus word. For example, there could be a nonlexical route in the model; that is, direct connections from input phonemes (e.g., /k/, /ae/, and /t/, to their output counterparts). Hanley, Dell, Kay, and Baron (2004) added this route to the interactive two-step model, calling it the dual-route model, and Dell et al. showed that it could explain the good repetition of some patients who had poor naming.

In summary, the interactive two-step model attributes aphasic errors to low connection strengths in the lexical network that stores words, their meanings, and their sounds. The model can simulate much of the variability in naming deficits by assuming that patients vary in their s and p parameters, and it can use its characterization of naming to generate predictions about repetition. Because the model is computationally implemented, it is possible to understand the mechanisms behind the model's successes and, perhaps more importantly, locate the fault when it fails.

For example, recall that the model could not simulate the naming of a few patients who made many semantic errors. However, Schwartz et al. (2006) were able to attribute some of these failures to the model's rigid assumption that semantic representations are always intact. Similarly, the model's predictions about repetition were not always accurate. Again, because of the explicit nature of computational modeling, it was possible to identify and create an alternative model, the dual-route repetition model of Hanley et al. (2004). In both of these examples of the model's shortcomings, the model was too simple. It originally did *not* allow for a lesionable parameter to represent the strength of semantic input and it originally did *not* allow for a nonlexical route to augment repetition. Yet, these complications to the model may be necessary to explain the variability of aphasia.

The interactive two-step model is simple in another way. It assumes that all the connections of a particular type (e.g., lexical-semantic connections) have the same weight. Clearly, this is wrong. The strengths of connections should reflect differences in an individual's experiences with words. We know that lexical experience has strong effects on aphasic errors, as these errors are more likely on low-frequency and late-acquired words (e.g., Kittredge, Dell, Verkuilen, & Schwartz, in press). The remaining two models presented in this chapter address effects of experience because they include a learning component. In these models, the weights are set by exposing the network to training trials that simulate linguistic experience. One of these models—the next one that we discuss—also simulates word production, but is specific to the naming of visually presented objects.

A PARALLEL DISTRIBUTED PROCESSING MODEL OF NAMING ERRORS IN OPTIC APHASIA

The parallel distributed processing (PDP) model of Plaut and Shallice (1993a) is designed to mimic the impairment of *optic aphasia*. Patients with this disorder typically make errors when naming visually presented objects. Their mistakes are often semantically related to the target, or responses related to a previous target (perseverations). However, they are relatively unimpaired at naming objects presented in other modalities and on tests of visual object recognition. Unlike previous theories of optic aphasia, which have focused on the dissociation between visual object naming and other tasks, the optic aphasia model seeks to explain visual object naming errors. It takes its key architectural components and processing assumptions from a related PDP model of *deep dyslexia* (an impairment in accessing semantic representations from visual word forms; Hinton & Shallice, 1991; Plaut & Shallice, 1993b). To develop the optic aphasia model, Plaut and Shallice (1993a) modified the deep dyslexia model, lesioned it to simulate brain damage, and compared its responses to those of optic aphasics. We will discuss each of these steps in turn.

INITIAL MODEL ARCHITECTURE

The model assumes that optic aphasia, like deep dyslexia, stems from an impairment in accessing semantic representations from visual representations. To begin

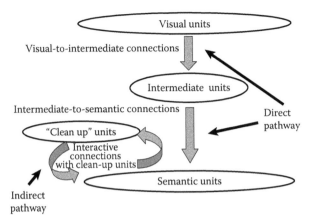

FIGURE 8.3   The optic aphasia model. A grey arrow between two layers shows that there are a randomly selected 25% of the potential trainable connections from all units at one layer to all units of the other layer.

with, Plaut and Shallice constructed a model that accesses semantic information in two stages. First, a rough approximation of the object's semantics is generated from its visual representation (the authors call this the model's *direct pathway*), and then this approximation is iteratively refined to the precise semantics of the object (via the *indirect pathway*). The direct pathway consists of a visual input layer, an intermediate layer, and a semantic output layer (see Figure 8.3). The visual layer is linked to the intermediate layer, and the intermediate layer to the semantic layer, by top-down, excitatory connections. In contrast to the interactive two-step model, representations in the optic aphasia model are *distributed*. For instance, the visual representation of "spoon" consists of a pattern of activity over many units in the visual layer, rather than the activation of a single node. The units of the input layer represent the visual information available from object recognition. Subgroups of these units code different visual features, such as the object's texture and color. For example, to indicate that a spoon has the properties "smooth" and "silver," the model shows a specific pattern of activity (shared by other smooth, silver objects) over the texture and color subgroups of the visual units, respectively. Similarly, the semantic output layer has subgroups of units that code different semantic features. The intermediate units mediate between the input and output layers. Since visually similar objects are not necessarily semantically similar to the same degree, these units provide a layer of abstraction that allows the model to map similar inputs to less similar outputs (Elman et al., 1996). The pattern of activation over the intermediate units for a given object is determined during a period of *training* in which the model learns to map an object's input pattern to its output pattern.

   An important property of distributed representations is that they naturally reflect similarity: Related objects will have similar patterns of activation over the model's units. If each unit's activation is treated as a separate dimension, all the units at a particular layer define a multidimensional space. A given object's visual representation is then a point in the visual-layer space, where more similar objects are closer to each other. The model's direct pathway generates an analogous point in semantic-layer space, representing the model's rough approximation to the object's semantics. However, this initial semantic representation does not correspond to any known object, and so the function of the indirect pathway is to move it closer to a known object. It does this by sending activation from the semantic layer along excitatory connections to a layer of "clean up" units, which then send activation back to the semantic layer. As a result of this interactive feedback loop, the model develops *basins of attraction* around points representing known objects in semantic space, areas that "pull" the initial activation towards an *attractor* (known object semantics). For instance, if the activation generated by the direct pathway falls into spoon's basin of attraction, it is biased to move toward the point in semantic space representing spoon.

TRAINING: SETTING THE MODEL'S LONG-TERM CONNECTION WEIGHTS

The model's architecture specifies the units and the potential connections between them, but the connection weights must be learned. Moreover, each connection is associated with a *long-term weight* (like the weights used in the interactive two-step model), as well as a *short-term weight* that reflects the model's recent experience (to induce perseverative behavior when the model is tested). The activation that is sent from one unit to another is a function of both the long-term and the short-term weights on the connection between them. During training, the visual input units were activated to correspond to an object (e.g., spoon). Activation flowed from the visual units to the intermediate units and on to the semantic units, and then looped from semantic units to the clean up units and back again. After a period of time, the activation of each semantic unit was compared to the desired activation (the activation it would have if the model had retrieved the correct object semantics). A learning rule computed the *error*, or difference between these activations and changed the network's connection weights appropriately. Error-based learning works such that if a semantic unit is much too active (a large error), the long-term weights on the connections leading to that semantic unit from intermediate units, and from visual units to those intermediate units, are greatly reduced; if the unit has a small error, the weights are reduced less. The training process was performed many times for each of 40 different objects from four semantic categories until the error on the semantic units was small. As for the short-term weights, they were set at the end of each object presentation to reflect the model's recent experience.

LESIONING AND TESTING THE MODEL

The underlying cause of optic aphasia is debated. Some have viewed it as a deficit in accessing semantic representations (e.g., Riddoch & Humphreys, 1987), and Plaut and Shallice instantiated this by removing a proportion of the connections (e.g., 20% would be a moderate lesion) between the visual layer and the intermediate layer. Because the goal of the modeling was to explore the underlying deficit, they administered a variety of lesion severities in this and in other layers.

An important property of networks with distributed representations is that of *graceful degradation*—when damaged, their performance is not catastrophically impaired but degraded proportionate to the amount of damage, like that of actual neuropsychological patients (Elman et al., 1996). So even when a lesion removed 20% of the connections previously relied on for semantic access, the model could still correctly name objects about 50–80% of the time.

After being lesioned, the model was tested in the following way: A prime object (e.g., spoon) was presented, after which the short-term weights were set to reflect this recent experience. The model was then presented with a target object (e.g., fork), and the model's activation over the semantic output units was coded as one of several response types. To avoid being classified as an *omission* (lack of response), the output had to be sufficiently close to one known object, as well as sufficiently far away from all other known objects in semantic space. If the output met these criteria, the response was considered to be either correct (e.g., closest known object was fork, the target) or an error (e.g., closest known object was knife, not the target). If the response was an error (e.g., knife) it was categorized as a *visual* error if the target and error were sufficiently close in visual space, *semantic* if they were close in semantic space, or *mixed* if (like knife) it was close in both respects. Furthermore, an error was deemed to have a perseverative component to it if it was related to the prime (e.g., spoon).

COMPARING MODEL BEHAVIOR WITH PATIENT PERFORMANCE

Unlike Schwartz et al. (2006), Plaut and Shallice did not calculate numerical measures of the model's fit to empirical data, but instead compared the overall pattern of errors produced by the model with that of optic aphasic patients. If the model mimicked the patient data, the authors' goal was to explain why the model behaved as it did, and apply this explanation to the deficit in optic aphasia. The model's rates of making different error types were compared to a "chance rate" (a random pairing of errors with other objects), to assess the influence of visual and semantic similarity and perseveration in the model. If we ignore perseverative influence for the moment and focus on the error's relation to the target, previous studies have found that optic aphasics make about twice as many semantic errors as visual errors (Iorio, Falanga, Fragassi, & Grossi, 1992), and that mixed errors are also common (Lhermitte & Beauvois, 1973). Across lesion types that yielded a 20–80% error rate, the model produced a similar pattern of results: Mixed errors were the most frequent, followed by semantic errors, and the rate of both of these error types exceeded chance. By contrast, visual errors occurred at a rate closer to chance.

Why does the model make mainly semantic and mixed errors? Plaut and Shallice attribute this result to attractors. Recall that basins of attraction "capture" the first-pass activity generated by the direct pathway and move it toward an attractor in semantic space. Mapping visual object representations to semantic representations is a relatively systematic process: Objects with similar visual features will tend, on average, to have fairly similar semantic features (consider "fork" and "knife"). This means that the direct pathway will map the visual representation of fork to an area of semantic space somewhere near fork, and so if the network is damaged this first-pass semantics may be captured by a nearby attractor basin for knife, for example. Thus, attractors bias the model toward semantic or mixed errors, with the consequence that purely visual errors are relatively rare.

We mentioned before that optic aphasics make many perseverations, which can be exact reproductions of a previous target (some semantically related to the current target) or words related to a previous target. Looking at the model's performance across lesions that yielded 20–80% overall accuracy, it produced exact perseverations and perseverations semantically related to the target at rates well above chance, and fewer perseverations semantically related to the prime. The fact that the model perseverates is not surprising, because the short-term weights were included in the model specifically to produce this behavior. However, the fact that a strong combined influence of perseveration and semantic relatedness is also seen in the errors of patients supports the use of short-term weights and attractors to model optic aphasia.

Like Schwartz et al. (2006), Plaut and Shallice used the model's responses given different lesion locations and severities to better understand the deficits of individual patients, as well as to derive additional support for the model. In particular, they focus on patients whose behavior deviates from the majority of optic aphasics. For instance, one patient described by Coslett and Saffran (1989) made many unrelated errors (in contrast to most optic aphasics, who make mostly mixed, semantic, and perseverative errors), despite demonstrating good performance on nonverbal tests of semantic comprehension (e.g., object categorization). In the model, severe lesions produced an error profile with many responses unrelated to the target or prime. Even with such a severe impairment, the seemingly unrelated responses of the model, though, were still semantically/visually closer to the target than chance. The authors argue that because nonverbal tests of semantic comprehension require less precise access of semantic representations, good nonverbal comprehension can be accommodated in the same model as severely impaired visual object naming. Plaut and Shallice also discuss the moderately impaired patient of McCarthy and Warrington (1986), who made many omissions (but whose remaining errors were semantic) and did not perform well on nonverbal tests of semantic comprehension. In the model, lesions to the indirect pathway yielded many omissions, because the damaged feedback loop could not move the initial activity close enough to a real word. Also, the errors that the model does produce given this type of lesion are almost all semantic ones, so the entire error pattern is similar to that of McCarthy and Warrington's patient. Plaut and Shallice argue that this error pattern is also expected under lesions to the semantic units themselves, and thus a semantic lesion could explain both a preponderance of omissions in visual object naming and poor performance on nonverbal semantic tasks.

SUMMARY: STRENGTHS AND LIMITATIONS

The optic aphasia model successfully simulates the errors made by optic aphasics in visual object naming. It does this by storing visual and semantic representations of objects in a distributed manner and allowing the mappings between these representations to develop in a way that minimizes error, rather than imposing mappings according to a particular theory. The model's use of separate direct and indirect pathways leads to the development of attractors that move representations away from visual similarity and toward semantic similarity. This allows one lesion anywhere in the model to cause naming errors with both visual and semantic similarity to the target object. The use of two pathways is also theoretically significant in that it separates semantic access into two steps: Mapping visual input to semantics, and searching within semantic space for exact meanings. The authors are able to simulate variability in optic aphasic performance by applying lesions of different severities in a variety of locations. More generally, the optic aphasia model is one in a line of models that provide support for the connectionist processing and architectural assumptions leading to their behavior. These models' distributed representations, attractors, and weights acquired through error-based learning have successfully simulated aspects of deep dyslexia, optic aphasia, perseveration in linguistic aphasia, and normal subjects' reading of degraded input (Gotts & Plaut, 2004; McLeod, Shallice, & Plaut, 2000; Plaut & Shallice, 1993a; Plaut & Shallice, 1993b).

Like the interactive two-step model, the explicit computational implementation of the optic aphasia model allows a better understanding of the mechanisms that lie behind the deficit. Recall that when faced with a patient who exhibited many omissions and whose existing errors were semantic, the model was able to associate this with a particular type of deficit (damage to the indirect pathway). However, this same example made clear the limitations of the model and directions for future research. Although Plaut and Shallice say that damaging the indirect pathway is analogous to damaging semantic units, they do not offer a simulation proof. The model also only simulates one task performed by optic aphasics, and so is unable to assess whether the damaged semantic units posited to explain this patient's visual object naming performance would also lead to poor object recognition. These limitations were recently addressed by Plaut's (2002) extension of the optic aphasia model to simulate performance on nonverbal comprehension tasks.

Although the optic aphasia model is more realistic than the interactive two-step model in its incorporation of learning, the tests of its empirical validity are more limited. Plaut and Shallice compare the model's performance to fewer patients— and their comparisons are more qualitative than quantitative. Perhaps more importantly, the model's predictions were not systematically tested. Also, this model only simulates one kind of aphasia, and so it is only in conjunction with other simulations that it moves toward the "holy grail" of developing a single computational framework that can account for a variety of aphasic data. Another aspect of the computational holy grail is to account for aphasic behavior beyond that of a single-word naming trial. Plaut and Shallice's inclusion of short-term perseverative influences in their model represents a step in that direction. The third and final model we consider takes on this challenge more directly by trying to simulate the production of multiword utterances.

APHASIC LEXICAL ACCESS IN SENTENCE PRODUCTION

Compared to the two previous models, our last model, the *division of labor* (DoL) model (Gordon & Dell, 2003), is quite modest in both its aims and its accomplishments. It is noteworthy, though, as one of the few connectionist models of aphasia that actually attempted to simulate the production of sentences as opposed to single words. The impetus for the model was a study of sentence production by Breedin, Saffran, and Schwartz (1998) that contrasted sentences with semantically simple verbs such as *go*, and complex verbs such as *fly* (see also Barde, Schwartz, & Boronat, 2006). The simple verb *go* is semantically primitive; it can be associated with a single feature (e.g., *motion*). The verb *fly* also has the *motion* feature, but it is more complex because it includes a feature for the manner of motion (e.g., *through_air*).

Breedin and colleagues gave aphasic subjects brief stories that included sentences such as "Carl makes boats." Each sentence had either a simple verb like *make* or a more complex verb such as *build* (to build something is to make something in a particular way). Then the patients were prompted with a question (e.g., "What does Carl do?") to produce each sentence. Accuracy in retrieving the verb was the principal measure. Breedin et al. also assessed patient use of simple and complex verbs in narrative speech.

It turned out that the influence of verb complexity on patient performance depended on the distinction between agrammatic and anomic aphasia. Agrammatic speech is disfluent, ungrammatical, and lacking in function morphemes (function words and grammatical affixes), while anomic speech is mostly fluent and grammatical, but lacks content words, particularly nouns. Breedin et al. found that agrammatic individuals had more difficulty with simple than complex verbs. For example, only 9% of agrammatic subject SS's verbs in narrative speech were simple, and in the question–answering task SS tended to replace simple verbs with complex ones, saying, for example, "build ... build boats" for the target "Carl makes boats," (17 complex-for-simple substitutions, but only 5 simple-for-complex substitutions). The anomic subjects exhibited the opposite dissociation. For example, the verbs in anomic subject VP's narrative speech were simple 85% of the time, and complex-to-simple substitutions outnumbered simple-to-complex ones by 29 to 5.

Why is agrammatism, which presumably results from a syntactic deficit, associated with a difficulty in producing simple verbs, while anomia, which is a lexical deficit, is associated with greater difficulty with complex verbs? That is the question that the DoL model tried to answer. According to the model, the double dissociation between simple and complex verbs has to do with the relative contributions of syntax and semantics to verb retrieval. To see how this works, we first have to consider how lexical, syntactic, and semantic information are represented in the model's network (Figure 8.4). The network contains three kinds of units: semantic features, syntactic-sequential states, and lexical units. The semantic-feature units serve as input, much as the semantic features in the interactive two-step model do. Only here, they represent the meaning of the intended sentence, rather than a

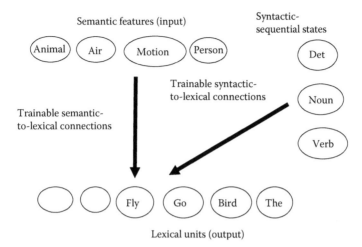

FIGURE 8.4   The division of labor model.

single word. The lexical units are the model's output and must be retrieved one at a time in the correct order. For example, if the sentence is "The bird flies," semantic-feature units for the bird concept (*winged, animal*) and the flying concept (*motion, through_air*) would be activated and these would remain active throughout the production of the sentence. The network's task is then to activate, first, the lexical unit *the*, then *bird*, and then finally *fly*. (The model did not implement the inflectional morphology associated with verb agreement).

Because the semantic features remain active throughout the incremental generation of the sentence, the model needs something to keep track of where it is in the sentence. This is the function of the syntactic-sequential state units. Their activation changes throughout the production process, thus providing a signal that the network can use to tell where it is. If we wanted to produce "The bird flies," there would have to be at least three syntactic-sequential state units, one representing when *the* should be retrieved (e.g., a state that can be called DET for determiner), one representing that it is time for the subject noun (NOUN), and one for the main verb (VERB). Specifically, at the start of the sentence, all the semantic features would be on, but only the syntactic-sequential state associated with the beginning of the sentence (here, DET) would be active. With these semantic and syntactic inputs, the model should activate the output unit for *the*. After *the* has been chosen, DET will turn off and NOUN will become active, which should lead to the retrieval of *bird*. And finally, NOUN will turn off and VERB will turn on, enabling retrieval of *fly*. In short, the model generates a sequence of states: DET, then NOUN, then VERB, and the activation of these units combines with activation from semantics to ensure that the right word is retrieved at the right time.

But how does the network know what word to retrieve at what time? It has to learn this. That is, the model has to experience training sentences and, based on this experience, adjust its connection weights so that semantically appropriate words become active at the right point in the sentence. Two sets of connection weights are critical: those between semantic features and words (*semantic weights*), and those between syntactic-sequential states and words (*syntactic weights*). Let us look at some of the values for these weights after the model has been trained to say sentences such as "The bird flies." A word such as *bird* acquires strong, excitatory connections from both semantic features and appropriate syntactic-sequential states. The learned weight from the feature *animal* to the word *bird* was +1.3; the weight from the NOUN state to *bird* was also +1.3. In other words, the responsibility for activating the unit for *bird* falls on both semantic and syntactic weights. The semantics and the syntax thus "divide the labor" of word retrieval, with the semantic weights telling the lexical system what words are good matches to the sentence meaning and the syntactic weights telling it where the grammar allows for that word to be positioned.

What about verbs? In the model, their retrieval also depends on both semantic and syntactic weights. But differences in the semantic complexity of the verbs affect the division of labor between the two types of weights. The complex verb *fly* (*motion* and *through_air*) is very much retrieved through semantics. For example, it has a strong weight from *through_air* (+1.1), but only a weak weight from the relevant syntactic-sequential state, VERB (+0.4). The simple verb *go* (*motion*) exhibits the opposite pattern. The syntactic weight from VERB is strong (+1.3), but the weight from its only semantic feature *motion* is weak (+0.5). In short, the model learns to treat simple verbs as more syntactic and complex ones as more semantic.

Why does the model's learning process create a different division of labor for simple and complex verbs? Like in the optic aphasia naming model, the weights are changed by error-based learning. For example, if the word *plane* is activated when *bird* is sought, the weights from the features of *bird* (e.g., *animal*) to the *bird* unit are increased while those to *plane* are decreased. Error-based learning creates cue competition, the tendency for inputs to compete with one another to control output. The weights from two inputs that are both associated with the same output will compete so that if one weight becomes strong, the other will remain weak. When one input is primarily responsible for retrieving the output, the other input's weight cannot get stronger, even though it may be predictive of the output.

Cue competition between the semantic and the syntactic weights leads to a greater reliance on syntax for the simple verbs. Because a simple verb does not have strong semantic cues (e.g., the feature *motion* is predictive of many verbs other than *go*), the syntactic weights (e.g., from VERB to *go*) have to grow strong to pick up the slack. Complex verbs, in contrast, have strong, predictive semantic cues (e.g., *through_air* is a strong predictor of *fly*). Because of the competition from these strong cues, though, the syntactic weights to the complex verbs will be weak and the retrieval of these verbs will depend less on the syntax.

If agrammatic aphasia is attributed to a loss of syntactic weights, and anomic aphasia to a loss of semantic weights (like low *s* weights in the interactive two-step model), the differences in verb retrieval found by Breedin et al. can be explained. Let us first consider the model's ability to mimic agrammatic production in this study. Reducing the syntactic weights led to the predicted superiority of complex verbs: 35% of complex verbs were retrieved, but only 21% of simple verbs.

Moreover, the model's output exhibited other features of agrammatism, such as the tendency for short, ungrammatical utterances lacking function words. "The bird goes" might be spoken as "bird flies" or just "bird." The tendency to omit words arises because the agrammatic lesion reduces the syntactic input to target words, leaving them severely underactivated. This was particularly true for function words such as "the." Like the simple verbs, function words have few semantic features. In fact, in Gordon and Dell's implementation, *the* had no semantic features at all. Consequently, the model's learning rule assigned all of the responsibility for retrieving *the* to the syntactic weights—a huge +3.4 syntactic weight from the DET state. Thus, a syntactic lesion selectively impairs function words and content words with less semantic content such as simple verbs.

Reducing the semantic weights in the model created behavior that is similar to that in fluent aphasia (e.g., anomic or Wernicke's aphasia). As in Breedin et al.'s data from anomic patients, simple verbs were more easily retrieved than complex ones: 38% for simple verbs and 6% for complex verbs. Moreover, with this lesion, the model's speech was classically anomic. Difficulty was confined to the retrieval of content words and the resulting sentences were otherwise grammatical. For example, instead of "The bird flies," the model might produce "The plane goes." Notice that the substituted words (*plane* for *bird*; *go* for *fly*) preserve the grammatical structure of the sentence. Also, the underactivation of words that was characteristic of a syntactic lesion in the model was not present with the semantic lesion. If anything, incorrect semantically related words were *more* active than they should be with this lesion. The reason for this overactivation is that inhibitory (negative) weights are an important aspect of the model's semantic connections. For example, after the model has learned its weights, the word *plane* is strongly inhibited by the feature *animal*. This is because the model has to learn to suppress *plane* when it wants to retrieve *bird*. Damaging these inhibitory weights in a semantic lesion thus leads to overactivation of the semantic neighbors of a target word and ultimately to semantic errors.

The DoL model's association between agrammatic lesions with underactivation and anomic lesions with overactivation echoes another important connectionist characterization of aphasia, the model of lexical input processing by McNellis and Blumstein (2001). According to this model, successful word processing requires that the network units' resting activation levels exist within a certain range. If the resting activations are too low, the resulting underactivation of word units prevents the system from computing relations between words. If the resting activations are too high, the system is overwhelmed with extraneous information. Moreover, McNellis and Blumstein propose that the distinction between Broca's and Wernicke's aphasia corresponds to these underactivation and overactivation states, respectively. Studies of lexical and semantic priming with aphasic subjects have generally supported this proposal (see Blumstein & Milberg, 2000 for a review) and theorists (e.g., Goldstein, 1948) have long attempted to associate aphasia, and particularly the distinction between fluent and nonfluent aphasia, with notions of under- or overactivation (or, correspondingly, too much or too little inhibition). Connectionist models such as the DoL model or that of McNellis and Blumstein allow for these proposals to be made concrete.

SUMMARY AND CONCLUSIONS

It should be clear from our review that we are far from the computational holy grail—a unified model of aphasia. The models are as diverse as the data. Some models (e.g., DoL model) appeal to connectionist learning principles to explain the data. Others (e.g., the interactive two-step model) attribute error effects to interactive spreading activation. And some do both (e.g., the optic aphasia model). The models also differ in how they represent linguistic knowledge, with the optic aphasia model emphasizing distributed representations of lexical knowledge and the other two models using localist representations of words.

Despite these differences, the connectionist approaches share what can be called a *cooperative* view of language processing. Although the models have separate network levels that correspond to distinct representational types, such as phonology or semantics, the levels work together to explain empirical phenomena. We might describe an error as "semantic" or "phonological," but that does not mean that responsibility for the error lies within a single level. On the contrary, connectionist treatments of language propose that multiple levels conspire to generate both correct and errorful behavior. We see these multilevel effects in models with a bidirectional or interactive flow of activation, such as the optic aphasia model's account of mixed visual-semantic naming errors, or the interactive two-step model's explanation for form-related word errors in production. Connectionist models also allow for multiple levels to affect processing through learning. For example, the learned weights from syntactic states in the DoL model depend on the semantic complexity of verbs, and the weights in the optic aphasia model reflect both semantic and visual similarity.

We claim that the cooperative view of language processing has much to offer research on communication disorders. The diversity of symptoms and syndromes, the multilevel nature of errors, and the often impenetrable relation between behavior and lesion loci argue for models that respect the interactions among processing components. Despite lacking our present day computational tools, Lichtheim no doubt recognized this when he made the first diagrammatic "model" of aphasia in 1885. We like to think that modern connectionist models are just continuing a tradition.

ACKNOWLEDGMENT

Preparation of this chapter was supported by the NIH (HD-44458 and DC-00191).

REFERENCES

Barde, L. H. F., Schwartz, M. F., & Boronat, C. B. (2006). Semantic weight and verb retrieval in aphasia. *Brain and Language, 97*(3), 266–278.
Blumstein, S. E., & Milberg, W. P. (2000). Language deficits in Broca's and Wernicke's aphasia: A singular impairment. In Y. Grodzinsky et al. (Eds.), *Language and the brain: Representation and processing* (pp. 167–184.) New York, NY: Academic Press.

Breedin, S. D., Saffran, E. M., & Schwartz, M. F. (1998). Semantic factors in verb retrieval: An effect of complexity. *Brain and Language, 63*(1), 1–31.

Chang, F. (2002). Symbolically speaking: A connectionist model of sentence production. *Cognitive Science, 26*(5), 609–651.

Coslett, H. B., & Saffran, E. M. (1989). Preserved object recognition and reading comprehension in optic aphasia. *Brain, 112*, 1091–1110.

Cottrell, G. (1985) Implications of connectionist parsing for aphasia. *Proceedings of the Ninth Annual Symposium on Computer Applications in Medical Care,* Baltimore, MD, Aug. 18–23. (pp. 237–241)

Dell, G. S., Martin, N., & Schwartz, M. F. (2007). A case-series test of the interactive two-step model of lexical access: Predicting word repetition from picture naming. *Journal of Memory and Language, 56*(4), 490–520.

Dell, G. S., Schwartz, M. F., Martin, N., Saffran, E. M., & Gagnon, D. A. (1997). Lexical access in aphasic and nonaphasic speakers. *Psychological Review, 104*(4), 801–838.

Elman, J. L., Bates, E. A., Johnson, M. H., Karmiloff-Smith, A., Parisi, D., & Plunkett, K. (1996). *Rethinking innateness: A connectionist perspective on development.* Cambridge, MA: The MIT Press.

Goldstein, K. (1948). *Language and language disturbances: Aphasic symptom complexes and their significance for medicine and theory of language.* New York, NY: Grune & Stratton.

Gordon, J. K., & Dell, G. S. (2003). Learning to divide the labor: An account of deficits in light and heavy verb production. *Cognitive Science, 27*(1), 1–40.

Gotts, S. J., & Plaut, D. C. (2004). Connectionist approaches to understanding aphasic perseveration. *Seminars in Speech and Language, 25*, 323–334.

Graves, R. E. (1997). The legacy of the Wernicke-Lichtheim model. *Journal of the History of the Neurosciences, 6*(10), 3–20.

Hanley, J. R., Dell, G. S., Kay, J., & Baron, R. (2004). Evidence for the involvement of a nonlexical route in the repetition of familiar words: A comparison of single and dual route models of auditory repetition. *Cognitive Neuropsychology, 21*(2–4), 147–158.

Harley, T. A. (1993). Phonological activation of semantic competitors during lexical access in speech production. *Language and Cognitive Processes, 8*(3), 291–309.

Harley, T. A. (1996). Connectionist modeling of the recovery of language functions following brain damage. *Brain and Language, 52*(1), 7–24.

Hinton, G. E., & Shallice, T. (1991). Lesioning an attractor network: Investigations of acquired dyslexia. *Psychological Review, 98*(1), 74–95.

Iorio, L., Falanga, A., Fragassi, N. A., & Grossi, D. (1992). Visual associative agnosia and optic aphasia: A single case study and review of the syndromes. *Cortex, 28*, 23–37.

Kittredge, A. K., Dell, G. S., Verkuilen, J., & Schwartz, M. F. (in press). Where is the effect of lexical frequency in word production? Insights from aphasic picture naming errors. *Cognitive Neuropsychology, 25*, 583–608.

Laine, M., Tikkala, A., & Juhola, M. (1998). Modelling anomia by the discrete two-stage word production architecture. *Journal of Neurolinguistics, 11*(3), 275–294.

Lhermitte, F., & Beauvois, M. F. (1973). A visual-speech disconnexion syndrome: Report of a case with optic aphasia, agnosic alexia and colour agnosia. *Brain, 96*, 695–714.

Lichtheim, L. (1885). On aphasia. *Brain, 7*, 433–484.

Martin, N., Dell, G. S., Saffran, E. M., & Schwartz, M. F. (1994). Origins of paraphasias in deep dyslexia: Testing the consequences of a decay impairment to an interactive spreading activation model of lexical retrieval. *Brain and Language, 47*(4), 609–660.

Martin, N., Saffran, E. M., & Dell, G. S. (1996). Recovery in deep dysphasia: Evidence for a relation between auditory-verbal STM capacity and lexical errors in repetition. *Brain and Language, 52*(1), 83–113.

McCarthy, R., & Warrington, E. K. (1986). Visual associative agnosia: A clinico-anatomical study of a single case. *Journal of Neurology, Neurosurgery and Psychiatry, 49*, 1233–1240.

McLeod, P., Shallice, T., & Plaut, D. C. (2000). Attractor dynamics in word recognition: Converging evidence from errors by normal subjects, dyslexic patients and a connectionist model. *Cognition, 74*(1), 91–113.

McNellis, M. G., & Blumstein, S. E. (2001). Self-organizing dynamics of lexical access in normals and aphasics. *Journal of Cognitive Neuroscience, 13*(2), 151–170.

Plaut, D. C. (1996). Relearning after damage in connectionist networks: Toward a theory of rehabilitation. *Brain and Language, 52*(1), 25–82.

Plaut, D. C. (2002). Graded modality specific specialisation in semantics: A computational account of optic aphasia. *Cognitive Neuropsychology, 19*(7), 603–639.

Plaut, D. C., & Shallice, T. (1993a). Perseverative and semantic influences on visual object naming errors in optic aphasia: A connectionist account. *Journal of Cognitive Neuroscience, 5*(1), 89–117.

Plaut, D. C., & Shallice, T. (1993b). Deep dyslexia: A case study of connectionist neuropsychology. *Cognitive Neuropsychology, 10*(5), 377–500.

Rapp, B., & Goldrick, M. (2000). Discreteness and interactivity in spoken word production. *Psychological Review, 107*(3), 460–499.

Riddoch, M. J., & Humphreys, G. W. (1987). Visual object processing in optic aphasia: A case of semantic access agnosia. *Cognitive Neuropsychology, 4*(2), 131–185.

Schwartz, M. F., Dell, G. S., Martin, N., Gahl, S., & Sobel, P. (2006). A case-series test of the interactive two-step model of lexical access: Evidence from picture naming. *Journal of Memory and Language, 54*(2), 228–264.

Weems, S. A., & Reggia, J. A. (2006). Simulating single word processing in the classic aphasia syndromes based on the Wernicke-Lichtheim-Geschwind theory. *Brain and Language, 98*(3), 291–309.

Wright, J. F., & Ahmad, K. (1997). The connectionist simulation of aphasic naming. *Brain and Language, 59*(2), 367–389.

9 Modeling the Attentional Control of Vocal Utterances: From Wernicke to WEAVER++

Ardi Roelofs

INTRODUCTION

In *Die Sprache*, Wundt (1900) criticized the now classic model of normal and aphasic utterance production of Wernicke (1874, 1885, 1886) by arguing that producing verbal utterances is an active goal-driven process rather than a passive associative process proceeding from stimulus to vocal response, as held by the model. According to Wundt (1900, 1904), an attentional process located in the frontal lobes of the human brain actively controls an utterance perception and production network located in perisylvian brain areas, described by the Wernicke model. Modern models of vocal utterance production such as WEAVER++ (Levelt, Roelofs, & Meyer, 1999; Roelofs, 1992, 1997, 2003) build in many respects on the Wernicke model, but also address Wundt's critique by implementing assumptions on how the production–perception network is controlled. Characteristics of vocal utterance production, such as production onset latencies, errors, and corresponding brain activity, arise from the interplay of the production–perception network and the attentional control system. For example, patterns of speech errors by normal and aphasic speakers seem to be determined, at least in part, by self-monitoring, which is an important attentional control function (Roelofs, 2004). Models can benefit aphasia therapy. As Basso and Marangolo (2000) stated, "Clearly articulated and detailed hypotheses about representations and processing of cognitive functions allow rejection of all those strategies for treatment that are not theoretically justified. The more detailed the cognitive model, the narrower the spectrum of rationally motivated treatments" (p. 228).

The remainder of this chapter is organized as follows. I start by describing some of the key characteristics of the classic Wernicke model and outline Wundt's critique that the model lacks attentional control mechanisms. According to Wundt, understanding attentional control is important for aphasia therapy, because control processes may partly compensate the negative effects of lesions on language performance. Next, I describe vocal utterance production and perception in the WEAVER++ model (Levelt et al., 1999; Roelofs, 1992, 1997, 2003) as well as the model's assumptions on attentional control. I then review brain imaging evidence on the attentional control of word production, which has confirmed Wundt's suggestion that control processes are localized in the frontal lobes. Controversy exists about the role of one of the frontal areas, the anterior cingulate cortex (ACC). Researchers generally agree that the ACC plays a role in the contextual regulation of nonverbal vocal utterances, including monkey calls and human crying, laughing, and pain shrieking. However, no agreement exists on the role of the ACC in spoken word production. Some researchers deny any role for the ACC in word production (e.g., Jürgens, 2002), while others assume involvement of the human ACC but disagree on whether the ACC plays a regulatory role (Posner & Raichle, 1994; Posner & Rothbart, 2007; Roelofs & Hagoort, 2002) or a role in detecting conflict or predicting error likelihood (Brown & Braver, 2005; Miller & Cohen, 2001; Sohn, Albert, Jung, Carter, & Anderson, 2007). I review brain imaging evidence from my own laboratory for a regulatory role of the human ACC in attentional control. Finally, avenues for future research are indicated.

WERNICKE'S MODEL AND WUNDT'S CRITIQUE

In a small monograph published in 1874, called *The aphasia symptom-complex: A psychological study on an anatomical basis.* Wernicke presented a model for the functional neuroanatomy of vocal utterance production and comprehension. During the past century, the model has been extremely influential in directing and organizing research results on aphasic and normal language performance. According to Wernicke (1874), verbal vocal utterances require both cortical and brainstem mechanisms, whereas nonverbal vocal utterances, such as crying, only need brainstem circuits. Figure 9.1 illustrates the structure of the model.

At the heart of the model, auditory images for words are linked to motor images for words. The auditory images were presumed to be stored in what is today called Wernicke's area, which includes the left posterior superior temporal lobe. The motor images were assumed to be stored in Broca's area, which consists of the left posterior inferior frontal lobe. The model assumes that when a word is heard (Wernicke used the example of hearing the word BELL), auditory signals from sensory brainstem nuclei travel to the primary auditory cortex and then activate the auditory images for words. The auditory images activate associated concept images, which include sensory images of the visual and tactile impressions of the corresponding object. This leads to comprehension of the word. In repeating a heard word, the auditory images activate the corresponding motor images in Broca's area, which then activate the motor nuclei in the brainstem via primary motor cortex. In naming a pictured bell, concept images corresponding to the bell are activated, which then activate the motor images. The motor image activates the auditory image for the word, which in turn activates the motor image. This reverberation of activation stabilizes the activation of the motor images, which serves a monitoring function.

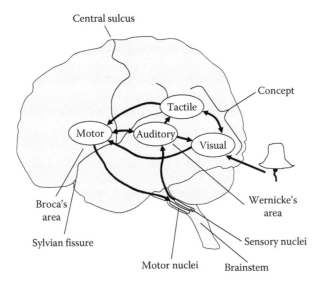

FIGURE 9.1 Illustration of the functional neuroanatomy for vocal utterance production and perception assumed by Wernicke's model. Concept, auditory, and motor images are located in a left-lateralized perisylvian network of brain areas.

Wernicke (1874, 1885, 1886) developed the model to explain various types of aphasia, which were presumed to be the result of different loci of brain damage. For example, according to the model, damage to the auditory images gives rise to speech comprehension deficits (today called Wernicke's aphasia), whereas damage to the motor images gives rise to deficits in speech production (Broca's aphasia). The reverberation of activation between motor and auditory images in speech production explains why brain-damaged patients with speech recognition deficits (people with Wernicke's aphasia) often have fluent but phonemically disordered speech production. When the auditory word images are lesioned, activity of the motor images no longer sufficiently stabilizes, explaining the phonemic paraphasias.

It is outside the scope of the present chapter to evaluate the scientific merits of Wernicke's model. For a description of the impact of the model during the past century, I refer to Shallice (1988). Overviews of modern theorizing on aphasia may be found in, for example, Caplan (1992), Martin (2003), Nickels (1997), and Rapp (2001). Relevant for the present chapter is the critique on the model advanced by Wundt (1900). According to Wundt, the retrieval of words from memory is an active goal-driven process rather than a passive associative process, as held by Wernicke's model. In particular, an attentional process located in the frontal lobes of the human brain controls the word perception and production network located in perisylvian brain areas, described by the Wernicke model. Consequently, characteristics of normal and impaired vocal performance arise from interactions between the production–perception network and the attentional control system.

Wundt (1900) maintained that such interactions may partly compensate the negative effects of lesions on language performance. In support of this claim, he describes an anomic patient who used the strategy of naming objects by first writing the object name down and then reading the written name aloud (today, recognized as a common compensatory strategy, cf. Nickels, 2002). Furthermore, the patient failed to name attributes of objects both when asked for the attribute ("what is the color of blood?") and when the attribute was shown (a red patch) but not when he actively got hold of the object together with the attribute (i.e., a drop of blood). This suggests that actively going after an enriched input may help remedy word retrieval problems. Wundt speculated that the strategic use of alternative routes through the perception-production network could lead to new network associations substituting the damaged ones. He recommended extended practice on using the alternative route as a form of aphasia therapy. Today, this is one of the approaches to therapy for naming disorders (e.g., Nickels, 2002). Studies of phenomena such as central nervous system repair, cortical reorganization after brain damage, and the improvement of language function by behavioral therapy, support the view that patients may regain lost capabilities by extensive training (e.g., Taub, Uswatte, & Elbert, 2002). Surprisingly, although Wundt's critique on Wernicke's model seems fundamental, assumptions about attentional control have typically not been part of computational models of word production and perception that have been developed during the past century (e.g., Coltheart, Rastle, Perry, Langdon, & Ziegler, 2001; Dell, Schwartz, Martin, Saffran, & Gagnon, 1997; Rapp & Goldrick, 2000).

In a review of the literature on treatment for word-retrieval disorders, Nickels (2002) concludes that

> There can be no doubt that therapy for word-retrieval impairments can be highly successful, resulting in long-term improvements which can be of great communicative significance for the individual with aphasia. However, predicting the precise result of a specific treatment task with a specific individual with certainty is still not possible. (p. 935)

According to her, "If one is ever to achieve (or even attempt) prediction in treatment, between task and impairment, a clearly articulated theory of the levels of processing that can be impaired is essential" (p. 955). One such theoretical effort is reviewed next.

THE WEAVER++ MODEL

In a seminal article, Norman and Shallice (1986) made a distinction between "horizontal threads" and "vertical threads" in the control of perception and action. Horizontal threads are strands of processing that map perceptions onto actions and vertical threads are attentional influences on these mappings. Behavior arises from interactions between horizontal and vertical threads. WEAVER++ (Roelofs, 1992, 1997, 2003, 2004, 2007) is a model that computationally implements specific claims about how the horizontal and vertical threads are woven together in the planning and comprehending of spoken words. Different from Wernicke's model, WEAVER++ was designed to explain evidence from word production latencies (see Levelt et al., 1999, for a review). I first describe the functional claims of the model, and then the presumed neuroanatomical correlates, as assessed by functional brain imaging studies rather than lesion-deficit analyses.

FUNCTIONAL ASPECTS

Whereas the Wernicke model assumes an associative network of concept, auditory, and motor images for words, WEAVER++ distinguishes concepts, lemmas, morphemes, phonemes, and syllable motor programs, as illustrated in Figure 9.2. For example, naming a pictured bell involves the activation of the representation of the concept BELL(X), the lemma of *bell* specifying that the word is a noun (for languages such as Dutch, lemmas also specify grammatical gender), the morpheme <bell>, the phonemes /b/, /e/, and /l/, and the syllable motor program [bel]. In the model, activation spreads from level to level, whereby each node sends a proportion of its activation to connected nodes. Consequently, network activation induced by perceived objects decreases with network distance. The activation

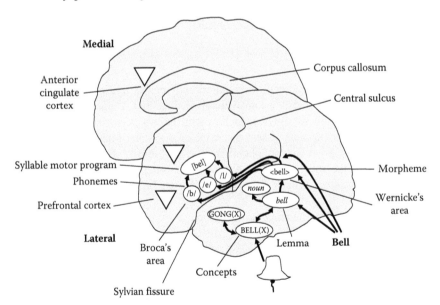

FIGURE 9.2   Illustration of the functional neuroanatomy for vocal utterance production and perception assumed by the WEAVER++ model. Only cortical areas are shown. Representations of concepts (e.g., BELL(X)), lemmas (e.g., *bell* specifying that the word is a noun), morphemes (e.g., <bell>), phonemes (e.g., /b/, /e/, and /l/), and syllable motor programs (e.g., [bel]) are located in a left-lateralized perisylvian network of brain areas. An attentional control system located in anterior cingulate cortex and in ventro- and dorsolateral prefrontal cortex (indicated by triangles) exerts regulatory influences over the lexical network.

flow from concepts to phonological forms is limited unless attentional enhancements are involved to boost the activation (Roelofs, 1992, 2003).

Following Wernicke's model, WEAVER++ assumes that perceived objects have direct access to concepts (e.g., BELL(X)) and only indirect access to word forms (e.g., <bell> and /b/, /e/, /l/), whereas perceived spoken and written words have direct access to word forms and only indirect access to concepts (cf. Roelofs, 1992, 2003, 2005, 2006, 2007). Consequently, naming objects requires concept selection, whereas spoken words can be repeated without concept selection. The latter is achieved by mapping input word-forms (e.g., the input phonological or orthographic form of BELL) directly onto output word-forms (e.g., <bell> and /b/, /e/, /l/), without engaging concepts and lemmas, as illustrated in Figure 9.2.

Whereas Wernicke's model lacks attentional control mechanisms, these are present in WEAVER++. In particular, a goal-driven selection of information from the lexical network in WEAVER++ is regulated by a system of condition-action rules. When a goal is placed in working memory, word planning is controlled by those rules that include the goal among their conditions. For object naming, a rule would specify that:

> IF the goal is to say the name of the object,
> and the concept corresponds to the object,
> THEN select the concept,
> and enhance its activation.

The activation enhancements are required until appropriate syllable motor programs have been activated above an availability threshold. The attentional control system determines how strongly and for how long the enhancement occurs (Roelofs, 2003, 2007). A speaker may assess the required duration of the enhancement by monitoring the progress on word planning (Roelofs, 2004, 2007). Condition-action rules allow for the specification of alternative naming routes. For example, the compensatory writing strategy discussed earlier may be specified as:

> IF the goal is to say the name of the object,
> and naming fails,
> THEN set the goal to write the name of the object,
> and read aloud the written name.

A compensatory strategy that has been studied in much detail is letter-by-letter reading in pure alexia (e.g., Cohen et al., 2004; Henry et al., 2005; Shallice, 1988), which is a frequent consequence of left occipitotemporal cortex damage. This area seems to implement the abstract identity of strings of letters. Pure alexic patients often retain single letter recognition abilities, and develop an effortful letter-by-letter strategy, which is the basis of most rehabilitation techniques. The strategy consists of silently sounding out the letters of the word from left to right. Consequently, word reading latency increases linearly with the number of letters in the word. Using brain imaging, Cohen et al. (2004) observed increased activation of the right occipitotemporal cortex in reading by a pure alexic patient compared to healthy controls, suggesting that letters were identified in the right rather than the left hemispheric area, as is normally the case. Moreover, the patient showed stronger than normal activation in left frontal and parietal areas that are implicated in phonological recoding and working memory, suggesting that the letter-by-letter strategy more strongly engages these functions. Examination of the patient 8 months later revealed decreased word reading latencies and decreased activation in the right occipitotemporal cortex (Henry et al., 2005), suggesting that the area became better at identifying letters with practice. The work of Cohen et al. (2004) and Henry et al. (2005) demonstrates the utility of functional brain imaging in assessing the effect of strategy use. Moreover, it provides some evidence for Wundt's conjecture that compensatory strategies may establish new routes through the perception-production network.

NEUROANATOMICAL ASPECTS

Following Wernicke's model, WEAVER++ assumes that the activation of representations underlying object naming proceeds from percepts in posterior cortical areas to articulatory programs in anterior areas, as illustrated in Figure 9.2. Using WEAVER++ as framework, Indefrey and Levelt (2004) performed a meta-analysis of 82 neuroimaging studies on word production, which suggested that the following cortical areas are involved. Information on the time course of word production in relation to these areas came from magnetoencephalographic studies. The meta-analysis included object naming (e.g., say "bell" to a pictured bell), word generation (producing a use for a noun, e.g., say "ring" to the spoken or written word BELL), word repetition or reading (e.g., say "bell" to BELL), and pseudoword repetition or reading (e.g., say "bez" to BEZ). Activation of percepts and concepts in object naming happens in occipital and inferiotemporal regions of the brain. The middle part of the left middle temporal gyrus seems to be involved with lemma retrieval. When the total object naming time is about 600 ms, activity in these areas occurs within the first 275 ms after an object is presented. Next, activation spreads to Wernicke's area, where the morphological code (i.e., lexical phonological code) of the word seems to be retrieved. Activation is then transmitted to Broca's area for phoneme processing and syllabification, taking some 125 ms. During the next 200 ms, syllable motor programs are accessed. The sensorimotor areas control articulation. Word repetition and reading may be accomplished by activating the areas of Wernicke and Broca for aspects of form encoding, and motor areas for articulation.

Neuroimaging studies on word planning have confirmed Wundt's (1900, 1904) suggestion that the perisylvian production-perception network is controlled by attentional control mechanisms located in the frontal lobes. In particular, attentional control processes engage the lateral prefrontal cortex (LPFC) and the ACC, as illustrated in Figure 9.2. The ACC and LPFC are more active in word generation (say "ring" to BELL) when the attentional control demands are high than in word repetition (say "bell" to BELL) when the demands are much lower (Petersen, Fox,

Posner, Mintun, & Raichle, 1988; Thompson-Schill, D'Esposito, Aguirre, & Farah, 1997). The increased activity in the frontal areas disappears when word selection becomes easy after repeated generation of the same use to a word (Petersen, van Mier, Fiez, & Raichle, 1998). Moreover, activity in the frontal areas is higher in object naming when there are several good names for an object so that selection difficulties arise than when there is only a single appropriate name (Kan & Thompson-Schill, 2004). Also, the frontal areas are more active when retrieval fails and words are on the tip of the tongue than when words are readily available (Maril, Wagner, & Schacter, 2001). Frontal areas are also more active in naming objects with semantically related words superimposed (e.g., naming a pictured bell combined with the word GONG) than without word distractors, as demonstrated by de Zubicaray, Wilson, McMahon, and Muthiah (2001). Thus, the neuroimaging evidence suggests that medial and lateral prefrontal areas exert attentional control over word planning. Along with the increased frontal activity, there is an elevation of activity in perisylvian areas (e.g., de Zubicaray et al., 2001; Raichle et al., 1994; Snyder, Abdullaev, Posner, & Raichle, 1995).

Evidence for the involvement of frontal areas in the attentional control of word production also comes from impaired performance. Semantic retrieval problems due to lesions of temporal areas of the human brain typically preserve the ability to generate category terms. For example, a patient may be able to say "instrument" to a bell, without being able to say "bell." Humphreys and Forde (2005) reported evidence on a patient with combined frontal-temporal damage, who had, instead, a specific impairment of generating category terms. According to Humphreys and Forde, the unusual impairment resulted because categorizing requires the attentional control provided by the frontal lobes.

Although both the ACC and LPFC are involved in the attentional control of word planning, the areas seem to play different roles. Evidence suggests that the dorsolateral prefrontal cortex (DLPFC) is involved in maintaining goals in working memory (for a review, see Kane & Engle, 2002). WEAVER++'s assumption that abstract condition-action rules mediate goal-oriented retrieval and selection processes in prefrontal cortex is supported by evidence from single cell recordings and hemodynamic neuroimaging studies (e.g., Bunge, 2004; Bunge, Kahn, Wallis, Miller, & Wagner, 2003; Wallis, Anderson, & Miller, 2001). Moreover, evidence suggests that the ventrolateral prefrontal cortex play a role in selection among competing response alternatives (Thompson-Schill et al., 1997), the control of memory retrieval, or both (Badre, Poldrack, Paré-Blagoev, Insler, & Wagner, 2005). The ACC seems to exert regulatory influences over these processes.

In the light of Darwin's continuity hypothesis (i.e., new capabilities arise in evolution by modification and extension of existing ones), the involvement of the ACC in the attentional control of spoken word production seems plausible, because the area also controls nonverbal vocal utterances, considered by many to be the evolutionary forerunner of speech (e.g., Deacon, 1989, 1997; Jürgens, 1998; Ploog, 1992). Vocal utterances of nonhuman primates (monkeys and apes) consist of innate emotional vocalizations, such as fear, aggression, alarm, and contact calls. The two most stereotypical innate vocalizations in humans are cry-ing and laughing (e.g., Newman, 2007). Evidence suggests that the ACC plays a critical role in the voluntary initiation and suppression of these nonverbal vocal utterances (e.g., Aitken, 1981). The area does so by sending regulatory signals to the periaqueductal gray in the caudal midbrain. The periaqueductal area links emotional signals from the amygdala and other areas to the corresponding vocal responses. Also, the area links sensory stimuli, such as a heard vocal utterance, to corresponding vocal motor programs, thereby providing a low-level audio-vo-cal interface. Neighboring areas in the midbrain contain sensorimotor-orienting circuits underlying the automatic shift of gaze and attention and the turning of the head toward the sensory stimuli. The ACC signals the periaqueductal gray to initiate or withhold the motor program, depending on the context. The motor programs are embodied by premotor and motor nuclei in the lower brainstem and spinal cord (as assumed by Wernicke). The premotor nuclei coordinate the activity of the motor nuclei controlling the larynx, respiratory apparatus, and supralaryngeal tract. The three levels of vocal control (ACC, periaqueductal gray, lower brainstem nuclei) seem to be present in mammalian species as differ-ent as the cat and the bat (see Jürgens, 2002, for a review). For example, the ACC exerts control over the echolocation of bats (Duncan & Henson, 1994; Gooler & O'Neill, 1987), showing that the area also regulates noncommunicative use of the voice.

In the human speech system, the motor region of the posterior ventrolateral cortex directly projects onto the brainstem premotor and motor nuclei for the con-trol of the oral, vocal, and respiratory muscles, bypassing the periaqueductal gray. Still, the ACC may exert regulatory influences over the speech system through its connections with ventrolateral prefrontal, premotor, and motor cortex (Deacon, 1997; Jürgens, 2002; Paus, 2001). The ACC seems implicated in enhancing the activation of target representations in the ventrolateral frontal areas until retrieval and selection processes have been accomplished in accordance with the goals maintained in DLPFC (Roelofs, van Turennout, & Coles, 2006). According to this view, the ACC plays a role in the regulation of both verbal and nonverbal vocal utterances (cf. Deacon, 1989, 1997; Posner & Raichle, 1994), although through different neural pathways, as illustrated in Figure 9.3.

The activation enhancements provided by the ACC constitute a kind of driv-ing force behind vocal utterance production. This fits with the idea that for action control, it is not enough to have goals in working memory, but one should be motivated to attain them. Anatomically, the ACC is in a good position to provide such a driving force (cf. Paus, 2001). The necessary arousal may be provided through the extensive projections from the thalamus and reticular brainstem nuclei to the ACC. The information on what goals to achieve may be provided through the extensive connections between the ACC and dorsolateral prefrontal cortex. Access to the motor system by the ACC is provided by the dense projections of the motor areas of the cingulate sulcus onto the brainstem and motor cortex. The idea that the ACC provides a kind of driving force behind vocal utterance produc-tion agrees with the effect of massive damage to the ACC.

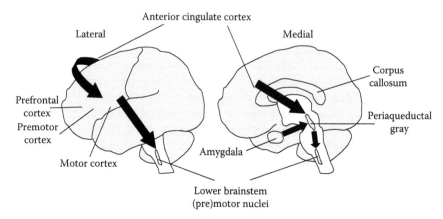

FIGURE 9.3 Illustration of the regulatory pathways of the anterior cingulate cortex in verbal (lateral view) and nonverbal vocal utterances (medial view). In verbal utterances, the ACC exerts control over lateral prefrontal, premotor, and motor cortex, which directly controls the pontine and medullary (pre)motor nuclei. In nonverbal utterances, the ACC exerts control over the periaqueductal gray.

Damage of the medial frontal cortex including the ACC typically results in transient akinetic mutism, which is characterized by reduced frequency of spontaneous speech with a preserved ability to repeat what is said (i.e., when externally triggered). The mutism arises with left or bilateral medial lesions, but damage to the right ACC may also result in transient speech aspontaneity (Chang, Lee, Lui, & Lai, 2007). Jürgens and von Cramon (1982) reported a case study of a patient with a lesion to the medial frontal cortex on the left side, which included damage to the ACC. The patient first exhibited a state of akinetic mutism during which no spontaneous vocal utterances were produced. After a few months, the patient could whisper but not produce voiced verbal utterances, which was restored only later. During the following months, the frequency of spontaneous utterances increased, but emotional intonation (e.g., an angry voice) remained impaired. A patient reported by Rubens (1975) presented with voiceless laughing and crying in the initial phase of mutism. Later, the ability to produce voiced verbal utterances was regained, but the intonation remained monotonous. According to Jürgens and von Cramon (1982), these findings indicate a role for the ACC in the volitional control of the emotional aspect of spoken utterances, but not their verbal aspect.

ROLE OF THE ACC IN ATTENTIONAL CONTROL

Although the role that I proposed for the ACC in the attentional control of both verbal and nonverbal vocal utterances seems plausible, this claim is controversial. Whereas researchers generally agree that the ACC plays a role in the attentional control of nonverbal vocal utterances, they have found no agreement on the role of the human ACC in the production of verbal vocal utterances. Some researchers deny any role for the ACC in spoken word production except for emotional aspects (e.g., Jürgens, 2002). Other researchers assume involvement of the human ACC in attentional control but disagree on whether the ACC plays a regulatory role (Posner & Raichle, 1994; Posner & Rothbart, 2007; Roelofs & Hagoort, 2002), as in call production, or a role in detecting conflict or predicting error-likelihood (Brown & Braver, 2005; Miller & Cohen, 2001; Sohn et al., 2007). I discuss the different views on the role of the human ACC in attentional control, and review brain imaging evidence from my own laboratory supporting a regulatory role of the human ACC.

EMOTIONAL VOCALIZATION

Based on three decades of electrophysiological studies of monkey vocalization, Jürgens and colleagues developed a model of the role of the ACC in vocal utterances (see Jürgens, 1998, 2002, 2009, for reviews), which has become a leading model in the literature on mammalian vocalization. This work has shown that the anterior cingulate is the only cortical area that is directly involved in call production by monkeys. Although extensive connectivity between the ACC and lateral prefrontal, premotor, and motor cortex is acknowledged (e.g., Jürgens, 2002), a role of the ACC in the control of speech is denied (Jürgens, 2002, 2009). The extensive connectivity between the ACC and lateral frontal cortex may serve functions unrelated to speech. For example, the ACC is implicated in the voluntary initiation of swallowing (Maeda et al., 2006; Watanabe, Abe, Ishikawa, Yamada, & Yamane, 2004).

However, given the neuroimaging evidence on word production reviewed above, it seems difficult to maintain that the ACC plays no role in spoken word production. Vocalization, like swallowing, requires the coordinated activity of the oral, vocal, and respiratory muscles. Since swallowing and breathing are exclusive activities, the larynx plays a critical role in gating access to the respiratory tract. MacNeilage (1998) suggested that ingestion-related capabilities in lateral frontal cortex associated with chewing, sucking, and licking were modified in human evolution to serve a role in speaking. The extensive connectivity between de ACC and lateral frontal cortex, including Broca's area and the larynx motor cortex, may have become exploited in the control of speech production (cf. Ploog, 1992). Clearly, the ACC is involved in speech production only under certain circumstances, namely when utterance production requires attentional control. However, a circumscribed role of the ACC is also observed in call production, where the area plays a role only in the contextual regulation of vocalization, but not in their production per se.

REGULATION VERSUS CONFLICT DETECTION

Whereas Jürgens (2002, 2009) denies any role for the ACC in spoken word production, other researchers assume involvement of the human ACC but disagree on whether the area plays a regulatory role (Posner & Raichle, 1994; Posner & Rothbart, 2007; Roelofs & Hagoort, 2002) or a role in detecting conflict or predicting error-likelihood. According to the latter view, the ACC is involved in performance monitoring (Miller & Cohen, 2001). In particular, ACC activity reflects the detection of response conflict and acts as a signal that engages attentional control processes subserved by LPFC.

In a review of the monkey literature on the control of gaze by the frontal lobes, Schall and Boucher (2007) conclude that neurons in the supplementary eye field (part of the medial frontal cortex) exhibit activity specifically related to response conflict, but neurons in the ACC do not. The ACC neurons only reflect the amount of control exerted. This conclusion was surprising given that the conflict detection hypothesis is the dominant view on ACC function in the literature on humans. According to Schall and Boucher, the difference between monkeys (control-related activity but no conflict-related activity in the ACC) and humans (ACC conflict detection) may reflect differences in species, tasks, or effectors. For example, monkey studies have typically employed saccadic stop-signal tasks, in which conflict is evoked by infrequently presenting a stop signal while preparation of a saccade is in progress. In contrast, human studies have typically employed Stroop-like tasks with vocal or manual responding. For example, in the color-word Stroop task, participants name the ink color of congruent or incongruent color words (e.g., the word RED printed in green), whereby vocal responding is slower in the incongruent than the congruent condition. In the arrow-word version of this task, the stimuli consist of incongruent and congruent combinations of left- or right-pointing arrows and the words LEFT or RIGHT, and the participants respond by pressing a left or right response button. According to Schall and Boucher, it is possible that the saccadic responses in monkey studies yielded less conflict than the vocal and manual responses in human studies, explaining the difference in results between monkeys and humans.

However, it is also possible that the difference in results between monkeys and humans has another ground, namely a confound between conflict and control in the human studies. Incongruent and congruent stimuli not only differ in the amount of conflict they evoke, but also in the amount of attentional control required by the corresponding responses. Thus, the conflict-related activity in Stroop-like tasks is compatible with both the regulative and conflict detection hypotheses on ACC function. It is possible to discriminate between the two hypotheses empirically by using neutral stimuli. A critical prediction made by the conflict hypothesis is that ACC activity should be increased only when conflicting response alternatives are present (e.g., in responding to the word LEFT combined with a right-pointing arrow). ACC activity should not differ between congruent trials (e.g., the word LEFT combined with a left-pointing arrow) and neutral trials (e.g., the word LEFT only), because competing response alternatives are absent on both trial types. In contrast, the regulatory hypothesis (Posner & Raichle, 1994; Posner & Rothbart, 2007; Roelofs & Hagoort, 2002) not only predicts more ACC activity on incongruent than on neutral trials, but also less ACC activity on congruent than on neutral trials. Less ACC activity is predicted because the correct response (left) is already activated by the distractor (a left-pointing arrow) on congruent trials and therefore less enhancement of the target is required.

To test between the conflict detection and regulation hypotheses about ACC function, Roelofs et al. (2006) conducted a functional magnetic resonance imaging (fMRI) study. Participants were scanned while they were presented with arrow-word combinations. The participants were asked to communicate the direction denoted by the word by pressing a left or right button using the index and middle fingers of their left hand. A meta-analysis of the existing neuroimaging literature and the results from a new neuroimaging experiment by Barch et al. (2001) has shown that Stroop-like tasks activate the dorsal ACC regardless of whether the direction of the word is communicated through a spoken or manual response. On incongruent trials in the experiment of Roelofs et al. (2006), the word and the arrow designated opposite responses. On congruent trials, the word and arrow designated the same response. On neutral trials, a word was presented in combination with a straight line, so only one response was designated by the stimulus. Congruent, incongruent, and neutral trials were presented rapidly in a randomly intermixed order. The response time data showed that, consistent with earlier findings (e.g., Roelofs, 2003 for a review), responses to the words were much slower on incongruent than on neutral trials and fastest on congruent trials. The neuroimaging data demonstrated that activity in the ACC was larger on incongruent than on congruent trials. The same held for activity in the LPFC. Importantly, ACC activity was larger for neutral than for congruent stimuli, in the absence of response conflict. This result demonstrates the engagement of the ACC in the regulation of communicative responses. This conclusion was corroborated by successful WEAVER++ simulations of the chronometric and neuroimaging findings (Roelofs et al., 2006).

ANTICIPATORY ADJUSTMENTS

People are often faced with circumstances in which certain vocal behaviors are inappropriate, such as laughing at a funeral or talking aloud in a library. This raises the question whether the ACC is also involved in adjusting the control settings for responding (e.g., raising the response thresholds) depending on the communicative situation. Sohn et al. (2007) proposed that the ACC plays a role in signaling upcoming response conflict. Brown and Braver (2005) argued that the ACC signals upcoming error likelihood, independent of response conflict. More generally, environmental cues may provide information about which type of stimulus is coming and, as a consequence, about which control setting is most appropriate for responding to the stimulus. However, these contextual cues do not necessarily have to predict response conflict or error likelihood. This raises the question whether anticipatory activity in the ACC may be obtained independent of upcoming conflict or error likelihood. Aarts, Roelofs, and Van Turennout (2008) conducted an fMRI experiment that examined this issue.

As in the study of Roelofs et al. (2006), participants were scanned while they were presented with arrow-word combinations. Again, the index and middle fingers of the left hand were used for responding. On each trial, the participants were now informed about the arrow-word stimulus conditions by means of symbolic cues, which were presented well before the arrow-word stimulus. The cue was a colored square that indicated whether the upcoming arrow-word stimulus was congruent, incongruent, or neutral, or the cue provided no information about the upcoming condition. Green squares were always preceding congruent stimuli, red squares preceded incongruent stimuli, and yellow squares preceded neutral stimuli. The uninformative cues were grey squares, which could be followed by any of the stimulus types.

If the ACC plays a role in anticipatory adjustments in control, ACC activity should be higher in response to informative cues than to uninformative cues. If the adjustments are independent of response conflict or error likelihood, enhanced ACC activity should be obtained for cues preceding congruent stimuli. Adjustments are expected in premotor cortex, where response rules are implemented (Wallis & Miller, 2003). An informative cue preceding an incongruent stimulus might encourage participants to weaken the connections between the arrows and their responses, because the arrows elicit the wrong response. However, an informative cue preceding a congruent target might encourage participants to strengthen the connections between the arrows and the corresponding responses, because the arrows now elicit the correct response. In WEAVER++, the adjustments may be achieved by condition-action rules specifying that,

> IF the goal is to indicate the direction denoted by the word,
> and the cue is green,
> THEN strengthen the connection between arrows and responses.

If such advance adjustments are successful, ACC activity should exhibit smaller differences among target conditions in response to the arrow-word stimuli after informative cues (when control was adjusted in advance) than following uninformative cues (when control was not adjusted in advance).

Aarts et al. (2008) observed that participants responded faster to the arrow-word stimuli after informative than uninformative cues, indicating cue-based adjustments in control. Moreover, ACC activity was larger following informative than uninformative cues, as would be expected if the ACC is involved in anticipatory control. Importantly, this activation in the ACC was observed for informative cues even when the information conveyed by the cue was that the upcoming arrow-word stimulus evokes no response conflict and has low error likelihood. This finding demonstrates that the ACC is involved in anticipatory control processes independent of upcoming response conflict or error likelihood. Moreover, the response of the ACC to the target stimuli was critically dependent upon whether the cue was informative or not. ACC activity differed among target conditions after uninformative cues only, indicating ACC involvement in actual control adjustments. Taken together, these findings argue strongly for a role of the ACC in anticipatory control independent of anticipated conflict and error likelihood, and also show that such control can eliminate conflict-related ACC activity during target processing.

Premotor cortex activity should reflect the operation of control in response to informative cues. Therefore, we expected a positive correlation between cue-related ACC and premotor activity. The correlation should be confined to the right premotor cortex, contralateral to the response hand. Correlation analyses confirmed that cue-based activity in the ACC was positively correlated with activity in the dorsal premotor cortex and the supplementary motor area contralateral to the response hand. Although several other frontal areas were active in response to the cues, no correlations between cue-based ACC activity and the other regions were found. These results provide evidence for a direct influence of the ACC over premotor cortex (cf. Figure 9.3).

SUMMARY AND CONCLUSIONS

This chapter outlined the classic model of Wernicke (1874) for the functional neuroanatomy of vocal utterance production and comprehension, and Wundt's (1900, 1904) critique that the model lacks attentional control mechanisms, which he localized in the frontal lobes. Next, the WEAVER++ model (Roelofs, 1992, 2003, 2007) was described, which builds in many respects on Wernicke's ideas but also addresses Wundt's critique by implementing assumptions on attentional control. Characteristics of utterance production by healthy and brain-damaged individuals arise from the interplay of a perisylvian production-perception network and the frontal attentional control system. I indicated that controversy exists about the role of one of the frontal areas, the ACC. Whereas some researchers deny any role for the ACC in spoken word production, other researchers assume involvement of the area but disagree on whether it plays a regulatory role, as in call production, or a role in detecting conflict or predicting error-likelihood. I reviewed evidence for a regulatory role of the ACC.

Aphasiologists agree that a good theoretical model is important for therapy (e.g., Basso & Marangolo, 2000; Nickels, 1997, 2002). However, according to Nickels (2002), "One of the limitations remains that while theories of language processing are becoming increasingly specified (e.g., Levelt et al., 1999), how these models will function once damaged is not at all clear (but see Dell et al., 1997, for a computationally implemented theory that has investigated the effects of "lesioning"" (p. 955). Given the importance of modeling for therapy, future research should further theoretically analyze and model vocal utterance production and its attentional control, impairments, and their interactions. I hope this chapter has provided some helpful hints for this research and for clinical practice.

ACKNOWLEDGMENT

The preparation of the chapter was supported by a VICI grant from the Netherlands Organisation for Scientific Research (NWO).

REFERENCES

Aarts, E., Roelofs, A., & Van Turennout, M. (2008). Anticipatory activity in anterior cingulate cortex can be independent of conflict and error likelihood. *Journal of Neuroscience, 28*, 4671–4678.

Aitken, P. G. (1981). Cortical control of conditioned and spontaneous vocal behavior in rhesus monkeys. *Brain and Language, 13*, 171–184.

Badre, D., Poldrack, R. A., Paré-Blagoev, E., Insler, R. Z., & Wagner, A. D. (2005). Dissociable controlled retrieval and generalized selection mechanisms in ventrolateral prefrontal cortex. *Neuron, 47*, 907–918.

Barch, D. M., Braver, T. S., Akbudak, E., Conturo, T., Ollinger, J., & Snyder, A. (2001). Anterior cingulate cortex and response conflict: Effects of response modality and processing domain. *Cerebral Cortex, 11*, 837–848.

Basso, A., & Marangolo, P. (2000). Cognitive neuropsychological rehabilitation: The emperor's new clothes? *Neuropsychological Rehabilitation, 10*, 219–230.

Brown, J. W., & Braver, T. S. (2005). Learned predictions of error likelihood in the anterior cingulate cortex. *Science, 307*, 1118–1121.

Bunge, S. A. (2004). How we use rules to select actions: A review of evidence from cognitive neuroscience. *Cognitive, Affective, & Behavioral Neuroscience, 4*, 564–579.

Bunge, S. A., Kahn, I., Wallis, J. D., Miller, E. K., & Wagner, A. D. (2003). Neural circuits subserving the retrieval and maintenance of abstract rules. *Journal of Neurophysiology, 90*, 3419–3428.

Caplan, D. (1992). *Language: Structure, processing, and disorders.* Cambridge, MA: MIT Press.

Chang, C.-C., Lee, Y. C., Lui, C.-C., & Lai, S.-L. (2007). Right anterior cingulate cortex infarction and transient speech aspontaneity. *Archives of Neurology, 64*, 442–446.

Cohen, L., Henry, C., Dehaene, S., Martinaud, O., Lehéricy, S., Lemer, C., & Ferrieux, S. (2004). The pathophysiology of letter-by-letter reading. *Neuropsychologia, 42*, 1768–1780.

Coltheart, M., Rastle, K., Perry, C., Langdon, R., & Ziegler, J. (2001). DRC: A dual route cascaded model of visual word recognition and reading aloud. *Psychological Review, 108*, 204–256.

Deacon, T. W. (1989). The neural circuitry underlying primate calls and human language. *Human Evolution, 4*, 367–401.

Deacon, T. W. (1997). *The symbolic species: The co-evolution of language and the brain.* New York, NY: Norton.

Dell, G. S., Schwartz, M. F., Martin, N., Saffran, E. M., & Gagnon, D. A. (1997). Lexical access in aphasic and nonaphasic speakers. *Psychological Review, 104*, 801–838.

de Zubicaray, G. I., Wilson, S. J., McMahon, K. K., & Muthiah, S. (2001). The semantic interference effect in the picture-word paradigm: An event-related fMRI study employing overt responses. *Human Brain Mapping, 14*, 218–227.

Duncan, G. E., & Henson, O. W. (1994). Brain activity patterns in flying, echolocating bats (*Pteronotus parnellii*): Assessed by high resolution autoradiographic imaging with [³H]2-deoxyglucose. *Neuroscience, 59*, 1051–1070.

Gooler, D. M., & O'Neill, W. E. (1987). Topographic representation of vocal frequency demonstrated by microstimulation of anterior cingulate cortex in the echolocating bat, *Pteronotus parnelli parnelli*. *Journal of Comparative Physiology A, 161*, 283–294.

Henry, C., Gaillard, R., Volle, E., Chiras, J., Ferrieux, S., Dehaene, S., & Cohen, L. (2005). Brain activations during letter-by-letter reading: A follow-up study. *Neuropsychologia, 43*, 1983–1989.

Humphreys, G. W., & Forde, E. M. E. (2005). Naming a giraffe but not an animal: Basic-level but not superordinate naming in a patient with impaired semantics. *Cognitive Neuropsychology, 22*, 539–558.

Indefrey, P., & Levelt, W. J. M. (2004). The spatial and temporal signatures of word production components. *Cognition, 92*, 101–144.

Jürgens, U. (1998). Speech evolved from vocalization, not mastication. *Behavioral and Brain Sciences, 21*, 519–520.

Jürgens, U. (2002). Neural pathways underlying vocal control. *Neuroscience and Biobehavioral Reviews, 26*, 235–258.

Jürgens, U. (2009). The neural control of vocalization in mammals: A review. *Journal of Voice, 23*, 1–10.

Jürgens, U., & von Cramon, D. (1982). On the role of the anterior cingulate cortex in phonation: A case report. *Brain and Language, 15*, 234–248.

Kan, I. P., & Thompson-Schill, S. L. (2004). Effect of name agreement on prefrontal activity during overt and covert picture naming. *Cognitive, Affective, & Behavioral Neuroscience, 4*, 43–57.

Kane, M. J., & Engle, R. W. (2002). The role of prefrontal cortex in working-memory capacity, executive attention, and general fluid intelligence: An individual-differences perspective. *Psychonomic Bulletin and Review, 9*, 637–671.

Levelt, W. J. M., Roelofs, A., & Meyer, A. S. (1999). A theory of lexical access in speech production. *Behavioral and Brain Sciences, 22*, 1–38.

MacNeilage, P. F. (1998). The frame/content theory of evolution of speech production. *Behavioral and Brain Sciences, 21*, 499–511.

Maeda, K., Takashi, O., Shinagawa, H., Honda, E., Kurabayashi, T., & Ohyama, K. (2006). Role of the anterior cingulate cortex in volitional swallowing: An electromyographic and functional magnetic resonance imaging study. *Journal of Medical and Dental Sciences, 53*, 149–157.

Maril, A., Wagner, A. D., & Schacter, D. L. (2001). On the tip of the tongue: An event-related fMRI study of semantic retrieval failure and cognitive conflict. *Neuron, 31*, 653–660.

Martin, R. C. (2003). Language processing: Functional organization and neuroanatomical basis. *Annual Review of Psychology, 54*, 55–89.

Miller, E. K., & Cohen, J. D. (2001). An integrative theory of prefrontal cortex function. *Annual Review of Neuroscience, 24*, 167–202.

Newman, J. D. (2007). Neural circuits underlying crying and cry responding in mammals. *Behavioural Brain Research, 182*, 155–165.

Nickels, L. (1997). *Spoken word production and its breakdown in aphasia.* Hove, UK: Psychology Press.

Nickels, L. (2002). Therapy for naming disorders: Revisiting, revising, and reviewing. *Aphasiology, 16*, 935–979.

Norman, D. A., & Shallice, T. (1986). Attention to action: Willed and automatic control of behavior. In R. J. Davidson, G. E. Schwarts, & D. Shapiro (Eds.), *Consciousness and self-regulation: Advances in research and theory* (pp. 1–18). New York, NY: Plenum Press.

Paus, T. (2001). Primate anterior cingulate cortex: Where motor control, drive and cognition interface. *Nature Reviews Neuroscience, 2*, 417–424.

Petersen, S. E., Fox, P. T., Posner, M. I., Mintun, M., & Raichle, M. E. (1988). Positron emission tomographic studies of the cortical anatomy of single-word processing. *Nature, 331*, 585–589.

Petersen, S. E., van Mier, H., Fiez, J. A., & Raichle, M. E. (1998). The effects of practice on the functional anatomy of task performance. *Proceedings of the National Academy of Sciences USA, 95*, 853–860.

Ploog, D. W. (1992). The evolution of vocal communication. In H. Papoušek, U. Jürgens, & M. Papoušek (Eds.), *Nonverbal vocal communication: Comparative and developmental approaches* (pp. 6–30). Cambridge, UK: Cambridge University Press.

Posner, M. I., & Raichle, M. E. (1994). *Images of mind.* New York, NY: W. H. Freeman.

Posner, M. I., & Rothbart, M. K. (2007). *Educating the human brain.* Washington, DC: APA Books.

Raichle, M. E., Fiez, J. A., Videen, T. O., MacLeod, A.-M. K., Pardo, J. V., Fox, P. T., & Petersen, S. E. (1994). Practice-related changes in human brain functional anatomy during nonmotor learning. *Cerebral Cortex, 4*, 8–26.

Rapp, B. (Ed.). (2001). *What deficits reveal about the human mind/brain: A handbook of cognitive neuropsychology.* Philadelphia, PA: Psychology Press.

Rapp, B., & Goldrick, M. (2000). Discreteness and interactivity in spoken word production. *Psychological Review, 107*, 460–499.

Roelofs, A. (1992). A spreading-activation theory of lemma retrieval in speaking. *Cognition, 42*, 107–142.

Roelofs, A. (1997). The WEAVER model of word-form encoding in speech production. *Cognition, 64*, 249–284.

Roelofs, A. (2003). Goal-referenced selection of verbal action: Modeling attentional control in the Stroop task. *Psychological Review, 110*, 88–125.

Roelofs, A. (2004). Error biases in spoken word planning and monitoring by aphasic and nonaphasic speakers: Comment on Rapp and Goldrick (2000). *Psychological Review, 111*, 561–572.

Roelofs, A. (2005). The visual-auditory color-word Stroop asymmetry and its time course. *Memory & Cognition, 33*, 1325–1336.

Roelofs, A. (2006). Context effects of pictures and words in naming objects, reading words, and generating simple phrases. *Quarterly Journal of Experimental Psychology, 59*, 1764–1784.

Roelofs, A. (2007). Attention and gaze control in picture naming, word reading, and word categorizing. *Journal of Memory and Language, 57*, 232–251.

Roelofs, A., & Hagoort, P. (2002). Control of language use: Cognitive modeling of the hemodynamics of Stroop task performance. *Cognitive Brain Research, 15*, 85–97.

Roelofs, A., van Turennout, M., & Coles, M. G. H. (2006). Anterior cingulate cortex activity can be independent of response conflict in Stroop-like tasks. *Proceedings of the National Academy of Sciences USA, 103*, 13884–13889.

Rubens, A. B. (1975). Aphasia with infarction in the territory of the anterior cerebral artery. *Cortex, 11*, 239–250.

Schall, J. D., & Boucher, L. (2007). Executive control of gaze by the frontal lobes. *Cognitive, Affective, & Behavioral Neuroscience, 7*, 396–412.

Shallice, T. (1988). *From neuropsychology to mental structure.* Cambridge, UK: Cambridge University Press.

Snyder, A. Z., Abdullaev, Y. G., Posner, M. I., & Raichle, M. E. (1995). Scalp electrical potentials reflect regional cerebral blood flow responses during processing of written words. *Proceedings of the National Academy of Sciences USA, 92*, 1689–1693.

Sohn, M.-H., Albert, M. V., Jung, K., Carter, C. S., & Anderson, J. R. (2007). Anticipation of conflict monitoring in the anterior cingulate cortex and the prefrontal cortex. *Proceedings of the National Academy of Sciences USA, 104,* 10330–10334.

Taub, E., Uswatte, G., & Elbert, T. (2002). New treatments in neurorehabilitation founded on basic research. *Nature Review Neuroscience, 3,* 228–236.

Thompson-Schill, S. L., D'Esposito, M., Aguirre, G. K., & Farah, M. J. (1997). Role of left inferior prefrontal cortex in retrieval of semantic knowledge: A reevaluation. *Proceedings of the National Academy of Sciences USA, 94,* 14792–14797.

Wallis, J. D., & Miller, E. K. (2003). From rule to response: Neuronal processes in the premotor and prefrontal cortex. *Journal of Neurophysiology, 90,* 1790–1806.

Wallis, J. D., Anderson, K. C., & Miller, E. (2001). Single neurons in prefrontal cortex encode abstract rules. *Nature, 411,* 953–956.

Watanabe, Y., Abe, S., Ishikawa, T., Yamada, Y., & Yamane, G. (2004). Cortical regulation during the early stage of initiation of voluntary swallowing in humans. *Dysphagia, 19,* 100–108.

Wernicke, C. (1874). *The aphasia symptom-complex: A psychological study on an anatomical basis.* Breslau, Germany: Cohn & Weigert.

Wernicke, C. (1885). Some new studies on aphasia. *Fortschritte der Medizin, 3,* 824–830.

Wernicke, C. (1886). Some new studies on aphasia. *Fortschritte der Medizin, 4,* 371–377, 463–469.

Wundt, W. (1900). *Language.* Leipzig, Germany: Verlag von Wilhelm Engelmann.

Wundt, W. (1904). *Principles of physiological psychology.* London, UK: Swan Sonnenschein.

10 Theories of Semantic Processing

John Shelley-Tremblay

INTRODUCTION

Semantics, broadly defined refers to meaning. The study of semantics has been important in the fields of linguistics, rhetoric, law, philosophy, and political science as far back as the ancient Greeks. For the modern student of communication disorders, the study of semantics is critical for understanding the nature of any given language deficit. Why is this? It is because the intention of any communicative act ultimately is to convey meaning. The most common way that semantics impact communication disorders is that in both developmental and acquired disorders of language, there can be observed some abnormality with either the structure of, or access to, concepts or their interconnections. The semantic system is one way that humans store information in memory, and as such semantic problems are memory problems. This chapter will review the most influential and widely researched theories of semantic representation. By the end of this chapter you will be familiar with local and distributed models as well as the concept of spreading activation. Further reading (e.g., Chapters 6, 11, and 12) will show that problems with semantics have been implicated in many of the most common disorders that a speech pathologist or other communication disorders professional will have to deal with on a regular basis, including the aphasias and Alzheimer's disease (AD).

Semantic memory has been conceptualized as a system for representing general world knowledge, linguistic skill, and aspects of vocabulary (Collins & Loftus, 1975; Moss, Tyler, & Jennings, 1997; Zurif, Caramazza, Myerson, & Galvin, 1974). This can be contrasted with episodic memory, which can be thought of as autobiographical memory for contextually specific events (Heilman & Valenstein, 1993; Tulving, 1984; Tulving & Thomson, 1973). Semantic memory is often thought of as the end result of a person's abstracting the relevant information from multiple learning experiences. For example, as a young child encounters dogs for the first time, she may begin to notice that all dogs have certain visual, structural, and functional features in common. She may also notice that dogs occur in certain contexts, emit specific noises, and may be associated with some of the goals of the child, such as throwing Frisbees or taking a walk. All of this information may become incorporated into different aspects of semantic memory, but the emphasis would not be on what specific dog could catch Frisbees or when this dog was first seen. Instead the semantic system would specialize in storing the information about dogs, in general, and how they are related to the rest of the world.

In his introduction to a special issue of *Brain and Language* on the investigation of lexical semantic representation in AD, Henderson (1996) states that four general issues are of central importance to the current study of lexical semantic representation: (1) What are the processes by which semantic information comes to be stored in the lexicon? (2) How is meaning represented in the lexicon (what is its nature)? (3) How is this knowledge accessed and retrieved? (4) How do other cognitive operations affect these lexical semantic processes? It is the purpose of this chapter to address the state of the understanding of these issues, with a focus on issue number 2, as it bears most strongly on all others. Semantic priming is the most common technique for investigating issues number 2 and 3. This chapter will examine local- and feature-based models first and conclude with a discussion of distributed models of semantics.

THE LEXICON VERSUS THE SEMANTIC SYSTEM

Often times in published research the terms lexical and semantic are used interchangeably, and/or indiscriminately (Brown & Hagoort, 1993; Deacon, Hewitt, Yang, & Nagata, 2000; Holcomb, 1993). The reason for this seems to be an insufficient empirical basis upon which to discriminate between these closely related constructs. The lexicon refers specifically to a dictionary-like cognitive information structure that contains a person's vocabulary, including the morphology, argument structure, thematic role, and "meaning" of a vocabulary item. A conceptualization of the place of the lexicon in relationship to the rest of the language system is shown in Figure 10.1.

The difficulty with saying that any lexical item contains the meaning of a concept is that all meanings are dependent upon their relationships to other concepts. Thus the lexical "definition" of any concept may best be thought of as an organized system of "pointers" to other concepts, or alternately, as the convergence of multiple concepts to form a unique reference. For example, one would not normally be said to know about the concept "dog" without an understanding of some of the critical components of a dog, including: four legs, a tail, teeth, and so on. While "dog" is more than a collection of other concepts (a dog is not just a large cat with hair instead of fur, even though they are related and share many features), an understanding of "dog" rests on an understanding of its components. This notion is explored more below, in the section that critiques featural theories of meaning.

For the discussion that follows on local semantic systems, lexical and semantic may be interchangeable because any test of the semantic system must necessarily be carried out through access to the lexicon. As yet, I am unaware of any experimental manipulation that can achieve semantic access without lexical access first occurring. Even in the case of shapes or pictures serving as primes (Rock & Gutman, 1981), it is possible that the priming observed is a result of the pictorial codes activating the propositional codes stored in the lexical system. This is only a concern if one takes the "dual code" stance on the issue of multiple codes versus a unitary code for information storage in cortex (Kosslyn, 1981). If one takes the

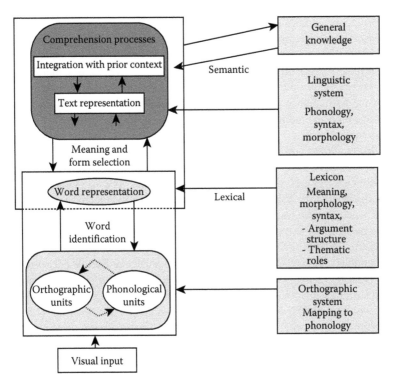

FIGURE 10.1 A schematic representation of the reader. The left column represents a sequential stream of hypothesized processing and representational stages as the language system processes a visually presented word. The right column refers to the general cognitive system that is subserved by the stages on the left. (Based on Perfetti, 2000, in Brown, C., and Hagoort, P., Eds., *The Neurocognition of Language*. Oxford.)

position that all information is represented in an elaborated propositional format (Paivio, 1991), then the idea of pictorial, auditory, and even somatosensory stimuli all converging on a single lexical system that serves to index semantic relationships is unproblematic.

MODELS OF SEMANTIC MEMORY

The dominant models of semantic memory that have appeared over the last four decades can be roughly divided into one of two types: local or distributed. These terms have been applied to a wide variety of models of semantic memory, and as a result it is possible to become confused about what stands as the defining features of these two types. At the most elementary level, local models are defined as ones in which each "concept" in semantic memory has a unique location, or "node" in memory, while distributed systems posit that the same representational structures subserve multiple "concepts." Concepts, as defined in Collins and Loftus's (1975) local theory, are "particular senses of words or phrases." For example, "car," "driving a car," and "the particular car that I own" could all be thought of as concepts. Certainly this is an extremely flexible and underspecified notion of a concept. At the core of both local and distributed models (which make few revisions to the construct of "concept") is a poor operational definition of a key aspect of the theory. This situation is similar, by analogy, to a theory of chemistry that makes no distinction between atoms and molecules, or acknowledges a distinction, but makes no attempt to look for functional differences between basic and conglomerated units.

A discussion of how this definitional deficiency may be addressed follows in the next section of the chapter. For now, setting aside this issue, an attempt to further delineate these classes of theory must be made. The whole notion of local versus distributed representation of information has a long history, and within the neurosciences can be traced back to the early aphasiologists. The heart of the difference between these types lies in the debate between the localizationists (Gaul & Spurzheim, 1810–1819; Geschwind, 1965) and those who adhere to the doctrine of mass action (Lashley, 1938). Localizationists, in particular Barlow (1972) generally believe that individual neurons are capable of a high degree of coding specificity, such that a single neuron, or small group of neurons, would fire in response to a particular stimulus, and no other. The ubiquitous example of this doctrine is the notion of a "grandmother cell," which is sensitive only to the face of one's own grandmother. While this particular cell has not been found, similar instances of neuronal specificity have been discovered, such as a "monkey-hand cell," which responds most strongly to the image of a hand from its own species (Hinton, Anderson, Hinton, & Anderson, 1989). This example may be instructive of the way that the brain can represent so many unique concepts. It seems that the cortex is structured to create fairly specific coding mechanisms for the different basic stimuli that are encountered frequently, and that have a high survival value to the organism, such as the orientation sensitive cells described in cat visual cortex by Hubel and Wiesel (1979). This does not imply, however, that the majority of abstract semantic concepts would have their own neuron population assigned to them.

LOCAL MODELS

In discussing local semantic models, such as the most well-known version proposed by Collins and Quillian (1969) and Collins and Loftus (1975), the basic idea of a "node" may be somewhat incompatible with current conceptions of neuroanatomy/ physiology. To the extent that Collins and Loftus (1975) is a Human Information Processing model (Neisser, 1967) that seeks only to provide a functional description of how the mind processes symbols, this discrepancy is unproblematic. However, if any modern theory wishes to employ models that can accommodate and integrate data from a wide range of sources, including the neurosciences, then the local models deserve a considerable revisiting. Such examination of the tenets of local theories has been attempted for the purposes of computational simulation Fahlman, Hinton, and Anderson (1989), and word recognition (Rumelhart & McClelland, 1986), but few authors have systematically attempted to create a local model that is

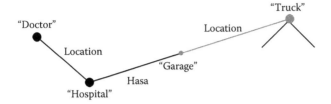

FIGURE 10.2   A portion of a local neural network. Words in parentheses indicate concepts that are represented in nodes (circles). The lines associate connections of the sort indicated by the labels, such as "DOCTOR" and "HOSPITAL" are related in that a doctor is found at the location, hospital. Strongly associated words are usually depicted as being closer together in the network. (Based on Collins, A. M. and Loftus, E. F., *Psychol. Rev.*, 82, 407–428, 1975.).

both functionally descriptive of the vast body of experimental literature, as well as biologically plausible.

Perhaps the real appeal of the local models is in their conceptual and diagrammatic simplicity. As seen in Figure 10.2, concepts are represented as circles, which depict a unique informational location or node. These nodes are then connected through links that determine the strength, as well as the type, of the relationship between the nodes. The Collins and Quillian formulation of a semantic network allowed for five basic types of relationships, as well as for viewing links as a type of node, or concept, in themselves. Again, the advantage is flexibility, but the disadvantage is that it is difficult to conceive of experiments that could disconfirm such a flexible theory in a way that would require it to be discarded. Perhaps the best candidate for such experiments to date has been those involving the interposition of an unrelated intervening item between the first and second stimuli in a semantic priming paradigm. These studies will be discussed in detail below, but unfortunately have yielded highly mixed results.

In addition to the Collins and Loftus (1975) model and the Posner and Snyder (1975) model that introduced the element of controlled processing into semantic network theory, the models of J. R. Anderson (1974, 1976, 1983; Anderson & Reder, 1999) were based on the assumption of spreading activation through a local network. Anderson's main finding was that a "fan effect" occurred in which the ease of recognition of a target item was inversely related to the number of concepts that it was associated to during a study phase. This effect, expressed most completely in the Adaptive Control of Thought (ACT; J. R. Anderson, 1983) and ACT-R (J. R. Anderson, 1993) theories, provided support for the notion that when a word stimulus is presented, then its corresponding representation becomes activated. This activation is finite, similar to an electrical charge, and it then spreads out to all related concepts automatically. According to ACT, because the activation is of finite level and duration, the larger the number of related concepts, the smaller amount of activation any one related concept would receive. This proposition is expressed most basically as:

$$A_i = B_i + 3W_jS_{ji}.$$

Where latency to retrieve any piece of information from memory is determined by its current activation level, A_i, which is equal to the base level of activation B_i (determined by factors including recency and frequency of study), plus the sum of j concepts that make up the probe stimulus. The W_j indicates the amount of attention given any one source of information in the probe, and S_{ji} equals the strength of association between source j and piece of information i. This equation is best illustrated in the simple propositional statements often used by Anderson, such as "A hippie is in the park." When hippie is paired with park, house, and bank (3 pairs) during study, it takes longer to retrieve than if it was presented as paired with park alone (1 pair).

The utility of this mathematical formulation is that it has allowed Anderson and others (M. C. Anderson & Spellman, 1995; Radvansky, Spieler, & Zacks, 1993) to test their reaction time and accuracy results against both the qualitative and quantitative predictions of the model. The results of such analyses over multiple experiments have lead, generally, to a confirmation of the feasibility of spreading activation as a mechanism for explaining relationships between items in associative memory (J. R. Anderson & Reder, 1999). In a recent series of articles, M. C. Anderson and his associates have proposed that the fan effect can be equally well explained in terms of inhibitory processes (see M. C. Anderson & Spelman, 1995 for a summary), as opposed to a simple dilution of facilitation across multiple items. In a paradigm similar to the typical study-and-test method of Anderson, these authors had participants practice particular associations to a category heading, for example, study "blood" and "tomato" for the category "red." One of the associates received more practice (here, blood), and subjects demonstrated an (unsurprising) boost in recall for that item. Interestingly, the less studied item (here, tomato) not only yielded poorer recall performance, but novel members of the same category as the less studied item also showed a recall decrement at test. For instance, the red food "strawberry" was more difficult to recall than another food (crackers) that did not fit into the category of red. While ACT-R did not predict such an effect, the presence of inhibition is in no way incompatible with spreading activation, assuming that the locus of the inhibition can be shown to operate in a manner that modulates, not replaces, automatic spreading of activation. Anderson and Reder (1999) argue that their model can accomplish this theoretical feat with a minimum of adjustment. While the last 30 years have produced relatively little change in the basic conceptualization of the local semantic network as a series of nodes over which activation spreads, the field has been rife with alternative explanations for the priming effect that has been the primary tool for the study of semantic networks.

WORD IDENTIFICATION AND MODELS OF SEMANTIC PRIMING

Semantic information can be thought of as just another type of data that is processed by the human brain on a regular basis. Thus there is the input of semantic information from the environment, most often in the form of written or spoken words, as well as the storage of semantic information, and the use of semantics by output systems to create meaningful writing and speech. It is to the first task of identifying words and extracting their meaning that we now turn our attention. Researchers have used a single experimental technique above all others in the past 35 years to investigate the process of word recognition: semantic priming.

Semantic priming refers to the processing advantage that occurs when a word (the target) is preceded by another word (the prime) when it is related in meaning to the target. The nature of the meaning relationship can be one or more of the following, but is not limited to: shared physical, functional, or visual features, membership in the same semantic category, or a simple associative relationship, such as ice cream scoop. An example of a typical semantic priming sequence is presented in Figure 10.3.

The phenomenon of priming has become ubiquitous with cognitive psychology, and the existence of positive semantic priming has been solidly established. The nature of the operations behind semantic priming, on the other hand, is far from completely understood. What one believes is taking place during semantic priming depends on one's view of the nature of semantic representation, as well as what operations are believed to be going on during the specific task that the subject is required to do. This is because the strength and direction of priming effects vary greatly with the subject's task, as well as the stimulus and display parameters involved in task presentation. With that in mind, we can begin to review some of the most influential theories of priming, and then discuss the most common parameters that have been found to influence priming in meaningful ways.

As mentioned above, perhaps the best known theory of semantic priming is that of Collins and Loftus (1975). Their explanation of semantic priming rested

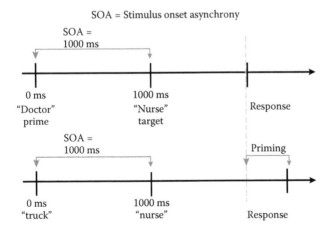

FIGURE 10.3   The target word, "NURSE", is preceded by a related prime, "DOCTOR", in the top time line. In the bottom time line, the target word is preceded by an unrelated prime, "TRUCK." The subject is asked to make a speeded response to the target word. A reduction in RT to the target is taken as an indication of the primes facilitative effect on the target.

on (1) their proposal that semantic information is best described as being organized as a local network (see above), and (2) their notion of how the search of
this network takes place. When a word is presented to a subject, for instance the
prime "DOCTOR," then the activation generated by the lexical identification of
the stimulus begins to radiate out to all related concepts through the series of
associative links described above. These authors proposed that, in addition to the
nodes and links just described, a system of "tags" should be included that function to mark the path that spreading activation follows. As spreading activation
travels, it leaves behind a trace (tag) that indicates not only its node of origin, but
the last node that it had just passed through.

When the target is presented, the subject is supposed to initiate a search of
their semantic memory in order to find the lexical entry of the word, in the case
of a lexical decision task, or in order to find the word's semantic properties, such
as its associates, in the case of a semantic relatedness judgment task. This theory
was designed to account for data in semantic verification tasks of the sort, "All
apples are fruit." In order to check for the truth of this proposition, the subject is
supposed to initiate a memory search to compare the information about these two
items. If the word Macintosh had been presented prior to the to-be-verified proposition, then all of its associatively related concepts, including "apple," will recently
have had activation tags placed along their network. The result of this is that when
the spreading activation from related tags "intersects"; that is, tags from the two
concepts are found in the same place, then an evaluation process is said to occur
in which each path is traced back to its start. If the concepts link up, then they are
judged to be related. If they do not link up, they are said to be unrelated.

In the case of the lexical decision task, targets that are merely letter strings
are nonetheless still afforded some space in memory, albeit in a very infrequently
accessed portion of memory. This aspect of the theory at first seems untenable
because of its notion that every nonsense string would for some reason have representation in memory. However, the presence of priming effects, both behavioral
and in event-related potential (ERP) studies for morphologically legal nonwords
suggests that there may be some utility to this notion (Rugg, 1985). It may well
be that every nonsense string is not uniquely represented, but is simply evaluated
based on its physical proximity to the nearest real word, for instance "BEEG,"
might elicit much the same pattern of activation as "BEEF." Essentially, the priming advantage for lexical decision tasks has been hypothesized to arise from a
process of comparison in which the memory search says, "Oh, BEEF has semantic associates, as indicated by this tag-related processing advantage, so if it has
associates, it must be a word. Let's press the 'word' button more quickly."

With this in mind, it is important to note that the process thought to be in
operation during these tasks is word identification. A great deal of effort has been
spent to try and isolate the nature of the processes underlying word identification,
and the evidence tends now to point to the notion that it can, but doesn't normally
proceed without attention (Besner & Stolz, 1998). The first authors to popularize
the distinction between automatic and controlled processes in word identification
were Posner and Snyder (1975), who described studies that revealed that priming

was greatly influenced by the length of delay between prime and target (see Synder, 1975). At short delays, or stimulus onset asynchronies (SOA) of less than 250 msec, only facilitatory effects were found, while at long SOAs, greater than about 750 msec, both facilitation and inhibition were possible. It was theorized in addition to the automatic spreading activation already described; when subjects were given ample time they would use controlled processes as well.

The two most often discussed types of controlled processes are expectancy generation, and various forms of postlexical matching processes (de Groot, 1983; de Groot, Thomassen, & Hudson, 1982). These matching processes are referred to as postlexical because they are thought to occur after the word form and meaning of a word stimulus have been accessed, and the priming advantage is theorized to occur somewhere between meaning access and the motor response. This dichotomy is somewhat misleading, in that even in the original Collins and Quillian (1969) formulation of spreading activation in a local network, the priming effect produced by the system of activation tags was not realized until after activation had spread through the network and the paths were evaluated in a memory search process.

The matching mechanism was formulated as an explanation for the results obtained in a study by deGroot (de Groot, 1983; de Groot et al., 1982), who used a combination of masked and unmasked primes to test the limits to which activation spreads in a network. DeGroot was interested in determining whether activation could be shown to spread to all immediately related concepts of a prime word, and beyond that, how many more distantly associated concepts would receive automatic facilitation. Recall that Collins and Loftus's theory predicted automatic spreading activation through all related nodes in a network, with this activation spreading first to all immediate associates (one-step pairs), and after that to more distant associates. Consider the pair Lion–Zebra (two-step pairs), which may not appear associatively related upon first inspection. Consider then the interposition of Tiger between Lion and Zebra, and the shared association of stripes becomes apparent. Thus pairs like Lion–Tiger, as well as pairs like Lion–Zebra were tested under unmasked and masked conditions. Under unmasked conditions, only Lion–Tiger pairs received clear-cut facilitation in terms of decreased RT time on a go/ no-go type of lexical decision task.

DeGroot speculated, however, that the failure to find reliable priming for second degree primes may have been due to a controlled checking strategy. Essentially she suggested that subjects always look for a meaningful relationship between a prime and target after the recognition of both had occurred, and after a "Yes" response had been planned for the target in the case that it was a word. If subjects are presented with unrelated pairs, then somewhere between response planning and response execution they attempt to process the meaning of the pair until their discrepancy can be resolved. This is said to happen because readers are trained to expect that words in a normal text will be coherent, and contextually related as a rule. Violations of this rule lead to increased processing time. She proposed that such a process, if in operation, could preclude the detection of any automatic priming effects, as they would act to delay the decision process to a point where automatic facilitation would have dissipated. In further experiments, DeGroot

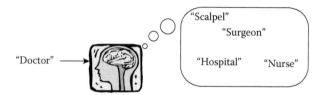

FIGURE 10.4 A schematic representation of the semantic expectancy generation process. After viewing "DOCTOR," the subject begins to produce candidate targets based on the expectation of semantic relatedness. If one of the generated possibilities is "NURSE," then response time will be shortened.

found that when her stimuli were masked, in an effort to limit conscious word identification and hence controlled meaning processing, no two-step priming was produced. Therefore, she concluded that no spreading activation was occurring beyond the one-step associate.

As a result of her failure to find spreading activation beyond the first associate, she suggested a model in which the semantic network is composed of clusters of concepts, with a central concept (DOG) surrounded by its core associates (CAT). Activation may spread automatically between these concepts. However, she proposed that no direct associative links exist between central concepts and more peripheral ones, so that any priming that occurs between those concepts would be due to a postlexical process involving a search of already active concepts. To date, this theory has received mixed support, but has not been conclusively disconfirmed.

The other mechanism that has been thought to be active at long SOAs is that of semantic expectancy. Here, when subjects have been exposed to an experimental situation in which the prime is somewhat predictive of the target, then it is thought that they begin to actively generate a set of possible targets after the appearance of the prime. This process is illustrated in Figure 10.4. Generally, when the proportion of primes and targets is relatively high ($\exists$ .50), it would be reasonable to adopt such a strategy. If the subject happens to generate the target as part of his or her expectancy set, then the response to that target should be facilitated due to its prior activation by the expectancy mechanism.

While this strategy occurs after the prime has been processed, it does occur before the meaning of the target word has been processed, and so in that sense is a controlled process that is not postlexical. In other words, it is distinct from expectancy generation because its effect is to change the level of activation of the target before it is actually encountered as a stimulus, not to facilitate a matching process after lexical activation. All of the mechanisms discussed in this section have been proposed to account for experimental data in local conceptions of a semantic network, but other possibilities for lexical–semantic organization exist.

FEATURE-BASED SEMANTIC MODELS

While the paradigms thus far have assumed that concepts are relatively unitary constructions that are linked together through some sort of associative connections, other models have been proposed that view concepts as an aggregate of features. One of the best known of these models is that of Smith, Shoben, and Rips (1974). In their theory, concepts are composed of both defining and characteristic features. The former are thought to be those elements of a concept that are necessary and sufficient for the basic definition of the concept, while the latter may often be associated with, but not critical to, a concept's meaning. While not grouped by Smith et al., modern featural theory researchers have divided the majority of features into structural and functional features, with the structural features composed of both sensory aspects (square-shaped), and material qualities (made of clay; Moss et al., 1997). Functional features would permit the comparison of "spoon" and "shovel," because both can be used to scoop. Like Collins and Loftus's model, this model was designed to account for performance on a sentence verification task where subjects are asked to indicate the truth of a statement such as "All robins are birds." Memory access is accomplished through a two-stage search process in which (1) a set of category names are retrieved that contains the names of all categories that have some members in common with the category of the predicate noun (bird in the previous example), and (2) a feature by feature comparison process occurs in which the attributes of the subject and predicate of the sentence are checked for a match.

A major advantage of such a model is that it permits a detailed mapping of semantic space, such that the distances between concepts can be determined along empirically derived continua. This was accomplished by Smith et al. by the use of typicality ratings as the dependent measure used in a factor analysis technique. Such a semantic space allows for the predictions to be made about the typicality of any new instance of a concept that is introduced to such a space. Network models must suppose the existence of a new node, not only for new concepts, but for even slightly different senses of an existing concept. For instance, the notion of a "Coke" and that of a "large Coke" would have separate representations in a local network, while a feature model would need only to change the weight on the dimension of size to encode this second concept. This seems to be a more precise and economical format for information storage.

Another advantage of such a conception of semantic representation is in its ability to specify what elements are included in the definition of any concept. For instance, "dog" in a local network for one researcher may not be exactly the same for another. In practice, however, this is enormously difficult due to several factors. In the first place, it may be impossible to determine what constitutes a necessary feature for any category. For example, the concept of "furniture" may typically include tables and chairs, which share four legs and the ability to hold other items on top of them. On the other hand, "furniture" may contain beanbag chairs, with no legs, and grandfather clocks that do not hold other objects. Second, there may be a great deal of difference between the featural composition of a concept between individuals. While two people may be able to agree that the fury creature standing before them should be labeled "dog," this does not mean that they have the same set of key attributes in their representations of dog.

The model of Smith et al. (1974) was criticized so effectively by Collins and Loftus (1975) that it lost a good deal of influence in the field of semantic research. Besides the difficulty in distinguishing defining from characteristic features, the Smith et al. model proposed that people do not search the superordinate category when making category judgments. Often times, as stated in Collins and Loftus, people must decide upon category membership not based on defining features, but simply on whether they had learned explicitly that "X was a Y." The example given by Collins and Loftus was of a person being uncertain of the properties of a sponge, but still being able to correctly categorize it as an animal due to their explicit learning of that fact. One way to view the critical difference between these types of theories is that featural theories permit a sort of calculation of the semantic status of each concept online, based on the evidence of its featural composition. Local network theories seem to propose that what gets stored and linked together are the outputs of processes. In other words, while features may be used to construct and judge instances of categories, local nodes are the output of such constructive or wrote learning processes.

DISTRIBUTED MODELS

The doctrine of mass action stands somewhat at odds with local models. In this way of thinking, a relatively large proportion of all neurons are involved in the representation of every concept that is being processed during one operation. Perhaps the most cogent formulation of such a model for use with semantic memory is that of Masson (1995; Masson & Borowsky, 1998). This model is truly "distributed" in that it postulates that every concept is represented over a large array of processing units that are generally the same within any on module of the system. Such an array is generally thought to consist of multiple layers, or levels, starting with an input unit, followed by some number of hidden layers, and finally an output layer. This arrangement is illustrated in Figure 10.5.

Masson's model proposes the division of the neural network into three main subnetworks based on their representational content: orthographic units, phonological units, and meaning units. These subsystems are completely interconnected though feed forward and feedback pathways, thus allowing the output of semantic and phonological analyses to influence the activity state of the orthographic units. This feature allows the network to account for such basic phenomenon as the word-superiority effect (Reicher, 1969), where word identification is faster than an equivalent nonword string. Here, lexical level information would actually bias orthographic processing units, causing a more rapid identification of previously encountered (legal) word forms.

If a word is presented visually, the orthographic system takes the word form as its input, then the input is transduced into values that are passed to an unspecified number of intermediate units, and finally these values are passed as output to a higher level subsystem. Orthographic output is proposed to pass either directly to the semantic unit, or by way of the phonological unit to the semantic unit. This architecture is necessary to account for evidence suggesting that while a phonological

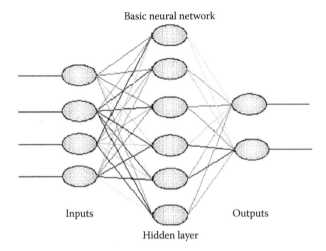

FIGURE 10.5   A basic three-level neural network model with parallel, distributed connections between each of the processing units. Activation levels of each node, on their own, represent no concepts. But, when taken together the unique activity of the output level is suggested to be able to code for any unique concept. (Adapted from www.e-orthopaedics.com/sakura/ images/neural.gif.)

activation may be the default result of an orthographic analysis, meaning activation can take place in the absence of concomitant phonological analysis (Jared & Seidenberg, 1991). Whenever input enters one of the distributed processing subsystems, it is cycled through repeatedly, with output being fed back into the input channel until the most stable pattern of activation is found. In this sense, "identification" at any processing level means the point at which error between input and outpoint is minimized.

The basic explanation for semantic priming in a distributed model is that when a prime appears, it causes the processing units to take on the values associated with that word at each level of analysis. Because the processing units can only hold one value at a time, if a related target appears it will find the current pattern of semantic activation to be similar to its own. Thus the time necessary for the target to reach a stable level of representation will be shortened. Unrelated words require a resetting of the units, while neutral stimuli would leave the network in a relatively unbiased state. Thus, RT for tasks requiring word identification should be slowest for unrelated, moderate for neutral, and quickest for related. In this way, distributed models can account for the same findings of inhibition for unrelated words at long SOAs that were discussed earlier in the work of Posner and Snyder (1975).

As alluded to above, distributed models can be viewed as having the advantage that they resemble, in function and somewhat in structure, the populations of neurons thought to be responsible for all cognition. However, as discussed in Masson (1995), the primary test of the utility of such models is in their ability to account for existing data parsimoniously, and to make unique predictions. The primary experimental evidence for the distributed model discussed by Masson concerns its ability to accurately predict the magnitude and direction of semantic priming effects in a situation in which an unrelated item is interposed between a related prime and target. Similar to the paradigm utilized by deGroot (above), the intervening item manipulation compares the RT results from two critical conditions: a prime followed by a related target (DOG–CAT), as opposed to a prime followed by an intervening item and then a target (DOG–ROCK–CAT).

The original formulation of local network models predict that an intervening item should have no effect on the strength of priming effects because activation is thought to spread automatically to all nodes in the network. Presenting an intervening item should just serve to add another source of activation to the network, but not disrupt the initial activation. Because distributed networks can represent only one concept at a time in their processing units, the intervening item should disrupt priming to the extent that it is different from the activation pattern of the prime and target. Thus unrelated intervening items should disrupt priming the most, and neutral stimuli (like "XXXX") should have a marginally disruptive influence.

Masson reports two studies designed to test these predictions. Study 1 presented subjects with a prime, intervening item on some trials, and target for 200 msec each, with an SOA of 400 msec. The subject's task was to name the target as quickly as possible. As predicted by his model, Masson found that the unrelated intervening item significantly disrupted priming when compared to the condition where the target followed the prime directly. Masson performed a second study in which priming across trials was assessed. In this experiment he lengthened both the duration and SOA of the stimuli and arranged the items so that the target of one pair would serve as a prime to the next pair. He predicted that under these conditions the disruption of priming seen in experiment 1 would diminish because the degree of disruption should be proportional to the amount of processing devoted to the intervening item, relative to the prime. In a sense, the pattern set up when processing the intervening item is more likely to disrupt priming if (1) the prime's pattern is less established, and (2) the intervening item's pattern is allowed to completely stabilize in the system. While the complexity of his results renders them prohibitively large to report in detail, he found that the intervening item disruption diminished as predicted.

The purpose of Masson's paper was to provide support for the plausibility of an alternative representational scheme to the local network. In this endeavor he was initially successful. On the other hand, he pointed out that the model was incomplete in that it did not provide mechanisms to account for many of the common strategic processing factors encountered in priming research, including: proportion of related to unrelated prime–target pairs (so-called relatedness proportion, or RP), proportion of nonwords, and semantic expectancy strategies. It also lacked an ability to account for a "learning effect" apparent in a comparison of the two studies. Briefly, when a legal word is used as the intervening item ("Ready"), subjects slowly become habituated to it, and the pattern of disruption changes. The failure of any of these models to account for how the semantic system can be restructured to permit new word learning is a serious shortcoming, as word learning is one of the hallmarks of human linguistic behavior.

SUMMARY AND CONCLUSION

We have reviewed the most common theories of semantic representation that have emerged in the last 35 years. The models consisted of local theories, feature-based theories, and distributed models. The advantage of local theories was that they were extremely flexible and powerful, and can model almost any experimental result. This was particularly true of Anderson's ACT models, which were so flexible that they may not be falsifiable. A theory that cannot be proven wrong is problematic for science, because it proves difficult to know when to discard it in favor of a better theory. Nonetheless, local models that operate using spreading activation have been the most influential and widely investigated since the 1970s.

Feature-based theories had the advantage of allowing the most precise and economical mapping of semantic knowledge, but suffered from the problem of finding good "critical" or defining features that would be necessary to differentiate one concept form from another. Powerful theories of semantic representation, like those of Anderson, include aspects both of local network and feature-based theories. Distributed models offered the distinct advantage of being more biologically plausible. Remember that our brains are composed of billions of highly flexible units (neurons) that may be reconfigured to complete many processing tasks, and that each neuron may be involved in the representation of many different pieces of semantic information. Distributed models were furthermore able to account for the intervening item phenomenon that was problematic for standard local spreading activation models.

In summary, the study of semantic representation has made great strides in accounting for the richness and complexity of human knowledge in the past 40 years. Elements of these theories still figure prominently in the twenty-first-century language studies, and they continue to provide a means to account for normal word recognition. Chapter 30 in this volume will examine how these models play a central role in understanding what breaks down in some common communication disorders.

REFERENCES

Anderson, J. R. (1974). Retrieval of propositional information from long-term memory. *Cognitive Psychology, 6*, 451–474.

Anderson, J. R. (1976). *Language, memory, and thought.* Potomac, MD: Lawrence Erlbaum.

Anderson, J. R. (1983). Spreading activation theory of memory. *Journal of Verbal Learning & Verbal Behavior, 22*, 261–295.

Anderson, J. R. (1993). Problem solving and learning. *American Psychologist, 48*, 35–44.

Anderson, J. R., & Reder, L. M. (1999). The fan effect: New results and new theories. *Journal of Experimental Psychology: General, 128*, 186–197.

Anderson, M. C., & Spellman, B. A. (1995). On the status of inhibitory mechanisms in cognition: Memory retrieval as a model case. *Psychological Review, 102*, 68–100.

Barlow, H. B. (1972). Single units and sensation: A neuron doctrine for perceptual psychology? *Perception, 1*, 371–394.

Besner, D., & Stolz, J. A. (1998). Unintentional reading: Can phonological computation be controlled? *Canadian Journal of Experimental Psychology, 52*, 35–42.

Brown, C., & Hagoort, P. (1993). The processing nature of the N400: Evidence from masked priming. *Journal of Cognitive Neuroscience, 5*, 10.

Collins, A. M., & Loftus, E. F. (1975). A spreading activation theory of semantic processing. *Psychological Review, 82*, 407–428.

Collins, A. M., & Quillian, M. R. (1969). Retrieval time from semantic memory. *Journal of Verbal Learning and Verbal Behavior, 8*, 240–248.

de Groot, A. M. (1983). The range of automatic spreading activation in word priming. *Journal of Verbal Learning & Verbal Behavior, 22*, 417–436.

de Groot, A. M., Thomassen, A. J., & Hudson, P. T. (1982). Associative facilitation of word recognition as measured from a neutral prime. *Memory & Cognition, 10*, 358–370.

Deacon, D., Hewitt, S., Yang, C.-M., & Nagata, M. (2000). Event-related potential indices of semantic priming using masked and unmasked words: Evidence that the N400 does not reflect a post-lexical process. *Cognitive Brain Research, 9*(2), 137–146.

Fahlman, S. E., Hinton, G. E., & Anderson, J. A. (1989). Representing implicit knowledge. In *Parallel models of associative memory* (updated ed., pp. 171–185). Hillsdale, NJ, England: Lawrence Erlbaum Associates, Inc.

Gaul, F., & Spurzheim, G. (1810–1819). *The anatomy and physiology of the nervous system in general and the brain in particular* (Vol. 1–4). Paris, France: F. Schoell.

Geschwind, N. (1965). Disconnection syndromes in animals and man. *Brain, 88*, 237–294.

Heilman, K., & Valenstein, E. (Eds.). (1993). *Clinical neuropsychology* (3rd ed.). New York, NY: Oxford University Press.

Henderson, V. W. (1996). The investigation of lexical semantic representation in Alzheimer's disease. *Brain & Language, 54*, 179–183.

Hinton, G. E., Anderson, J. A., Hinton, G. E., & Anderson, J. A. (1989). *Parallel models of associative memory* (updated ed.). Hillsdale, NJ, England: Lawrence Erlbaum Associates, Inc.

Holcomb, P. J. (1993). Semantic priming and stimulus degradation: Implications for the role of the N400 in language processing. *Psychophysiology, 30*(1), 47–61.

Hubel, D. H., & Wiesel, T. N. (1979). Brain mechanisms of vision. *Scientific American, 241*(3), 150–162.

Jared, D., & Seidenberg, M. S. (1991). Does word identification proceed from spelling to sound to meaning? *Journal of Experimental Psychology: General, 120*, 358–394.

Kosslyn, S. M. (1981). The medium and the message in mental imagery: A theory. *Psychological Review, 88*(1), 46–66.

Lashley, K. S. (1938). Factors limiting recovery after central nervous system lesions. *Journal of Mental and Nervous System Disorders, 888*, 733–755.

Masson, M. E. J. (1995). A distributed model of semantic priming. *Journal of Experimental Psychology: Learning, Memory, & Cognition, 21*, 3–23.

Masson, M. E. J., & Borowsky, R. (1998). More than meets the eye: Context effects in word identification. *Memory & Cognition, 26*, 1245–1269.

Moss, H. E., Tyler, L. K., & Jennings, F. (1997). When leopards lose their spots: Knowledge of visual properties in category-specific deficits for living things. *Cognitive Neuropsychology, 14*, 901–950.

Neisser, U. (1967). *Cognitive psychology*. East Norwalk, CT: Appleton-Century-Crofts.

Paivio, A. (1991). *Images in mind: The evolution of a theory*. Hertfordshire, England: Harvester Wheatsheaf.

Posner, M. I., & Snyder, R. R. (1975). Attention and cognitive control. In R. L. Solso (Ed.), *Information processing and cognition: The Loyola symposium* (pp. 55–85). New York, NY: John Wiley, & Sons.

Radvansky, G. A., Spieler, D. H., & Zacks, R.T. (1993). Mental model organization. *Journal of Experimental Psychology: Learning, Memory, & Cognition, 19*, 95–114.

Reicher, G. M. (1969). Perceptual recognition as a function of meaningfulness of stimulus material. *Journal of Experimental Psychology: General, 81*, 275–280.

Rock, I., & Gutman, D. (1981). The effect of inattention on form perception. *Journal of Experimental Psychology: Human Perception and Performance, 7*(2), 275–285.

Rugg, M. D. (1985). The effects of semantic priming and word repetition on event-related potentials. *Psychophysiology, 22*, 642–647.

Rumelhart, D. E., & McClelland, J. E. (1986). *Parallel distributed processing: Explorations in the microstructure of cognition* (Vol. 1. Foundations). Cambridge, MA: MIT Press.

Smith, E. E., Shoben, E. J., & Rips, L. (1974). Structure and process in semantic memory: A featural model for semantic decisions. *Psychological Review, 81*, 214–241.

Snyder, P. (1975). *Facilitation and inhibition in the processing of signals* (Vol. V). New York, NY: Academic Press.

Tulving, E. (1984). Précis of elements of episodic memory. *Behavioral & Brain Sciences, 7*, 223–268.

Tulving, E., & Thomson, D. M. (1973). Encoding specificity and retrieval processes in episodic memory. *Psychological Review, 80*, 359–380.

Zurif, E. B., Caramazza, A., Myerson, R., & Galvin, J. (1974). Semantic feature representations for normal and aphasic language. *Brain and Language, 1*, 167–187.

11 Language Comprehension: A Neurocognitive Perspective

Catherine Longworth and
William Marslen-Wilson

INTRODUCTION

Within milliseconds of perceiving speech or text we recognize individual words from the tens of thousands we have learned, gain access to their linguistic properties, and integrate their meaning with that of the preceding words to compute an interpretation of the intended message. Language comprehension seems so rapid and effortless for most of us that the question hardly seems to arise of how this astonishing decoding operation is actually carried out. Nevertheless, common neurological conditions, such as stroke or forms of dementia, very often disrupt both general and specific aspects of the comprehension process, indicating the complexity of its cognitive and neural foundations. A complete understanding of language comprehension must therefore provide an account not only of the mental representations of language and the processes that operate upon them, but also of how these relate to the brain and to the breakdown of function following brain damage (i.e., a *neurocognitive* account). This chapter provides a historical overview of the ways in which the language comprehension system has been investigated and outlines the basis of our neurocognitive approach to language comprehension, illustrated by a clinical example.

HISTORICAL OVERVIEW

The classic neurological account of language, the Wernicke–Lichtheim model, proposed that language depends upon a left lateralized network of discrete brain regions connected by white matter tracts. In this network the posterior left superior temporal gyrus (Wernicke's area) was thought to be critical for comprehension, whereas the anterior left inferior frontal gyrus (LIFG) (Broca's area) was critical for production and the arcuate fasciculus allowed information to flow between the two regions (see Figure 11.1). Thus damage to Wernicke's area should result in comprehension failure as opposed to damage to Broca's area, which should

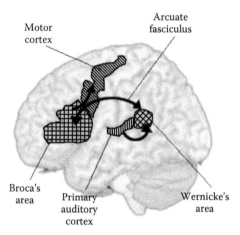

FIGURE 11.1   The classic Wernicke–Lichtheim model of language in the brain. (Reprinted from Tyler, L. K. and Marslen-Wilson, W. D., *Phil. Trans. R. Soc. B* 363, 1493, 1037–1054, 2008. With permission.)

result in difficulties with language production. This model is often still used today to describe the aphasic syndromes associated with damage to these two regions (e.g., Broca's and Wernicke's aphasias). It relies on a methodology of lesion-deficit associations, by which observed language deficits were assumed to be related to brain lesions. At the time these lesions could only be identified at postmortem, but the methodology has been updated with the advent of structural brain scanning and today we can visualize brain lesions *in vivo* and pinpoint their location using voxel-based morphometry (VBM; Ashburner & Friston, 2000). It is risky, none-theless, to assume a simple mapping between comprehension deficits and observable lesions, since deficits may reflect neural disruption that cannot be visualized in standard neuroimaging or in distant regions that rely on the damaged area. Lesion-deficit mapping must be combined with other methodologies to build up a full picture of how abilities such as language comprehension are instantiated in the brain. It is also necessary to specify those representations or processes that are associated with a particular lesion, rather than trying to localize comprehension as a whole.[*]

The cognitive revolution of the 1960s onward addressed this omission by seeking to identify the mental processes and representations underlying human abilities, such as language comprehension, typically through the use of speeded experimental paradigms. Priming, for example, is an experimental paradigm in

---

[*] It is also important to remember that the classic lesion-deficit approach will be effectively blind to linguistic (or other communicative) functions whose neural substrate is more distributed and represented in both hemispheres. Thus, while the classic Wernicke–Lichtheim model successfully picked out the left-hemisphere fronto-temporal network that is critical to certain key linguistic functions, it fails to capture more distributed bihemispheric aspects of communicative function— and even failed to detect the major left hemisphere "ventral" pathway, running down the superior and middle temporal lobe to connect with inferior frontal structures (as discussed next).

which responses to target words are facilitated by prior presentation of related words or primes. By manipulating the relationship between primes and targets it has been possible to investigate how words are represented in the mind (e.g., Marslen-Wilson, Tyler, Waksler, & Older, 1994) and the time course with which we access their meanings (e.g., Moss, McCormick, & Tyler, 1997; Tyler, Moss, Galpin, & Voice, 2002). The evidence gathered using methods such as these resulted in cognitive theories, such as the cohort theory of spoken word recognition, focusing on the critical early stages of relating sound to lexical form and meaning during language comprehension (Gaskell & Marslen-Wilson, 1997; Marslen-Wilson, 1987; Marslen-Wilson & Welsh, 1978).

In its classic formulation, the cohort theory suggests that spoken word recognition has three stages: lexical access, selection, and integration. The first two of these stages occur before a word can be identified, and the last stage occurs after word recognition, or postlexically. During the access stage, mental representations of all the lexical forms matching the speech input (the "cohort") are activated in parallel, together with their associated meanings. The extent to which these forms continue to match the incoming signal is mirrored in their level of activation. In the selection stage the form with the greatest level of activation (i.e., that which most closely matches the perceptual evidence) is identified as the best match to the speaker's intention and recognition occurs. Finally, during the integration stage the semantic and syntactic properties of the identified form are integrated with higher order representations of the message. The whole process occurs within a fraction of a second.

Cognitive science has helped to specify the representations and processes involved in language comprehension but does not tell us how these relate to their neural instantiation. For this reason many researchers have turned to cognitive neuroscience, which complements information about language pathology using lesion-deficit mapping, with information about the healthy language system using electrophysiological (EEG and MEG) methods (e.g., Hauk, Davis, Ford, Pulvermuller, & Marslen-Wilson, 2006) and functional neuroimaging (fMRI, PET) methods (e.g., Bozic, Marslen-Wilson, Stamatakis, Davis, & Tyler, 2007). For example, fMRI can be used to confirm that the brain-behavior associations implied by lesion-deficit mapping are present in the healthy brain. Two main methods of analysis are used. Subtractive analyses identify the brain regions in which activity increases during an experimental task, in contrast to a control condition. This identifies all the regions active for a given task, but does not establish those regions that are essential for this task or how the activity in different regions relates to each other. Connectivity analyses, on the other hand, allow us to identify how activity in a given region relates to activity elsewhere and thus can be used to develop maps of the neural systems underlying components of language comprehension. Electrophysiological techniques complement neuroimaging by providing a direct window onto the millisecond timecourse of language comprehension in the brain.

In addition to examining human abilities directly, cognitive neuroscience also makes use of primate research to investigate the nonhuman precursors for our major cognitive systems. In the case of language this has involved examining the extent to which knowledge of primate auditory processing informs our understanding of human speech processing. Research suggests that the differentiation of sensory processing into dorsal and ventral processing streams, previously established for primate visual processing (Ungerleider & Mishkin, 1982), also applies to primate auditory processing. Auditory information is initially processed in auditory cortex and then travels either via a dorsal stream leaving the auditory cortex posteriorly and looping round to the inferior frontal cortex or via a ventral stream linking to the inferior frontal cortex anteriorly (Kaas & Hackett, 1999; Rauschecker & Tian, 2000). Research on macaques has proposed that, the ventral route processes the identity of the sound (i.e., a "what" pathway) whereas the dorsal route processes the location of the sound (i.e., a "where" pathway; Kaas & Hackett, 1999; Rauschecker & Tian, 2000). This differentiation of the primate auditory system is echoed in suggestions that the language system in humans divides into multiple processing pathways (Hickok & Poeppel, 2004; Scott & Johnsrude, 2003; Figure 11.2). For example, in contrast to the simplified left hemisphere system proposed by the classic model of language, current neurocognitive models propose that language comprehension is instantiated in the brain through two neural pathways, each with distinct functions and with contributions made by both cerebral hemispheres.

A NEUROCOGNITIVE APPROACH TO LANGUAGE COMPREHENSION

Language conveys two types of information between sender and receiver: semantic information about meanings in the world and syntactic information about the grammatical properties of lexical forms (e.g., tense, number, aspect, etc.) and how they combine to form sentences. This information is associated with specific entries within a store of lexical representations known as the "mental lexicon." As we listen to speech or read text we match spoken or written inputs to lexical representations and access their meanings and grammatical properties.

LEXICAL REPRESENTATION AND MORPHOLOGY

It is often assumed that the basic unit of language is the word. It is not clear, however, that this is the fundamental unit of representation in the mental lexicon, since linguistics recognizes an even smaller unit, the morpheme. This has been defined as "the smallest meaningful unit" of language (Bloomfield, 1933) or "the smallest unit of grammatical analysis" (Lyons, 1968). In English many morphemes occur as individual words, or monomorphemes, associated with specific semantic or syntactic information (e.g., *the frog*). However, there are also many morphologically complex words, formed by adding bound morphemes to word stems. Bound morphemes (e.g., *pre-, -un, -ing, -ness, -ed*), or affixes, occur only in combination with stems. English has two means of generating these combinations: inflectional and derivational morphology. Inflectional affixes convey syntactic information that makes words appropriate for their role in a sentence, while maintaining their

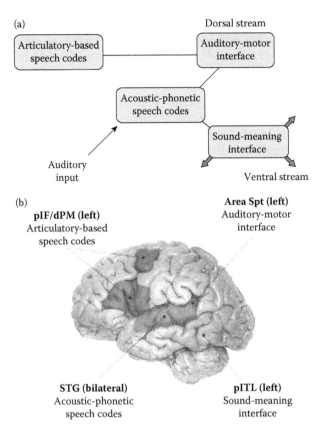

(a)   Dorsal stream

Articulatory-based   ——————   Auditory-motor
  speech codes   interface

                  Acoustic-phonetic
                    speech codes

                                          Sound-meaning
                                             interface

        Auditory
         input   Ventral stream

(b)   **Area Spt (left)**
      pIF/dPM (left)   Auditory-motor
     Articulatory-based   interface
       speech codes

      STG (bilateral)   **pITL (left)**
      Acoustic-phonetic   Sound-meaning
        speech codes   interface

FIGURE 11.2   Hickok and Poeppel's model of language in the brain featuring dorsal and ventral processing streams. Panel (a) presents a schematic diagram of the two pathway model, with an auditory-motor dorsal stream and sound-meaning ventral stream. Panel (b) shows how these two streams map onto specific brain areas (pIF/dPM = posterior Inferior Frontal/dorsal Premotor cortex, STG = Superior Temporal Gyrus, Area Spt = Sylvian–parietal–temporal, an area of the Sylvian fissure at the boundary of the temporal and parietal lobes, pITL = posterior Inferior Temporal Lobe). (Reprinted from Hickok, G. and Poeppel, D., *Cognition*, 92, 67–99, 2004. With permission.)

meaning and word class. Derivational affixes change the meaning or word class of a stem morpheme, generating new entries in the mental lexicon.

INFLECTIONAL MORPHOLOGY

A series of studies indicates that lexical access to words made up of stems and inflectional affixes differs from lexical access to words without an internal structure and relies on a different neurocognitive processing stream. In one such study (Marslen-Wilson & Tyler, 1997; Tyler et al., 2002a) we used auditory morphological priming to contrast lexical access to regular and irregular past tense forms.

This allowed us to compare the processing of inflected forms with an internal structure divisible into component morphemes (e.g., *jump-ed*) and unstructured forms that must be processed as whole forms (e.g., *taught*). Both past tense conditions were compared to a semantic priming condition (e.g., *swan/goose*) and a phonological control condition (e.g., *tinsel/tin*).

A group of healthy volunteers showed a pattern of response facilitation to target words that were preceded by morphologically related prime words (e.g., *jumped/ jump, taught/teach*) relative to unrelated control words (e.g., *played/jump, bought/ teach*) for both regular and irregular verbs. They also showed response facilitation to targets preceded by semantically related words (semantic priming, e.g., *swan/goose*) but no facilitation of words related only by form (e.g., *gravy/grave*). Nonfluent (or Broca's) aphasics, in contrast, showed normal priming for irregular verbs and semantically related words, but no priming from the regular past tense (Figure 11.3). Neuroimaging indicated that their brain damage was confined to left perisylvian regions (e.g., LIFG and superior temporal gyrus). Two further patients showed a converse pattern, with priming from regular verbs and semantically related words, but no facilitation for irregular past tense forms (Marslen-Wilson & Tyler, 1997, 1998). One of these patients was a nonfluent aphasic with bilateral lesions, including damage to the right temporal lobe and the other suffered from semantic dementia, which is associated with temporal lobe atrophy.

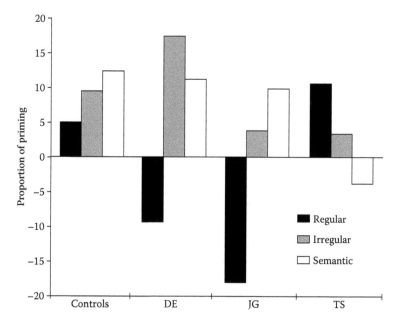

FIGURE 11.3   The double dissociation between regular and irregular past tense priming across patients. The labels DE and JG are the initials of two non-fluent left hemisphere patients; TS is a third patient with bilateral damage. The Controls are healthy individuals matched for age and education. (Reprinted from Marslen-Wilson, W. D. and Tyler, L. K., *Trends in Cognitive Science*, 2, 428–436, 1998. With permission.)

This double dissociation between regular and irregular past tense priming suggests the existence of two language processing routes through the brain: a dorsal route decomposing the words into stems and affixes and a ventral route recognizing unstructured words (and processing whole forms and stems).

A second study strengthens the evidence for a decompositional dorsal route (Longworth, Marslen-Wilson, Randall, & Tyler, 2005). This compared auditory semantic priming from regular and irregular verb stems and their past tense forms (e.g., *blame/accuse, blamed/accuse, teach/learn, taught/learn*). Nonfluent aphasic patients showed preserved semantic priming from verb stems and irregular forms, as did healthy volunteers, indicating an intact ability to map unstructured forms onto meaning. In contrast, however, they showed an absence of normal semantic priming following regular past tense forms (Figure 11.4). The mapping of form onto meaning appears to be disrupted by their impairment in processing words with a complex internal structure. This indicates that rather than being stored in the mental lexicon in their own right, in the same way as stems and irregular past tenses, regular past tense forms must be decomposed into their component parts in order to identify the stem and access its meaning and to process the syntactic implications of the past tense affix.

A third study indicates that the decomposition of inflected forms into stems and affixes is an early, obligatory stage of processing. This study used an auditory same–different task to contrast the processing of regular and irregular past tense forms and words and nonwords matched to their phonology. Nonfluent aphasics and a group of age-matched healthy volunteers were asked whether the second of two spoken stimuli, either two words or two nonwords spoken in

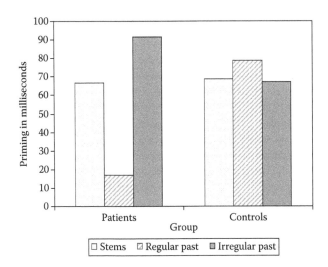

FIGURE 11.4   The failure of semantic priming from the regular past tense in patients with Broca's aphasia. (Reprinted from Longworth, C. E., Marslen-Wilson, W. D., Randall, B., and Tyler, L. K. *Journal of Cognitive Neuroscience,* 17, 7, 1087–1097, 2005. With permission.)

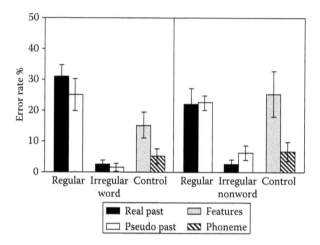

FIGURE 11.5 Patient error rates for words and nonwords in the same-different task. (Reprinted from Tyler, L. K. et al. *Neuropsychologia*, 40(8), 1154–1166, 2002. With permission.)

a male and a female voice, was the same as the first (Tyler et al., 2002b). For healthy volunteers this is an easy task, yet the patients not only had difficulties with regularly inflected word pairs (e.g., *played/play*) but also, crucially, with any word or nonword pair that ended in the phonetic hallmark of the regular past tense (e.g., *trade/tray, snade/snay*), which we have termed the English inflectional rhyme pattern (IRP). The IRP, characteristic not only of the regular past tense but also of the English "s" inflection, consists of a final coronal consonant (d, t, s, z) that agrees in voicing with the preceding consonant. The experiment compared performance on regular verbs (*played/play*) with other stimuli with the IRP: pseudoregular pairs (*trade/tray*), where the first word has the IRP and could potentially be a past tense of the second word; and nonwords matched to real and pseudoregular pairs (*snayed/snay*). These conditions were contrasted with performance in "additional phoneme" conditions, in which the stimuli were matched to the consonant vowel structure of the other conditions, so that the final consonant was dropped in the second of each pair, but this consonant was not a potential English inflection (e.g., *claim/clay, blane/blay*). The patients performed worst on regular verb pairs, confirming their impairment in decomposing inflected forms into morphemes. However, they also performed very poorly on pseudoregular and nonword regular pairs, despite near normal performance on the additional phoneme pairs (see Figure 11.5). This suggests that the patients have an impairment of a decompositional process triggered automatically by the presence of the IRP, irrespective of whether the input is a real regular past tense or not.[*]

---

[*] For an expansion of this line of research to unimpaired young adults, see Post, Marslen-Wilson, Randall, and Tyler, 2008.

These studies form part of a well-known debate in cognitive science on the extent of differentiation within the cognitive language system. The "Words and Rules" debate contrasts single route accounts, which argue that all words are accessed as whole forms in terms of learned associations between sensory inputs and representations of form and meaning (McClelland & Patterson, 2002; Rumelhart & McClelland, 1986) and dual route accounts, which claim that there is differentiation within the language processing system, with the form and meaning of some inputs computed from their component parts (Pinker & Prince, 1988; Pinker & Ullman, 2002). The studies summarized above provide evidence for differentiation within the language system in that regular inflectional morphology appears to engage a separate processing system than uninflected stems or irregular forms that are not analyzable into a stem and a regular inflectional affix.

In response to studies such as these, single route theorists argued that regular and irregular past tense deficits in language comprehension do not reflect impairments of decompositional and whole word access procedures, but difficulties with phonology or semantics, respectively (Joanisse & Seidenberg, 1999). Processing regular verbs was argued to depend on general phonological processing since the regular past tense differs from its verb stems by a single phoneme, which might be difficult to perceive. Processing irregular verbs were argued to depend on semantic processing due to the absence of a reliable phonological relationship between irregular past tense forms and their stems. It was argued that both phonological and semantic information are processed by an undifferentiated associative memory system. Such an account, however, makes the wrong predictions about patients with past tense deficits. As shown in the third study described, although nonfluent patients may have difficulties with words and nonwords matched to past tense phonology, their difficulties are greatest for regular past tense forms. In addition, dissociations have been reported between difficulties with the irregular past tense and semantic impairments (Miozzo, 2003; Tyler et al., 2004). Although these two types of deficit may co-occur, this is not necessarily the case, as demonstrated by patients with irregular past tense deficits but intact semantic processing (Miozzo, 2003).

However, perhaps the strongest evidence against the single route interpretation of past tense deficits comes from combining behavioral evidence with structural brain imaging. Tyler and colleagues (2005) correlated variations in behavioral performance with variations in MRI signal intensity to identify areas where abnormal performance is linked to neuroimaging evidence of damaged tissue. On MRI scans, differences in neural tissue integrity are reflected in characteristic variations in signal intensity, which can be visualized on a black–white scale. Relative to normative scan data, damaged areas of the brain often have lower signal intensity and appear darker on MRI scans. The Tyler et al. (2005) study correlated these variations in MRI signal intensity, across the whole brain, with variations in performance on the auditory morphological priming task for 22 neurological patients with a variety of different lesions and different cognitive deficits. The patients were not preselected on the basis of past tense deficits, but simply on the inclusion criteria of suitability for MRI and ability to perform the priming task.

Contrary to a single mechanism account, the results show double dissociations between the regular past tense and phonological conditions and between the irregular past tense and semantic conditions, in the regions found to be most critical for performance. This indicates that processing regular inflectional morphology is distinct from phonological processing and processing irregular past tense forms is distinct from semantic processing, because they rely on different brain regions.

The correlation between the regular past tense condition and signal intensity peaked in the LIFG at a standard threshold for statistical significance and extended to encompass the left superior temporal gyrus, Wernicke's area and the arcuate fasciculus at a more lenient threshold. In other words, the correlational procedure picked out just those areas of the brain thought to be critical for core grammatical (morpho-syntactic) functions in the normal brain. Performance on the phonological control condition, in contrast, did not show a statistically significant correlation in this area, and the two correlations were significantly different from one another. Instead the phonological condition correlated with signal intensity in a more medial brain area called the insula, with increased damage being associated with more disrupted performance. The insula is a region previously associated with phonological processing (Noesselt, Shah, & Jancke, 2003), and therefore likely to be involved in the phonological comparison processes on which performance here presumably depends. The regular past tense condition, however, did not correlate significantly with intensity in this region, consistent with the view that what drives performance here are factors to do with combinatorial linguistic analysis (elicited by the presence of an inflectional morpheme).

The correlation between the irregular past tense condition and signal intensity peaked at the left superior parietal lobule and extended to encompass surrounding areas at a more lenient threshold. These areas, which have been implicated in lexical access processes in other studies, are not only quite different from those seen in the regular past tense condition, but also quite different from those that correlate with performance in the semantic condition. This condition showed no significant correlation in the areas linked to irregular past tense performance, and instead correlated with signal intensity in the left medial fusiform gyrus (BA 37, hippocampus, and surrounding parahippocampal regions), extending to the left middle temporal gyrus (LMTG). These are areas found in other studies to play a role in linking phonological inputs to lexical semantic representations, and showed no correlation in this study with performance on the irregulars.

In subsequent investigations, we confirmed that the brain behavior relationships that had been implied by language pathology extended to the normal language system. To do this we used event-related fMRI to identify those brain regions that were active when healthy volunteers performed the same–different task described above (Tyler, Stamatakis, Post, Randall, & Marslen-Wilson, 2005). We also used connectivity analysis to investigate how activity in key regions correlated with activity elsewhere in the brain for the different conditions (Tyler & Marslen-Wilson, 2008). Healthy volunteers were asked to judge whether word pairs were the same or different while fMRI scans were conducted. The conditions allowed us to contrast the brain regions activated by regular verb pairs with those activated by pseudoregulars, irregular verbs, pseudoirregulars, pairs with an additional phoneme (e.g., claim-clay), and matching nonword conditions.

The results showed that the regular past tense condition and all other conditions containing the IRP (e.g., pseudo and nonword regulars) engaged significantly more activity in the LIFG and bilateral superior and middle temporal gyri, than either irregular past tense forms and stimuli matched to these (e.g., pseudo and nonword irregulars), or the additional phoneme conditions (e.g., real and nonword pairs with an additional phoneme). The increased temporal lobe activation may reflect processes operating on embedded lexical content (e.g., the *jump* in *jumped* and embedded *tray* in *trade*) since nonwords with or without the IRP, which by definition have no lexical content, did not differ in activation in these regions. In contrast, nonwords with the IRP (e.g., pairs like *snayed/snay*) activated the LIFG more strongly than nonwords without the IRP (e.g., *blane/blay*). Since neither condition has lexical content and they differ only in the presence of the IRP, the increased activation of the LIFG appears to reflect processes specific to the IRP. Finally, there was an interaction between regularity (regular versus irregular past tense) and word type (real versus pseudo) such that the real regular past tense condition, but not the pseudo or nonword regular past tense conditions, activated the left anterior cingulate more than real, pseudo, and nonword irregulars. This suggests that the left anterior cingulate is involved when, in addition to featuring embedded lexical content and the IRP, words can be genuinely segmented into stems and inflectional affixes.

A connectivity analysis (reported in Stamatakis, Marslen-Wilson, Tyler, & Fletcher, 2005) showed that activity in the LIFG and left anterior cingulate indeed covaried with activity in a third region, the left posterior middle temporal gyrus, to a greater extent for stimuli with the IRP, than they did for irregular past tense forms and words and nonwords matched to these. However, the covariance was stronger for real regular past tense forms than for pseudoregulars and nonwords matched to regular past tense forms (Stamatakis et al., 2005). Neuroimaging research suggests that the anterior cingulate may play a role in integrating information from different processing streams in frontal and temporal regions (Braver, Barch, Gray, Molfese, & Snyder, 2001; Fletcher, McKenna, Friston, Frith, & Dolan, 1999). It is possible that in the context of language comprehension, the anterior cingulate is differentially activated by real regular past tense forms due to the greater processing demands of integrating frontal systems supporting morpho-phonological segmentation with temporal processes involved in the access of the lexical content of their stems.

DERIVATIONAL MORPHOLOGY

The meaning and syntactic properties of regularly inflected words can be computed from the combination of their stems and affixes, making them fully compositional, and uniformly analyzed, as argued above, by cooperating left hemisphere fronto-temporal systems (Marslen-Wilson & Tyler, 2007).

Research on derived words, on the other hand, shows a more complex pattern of findings (Marslen-Wilson, 2007). This reflects the fact that derivational morphology creates new lexical entries, with their own meanings and syntactic properties, which vary in compositionality. In addition, responses to derived words are influenced by many properties of stems and affixes, such as the frequency with which stems are encountered in the language; the number of words sharing a stem morpheme (morphological family size); affix homonymy, or whether or not the form of the affix is associated with one meaning or several; and the degree of: semantic transparency in the relationship between the stem and derivational variants; allomorphy, or the phonetic or orthographic similarity between stem and derived form; and productivity, the extent to which an affix is used to create new words in the language. Many of these variables influence behavioral responses to derived words simultaneously, necessitating the use of multivariate approaches (for review, see Ford, Davis, & Marslen-Wilson, in press).

Despite the differences between inflectional and derivational morphology, research suggests that derived words engage an early, obligatory segmentation process, triggered by the presence of potential derivational affixes, in a similar manner to regularly inflected words. This research uses a paradigm known as visual masked priming, which involves presenting a written prime word so briefly that the reader is only aware of the subsequent target word, allowing us to investigate the earliest stages of visual word processing. Using this paradigm it has been found that derived words prime their stems in many different languages (e.g., Boudelaa & Marslen-Wilson, 2005; Deutsch, Frost, & Forster, 1998; Dominguez, Segui, & Cuetos, 2002; Marslen-Wilson, Bozic, & Randall 2008). Moreover, pseudoderived pairs that feature a potential derivational affix (e.g., *corner/corn*), but which are not themselves morphologically related also show priming (Rastle, Davis, Marslen-Wilson, & Tyler, 2000; Rastle, Davis, & New, 2005). Even nonwords composed of nonoccurring combinations of real stems and derivational affixes (e.g., *tallness*) have been found to prime their pseudostems (e.g., *tall*) as well as existing legal combinations (e.g., *taller*), suggesting that the priming reflects a prelexical segmentation process, blind to lexical status (Longtin, Segui, & Halle, 2003; Longtin & Meunier, 2005). An area of the left fusiform gyrus known as the visual word form area may be involved in this prelexical segmentation. An event-related fMRI study comparing masked priming effects in behavioral and neural responses to morphologically transparent (*teacher/teach*), semantically opaque (*department/depart*), and pseudoderived word pairs (*slipper/slip*) found that the visual word form area showed stronger priming for opaque and pseudoderived pairs than morphologically transparent pairs (Devlin, Jamison, Matthews, & Gonnerman, 2004).

In contrast to masked priming, however, overt priming—when the prime is presented for a long enough period for participants to become aware of its presence—is influenced by lexical properties and compositionality, and suggests that some derived words are stored as morphemes in a similar manner to regularly inflected words. For example, using cross-modal priming it has been found that spoken derived words facilitate responses to their visually presented stems when the relationship between the two is semantically transparent (*darkness/dark*) but not when it is opaque (*department/depart*; Marslen-Wilson et al., 1994). This finding was interpreted as indicating that the same underlying lexical representation of the stem (e.g., *dark*) is accessed by both prime (*darkness*) and target (*dark*) (Marslen-Wilson et al., 1994). Similarly, semantically transparent words sharing a derivational suffix (e.g., *darkness/toughness*) facilitate responses to each other in cross-modal priming, suggesting that the same lexical representation of the suffix (e.g., *–ness*) is accessed by both prime and target (Marslen-Wilson, Ford, Older, & Zhou, 1996). Moreover, related derived words with different suffixes (e.g., *darkness/darkly*) produce a phenomenon called suffix–suffix interference, argued to reflect interference between suffixes competing to link with the same representation of the stem (Marslen-Wilson et al., 1994). As with regular inflectional morphology, the LIFG appears to be involved in segmenting derived words to identify potential compositional representations in the mental lexicon. An event-related fMRI study using delayed priming found that both semantically transparent (*bravely/brave*) and opaque (*archer/arch*) pairs showed priming in the LIFG, whereas words with the same degree of semantic or orthographic relatedness showed no priming (Bozic et al., 2007).

SENTENCE-LEVEL SYNTACTIC AND SEMANTIC INFORMATION

So far we have considered how the language system in the brain is modulated by the nature of individual lexical representations. We have argued that accessing the lexical content of morphologically unstructured words (e.g., monomorphemic, irregularly inflected, or semantically opaque derived words) engages a ventral processing stream in the temporal lobes. Forms that are potentially compositional—in particular stimuli bearing the phonetic signature of the regular past tense form (the IRP)—engage a dorsal system that attempts to segment them into component morphemes, so that the syntactic properties of inflectional suffixes can be analyzed and the semantic content of stems or derivational affixes can be accessed by the ventral system. In addition, written stimuli with potential derivational affixes engage an obligatory prelexical process of segmentation that may involve a region of the brain known as the visual word form area.

We now turn briefly to the issue of how the language system is modulated by combinatorial processes operating at the level of the sentence (for a more detailed review see Tyler & Marslen-Wilson, 2008). In one recent study, this was investigated using an fMRI study contrasting responses to syntactic and semantic ambiguities (Rodd, Longe, Randall, & Tyler, 2004; Tyler & Marslen-Wilson, 2008). Healthy volunteers were presented with spoken sentences containing either a semantic or a syntactic ambiguity that was subsequently resolved (e.g., "She quickly learned that injured calves ... moo loudly" or "Out in the open, flying kites ... are liable to get tangled"). To make the task as naturalistic as possible volunteers listened passively to each sentence and were only then required to judge whether a visually presented word was related in meaning to the sentence. The degree of ambiguity was quantified by collecting ratings of the extent to which one reading of each ambiguous phrase was preferred over the other. Processing syntactic ambiguities engaged the LIFG, the LMTG extending forward into the anterior portion and backward into the inferior parietal lobule and the right superior temporal gyrus. Activity in these regions increased with increasing dominance, such that they were most strongly activated when the preferred reading was overturned by the continuation. This suggests that listeners developed a strong preference for a particular interpretation, which might then have to be overturned by subsequent information. Processing semantic ambiguities also engaged the LIFG and the LMTG. However, the LMTG activation was significantly less than that elicited by syntactic ambiguities and confined to the middle portion of the gyrus. The activation elicited by semantic ambiguities showed no effect of dominance, suggesting that both meanings of the ambiguous word were initially activated in parallel and only disambiguated later. A connectivity analysis showed further differences between the two conditions. Activation of the LIFG predicted activity in the left temporal pole, but in the case of the syntactic ambiguity condition the LIFG predicted temporal pole activation in the right hemisphere as well. In the syntactic ambiguity condition the LIFG also predicted activation in posterior regions, such as the posterior LMTG, inferior parietal gyrus, angular gyrus, and supramarginal gyrus of the left hemisphere. The posterior LMTG region identified was adjacent to that previously identified as covarying with activity in the LIFG and the left anterior cingulate for regular past tenses (Stamatakis et al., 2005). Thus it is possible that different types of combinatorial processes engage adjacent portions of the posterior LMTG.

A CLINICAL EXAMPLE

A clinical example exemplifies the consequences of damage to dorsal language processing pathways in the left hemisphere. Patient DE is a right-handed man who suffered a middle cerebral artery infarct following a road traffic accident at age 16, damaging the posterior inferior frontal gyrus and superior and middle temporal gyri of his left cerebral hemisphere. His language abilities have been investigated in depth in psycholinguistic research (Patterson & Marcel, 1977; Tyler, 1985, 1992; Tyler et al., 2002a, 2002b; Tyler, Moss, & Jennings, 1995; Tyler & Ostrin, 1994) and he participated in many of the studies that informed the neurocognitive model of language comprehension outlined in this chapter (Tyler et al., 2002a, 2002b, 2005). His acquired brain injury resulted in dysfluent speech and a number of selective deficits in combinatorial linguistic processing. For example, he has deep dyslexia, which is typified by morphological errors in reading aloud. Recent research confirms that these errors reflect the morphological status of words (Rastle, Tyler, & Marslen-Wilson, 2006) rather than other confounding linguistic features, such as word imageability or frequency as previously suggested (Funnell, 1987). DE also has impaired speech comprehension for morphologically complex words, as shown in his lack of morphological and semantic priming from regularly inflected words (Longworth et al., 2005; Tyler et al., 2002a) and high error rate in the regular past tense condition of the same-different task (Tyler et al., 2002b). At the sentence level, DE also shows agrammatic speech comprehension, again indicating impairment in the ability to combine linguistic units (Tyler et al., 2002a).

Connectivity analyses of fMRI data from DE reveal the unilateral nature of combinatorial linguistic processes. To examine his pattern of connectivity in the morphological domain, DE participated in the fMRI version of the same-different task (Tyler & Marslen-Wilson, 2008). For healthy age-matched volunteers, activity in the left inferior frontal cortex and anterior cingulate cortex predicted activity in the left posterior middle temporal gyrus. In contrast, DE showed a more right hemisphere pattern of connectivity, with increased activity in the inferior and middle temporal gyrus of the right hemisphere and bilateral anterior temporal lobes. His comprehension deficits for regularly inflected words suggest that this reorganization of function to the right hemisphere is insufficient to support combinatorial processes operating at the level of the word. He also participated in the fMRI study of semantic and syntactic ambiguity, allowing us to examine his pattern of connectivity in the syntactic domain. Syntactic ambiguities activated his left middle frontal gyrus and pre- and postcentral gyri and right inferior parietal lobule. A connectivity analysis showed that the peak of this left hemisphere activity predicted activation of posterior regions of the right hemisphere, in contrast to the left hemisphere posterior regions found in connectivity analyses of healthy volunteers. Again, despite this reorganization of function to the right hemisphere, his syntactic processing remains impaired, suggesting that a left hemisphere language processing stream is critical, not only for combinatorial processes at the level of lexical representation, but also at the level of the sentence. This contrasts with semantic processing, which remains seemingly intact in DE (Longworth et al., 2005) suggesting that comprehension of word meaning relied on primarily ventral pathways that function bihemispherically.

QUESTIONS AND ANSWERS

Why do we need a neurocognitive model of language comprehension?

Cognitive and neurological approaches to understanding language comprehension gain from the theoretical constraints provided by each other. Well-specified cognitive models of the mental representations and processes involved in language comprehension are necessary precursors to understanding how comprehension is instantiated in the brain. Equally, however, knowledge of the neural bases for language comprehension can be useful in distinguishing between competing cognitive models. Both domains of knowledge are required to understand how language comprehension occurs normally and breaks down after brain damage.

How does the current model differ from the classic Wernicke–Lichtheim model of language in the brain?

The classic model proposed a single, dorsal language processing pathway in the left hemisphere. In contrast, the current neurocognitive model posits at least two processing pathways: a unilateral dorsal pathway in the left hemisphere, required for combinatorial processes at the level of lexical representation and at the sentence level; and a bilateral ventral pathway required for processing unstructured lexical representations and semantic information.

How does the current model fit into broader theoretical debates?

The current model forms part of the "Words and Rules" debate in cognitive science, which asks whether language processing and by extension human cognition in general, shows evidence of differentiation or can be handled by an undifferentiated associative memory system. The neurocognitive model posits the existence of two distinct pathways for language comprehension, along the lines of dual route models of other primate systems.

What outstanding questions remain?

The neurocognitive model has implications for speech pathology. It suggests that combinatorial linguistic processes will be more vulnerable to brain damage than the processing of unstructured lexical representations and semantic information. Further research is required to assess the practical implications of this model for the assessment and rehabilitation of acquired language comprehension deficits.

REFERENCES

Ashburner, J., & Friston, K. J. (2000). Voxel-based morphometry: The methods. *Neuroimage, 11*(6/1), 805–821.

Bloomfield, L. (1933). *Language*. New York, NY: Holt.

Boudelaa, S., & Marslen-Wilson, W. D. (2005). Discontinuous morphology in time: Incremental masked priming in Arabic. *Language and Cognitive Processes, 20*, 207–260.

Bozic, M., Marslen-Wilson, W. D., Stamatakis, E., Davis, M. H., & Tyler, L. K. (2007). Differentiating morphology, form, and meaning: Neural correlates of morphological complexity. *Journal of Cognitive Neuroscience, 19*(9), 1464–1475.

Braver, T. S., Barch, D. M., Gray, J. R., Molfese, D. L., & Snyder, A. (2001). Anterior cingulate cortex and response conflict: Effects of frequency, inhibition and errors. *Cerebral Cortex, 11*, 825–836.

Deutsch, A., Frost, R., & Forster, K. I. (1998). Verbs and nouns are organized and accessed differently in the mental lexicon: Evidence from Hebrew. *Journal of Experimental Psychology: Learning, Memory, & Cognition, 24*, 1238–1255.

Devlin, J. T., Jamison, H. L., Matthews, P. M., & Gonnerman, L. (2004). Morphology and the internal structure of words. *Proceedings of the National Academy of Sciences, 101*, 14984–14988.

Dominguez, A., Segui, J., & Cuetos, F. (2002). The time-course of inflexional morphological priming. *Linguistics, 40*(2), 235–259.

Fletcher, P., McKenna, P. J., Friston, K. J., Frith, C. D., & Dolan, R. J. (1999). Abnormal cingulate modulation of fronto-temporal connectivity in schizophrenia. *Neuroimage, 9*, 337–342.

Ford, M. A., Davis, M. H., & Marslen-Wilson, W. D. (In press). Affix productivity promotes decomposition of derived words: Evidence from effects of base morpheme frequency. *Journal of Memory and Language*.

Funnell, E. (1987). Morphological errors in acquired dyslexia: A case of mistaken identity. *Quarterly Journal of Experimental Psychology, 39A*, 497–539.

Gaskell, M. G., & Marslen-Wilson, W. D. (1997). Integrating form and meaning: A distributed model of speech perception. *Language and Cognitive Processes, 12*(5–6), 613–656.

Hauk, O., Davis, M. H., Ford, M., Pulvermuller, F., & Marslen-Wilson, W. D. (2006). The *time* course of visual word-recognition as revealed by linear regression analysis of ERP data. *Neuroimage, 30*(4), 1383–1400.

Hickok, G., & Poeppel, D. (2004). Dorsal and ventral streams: A framework for understanding aspects of the functional anatomy of language. *Cognition, 92,* 67–99.

Joanisse, M. F., & Seidenberg, M. S. (1999). Impairments in verb morphology after brain injury: A connectionist model. *Proceedings of the National Academy of Sciences of the United States of America, 96*(13), 7592–7597.

Kaas, J. H., & Hackett, T. A. (1999). "What" and "where" processing in auditory cortex. *Nature Neuroscience, 2,* 1045–1047.

Longtin, C.-M., & Meunier, F. (2005). Morphological decomposition in early visual word processing. *Journal of Memory and Language, 53,* 26–41.

Longtin, C.-M., Segui, J., & Halle, P. A. (2003). Morphological priming without morphological relationship. *Language and Cognitive Processes, 18,* 313–334.

Longworth, C. E., Marslen-Wilson, W. D., Randall, B., & Tyler, L. K. (2005). Getting to the meaning of the regular past tense: Evidence from neuropsychology. *Journal of Cognitive Neuroscience, 17*(7), 1087–1097.

Lyons, J. (1968). *Introduction to theoretical linguistics.* Cambridge, UK: Cambridge University Press.

Marslen-Wilson, W. D. (1987). Functional parallelism in spoken word-recognition. *Cognition, 25*(1–2), 71–102.

Marslen-Wilson, W. D. (2007). Morphological processes in language comprehension. In G. Gaskell (Ed.), *Oxford handbook of psycholinguistics,* (pp. 175–193). Oxford, UK: OUP.

Marslen-Wilson, W. D, Bozic, M., & Randall, B. (2008). Early decomposition in visual word recognition: Dissociating morphology, form, and meaning. *Language and Cognitive Processes, 23*(3), 394–421.

Marslen-Wilson, W. D., Ford, M., Older, L., & Zhou, X. (1996). The combinatorial lexicon: Priming derivational affixes. In G. Cottrell (Ed.), *Proceedings of the 18th annual conference of the cognitive science society* (pp. 223–227). Mahwah, NJ: LEA.

Marslen-Wilson, W. D., & Tyler, L. K. (1997). Dissociating types of mental computation. *Nature, 387*(6633), 592–594.

Marslen-Wilson, W. D., & Tyler, L. K. (1998). Rules, representations and the English past tense. *Trends in Cognitive Science, 2,* 428–436.

Marslen-Wilson, W. D., & Tyler, L. K. (2007). Morphology, language and the brain: The decompositional substrate for language comprehension. *Philosophical Transactions of the Royal Society B: Biological Sciences, 362,* 823–836.

Marslen-Wilson, W.D. & Welsh, A. (1978), Processing interactions during word recognition in continuous speech. *Cognition 10,* 29–63.

Marslen-Wilson, W. D., Tyler, L. K., Waksler, R., & Older, L. (1994). Morphology and meaning in the English mental lexicon. *Psychological Review, 101*(1), 3–33.

McClelland, J., & Patterson, K. (2002). Rules or connections in past-tense inflections: What does the evidence rule out? *Trends in Cognitive Sciences, 6,* 465–472.

Miozzo, M. (2003). On the processing of regular and irregular forms of verbs and nouns: Evidence from neuropsychology. *Cognition, 87,* 101–127.

Moss, H. E., McCormick, S., & Tyler, L. K. (1997). The time course of activation of semantic information during spoken word recognition. *Language and Cognitive Processes, 12*(5/6), 695–731.

Noesselt, T., Shah, N., & Jancke, L. (2003). Top-down and bottom-up modulation of language related areas—an fMRI study. *BMC Neuroscience, 4,* 13.

Patterson, K., & Marcel, A. (1977). Aphasia, dyslexia and the phonological coding of written words. *Quarterly Journal of Experimental Psychology, 29,* 307–318.

Pinker, S., & Prince, A. (1988). On language and connectionism: Analysis of a parallel distributed-processing model of language-acquisition. *Cognition, 28*(1–2), 73–193.

Pinker, S., & Ullman, M. (2002). The past and future of the past tense. *Trends in Cognitive Sciences, 6,* 456–463.

Post, B., Marslen-Wilson, W. D., Randall, B., & Tyler, L. K. (2008). The processing of English regular inflections: Phonological cues to morphological structure. *Cognition, 109,* 1–17.

Rastle, K., Davis, M. H., Marslen-Wilson, W. D., & Tyler, L. K. (2000). Morphological and semantic effects in visual word recognition: A time-course study. *Language and Cognitive Processes, 15,* 507–537.

Rastle, K., Davis, M. H., & New, B. (2005). The broth in my brother's brothel: Morpho-orthographic segmentation in visual word recognition. *Psychonomic Bulletin, 11,* 1090–1098.

Rastle, K., Tyler, L. K., & Marslen-Wilson, W. D. (2006). New evidence for morphological errors in deep dyslexia. *Brain and Language, 97*(2), 189–199.

Rauschecker, J. P., & Tian, B. (2000). Mechanisms and streams for processing of 'what' and 'where' in auditory cortex. *Proceedings of the National Academy of Sciences, 97*(22), 11800–11806.

Rodd, J. M., Longe, O. A., Randall, B., & Tyler, L. K. (2004). Syntactic and semantic processing of spoken sentences: An fMRI study of ambiguity. *Journal of Cognitive Neuroscience, 16*(Suppl. C), 89.

Rumelhart, D. E., & McClelland, J. L. (1986). On learning the past tenses of English verbs. In D. E. Rumelhart, J. L. McClelland, & P. R. Group (Eds.), *Parallel distributed processing: Explorations in the microstructure of cognition* (Vol. 2). Cambridge, MA: MIT Press.

Scott, S. K., & Johnsrude, I. S. (2003). The neuroanatomical and functional organization of speech perception. *Trends in Neuroscience, 26,* 100–107.

Stamatakis, E. A., Marslen-Wilson, W. D., Tyler, L. K., & Fletcher, P. C. (2005). Cingulate control of fronto-temporal integration reflects linguistic demands: A three-way interaction in functional connectivity. *NeuroImage, 28,* 115–121.

Tyler, L. K. (1985). Real-time comprehension processes in agrammatism: A case-study. *Brain and Language, 26*(2), 259–275.

Tyler, L. K. (1992). *Spoken language comprehension: An experimental approach to disordered and normal processing.* Cambridge, MA: MIT Press.

Tyler, L. K., de Mornay-Davies, P., Anokhina, R., Longworth, C. E., Randall, B., & Marslen-Wilson, W. D. (2002a). Dissociations in processing past tense morphology: Neuropathology and behavioral studies. *Journal of Cognitive Neuroscience, 14,* 79–94.

Tyler, L. K., & Marslen-Wilson, W. D. (2008). Frontotemporal brain systems supporting spoken language comprehension. *Philosophical Transactions of the Royal Society of London B, 363*(1493), 1037–1054.

Tyler, L. K., Marslen-Wilson, W. D., & Stamatakis, E. A. (2005). Dissociating neuro-cognitive component processes: Voxel-based correlational methodology. *Neuropsychologia, 43,* 771–778.

Tyler, L. K., Moss, H. E., Galpin, A., & Voice, J. K. (2002). Activating meaning in time: The role of imageability and form-class. *Language and Cognitive Processes, 17*(5), 471–502.

Tyler, L. K., Moss, H. E., & Jennings, F. (1995). Abstract word deficits in aphasia: Evidence from semantic priming. *Neuropsychology, 9*(3), 354–363.

Tyler, L. K., & Ostrin, R. K. (1994). The processing of simple and complex words in an agrammatic patient: Evidence from priming. *Neuropsychologia, 32*(8), 1001–1013.

Tyler, L.K., Randall, B. & Marslen-Wilson, W.D. (2002b). Phonology and neuropsychology of the English past tense. *Neuropsychologia, 40*(8), 1154–1166.

Tyler, L. K., Stamatakis, E. A., Jones, R., Bright, P., Acres, K., & Marslen-Wilson, W. D. (2004). Deficits for semantics and the irregular past tense: A causal relationship? *Journal of Cognitive Neuroscience, 16,* 1159–1172.

Tyler, L. K., Stamatakis, E. A., Post, B., Randall, B., & Marslen-Wilson, W. D. (2005). Temporal and frontal systems in speech comprehension: An fMRI study of past tense processing. *Neuropsychologia, 43,* 1963–1974.

Ungerleider, L. G., & Mishkin, M. (1982). Two visual pathways. In D. J. Ingle, M. A. Goodale, & R. J. W. Mansfield (Eds.), *Analysis of visual behavior* (pp. 549–586). Cambridge, MA: MIT Press.

12 Formulaic Expressions in Mind and Brain: Empirical Studies and a Dual-Process Model of Language Competence

Diana Van Lancker Sidtis

INTRODUCTION

After a long period of neglect and misunderstanding, formulaic language has finally come into its own (Coulmas, 1994; Cowie, 1992; Kuiper, 2004; Pawley, 2001, 2007; Wray, 2002, 2008a). Neglect arose from the myopic perspective that the speech formulas, idioms, and other conventional expressions known to a language community take the form of a mundane look-up list of little interest to studies of grammar. As for misunderstanding, attempts to pin formulaic language down using generative linguistic approaches resembled, in the opinion of many today, trying to force a square peg into a round hole. These approaches not only failed to yield valid or useful descriptions; they also distorted the picture of a very large, very vibrant sector of language competence, which is worthy of examination on its own terms. Observations of formulaic language in diverse discourse contexts have greatly increased our perspective in the past decade, and theories have begun to mature. Much of this growth is attributable to the burgeoning interest in pragmatics—language use in everyday settings, and to the embracing of spoken text staunchly undertaken by sociolinguists (e.g., Schegloff, 1988; Tannen, 1989).

Our purpose in this article is to review progress in our understanding of formulaic language, beginning with a background discussion and continuing with a review of studies of normal use and incidence. Because many categories of formulaic language flourish in actual spontaneous language use, and because production material is the most difficult to capture and quantify, we focus on spoken texts, corpus studies, and discourse analyses, supplemented by formal studies that attempt to probe speech production. The overview will then examine formulaic language in disordered speech. In the conclusion, we propose a dual-process production model that accommodates both formulaic and novel language in a neurolinguistic context, whereby the accountable brain structures are described.

DEFINITIONS AND THEORY

Formulaic expressions carry meaning as whole units whose individual word parts do not necessarily reflect the meaning of the whole expression (Van Lancker Sidtis, 2004; Wray & Perkins, 2000). For example, the idiom "He put his foot in his mouth" has figurative meaning, as does the expression "That broke the ice." In the latter expression, the signifiers have more direct correspondence to the signified and so can be said to have more semantic transparency than the former expression. There are other forms of nonpropositional expressions that are more transparent in terms of literal meaning. One category is speech formulas, for example, "How are you?" or "After you" and such proverbs as "Better safe than sorry."

The best operational definition for formulaic expressions is an exclusionary one, applying "nonnovel" as the selection criterion; that is, formulaic expressions have in common that they are *not* newly created from the operation of grammatical rules on lexical items. They are holistically acquired and used in a language community based on shared knowledge of the stereotyped, canonical form, the conventionalized meaning, and conditions of use. The list of generally accepted categories has become well known: idioms (for which the lexical items do not carry their usual meanings: "She has him eating out of her hand"); speech formulas (conventional expressions used in specified conversational contexts: "I'll get back to you later"); proverbs, expletives and exclamations ("Oh, my God," "Wow"); pause fillers ("uh, um"), discourse particles ("well," "so," "then"), conventional expressions ("that being said"), sentence stems ("I think"), and indirect requests ("it's getting warm in here"). Some treatments of formulaic language include nonreversible dyads and triads ("salt and pepper," "red, white, and blue"), verb plus particle constructions ("back up" as in an argument), and specialized compound nouns ("truck driver"). These all have in common that they are not newly created but are produced and recognized by native speakers as unitary in form and meaning and conventionalized in usage. What remains to be further understood are the differences between these and other subtypes of formulaic language.

Stereotyped form, the first characteristic mentioned above, means that formulaic expressions, in their canonical form, contain precisely specified words in a certain word order spoken on a set intonation contour. Secondly, the meanings of formulaic expressions are conventionalized, which means the semantic aspects are idiosyncratic in various ways; they may be nonliteral, serve mainly as social signals, and/or they communicate a meaning that is greater than the sum of their parts—the special innuendos (Wray, 2002), which often deliver strong doses of affect and/or attitude. And third, as formulaic language lives in the realm of pragmatics, conditions of use constitute the third defining characteristic.

THE FLEXIBLE FORMULEME

A property of formulaic expressions that has wreaked havoc in linguistic circles is, paradoxically, their flexibility: many variants can and do appear. The canonical form can be, and usually is, altered in actual usage. We argue below that the goal to discover cogent and explanatory generalizations underlying these variations, which will hold for a large set of formulaic expressions, has not been especially enlightening; it is ruefully reminiscent of the previous "look-up table" approach to formulaic expressions. Instead, we assert the legitimacy of the view that references a canonical form or formuleme, and simultaneously allows for any alteration conforming to legal grammatical possibilities in the language, as long as the canonical form remains recognizable. People intend for formulaic utterances to be recognizable, and they can allude to them in many ways. In reviewing versions of formulaic utterances given as "unacceptable" ("starred") exemplars in Kuiper and Everaert (2000), we could imagine playful or creative contexts allowing any of these. To alter formulaic expressions is merely to engage in theme and variation, one of the oldest and most pervasive practices in art and culture.

Throughout this article, we argue that people are free to apply linguistic rules on formulaic expressions for any purpose: communication, verbal playfulness, performing a new twist on a conventionalized meaning, allusion to a previous instance of a formula, conflation of two formulas, and so on. The speaker's meaning under these situations will be determined by linguistic and social context, as has been found in earlier studies (Gibbs, 1981). It is the context bound, creative basis of formuleme variation that has led to inconsistent results in the quest for linguistic regularity underlying versions of idioms and other kinds of formulaic language. From anecdotal observation, we submit that "acceptability" parameters for formulaic expressions work from particularly soft constraints, meaning that acceptability judgments are highly subject to numerous linguistic and contextual effects (Sorace & Keller, 2005).

FORMULEME FAMILIARITY

As stated by Jackendoff (1995), a very large number of a broad range of formulaic expressions "are familiar to American speakers of English; that is, an American speaker must have them stored in memory" (p. 135). Formulaic expressions are "familiar" in the sense that a native speaker will recognize them as having this special status. For example, the sentence "He knew already a few days ago about the anniversary of the first actual moon landing" has probably not been said or heard before; this sentence has none of the properties of familiarity and predictability mentioned above (Pinker, 1995). On the other hand, the expressions "Leave me alone!" or "You've got to be kidding" or "You don't say!" (speech formulas); "David spilled the beans" or "She's a real snake in the grass" (idioms); and "A bird in the hand beats two in the bush" or "The early bird catches the worm" (proverbs) are all "familiar," in that native speakers recognize these utterances—they say that they do, and they demonstrate knowledge of their specialized meanings and appropriate contexts. This knowledge is demonstrated in more ways than can be enumerated here: ubiquitous allusions to formulaic expressions in the public media, echoing use in conversations, text, field and survey studies, and studies of word association. For example, people in a language community know not to say "See you later" on first entering a room; they do not give a "good morning" greeting twice in a row when passing in the hall to the same person. As an operational test, native speakers of a language accurately fill in blanks in such utterances, when key words are omitted (Van Lancker Sidtis & Rallon, 2004). Approximately a third of word association results is attributable to the "idiom effect," which means that given a target word, subjects produce words from a known formulaic expression (Clark, 1970).

Thus the effort to explain variants misses the main point: the stereotyped form (or "formuleme"), its conventional meaning, and its conditions of usage are known to the language community. Any grammatical alteration (passivizing, movement, insertion, and so on)—that could legally apply to the corresponding nonformulaic structure—is possible in the communicative context, so long as enough of the formuleme remains identifiable and the context allows for correct interpretation. The key feature of formulaic expressions is their personal familiarity: people know them. Their status as common knowledge in a linguistic community forms the major portion of their *raison d'être*. This is a matter of native speakers' intuitions, which stand as valid linguistic evidence (Devitt, 2006).

FUNCTIONS OF FORMULAIC LANGUAGE IN EVERYDAY DISCOURSE

The pervasive nature of these types of expressions in our daily repertoire of communication has been examined in studies documenting the function and frequency of formulaic language in conversations and in literary texts and films (Van Lancker Sidtis, 2004). In comparison to isolated novel expressions, an utterance that contains a formulaic expression imbues the communication with emotional and attitudinal weight (Van Lancker Sidtis, 2008). Certain function-based divisions of formulaic language reflect these features; for example, thanking, apologies, requests, and offers (Aijmer, 1996; Wray & Perkins, 2000). Others, falling under the heading of social interactions, include conversational maintenance and purpose (e.g., "How've you been?" "What's the occasion?" "I'm very sorry to hear that." "Really?" "No kidding!"). Formulaic expressions are used to achieve special purposes in communication (Tannen & Öztek, 1981), such as structuring talk (Fox Tree, 2006; Jucker, 1993) negotiating complaints (Drew & Holt, 1988); partnership solidarity (Bell & Healey, 1992; Bruess & Pearson, 1993), maintaining fluency in various contexts such as sport, weather forecasting, horse races, in the workplace, and auctions (Kuiper, 1991, 1992, 1996, 2000; Kuiper & Flindall, 2000; Kuiper & Haggo, 1985) and generally sounding like a native speaker of the language (Fillmore, 1979; Pawley & Syder, 1983; see review in Van Lancker Sidtis, 2004). Because they are not newly formed, formulaic expression free up resources in the speaker to look ahead to the next part of the encoding process (Kuiper, 2000; Wray & Perkins, 2000). Production of ready-made phrases allows for more consistent rates of speech and greater fluency. It might be said that formulaic expressions buy time during speech production.

Dissecting these types of expressions reveals that they are tools with a purpose that includes, but also transcends, the act of conveying factual information. Vivid examples of this quality can be found in the formulaic expressions identified, classified and validated by Van Lancker Sidtis and Rallon (2004) from the screen play *Some Like it Hot*: "Cut it out"; "I forgive you"; "I'm afraid not"; "Then hit'm with everything you've got"; "Quit stalling"; "It's gone to his head"; "They wouldn't be caught dead"; "You got a lot of nerve." We note their properties of stereotyped form, conventional meaning (including affective and attitudinal meanings), and restricted pragmatic conditions. Native speakers recognize them as familiar and know implicitly how they function in conversation.

QUANTITY OF FORMULAIC EXPRESSIONS IN EVERYDAY DISCOURSE

The actual number of these expressions is debated. Persons accumulating lists have not seen an upper limit. While experts trawling for formulaic expressions in the sea of language differ somewhat in how broadly to throw the net to establish formulaic categories, all agree that the number making up a typical speaker's repertory exceeds many tens of thousands, and some say the totals are upward of hundreds of thousands (K. Kuiper, personal communication, 2007). All kinds of formulaic expressions occur in daily speech a great deal of the time, but a compiled sum remains difficult to come by at the present time, in part because analytic efforts examining speech samples have been fragmented and piecemeal.

Naturalistic speech is a notoriously difficult beast. Yet to understand formulaic language, our interests turn to the kinds of expressions and how many of them; in what social and linguistic contexts do they appear, by whom are they spoken and how frequently do they appear, and with which themes and discourse styles are they associated. This requires qualitative and quantitative examination of natural speech. Some field studies of incidence have appeared. Jay (1980) tabulated use of cursing in specific populations (e.g., college students) and Gallahorn (1971) kept records of expletives emitted during team meetings of health care professionals on a psychiatric ward.

A brilliant contribution utilizing the fieldwork method came from Mathilde Hain (1951), who recorded over 350 proverbs in actual use among people who lived in a small German village, Ulfa, between the years of 1938 and 1943. Hain, a folklorist using sociolinguistic, field study methods, was interested in documenting veridical, spontaneous production of proverbs, and in simultaneously recording the linguistic and social contexts of these specialized utterances. In this way, she could concern herself with quantity—how many different proverbial utterances appeared in the years that she lived in the village performing field work, and quality: how was each utterance used to communicate in the unique context? She examined the time of appearance of a proverb in the conversational setting (early, late, toward the end) and how the utterance was dealt with by the speaker and the listener. She set about recording the function of proverbs in everyday life as well as their position in a discussion. Here are some speech situations from the Ulfa village life recorded by Hain (1951, pp. 26–27 (in translation). In the second example, the same proverb appeared in two settings (given in dialect, high German, and in the English translation):

1. The baptism of an infant with about 30 guests. ... Two older farmer women talk about the local young teacher, his performance in school and his meager salary. Mrs. X., especially, has a lot of information; she knows him and his modest means. X.: *Er ess hoard gscheit!* (er ist sehr klug) (Engl: he is very smart). At first K. listens pensively, then she responds slowly: *Aich saan als, wer de Hoawwern vedint hot, kritt en näid* (Engl.: I always say, those who deserve the oats don't get them). Mrs. X. energetically agrees: *Joa, so ess!* (That's for sure!). And so this topic has ended; the individual case has become part of the general understanding.

2. The old dirt farmer Ch., in his late 70s, who always has a joke at hand, tells an acquaintance from the city about his daughter-in-law's long illness, including how long they tried to heal her and how much money they spent! It would not have been necessary if she would have gone for x-rays in Giessen right away. B. says: One only knows in hindsight. As he is getting ready to leave, Ch. replies loudly, so that you can even hear it across the street: *Joa, wann's Kend gehowe ess, gitt's Gevadderleut* (ja, wenn das Kind aus der Taufe gehoben ist, gibt's Paten) (Engl: yes, when the child is baptized there will be godparents)!

I heard the same proverb in other situations. A dirt-farmer of about 50 years told me about her misfortune with her cows. When another one was infected with brucellosis the year before, she bought insurance for all animals. She ended her story calmly, almost wearily: *Wann's Kend gehowe ess, gitt's Gevadderleut!* In both situations the proverb offered a way out into a consoling generic situation.

Hain's labor-intensive study provides a rare record of ordinary usage of one particular category of formulaic expressions. From the examples provided throughout her fieldwork record, it is clear that each time a proverb is used, the speaker has an expectation that its stereotyped form and conventionalized meaning will be recognized by the listener(s) as part of their linguistic knowledge. Meanings were not glossed or explained. We reiterate three main facts about formulaic familiarity that must not be lost or ignored in any treatment: people know them; speakers using them expect listeners to know them, and to appreciate the meaning conveyed; and, indeed, mutual familiarity with the specialized expressions forms an essential part of the reason for using them.

In the past few decades, discourse samples, or corpora, have been examined, using spoken samples and written texts. With the benefit of computerized searching, various texts have been analyzed using different algorithms to count incidence of formulaic expressions. Using a mathematical standard only, Altenberg (1998) listed three-word combinations that occurred 10 times or more in the London-Lund Corpus (Greenbaum & Svartik, 1990). Other studies have utilized a human interface to classify utterance types. Some analyses have focused on a particular type of formula, such as proverbs. Cowie (1992) performed a study on "multiword lexical units" in newspaper language, differentiating idioms from collocations of various kinds. In an extensive treatment, Moon (1998) performed a descriptive study of formulaic expressions and idioms in an 18 million word corpus of contemporary English, the Oxford Hector Pilot Corpus (Glassman et al., 1992), augmenting her analysis from other text sources. Norrick (1985) reports only one complete proverb, plus a few proverbial allusions, in the 43,165 line corpus transcribed conversation published by Svartik and Quirk (1980). A comparative frequency count of proverbs in French and English conversational corpora is described by Arnaud and Moon (1993).

Some quantitative and qualitative data on formulaic expressions come from studies of literary texts, especially in oral literature (Kiparsky, 1976; Kuiper, 2000). Tilley (1950) counted proverbs in the plays of Shakespeare. Schweizer (1978) listed 194 idioms in 2876 pages of six novels of Günter Grass, yielding an average of 14.8 idioms per page. Lord (1960) analyzed formulaic language in the *Odyssey* and the *Iliad*. In his study of Homer's *Iliad*, Page (1959) estimates that about one-fifth of the poem is "composed of lines wholly repeated from one place to another" (p. 223), and that within the *Iliad*'s 28,000 lines, there are approximately 25,000 repeated phrases. In the screen play *Some Like it Hot* idioms, proverbs, and speech formulas constituted 25% of the total number of phrases in the text (Van Lancker Sidtis & Rallon, 2004). Much could be added concerning the qualitative contributions of formulas, such as the numerous literary devices throughout Grass's writings, which involve idiomatic forms and meanings, and the abundance of speech formulas utilized to artistic effect in the plays of Ionesco (Klaver, 1989).

PSYCHOLINGUISTIC STUDIES

Although this article is focused on production of formulaic expressions, a brief look at comprehension studies of idioms offers some understanding of what makes formulaic language special. Using idioms, speakers convey ideas and emotions using words that do not refer to their usual lexical meanings. "She's skating on thin ice" can be said without directly referring to skating, but to convey the idea of risky behavior. How the listener apprehends idiomatic meaning remains mysterious. Three models proposed to explain this process are literal-first (serial) processing, literal and idiomatic (parallel) processing, and direct access of idiomatic meaning (depending on the context). These models differ in their use of the notion of compositionality, as some are based on the assumption that idioms are not "composed," but are processed as cohesive unitary items. The foundation for this idea comes from studies showing that people remember idioms as chunks rather than composite forms (Horowitz & Manelis, 1973; Osgood & Hoosain, 1974; Pickens and Pollio, 1979; Simon, 1974), a result also shown for Chinese idioms (Simon, Zhang, Zang, & Peng, 1989).

The two models of noncompositionality are the Idiom List Hypothesis and the Lexical Representation Model. The Idiom List Hypothesis (Bobrow & Bell, 1973) proposes that idioms are lexical items stored in memory and that upon encountering an idiom, the comprehension device first attempts a literal interpretation. After failing, the idiom retrieval mode kicks in and the idiom is selected from the look-up list. Thus, serial processing predicts greater response time latencies for idioms than for literal utterances because literal interpretation is the first step in any language task. A number of later studies refuted these findings by showing that visual classification of idioms is faster than literal phrases, forming the basis for the Lexical Representation model. Originally formulated by Swinney and Cutler (1979), the Lexical Representation model suggests that idiomatic meaning is processed in parallel with literal meaning, and that idioms are stored and retrieved whole, accounting for the faster reaction times.

However, the question remains as to how idioms can undergo syntactic and semantic modifications and maintain their pragmatic identity. Different studies have addressed these two separate underlying issues: Are idioms stored and accessed as whole units, and/or are their individual words and syntactic form taken into account during the retrieval process? Experimental approaches to these questions involve measuring production errors, response time, accuracy in recall and recognition memory tasks, and various kinds of rating surveys. Fixed expressions that can undergo syntactic modifications yet maintain their conventional meaning are said to have syntactic flexibility (or productivity). For example, one could say "For years, she had been skating on really thin ice," and listeners, depending on context, could assume the nonliteral meaning. The notion "degree of compositionality," derived from native speakers' ratings, has been proposed to determine the flexibility of an idiom's comprehension (Gibbs & Gonzales, 1985; Gibbs, Nayak, Bolton, & Keppel, 1989). This finding is interesting although the reliability of the approach has been questioned (Cacciari & Tabossi, 1988; Titone & Conine, 1999). An idiom's "degree of compositionality" is likely not an all or none property, but instead viewed as a falling along a continuum, highly influenced by context. In addition, ratings in these surveys depend greatly on task instructions. Further, linguistic and situational contexts facilitate several aspects of nonliteral language comprehension, including how rapidly formulaic expressions (e.g., indirect requests and idioms) are processed, how they are interpreted (literally or figuratively), and how accurately and quickly they are retrieved from memory (Gibbs, 1980, 1981). Social context plays a major role in judgments or perceptions of lexical transparency and syntactic flexibility.

The various findings of syntactic and lexical flexibility have led to hybrid psycholinguistic models. The earliest example is the Configurational model (Cacciari & Tabossi, 1988), which integrates literal-first and idiomatic-only approaches.

This states that initially the idiom's potential literal meaning is activated until a key word is encountered that unlocks the idiom's figurative meaning. The idiom meaning is encoded within a specific word configuration that has weighted connections between its lexical nodes. Idioms are considered to have either high or low predictability, depending on how early the key occurs in the string.

Several creative approaches to the production mode have been designed. From studies using speech-error elicitation experiment (Cutting & Bock, 1997), the authors conclude that idioms are not frozen or devoid of information about their syntactic and semantic structure. Interference in the form of blending errors was more likely to occur between idioms sharing the same syntactic form, and the resultant word substitutions were in the same grammatical class. Another experiment showed that idiom production can result in activation of corresponding literal meaning. The authors put forth the argument that what is special about idioms is their relationship to a conceptual representation, which is a nonlinguistic entity, and that in normal language production, idioms are not special. Another study using a priming technique, in which a probe word is used to influence later online processing of a test word, also concluded that words in idioms stimulate word association networks as readily as words in literal sentences (Smolka, Rabanus, & Rösler, 2007).

We agree that syntactic and semantic operations can be performed on any formulaic expression, and that speakers can discern grammatical form and lexical meaning in these expressions. However, the additional properties of formulaic expressions reviewed above—among which are familiarity, stereotyped form, conventional, contextual-based meanings, and conditions of use are pragmatic-linguistic factors, which must be recognized in a veridical model of language competence. These are revealed in surveys, sentence completion studies, and association studies (Clark, 1970; Van Lancker Sidtis & Rallon, 2004). A series of idiom production experiments by Sprenger (2003) using a priming paradigm with response time measurement addressed this question, yielding the notion of superlemma, which corresponds to the idea proposed in this article of canonical form or formuleme. Similarly, analysis of speech errors involving idioms suggests that "idioms are both compositional and noncompositional at the same time, at different levels of processing" (Kuiper, van Egmond, Kempen, & Sprenger, 2007, p. 324). This superlemma or formuleme is stored and processed as a whole, but because it contains syntactic and semantic information of various kinds (as does any linguistic entity in the speaker's repertory), it can link to other parts of the lexicon and grammar.

The dual-process model of language competence, which has been previously mentioned and is proposed in this review, accommodates these findings (Van Lancker Sidtis, 2008; Wray and Perkins, 2000). The inconsistencies arising from idiom studies can be explained by the interplay of formulaic and novel processing. The dual-processing model states that formulaic expressions, which by definition have stereotyped form, conventionalized meanings, and are familiar in a language community (Kitzinger, 2000), exist in harmony with the grammar, which consists of rules and a lexicon. Formulaic expressions, depending on the intent and verbal creativity of the speaker and context, can be altered using standard grammatical processes. Because of this flexibility and context dependency, we submit that task demands in psycholinguistic approaches to the processing of formulaic expressions exert an overriding influence on the results. When subjects are involved in metalinguistic decisions about the interplay between formulaic and novel expressions, their performance will be highly influenced by contingencies of the experimental setting. The idiom studies do not lead to the conclusion that formulaic and novel language are processed in the same way, but rather show that grammar can operate on any legitimate utterance, and that standard lexical meanings can be discerned in any phrase. Again, the interesting point is not that formulaic expressions can be semantically transparent and composed and are therefore alterable, but that there is a *known entity to analyze and to alter.*

AUDITORY CONTRASTS OF IDIOMATIC AND LITERAL MEANINGS

Another set of studies highlights speakers' knowledge of differences between literal and idiomatic utterances. A series of studies using American English ditropic sentences, those having both idiomatic and literal meanings, such as "He was at the end of his rope," showed that listeners can distinguish between these kinds of meanings from the acoustic signal alone. Listening studies confirmed the discriminability of these utterance types, and acoustic measures of rate, pitch mean and variability, and terminal pitch revealed significantly contributory auditory cues. These observations implied that native speakers articulate literal and idiomatic utterances differently, formulating consistent and stable auditory-acoustic cues that listeners use to distinguish between the two meanings (Van Lancker, Canter, & Terbeek, 1981). Later studies examined utterances in French and Korean, revealing differences and similarities in the use of acoustic-phonetic cues to convey contrastively idiomatic and literal interpretations of ditropic sentences (Abdelli-Baruh, Yang, Ahn, & Van Lancker Sidtis, 2007). It was found that Parisian French and American English speakers utilized the same cues to distinguish the sentences, but in an opposite manner: French idioms were significantly longer, while for English, the literal versions were longer. Pitch was also differently utilized to signal the meaning differences. When Korean ditropic sentences were analyzed, it was seen that native speakers of Korean used duration, amplitude variations, and contrasting fundamental frequency in the last two words to mark utterances as either literal or idiomatic in Korean (Ahn, Yang, & Sidtis, 2010). Literal utterances have longer durations than idiomatic utterances, whereas idiomatic utterances are more varied in amplitude than literal utterances. Intonation contours differ for the two types of meanings: Literal utterances end more often with falling pitch whereas idiomatic utterances end with rising pitch. Thus formulaic and literal meaning contrasts, in utterances where the words and grammar do not differ, are successfully signaled by various acoustic-auditory cues known to the native speaker community.

In summary, many psycholinguistic studies have exploited the fact that formulaic expressions can be manipulated metalinguistically, but these studies have not yielded a consistently explanatory model. Demonstrating the interplay between formulaic and novel expressions using various performance tasks, some researchers have concluded that mental processes for these two types of utterances do not differ. As mentioned above, this conclusion misses the point of the status and value of formulaic expressions in everyday usage, and fails to acknowledge the dual-processing feature of language competence.

DISORDERED LANGUAGE IN NEUROLOGICAL CONDITIONS

A neurological account of formulaic language as a class of its own can be found in clinical observations of aphasic language (Espir & Rose, 1970). In clinical domains, the notion of formulaic language traces back to the well-known concept of "automatic speech" in aphasia, first identified and described by J. Hughlings Jackson (1874). Automatic speech includes "overlearned" utterances such as counting, speech formulas (salutations and conversational fillers), swearing, nursery rhymes, familiar lyrics and familiar songs, and other such expressions (Code, 1989; Van Lancker, 1993; Van Lancker & Cummings, 1999). Preservation of certain kinds of speech is dramatic when experienced in severe cases of language disturbance following left hemisphere stroke: the afflicted person cannot articulate a novel phrase or sentence, or can do so only with extreme effort and poor articulatory success. In contrast, he or she can fluently swear, count to 10, recite nursery rhymes, and produce a set of fixed expressions, such as "How are you," "Good-bye," "I don't know." This well-known fact remained anecdotally transmitted among clinicians until survey studies performed for English (Code, 1982, 1989), Chinese (Chung, Code, & Ball, 2004) and German speakers (Blanken & Marini, 1997), which systematically documented preserved expressions in severe aphasia.

Several group studies of production abilities in aphasia support impressions about preservation of formulaic expressions. Using three paired tasks, Lum and Ellis (1994) compared speech production in formulaic versus propositional contexts. First, counting was compared to naming Arabic numbers in nonconsecutive order; next, naming pictures with cues from formulaic expressions (e.g., Don't beat around the BUSH) was compared to naming pictures depicting novel phrases (Don't dig behind the BUSH); and third, formulaic and novel expressions were compared in a repetition task. Subjects performed better on formulaic subtests for number production and picture naming, with a slight advantage also for phrase repetition. A similar finding (Van Lancker & Bella, 1996) arose from comparing matched propositional and formulaic expressions in aphasic speakers also in the repetition and sentence completion tasks, again with weaker differences results in the repetition task.

It is clear that formulaic language has its most authentic presence in spontaneous speech. It is therefore desirable to examine the naturalistic speech of persons with left or right hemisphere damage due to stroke to determine the effect of localized damage on the use of formulaic expressions. Recently, a study of formulaic expressions in conversational speech of right hemisphere damaged subjects and left hemisphere damaged subjects compared to normal controls was undertaken (Van Lancker Sidtis & Postman, 2006). The incidence of formulaic language was significantly higher in left hemisphere damage resulting in aphasia than in matched normal control speakers, while in right hemisphere damage, formulaic expressions were significantly diminished in comparison to normal speech. A striking finding was the low percentage in right hemisphere damaged subjects' speech of pause fillers, *um* and *uh*, which serve semantic and pragmatic purposes in communication (Clark & Fox Tree, 2002). For left hemisphere damaged persons, these results suggest that formulaic expressions become a vehicle for communication in aphasia, and for right hemisphere damaged persons, who do not have phonological, syntactic, or linguistic–semantic deficits, these results may help clarify the clinical impression of abnormal pragmatics of communication.

Case studies and other limited observations in neurologically impaired speech have implicated subcortical structures in the brain. In one case report, a loss of formulaic speech production abilities followed damage in the basal ganglia, namely a right caudate stroke (Speedie, Wertman, Ta'ir, & Heilman, 1993). Another examination of two individuals with damage confined to subcortical nuclei, utilizing discourse obtained from structured interviews, revealed a significantly smaller proportion of formulaic expressions when compared to similar interview settings obtained from normal control speakers matched for education and age. In that same study, the aphasic speaker utilized a much greater proportion than all other groups (Van Lancker Sidtis, Canterucci, & Katsnelson, 2008). In another instance, which involved a motor speech disorder likely due to a subcortical stroke, a pathologically intrusive syllable (*sis*) occurred with greater frequency during recitation, counting, and other formulaic expressions than in novel speech (Van Lancker, Bogen, & Canter, 1983). Still other differences between formulaic and novel language production have been seen in analyses of speech samples from Parkinson's patients, who have diminished basal ganglia function, revealing reduced formulaic language expressions when speaking (Illes, Metterb, Hanson, & Iritanib, 1988). Further, in Parkinson speakers, acoustic measures of voice and articulation, as well as listeners' ratings, differ significantly for novel and formulaic vocalization tasks (Sidtis, Rogers, Katsnelson, & Sidtis, 2010).

The few functional brain imaging studies examining formulaic language have been inconsistent, and findings are not always in agreement with well-established information derived from clinical observations and lesion studies. Earlier studies of cerebral blood flow using SPECT methodology associated bilateral hemisphere activation with automatic speech (Larsen, Skinhoj, & Lassen, 1978; Ryding, Bradvik, & Ingvar, 1987), but with the proliferation of functional imaging of language studies, bilateral signal is reported for most language tasks, and the early SPECT results are no longer interpretable. Published studies of language processing in general typically report bilateral hemispheric blood flow responses, for reasons that are not yet well understood (Van Lancker Sidtis, 2006). More recently, Blank, Scott, Murphy, Warburton, and Wise (2002) reported bilateral activation for both propositional and automatic speech, which does not reveal an interesting contrast between the two language modes. Another study using PET imaging employed two automatic speech tasks: the months of the year and the Pledge of Allegiance (Bookheimer, Zeffiro, Blaxton, Gaillard, & Theodore, 2000), compared to tongue movements and consonant–vowel syllable production. Continuous production of the Pledge of Allegiance showed activation in traditional language areas; reciting the months of the year selectively engaged language Brodmann areas 44 and 22. These studies did not examine counting, which has been the most widely used task in cortical mapping, and is the most frequent type of preserved aphasic speech. Van Lancker, McIntosh, and Grafton (2003) reported that counting and word generation differed in brain activity, with only word generation showing activation in Broca's area, or the left anterior frontal area, and counting associated with more diffuse brain activity, including some subcortical sites.

A case study of a person with the diagnosis of "presenile dementia" was one of the first to suggest a special status for brain processing of formulaic expressions. A relative preservation of formulaic expressions was observed in a severely aphasic 59-year-old woman, who, after the onset of her illness, was never observed to produce a meaningful utterance, but could complete idioms and other familiar conventional expressions spoken to her with the last word missing (Whitaker, 1976). We studied an aphasic individual with a severe comprehension deficit and a diagnosis of transcortical sensory aphasia who was similarly unable to produce meaningful speech, but correctly completed 50% of idiomatic and other formulaic expressions presented verbally to him in a similar way (Van Lancker Sidtis, 2001). Idiom completion in another case of transcortical sensory aphasia was also reported by Nakagawa et al. (1993).

Like these cases described above, observations in Alzheimer speech tend to corroborate a role of the basal ganglia in production of formulaic expressions. It is commonly observed in the clinical setting that persons with considerable progression in the disease, with MiniMental State Examination scores as low as 7 (on a scale of 0–30), who have lost most cognitive capacity, continue to produce formulaic expressions, such as "Nice seeing you again," "Excuse me," and "Good-bye." Observations of conversational speech in Alzheimer's disease reveal a large proportion of formulaic expressions, although they are sometimes used inappropriately. An Alzheimer patient said "I haven't seen you for a while" to a stranger in the hallway while the two were waiting together for the elevator. In some speech samples, distortions of formulaic expressions appear, such as "But they were very good down there by me for," or a blend of two or more expressions, such as "put down my mind to it." The relative preservation of formulaic in comparison to novel expressions is likely attributable to the fact that Alzheimer's disease attacks the cortical layers, leaving the subcortical nuclei intact until very late in the disease, by which time the patient is mute.

Another example of preserved formulaicity in brain disease arises from observations of language behaviors in autism (Wray, 2008b). Clinicians and lay persons alike describe the frequent repetition of radio and television jingles taken from advertisements and serial shows by autistic and other developmentally delayed children (Bogdashina, 2005; Cohen, 2002; Cohen & Volkmar, 1997; Prizant & Duchan, 1981). Various forms of immediate and delayed echolalia, the repetition of verbal utterances of self or another speaker, are well known to occur in these children, alongside absent or severely impoverished spontaneous, novel speech production (Lord & Rhea, 1997). Prizant (1983) postulates that in many cases, echolalia becomes a communication strategy compensating for an inability to fully process language. On a more psychological level, stereotyped or excessively repetitive language may be the only means available for social contact (Howlin, 1997), which is often accompanied by similarly mechanical and ritualistic behaviors (Paul, 2004). Studies have shown that echoed utterances may have communicative functionality, similar to that seen for formulaic expressions (Dobbinson, Perkins, & Boucher, 2003). It has often been noted that many autistic spectrum disorder children exhibit a predominant development of holistic expressions with impoverished grammatical competence (Lord & Paul, 1997). Autistic echolalia has been referred to as the overuse of "gestalt language forms" that are normally seen in child language development (Prizant, Schuler, Wetherby, & Rydell, 1997). This perspective refers to a model of normal language development (e.g., Locke, 1993, 1995; Peters, 1977, 1983; Tomasello, 2003; Wong Fillmore, 1979) in which two modes of language acquisition, holistic and analytic, unfold in different but interactive maturational schedules. As Dobbinson et al. (2003, p. 305) suggest, "autistic formulaicity may be seen as the preferential use of a normative operation." In autistic children, the holistic process flourishes, while the mode of learning language that establishes grammatical competence is in varying degrees defective.

The relative preservation of formulaic expressions as Alzheimer's disease progresses to the severe state, while semantic functions and newly created spontaneous speech deteriorate, supports the notion of a dual-process model of language. Similarly, observations in autism reveal a more successful development of a holistic mode of language processing, in contrast to defective grammatical and semantic functions, again pointing toward the viability of a model of language that describes both holistic-configurational and analytic-compositional modes of processing in acquisition and use.

HOW ARE FORMULAIC EXPRESSIONS ACQUIRED?

Another provocative source that supports the dual-process model arises from developmental language studies, in infants' first and in adult second language acquisition. As mentioned above, researchers in child language document acquisition of holistic "chunks" of speech, which evolve into compositional structures (clark, 1974). While unitary utterances are utilized by children early on, acquisition of formulaic expressions at adult levels lags behind acquisition of grammatical competence (Kempler, Van Lancker, Marchman, & Bates, 1999). This suggests that the two processes, holistic and analytic, perform different roles at different stages of language acquisition, and, further that different maturational schedules are in play for novel versus formulaic language knowledge. Similarly, in adult second language acquisition, the difficulty posed by formulaic expressions is well known. It is likely that critical periods for native-like acquisition exist for various types of language competences, including for acquisition of formulaic expressions.

The question of acquisition of formulaic expressions in the native speaker has seldom been seriously posed. It is generally assumed that a major force in acquisition of formulaic expressions is frequency of exposure, such that many repetitions of a formulaic expression eventually make a lasting impression in the developing child's or adult's memory. A companion assumption is that, because our brains are finite, novel language is learned primarily by abstract rules. The point behind emphasizing the finiteness of our brains is that memory capacity is severely limited, when considering the very large set of phrases and sentences we command. We submit that both of these assumptions—frequency of exposure and limited memory capacity—are questionable, and fail to provide a basis for either a viable model or for empirical observations in formulaic language competence.

The "slow exposure" assumption is most likely wrong because, as mentioned above, the number of known expressions is very high. Native speakers acquire precise forms and complex semantic and pragmatic meanings of these expressions; unlike newly created sentences, they are all learned "by heart." If memory is poor for exact verbal replicas, then very many exposures of each expression are required. It is not a logical possibility that a sufficient number of repetitions of 100,000 (or, as some researchers say, 500,000) exact forms and contexts are provided for each language user, adequate to satisfy the requirements of the incremental learning process, leading to the huge repertory of pristinely stored formulemes.

It follows from this point, then, the "highly limited memory" assumption is also misguided. As the first bit of evidence, we point out again that people know tens of thousands of multiword expressions. Of interest here are recent findings by Gurevich, Johnson, & Goldberg, 2010 showing a successful verbatim memory for language. In these studies, participants reliably recognized and recalled full sentences that they were exposed to only once. It is likely that this fundamental ability to capture verbal material exactly is greatly heightened by the properties of formulaic language, and that this ability follows a unique maturational schedule. Similar and related findings are reported for incidental retention of voice identity information, such as gender (Geiselman, 1977; Geiselman & Crawley, 1976). For subjects listening to spoken words, voice attributes were clearly retained in memory (Goldinger, 1996). Using a memory model called the MINERVA 2, studies suggest that separate episodic memory traces are retained for each stimulus (Hintzman, 1986). These approaches reveal specificity of memory processes and allow for the possibility that brief exposures suffice to encode a large number of formulaic expressions. These expressions differ from novel expressions in their relationship to grammatical and semantic functions, social context, and use. These significant differences likely provide cues to signal a different type of encoding and retention process.

We propose that a specialized form of knowledge acquisition may be operative for formulaic expressions. For example, something comparable to one-trial learning, a special case in classic learning theory, should be considered. In this type of learning, rather than acquiring a piece of information over through repeated exposure or trials, organisms "learn" (acquire a conditioned response) immediately or very quickly as the result of a "strong contingency" reinforcement (Lattal, 1995). Another kind of instantaneous "learning" that is well studied is imprinting. Brain biochemistry and localization for imprinting have been extensively investigated in birds (Horn, 1985; Knudson, 1987). It is known that forebrain hemispheres with strong connections to striatal (subcortical) and brainstem structures are operative in imprinting, and these structures are also involved in visceral and endocrine functions as well as emotional expression (Horn, 1985, p. 243). Genetic determinants control the basic neuronal circuitry in some species studied, but flexibility allows for experience to shape the perceptual system (Knudsen, 1987). There are critical time windows but these sensitive periods are often labile and flexible (Marler, 1987, 1998). Also worth mentioning as a rapid memory process are "flash bulb memories," in which an unusual amount of experiential detail is retained in memory in association with receiving surprising information (Brown & Kulik, 1977). Features of the processes include arousal, surprise, and personal relevance, in addition to affect, attention, distinctiveness, and poststimulus elaboration (Christianson, 1992). It has been suggested that this function is part of an automatically preattentive mechanism (Neisser, 1976). Arousal levels may arise from hormonal or other chemical influences (Gold, 1992), which results in immediate and detailed acquiring of a stimulus.

Our perspective is that acquisition or learning of formulaic expression occurs according to a unique learning process comparable to the three relatively instantaneous types described above. We propose that throughout the early life span, formulaic expressions are acquired in a manner quite different from processes involved in learning the rules and lexicon that underlie generation of novel expressions. (In view of the difficulties encountered by adult second language learners, it is likely that the rapid acquisition ability diminishes with age.) These three examples of extraordinary learning and memory functions are offered to provoke new ways of looking at acquisition of formulaic expressions. These examples of near-instantaneous acquisition of information all demonstrate the coordinated roles of procedural, episodic, and declarative memory, as well as arousal and attention, rendering a special status to some kinds of knowledge acquisition. An alerting mechanism may be engaged by the fact that formulaic expressions pattern differently in the conversational setting and are tightly bound to social context. In summary, we propose that formulaic expressions, under specialized circumstances not yet understood, ascend quickly and suddenly into a native speaker's language competence.

DUAL-PROCESSING MODEL OF LANGUAGE COMPETENCE

Evidence for a dual-process model of language processing comes from several sources. Neurological damage can disturb, diminish, or enhance formulaic language. Novel and formulaic language are affected differently by different types of brain damage: left hemisphere damage leads to selective impairment of novel language and relative preservation of formulaic language, while right hemisphere and/or subcortical damage lead to selective impairment of formulaic language, sparing novel language (Van Lancker Sidtis & Postman, 2006). Enhancements or selective presentation of formulaic language use are seen in aphasia, Tourette's syndrome, and Alzheimer's disease, while diminution is observed in the right hemisphere and subcortical disease. It is likely that such differences will be more extensively and accurately documented as information about formulaic language is disseminated into clinical practice. Recognition of the important role of formulaic expressions in evaluation and recovery in aphasia and other neurological disorders has barely begun, despite the "automatic speech" tradition extending more than 100 years into the past.

The notion of two such processing modes has emerged from studies of learning and memory, comparing, for example, procedural and declarative knowledge (Mishkin, Malamut, & Bachevalier 1984; Squires, 1986). Subcortical structures have been associated with complex motor planning and execution (Baev, 1997; Lieberman, 2000; Marsden, 1982), "chunking of action repertoires" (Greybiel, 1998), and "habit learning" (Knowlton, Mangels, & Squire, 1996). These perspectives have been aligned with hierarchical levels of the central nervous system, such that automated motor gestures are accommodated by subcortical structures, which developed phylogenetically earlier in human evolution (Koestler, 1967). Correspondingly, it has been suggested that the origin of human language might be located in initial use of formulaic expressions (Code, 2005; Jaynes, 1976; Wray, 1998, 2000; Wray & Grace, 2007).

RELATIONSHIP OF FORMULAIC LANGUAGE TO ANIMAL VOCALIZATION AND ROLE IN EVOLUTION

The functional importance of subcortical nuclei in formulaic verbal behavior in humans is especially interesting when considering studies of animal vocalization. For many decades, investigations of the neurology of nonhuman animal vocalization have identified subcortical sites in the initiation and production of calls. While formulaic utterances and animal calls are obviously different in many ways, they are similar in being formal and conventionalized and in having essentially social and emotional functionality. In humans, stereotyped vocalizations have occurred when subcortical sites are electrically stimulated during stereotaxic surgical techniques, usually for treatment of epilepsy (Petrovici, 1980; Schaltenbrand, 1965). Hyperfunction of the basal ganglia/limbic system, as in persons with Tourette's syndrome, gives rise to semicompulsive emotive utterances (called coprolalia or "foul speaking"). Conversely, as mentioned above, subcortical hypofunction due to stroke or degenerative disease is associated with diminution of formulaic expressions.

A system of neuronal organization in the central nervous system emerges from studies of vocalization with higher level control in subcortical structures in nonhuman primates, and with cortical representation occurring only in humans. In humans, two levels of nervous system control for vocalization may be described: an older, subcortical system, which is capable of emotive and formulaic speech behavior; and a newer system that is cortical, unilateral, and involved in voluntary, novel, and planned speech (Jürgens, 2002; Ploog, 1975; Robinson, 1987). Formulaic expressions might be seen as an evolutionary counterpart of nonhuman vocal behavior. Some have proposed that this evolutionarily older system also continues to perform in the emotional and routinized vocal behaviors seen in formulaic expressions (Code, 2005; Jaynes, 1976; Jespersen, 1933; Patel, 2008; Wray, 2002).

Thus studies in primates and humans lend credence to the notion that formulaic language in humans emerges from a evolutionary history different from that proposed for novel language, and is differently structured and controlled in the brain.

CONCLUSION

The formulaic phrase has unique properties: it is cohesive and unitary in its canonical structure, while easily subject to variation. Like the phoneme, the morpheme, and the lexeme (abstract classes of sounds, units of meaning, and words, respectively), any emitted formulaic expression constitutes the instantiation of a formuleme. A formuleme may have aberrant grammatical form. It is often nonliteral or deviant in meaning properties and conveys a nuanced, connotational meaning that transcends the sum of its (lexical) parts. As an essentially pragmatic dimension of language, it is intimately tied to social context and has subtle specifications of usage. Most importantly, the canonical form of the expression, the formuleme, is known to native speakers. A formulaic expression functions differently in form, meaning, and use from a literal, novel, or propositional expression (Lounsbury, 1963).

Despite scattered attempts at treatments over the years, formulaic expressions have not found a niche in generative theory (Kuiper, 2000). Our view is that this failure arises from the fact that fixed, familiar, unitary expressions are informed by principles and properties that cause them to be essentially different from newly created sentences. They cannot be described by the same analytic apparatus. While there is no doubt that different types of formulaic utterances express the principles of formulaic language in different degrees, we reject the claim that formulaic and novel processes are processed in essentially the same manner in the language user (Gibbs, 1980, 1994; Gibbs et al., 1989). Instead, we have presented evidence that formulaic and novel language are more accurately characterized as two disparate modes of language competence. They have the ability to be in continuous interaction, and generative rules can operate on any formuleme, which can take any grammatically allowed variant providing it remains identifiable. Formulaic expressions are learned according to a distinctive maturational schedule that differs from learning principles that are operative for acquiring the rules of grammar, and they draw on instantaneous rather than incremental memory processes. These perspectives have relevance for models of language competence, language learning, and language loss in neurological disorders.

REFERENCES

Abdelli-Baruh, N., Yang, S.-Y., Ahn, J. S., & Van Lancker Sidtis, D. (2007, November, 15–17). Acoustic cues differentiating idiomatic from literal expressions across languages. *American Speech-Language Hearing Association*, Boston, MA.

Ahn, Ji Sook, Yang, Seung-yun, and Sidtis, D. (2010). The perception and acoustic features of Korean ditropic sentences. *Journal of the Acoustical Society of America*, 27 (3, Part 2), 1955.

Aijmer, K. (1996). *Conversational routines in English*. London, New York: Longman.

Altenberg, B. (1998). On the phraseology of spoken English: The evidence of recurrent word-combinations. In A. P. Cowie (Ed.), *Phraseology: Theory, analysis and application* (pp. 101–124). Oxford, UK: Clarendon Press.

Arnaud, P., & Moon, R. E. (1993). Frequency and use of English and French proverbs. In C. Plantin (Ed.), *Familiar phrases: Tropes, stereotyped expressions, and clichés* (pp. 323–341). Paris, France: Kime.

Baev, K. (1997). Highest level automatisms in the nervous system: A theory of functional principles underlying the highest forms of brain function. *Progress in Neurobiology, 51*, 129–166.

Bell, R. A., & Healey, J. G. (1992). Idiomatic communication and interpersonal solidarity in friends' relational cultures. *Human Communication Research, 3*, 307–335.

Blank, S. C., Scott, S., Murphy, K., Warburton, E., & Wise, R. (2002). Speech production: Wernicke, Broca and beyond. *Brain, 125*, 1829–1838.

Blanken, G., & Marini, V. (1997). Where do lexical speech automatisms come from? *Journal of Neurolinguistics, 10*, 19–31.

Bobrow, S., & Bell, S. (1973). On catching on to idiomatic expressions. *Memory and Cognition, 1*, 343–346.

Bogdashina, O. (2005). *Communication issues in autism and Aspergers syndrome. Do we speak the same language?* London, UK: Jessica Kingsley Publishers.

Bookheimer, S. Y., Zeffiro, T. A., Blaxton, T. A., Gaillard, P. W., & Theodore, W. H. (2000). Activation of language cortex with automatic speech tasks. *Neurology, 55*, 1151–1157.

Brown, R., & Kulik, J. (1977). Flashbulb memories. *Cognition, 5*, 73–93.

Bruess, C. J., & Pearson, J. C. (1993). 'Sweet pea' and 'pussy cat': An examination of idiom use and marital satisfaction over the life cycle. *Journal of Social and Personal Relationships, 10*, 609–615.

Cacciari, C., & Tabossi, P. (1988). The comprehension of idioms. *Journal of Memory and Language, 27*, 668–683.

Christianson, S.-Å. (1992). Do flashbulb memories differ from other types of emotional memories? In E. Winograd & U. Neisser (Eds.), *Affect and accuracy in recall: Studies of "flashbulb memories"* (pp. 191–211). Cambridge, UK: Cambridge University Press.

Chung, K. K. H., Code, C., & Ball, M. J. (2004). Lexical and non-lexical speech automatisms in aphasic Cantonese speakers. *Journal of Multilingual Communication Disorders, 2*, 32–42.

Clark, H. H. (1970). Word associations and linguistic theory. In J. Lyons (Ed.), *New horizons in linguistics* (pp. 271–286). Baltimore, MA: Penguin Books.

Clark, H. H., & Fox Tree, J. E. (2002). Using uh and um in spontaneous speaking. *Cognition, 84*(1), 73–111.

Clark, R. (1974). Performing without competence. *Journal of Child Language, 1,* 1–10.

Code, C. (1982). Neurolinguistic analysis of recurrent utterance in aphasia. *Cortex, 18,* 141–152.

Code, C. (1989). Speech automatisms and recurring utterances. In C. Code (Ed.), *The characteristics of aphasia* (pp. 155–177). London, UK: Taylor & Francis.

Code, C. (2005). First in, last out? The evolution of aphasic lexical speech automatisms to agrammatism and the evolution of human communication. *Interaction Studies, 6,* 311–334.

Cohen, D. J., & Volkmar, F. R. (Eds.). (1997). *Handbook of autism and pervasive developmental disorders.* New York, NY: Wiley & Sons.

Cohen, S. (2002). *Targeting autism: What we know, don't know, and can do to help young children with autism and related disorders.* Berkeley, CA: University of California Press.

Coulmas, F. (1994). Formulaic language. In R. E. Asher (Ed.), *Encyclopedia of language and linguistics* (pp. 1292–1293). Oxford, UK: Pergamon.

Cowie, A. P. (1992). Multiword lexical units and communicative language teaching. In P. Arnaud & H. Bejoint (Eds.), *Vocabulary and applied linguistics* (pp. 1–12). London, UK: Macmillan.

Cutting, J. C., & Bock, K. (1997). That's the way the cookie bounces: Syntactic and semantic components of experimentally elicited idiom blends. *Memory-Cognition, 25*(1), 57–71.

Devitt, M. (2006). Intuitions in linguistics. *British Journal for the Philosophy of Science, 57,* 481–513.

Dobbinson, S., Perkins, M. R., & Boucher, J. (2003). The interactional significance of formulas in autistic language. *Clinical Linguistics and Phonetics, 17*(4), 299–307.

Drew, P., & Holt, E. (1988). Complainable matters: The use of idiomatic expressions in making complaints. *Social Problems, 35,* 398–417.

Espir, L., & Rose, F. (1970). *The basic neurology of speech.* Oxford, UK: Blackwell Scientific Publications.

Fillmore, C. (1979). On fluency. In C. J. Fillmore, D. Kempler, & W. S.-Y. Wang (Eds.), *Individual differences in language ability and language behavior* (pp. 85–102). London, UK: Academic Press.

Fox Tree, J. E. (2006). Placing like in telling stories. *Discourse Studies: An Interdisciplinary Journal for the Study of Text and Talk, 8*(6), 723–743.

Gallahorn, G. E. (1971). The use of taboo words by psychiatric ward personnel. *Psychiatry, 34,* 309–321.

Geiselman, R. E. (1977). Incidental retention of a speaker's voice. *Memory and Cognition, 6,* 658–665.

Geiselman, R. E., & Crawley, J. M. (1976). Long-term memory for speaker's voice and source location. *Memory and Cognition, 4*(15), 483–489.

Gibbs, R. W. (1980). Spilling the beans on understanding and memory for idioms in conversation. *Memory and Cognition, 8*(2), 149–156.

Gibbs, R. W. (1981). Your wish is my command: Convention and context in interpreting indirect requests. *Journal of Verbal Learning and Verbal Behavior, 20,* 431–444.

Gibbs, R. W. (1994). *The poetics of mind: Figurative thought, language, and understanding.* New York, NY: Cambridge University Press.

Gibbs, R.W., Jr., & Gonzales, G. P. (1985). Syntactic frozenness in processing and remembering idioms. *Cognition, 20,* 243–259.

Gibbs, R. W., Jr., Nayak, N. P., Bolton, J. L., & Keppel, M. E. (1989). Speaker's assumptions about the lexical flexibility of idioms. *Memory and Cognition, 17*(1), 58–68.

Glassman, L., Grinberg, D., Hibbard, C., Meehan, J., Reid, L. G., & van Leunen, M.-C. (1992). Hector: Connecting words with definitions. SRC Report 92a. Palo Alto, CA: Digital Equipment Corporation Systems Research Center.

Gold, P. E. (1992). A proposed neurobiological basis for regulating memory storage for significant events. In E. Winograd & U. Neisser (Eds.), *Affect and accuracy in recall: Studies of "flashbulb memories"* (pp. 141–161). Cambridge, UK: Cambridge University Press.

Goldinger, S. D. (1996). Words and voices: Episodic trace in spoken work identification and recognition memory. *Journal of Experimental Psychology: Learning, Memory, and Cognition, 22*(5), 1166–1183.

Graybiel, A. M. (1998). The basal ganglia and chunking of action repertoires. *Neurobiology of Learning and Memory, 70*, 119–136.

Greenbaum, S., & Svartik, J. (1990). The London-Lund corpus of spoken English. In J. Svartik (Ed.), *The London-Lund corpus of spoken English: Description and research* (pp. 11–45). Lund, Sweden: Lund University Press.

Gurevich, O., Johnson, M.A., & Goldberg, A. (2010). Incidental verbatim memory for language. *Language and Cognition, 2–1*, 45–87.

Hain, M. (1951). Sprichwort und Volkssprache. English trans., In D. Sidtis & S. Mohr (Eds.), *Formulaic language in the field*. Anja Tachler, translator. Copyright. Giessen, Germany: Wilhelm Schmitz Verlag.

Hintzman, D. L. (1986). "Schema abstraction" in a multiple-trace memory model. *Psychological Review, 93*(4), 411–428.

Horn, G. (1985). *Memory, imprinting and the brain*. Oxford Psychology Series No. 10. Oxford, UK: Clarendon Press.

Horowitz, L. M., & Manelis, L. (1973). Recognition and cued recall of idioms and phrases. *Journal of Experimental Psychology, 100*, 291–296.

Howlin, P. (1997). *Autism: Preparing for adulthood*. New York, NY: Routledge.

Hughlings Jackson, J. (1874). On the nature of the duality of the brain. In J. Taylor (Ed.), *Selected writings of John Hughlings Jackson* (Vol. 2, pp. 129–145). London, UK: Hodder & Stoughton.

Illes, J., Metterb, E. J., Hanson, W. R., & Iritanib, S. (1988). Language production in Parkinson's disease: Acoustic and linguistic considerations. *Brain and Language, 33*, 146–160.

Jackendoff, R. (1995). The boundaries of the lexicon. In M. Everaert, E. van der Linden, A. Schenk, & R. Schreuder (Eds.), *Idioms: Structural and psychological perspectives* (pp. 133–166). Hillsdale, NJ: Lawrence Erlbaum Associates.

Jay, T. B. (1980). Sex roles and dirty word usage: A review of the literature and a reply to Haas. *Psychological Bulletin, 88*(3), 614–621.

Jaynes, J. (1976). *The origin of consciousness in the breakdown of the bicameral mind*. Boston, MA: Houghton Mifflin.

Jespersen, O. (1933). *Essentials of English grammar*. London, UK: George Allen and Unwin, Ltd.

Jucker, A. H. (1993). The discourse marker 'well': A relevance-theoretical account. *Journal of Pragmatics, 19*, 435–452.

Jürgens, U. (2002). Neural pathways underlying vocal control. *Neuroscience and Biobehavioral Reviews, 26*(2), 235–258.

Kempler, D., Van Lancker, D., Marchman, V., & Bates, E. (1999). Idiom comprehension in children and adults with unilateral brain damage. *Developmental Neuropsychology, 15*(3), 327–349.

Kiparsky, P. (1976). Oral poetry: Some linguistic and typological considerations. In B. A. Stolz & R. S. Shannon (Eds.), *Oral literature and the formula*. Ann Arbor, MI: Center for Coordination of Ancient and Modern Studies.

Kitzinger, C. (2000). How to resist an idiom. *Research on Language and Social Interaction, 33*, 121–154.

Klaver, E., (1989). The play of language in Ionesco's play of Chairs. *Modern Drama, 32*, 521–539.

Knowlton, B., Mangels, J., & Squire, L. (1996). A neostratal habit learning system in humans. *Science, 273*, 1399–1402.

Knudsen, E. I. (1987). Early experience shapes auditory localization behavior and the spatial tuning of auditory units in the barn owl. In J. P. Rauschecker & P. Marler (Eds.), *Imprinting and cortical plasticity* (pp. 3–7). New York, NY: John Wiley & Sons.

Koestler, A. (1967). *The ghost in the machine*. Chicago, IL: Henry Regnery Company.

Kuiper, K. (1991).The evolution of an oral tradition: Race-calling in Canterbury, New Zealand. *Oral Tradition, 6*, 19–34.

Kuiper, K. (1992). The English oral tradition in auction speech. *American Speech, 67*, 279–289.

Kuiper, K. (1996). *Smooth talkers: The linguistic performance of auctioneers and sportscasters*. Mahwah, NJ: Erlbaum Association Publishers.

Kuiper, K. (2000). On the linguistic properties of formulaic speech. *Oral Tradition, 15*(2), 279–305.

Kuiper, K. (2004). Formulaic performance in conventionalised varieties of speech. In N. Schmitt (Ed.), *Formulaic sequences: Acquisition, processing, and use* (pp. 37–54). Amsterdam, The Netherlands: John Benjamins.

Kuiper, K., & Everaert, M. (2000). Constraints on the phrase structural properties of English phrasal lexical items. In B. Roswadowska (Ed.), *PASE papers in language studies* (pp. 151–170). Wrocław, Poland: Aksel.

Kuiper, K., & Flindall, M. (2000). Social rituals, formulaic speech and small talk at the supermarket checkout. In J. Coupland (Ed.), *Small talk* (pp. 183–207). London, UK: Longman.

Kuiper, K., & Haggo, D. (1985). The nature of ice hockey commentaries. In R. Berry & J. Acheson (Eds.), *Regionalism and national identity: Multidisciplinary essays on Canada* (pp. 189–197). Australia and New Zealand, Christchurch: Association for Canadian Studies in Australia and New Zealand.

Kuiper, K., van Egmond, M., Kempen, G., & Sprenger, S. (2007). Slipping on superlemmas: Multi-word lexical items in speech production. *The Mental Lexicon, 2*(3), 313–357.

Larsen, B., Skinhoj, E., & Lassen, H. A. (1978). Variations in regional cortical blood flow in the right and left hemispheres during automatic speech. *Brain, 10*, 193–200.

Lattal, K. A. (1995). Contingency and behavior analysis. *Behavior Analyst, 24*, 147–161.

Lieberman, P. (2000). *Human language and our reptilian brain: The subcortical bases of speech, syntax, and thought*. Cambridge, MA: Harvard University Press.

Locke, J. L. (1993). *The child's path to spoken language*. Cambridge, MA: Harvard University Press.

Locke, J. L. (1995). Development of the capacity for spoken language. In P. Fletcher & B. MacWhinney (Eds.), *The handbook of child language* (pp. 278–302). Oxford, UK: Blackwell.

Lord, A. (1960). *The singer of tales*. Cambridge, MA: Harvard University Press.

Lord, C., & Paul, R. (1997). Language and communication in autism. In D. J. Cohen & F. R. Volkmar (Eds.), *Handbook of autism and pervasive developmental disorders* (pp. 195–225). New York, UK: John Wiley & Sons.

Lounsbury, F. G. (1963). Linguistics and psychology. In S. Koch (Ed.), *Psychology: Study of a science* (pp. 553–582). New York, NY: McGraw-Hill.

Lum, C. C., & Ellis, A. W. (1994). Is nonpropositional speech preserved in aphasia? *Brain and Language, 46,* 368–391.

Marler, P. (1987). Sensitive periods and the role of specific and general sensory stimulation in birdsong learning. In J. P. Rauschecker & P. Marler (Eds.), *Imprinting and cortical plasticity* (pp. 99–135). New York, NY: John Wiley & Sons.

Marler, P. (1998). Animal communication and human language. In G. Jablonski & L. C. Aiello (Eds.), *The origin and diversification of language.* Wattis Symposium Series in Anthropology (pp. 1–19). Memoirs of the California Academy of Sciences, No. 24, San Francisco, CA: California Academy of Sciences.

Marsden, C. D. (1982). The mysterious motor function of the basal ganglia: The Robert Wartenberg lecture. *Neurology, 32,* 514–539.

Mishkin, M., Malamut, B., & Bachevalier, J. (1984). Memories and habits: Two neural systems. In G. Lynch, J. L. McGaugh, & N. M. Weinberger (Eds.), *Neurobiology of learning and memory* (pp. 65–67). New York, NY: The Guilford Press.

Moon, R. E. (1998). Fixed expressions and text: A study of the distribution and textual behaviour of fixed expressions in English. *Oxford studies in lexicology and lexicography.* Oxford, UK: Clarendon Press.

Nakagawa, Y., Tanabe, H., Ikeda, M., Kazui, H., Ito, K., Inoue, N., . . . Shiraishi, J. (1993). Completion phenomenon in transcortical sensory aphasia. *Behavioural Neurology, 6*(3), 135–142.

Neisser, U. (1976). *Cognition and reality: Principles and implications of cognitive psychology.* San Francisco, CA: W. H. Freeman & Co.

Norrick, N. R. (1985). *How proverbs mean: Semantic studies in English proverbs.* Berlin, Germany: Mouton.

Osgood, C., & Hoosain, R. (1974). Salience of the word as a unit in the perception of language. *Perception and Psychophysics, 15,* 168–192.

Page, D. L. (1959). *History and the Homeric Iliad.* Berkeley, CA: University of California Press.

Patel, A. D. (2008). *Music, language, and the brain.* Oxford, UK: Oxford University Press.

Paul, R. (2004). Autism. In R. D. Kent (Ed.), *The MIT handbook of communication disorders.* Cambridge, MA: MIT Press.

Pawley, A. (2001). Phraseology, linguistics, and the dictionary. *International Journal of Lexicography, 14*(2), 122–134.

Pawley, A. (2007). Developments in the study of formulaic language since 1970: A personal view. In P. Skandera (Ed.), *Phraseology and culture in English* (pp. 3–45). Berlin, Germany: Mouton de Gruyter.

Pawley, A., & Syder, F. H. (1983). Two puzzles for linguistic theory: Nativelike selection and nativelike fluency. In J. C. Richards & R. Schmidt (Eds.), *Language and communication* (pp. 191–225). London, UK: Longman.

Peters, A. (1977). Language-learning strategies: Does the whole equal the sum of the parts? *Language, 53,* 560–573.

Peters, A. M. (1983). *The units of language acquisition.* Cambridge, UK: Cambridge University Press.

Petrovici, J.-N. (1980). Speech disturbances following stereotaxic surgery in ventrolateral thalamus. *Neurosurgical Review, 3*(3), 189–195.

Pickens, J. D., & Pollio, H. R. (1979). Patterns of figurative language competence in adult speakers. *Psychological Research, 40,* 299–313.

Pinker, S. (1995). *The language instinct.* New York, NY: Harper Collins.

Ploog, D. (1975). Vocal behavior and its 'localization' as prerequisite for speech. In K. J. Zülch, O. Creutzfeldt, & G. C. Galbraith (Eds.), *Cerebral localization*. Berlin, Germany: Springer-Verlag.

Prizant, B. M. (1983). Language acquisition and communicative behavior in autism: Toward an understanding of the 'whole' of it. *Journal of Speech and Hearing Disorders, 48,* 296–307.

Prizant, B. M., & Duchan, J. (1981). The functions of immediate echolalia in autistic children. *Journal of Speech and Hearing Disorders, 46,* 241–249.

Prizant, B. M., Schuler, A. L., Wetherby, A. B., & Rydell, P. (1997). Enhancing language and communication development: Language approaches. In D. J. Cohen & F. R. Volkmar (Eds.), *Handbook of autism and pervasive developmental disorders* (pp. 572–605). New York, NY: John Wiley & Sons.

Robinson, B. W. (1987). Limbic influences on human speech. *Annals of the New York Academy of Sciences, 280,* 761–771.

Ryding, E., Bradvik, B., & Ingvar, D. (1987). Changes of regional cerebral blood flow measured simultaneously in the right and left hemisphere during automatic speech and humming. *Brain, 110,* 1345–1358.

Schaltenbrand, G. (1965). The effects of stereotactic electrical stimulation in the depth of the brain. *Brain, 88,* 835–840.

Schegloff, E. (1988). Discourse as an interactional achievement II: An exercise in conversation analysis. In D. Tannen (Ed.), *Linguistics in context: Connecting observation and understanding* (pp. 135–158). Norwood, NJ: Ablex.

Schweizer, B.-M. (1978). *Sprachspiel mit Idiomen: eine Untersuchung am Prosawerk von Günter Grass*. Zürich, Switzerland: Juris Druk Verlag.

Sidtis, Diana, Canterucci, Gina, & Katsnelson, Dora. (2009). Effects of neurological damage on production of formulaic language. *Clinical Linguistics and Phonetics, 23* (15), 270–284.

Sidtis, D., Rogers, T., Godier,, V., Tagliati, M., & Sidtis, J.J. (2010). Voice and fluency changes as a function of speech task and deep brain stimulation. *Journal of Speech Language and Hearing Research,* to appear.

Simon, H. A. (1974). How big is a chunk? *Science, 183,* 482–448.

Simon, H. A., Zhang, W., Zang, W., & Peng, R. (1989). STM capacity for Chinese words and idioms with visual and auditory presentations. In H. A. Simon (Ed.), *Models of thought, II* (pp. 68–75). New Haven, CT and London, UK: Yale University Press.

Smolka, E., Rabanus, S., & Rösler, F. (2007). Processing verbs in German idioms: Evidence against the configuration hypothesis. *Metaphor and Symbol, 22*(3), 213–231.

Sorace, A., & Keller, F. (2005). Gradience in linguistic data. *Lingua, 115,* 1497–1524.

Speedie, L. J., Wertman, E., Ta'ir, J., & Heilman, K. M. (1993). Disruption of automatic speech following a right basal ganglia lesion. *Neurology, 43,* 1768–1774.

Sprenger, S. A. (2003). *Fixed expressions and the production of idioms*. Doctoral dissertation, University of Nijmegen.

Squires, L. R. (1986). Memory and the brain. In S. L. Friedman, K. A. Klivington, & R. W. Peterson (Eds.), *The brain, cognition, and education*. Orlando, FL: Academic Press.

Svartik, J., & Quirk, R. (1980). A corpus of English conversation. *Lund studies in English.* Lund, Sweden: CWK Gleerup.

Swinney, D. A., & Cutler, A. (1979). The access and processing of idiomatic expressions. *Journal of Verbal Learning and Verbal Behavior, 18,* 523–534.

Tannen, D. (1989). *Talking voices: Repetition, dialogue, and imagery in conversational discourse*. Cambridge, UK: Cambridge University Press.

Tannen, D., & Öztek, P. C. (1981). Health to our mouths: Formulaic expressions in Turkish and Greek. In F. Coulmas (Ed.), *Conversational routine. Explorations in standardized communication situations and prepatterned speech* (pp. 37–57). The Hague, The Netherlands: Mouton.

Tilley, M. P. (1950). *A dictionary of proverbs in England in the 16th and 17th centuries*. Ann Arbor, MI: University of Michigan Press.

Titone, D. A., & Conine, C. M. (1999). On the compositional and noncompositional nature of idiomatic expressions. *Journal of Pragmatics, 31*, 1655–1674.

Tomasello, M. (2003). *Constructing a language. A usage-based theory of language acquisition*. Cambridge, MA and London, UK: Harvard University Press.

Van Lancker, D. (1993). Nonpropositional speech in aphasia. In G. Blanken, J. Dittmann, J. Grimm, J. C. Marshall, & C,-W. Wallesch (Eds.), *Linguistic disorders and pathologies: An international handbook* (pp. 215–225). Berlin, Germany: Walter de Gruyter.

Van Lancker, D., & Bella, R. (1996). The relative roles of repetition and sentence completion tasks in revealing superior speech abilities in patients with nonfluent aphasia. *Journal of the International Neuropsychological Society, 2*, 6.

Van Lancker, D., Bogen, J. E., & Canter, G. J. (1983). A case report of pathological rule-governed syllable intrusion. *Brain and Language, 20*, 12–20.

Van Lancker, D., Canter, J., & Terbeek, D. (1981). Disambiguation of ditropic sentences: Acoustic and phonetic cues. *Journal of Speech and Hearing Research, 24*, 330–335.

Van Lancker, D., & Cummings, J. (1999). Expletives: Neurolinguistic and neurobehavioral perspectives on swearing. *Brain Research Reviews, 31*, 83–104.

Van Lancker, D., McIntosh, R., & Grafton, R. (2003). PET activation studies comparing two speech tasks widely used in surgical mapping. *Brain and Language, 85*, 245–261.

Van Lancker Sidtis, D. (2001). Preserved formulaic expressions in a case of transcortical sensory aphasia compared to incidence in normal everyday speech. *Brain and Language, 79*(1), 38–41.

Van Lancker Sidtis, D. (2004). When novel sentences spoken or heard for the first time in the history of the universe are not enough: Toward a dual-process model of language. *International Journal of Language and Communication Disorders, 39*(1), 1–44.

Van Lancker Sidtis, D. (2006). Has neuroimaging solved the problems of neurolinguistics? *Brain and Language, 98*, 276–290.

Van Lancker Sidtis, D. (2008). Formulaic and novel language in a dual-process model of language competence: Evidence from surveys, speech samples, and schemata. In R. Corrigan, E. Moravcsik, H. Ouali, & K. Wheatley (Eds.), *Proceedings of the 2007 University of Wisconsin-Milwaukee symposium on formulaic language*. Amsterdam, The Netherlands: John Benjamins.

Van Lancker Sidtis, D., & Postman, W. A. (2006). Formulaic expressions in spontaneous speech of left- and right-hemisphere damaged subjects. *Aphasiology, 20*(5), 411–426.

Van Lancker Sidtis, D., & Rallon, G. (2004). Tracking the incidence of formulaic expressions in everyday speech: Methods for classification and verification. *Language and Communication, 24*, 207–240.

Whitaker, H. (1976). A case of the isolation of the language function. In H. Whitaker & H. A. Whitaker (Eds.), *Studies in neurolinguistics* (Vol. 2, pp. 1–58). London, UK: Academic Press.

Wong Fillmore, L. (1979). Individual differences in second language acquisition. In C. J. Fillmore, D. Kempler, W. S.-Y. Wang (Eds.), *Individual differences in language ability and language behavior* (pp. 203–228). London, UK: Academic Press.

Wray, A. (1998). Protolanguage as a holistic system for social interaction. *Language and Communication, 18*, 47–67.

Wray, A. (2000). Holistic utterances in protolanguage: The link from primates to humans. In C. Knight, J. R. Hurford, & M. Studdert-Kennedy (Eds.), *The evolutionary emergence of language: Social function and the origins of linguistic form* (pp. 285–302). Cambridge, UK: Cambridge University Press.

Wray, A. (2002). *Formulaic language and the lexicon*. Cambridge, UK: Cambridge University Press.

Wray, A. (2008a). *Formulaic language: Pushing the boundaries*. Oxford, UK: Oxford University Press.

Wray, A. (2008b). Formulaic sequences in language disorder. In M. Ball, M. Perkins, N. Muller, & S. Howard (Eds.), *The handbook of clinical linguistics* (pp. 184–197). Oxford, UK: Blackwell Publishers Ltd.

Wray, A., & Grace, G. W. (2007). The consequences of talking to strangers: Evolutionary corollaries of socio-cultural influences on linguistic form. *Lingua, 117*(3), 543–578.

Wray, A., & Perkins, M. (2000). The functions of formulaic language: An integrated model. *Language and Communication, 20*, 1–28.

13 How Similarity Influences Word Recognition: The Effect of Neighbors

Mark Yates

INTRODUCTION

One of the most researched topics in the area of cognitive psychology has been the study of single-word recognition (Balota, Cortese, Sergent-Marshall, Spieler, & Yap, 2004). Of this research, one issue that has received considerable attention is how word processing is affected by orthographic and phonological similarity. The impetus for much of this research has been the predictions made by models of word recognition as to how similarity should influence word processing. A particular class of models that has been extremely influential along these lines are models that are characterized by *interactive activation and competition* (IAC). Models that embody the assumption of IAC are among some of the oldest models in psycholinguistics (e.g., McClelland & Elman, 1986; McClelland & Rumelhart, 1981; Rumelhart & McClelland, 1982). the IAC models consist of multiple hierarchical levels that are interconnected with excitatory and/or inhibitory connections. Within each level are nodes denoting the representation that is processed at that level (e.g., whole words or letters).

The seminal interactive activation model of McClelland and Rumelhart (1981) provides a good example of an IAC model. The interactive activation model was designed to explain letter perception and to provide an account of the word superiority effect (Reicher, 1969; Wheeler, 1970). The model consists of a visual feature level, letter level, and word level. The feature level feeds excitatory and inhibitory activation to the letter level. Likewise, the letter level passes both types of activation to the word level. For instance, if the node for the letter *L* occurring in the first position becomes active, it will increase the activation of any words beginning with the letter *L* (e.g., *LOVE*), and at the same time, it will inhibit the activation of any words *not* containing the letter *L* in the first position (e.g., *MAST*). Additionally, the word level feeds back activation, both excitatory and inhibitory, to the letter level. This means that as the word *LOVE* becomes active it will increase the activation of the *L* node and inhibit the other letter nodes. Finally, at each of the levels, there are within level inhibitory connections.

Given the current interest in IAC models and their predictions regarding the influence of similarity on word recognition, there are two goals of this chapter. The first is to review how orthographic and phonological similarity have been used to better understand both written and spoken word recognition. Specifically, I will focus on the effect of *neighbors*. There are various ways of determining whether two words are neighbors, but in general, a neighbor is simply a word that is similar to the target word in terms of spelling (i.e., an orthographic neighbor) or sound (i.e., a phonological neighbor). The second goal of this chapter is to explain the effects of neighbors within the context of models that have an IAC architecture. Although this chapter will concentrate on IAC models, this should not be taken as an indication that other types of models could not account for these effects. Another class of model that is common in word recognition are those that employ some type of learning algorithm (e.g., Harm & Seidenberg, 2004; Plaut, McClelland, Seidenberg, & Patterson, 1996; Seidenberg & McClelland, 1989), and some researchers have argued that these models can account for effects of similarity better than IAC models (Sears, Hino, & Lupker, 1995). Nevertheless, the reason for concentrating this chapter on IAC models is because these models have been studied extensively in relation to similarity effects.

ORTHOGRAPHIC NEIGHBORHOOD

Interest in orthographic neighbors was originally studied in relation to visual word recognition. As will be detailed below, exactly how orthographic neighbors influence processing has been a matter of some debate. Interestingly, in recent research, orthographic neighbors have been shown to influence auditory word recognition as well. In this section, I will cover the research dealing with orthographic neighborhood effects on both visual and auditory word recognition and relate this research to IAC models.

ORTHOGRAPHIC NEIGHBORHOOD EFFECTS ON VISUAL WORD RECOGNITION

The origins of orthographic neighborhood research can be traced to the work of Landauer and Streeter (1973) who reported that frequent words tended to have more orthographic neighbors than did infrequent words. Two words are said to be neighbors if they have the same number of letters and differ by one letter substitution. For example, *gate* and *game* are orthographic neighbors. Although Landauer and Streeter were the first to discuss orthographic neighbors, it was the work of Coltheart and colleagues (Coltheart, Davelaar, Jonasson, & Besner, 1977) that really sparked interest in the idea and led to a flurry of orthographic neighborhood studies. In fact, orthographic neighborhood is commonly referred to as Coltheart's N. Interestingly, Coltheart et al. (1977) failed to find an effect of orthographic neighborhood on lexical decisions to words. While Coltheart et al. (1977) failed to find an effect, subsequent research has shown that the size of the orthographic neighborhood is an important determinant of word recognition. The first researcher to do so was Andrews (1989) who demonstrated that words with a dense orthographic neighborhood (i.e., words having many neighbors) were verified more rapidly in a lexical decision task than were words having a sparse neighborhood (i.e., words with few neighbors). However, Andrew's results were quickly called into question by Grainger and Segui (1990) who noted that Andrew's stimuli were confounded with bigram frequency. To counter this criticism, Andrews (1992) showed that orthographic neighborhood facilitated lexical decisions even when bigram frequency was controlled. Later research in the area produced inconsistent results. Some researchers reported a facilitative effect of orthographic neighborhood density on lexical decisions (Balota et al., 2004; Forster & Shen, 1996; Huntsman & Lima, 2002; Sears et al., 1995), whereas others reported an inhibitory effect (Johnson & Pugh, 1994). It is worth noting that Johnson and Pugh's research differed from the other studies because their stimuli were blocked by orthographic neighborhood size. This means that participants saw all the high neighborhood words together in one block of trials and all small neighborhood words together in another block. As this experiment is the only one showing an inhibitory effect of orthographic neighborhood size, it seems likely that the inhibitory effect of orthographic neighborhood can be attributed to strategic factors that are employed when the words are blocked according to neighborhood size (Andrews, 1997).

An even more contentious issue concerns the nature of orthographic neighborhood frequency on lexical decisions. Grainger, O'Regan, Jacobs, and Segui (1989) demonstrated that words having at least one higher frequency neighbor were responded to more slowly than words without any higher frequency neighbors. Subsequent research also showed an inhibitory effect (Carreiras, Perea, & Grainger, 1997; Grainger, 1990; Grainger, O'Regan, Jacobs, & Segui, 1992; Huntsman & Lima, 1996; Perea & Pollatsek, 1998). Complicating matters, however, was additional research showing that orthographic neighborhood frequency facilitated lexical decisions, rather than inhibiting them (Sears et al., 1995). Unfortunately, it is not entirely clear why there is this discrepancy between the results generated from different labs, though at least two explanations have been suggested. One has to do with the different languages used in the various studies. Experiments demonstrating facilitation have been conducted with English words, whereas those reporting inhibition have typically used other languages (Andrews, 1997). One interesting hypothesis for this discrepancy is that English word recognition is more influenced by body neighbors (i.e., the vowel plus remaining consonants) and that body neighbors have a facilitative effect on processing (Ziegler & Perry, 1998). However, for other languages, body neighbors do not affect processing to the same degree as in English. Consequently, inhibitory effects emerge in these languages. The second potential reason for the equivocal pattern of orthographic neighborhood results has to do with the confounding of orthographic neighborhood and phonological neighborhood (Yates, Locker, & Simpson, 2004). In visual word recognition, phonological neighbors are defined as two words that differ by one *phoneme* substitution. For example, *gate* has *bait* and *game* as two of its neighbors. Because a one letter change is often the same as a one phoneme change (cf. *gate* and *game*), many neighbors that are orthographic neighbors will also be phonological neighbors. Yates et al. (2004) showed that past studies investigating orthographic neighborhood have been significantly confounded with phonological neighborhood, making it difficult to tell exactly what the effect of orthographic neighborhood really is. In fact, there is some evidence that when phonological neighborhood is controlled there is no effect of orthographic neighborhood on visual word recognition (Mulatti, Reynolds, & Besner, 2006).

In contrast to the debate regarding the influence of orthographic neighbors on lexical decisions, their influence in the naming task appears to be relatively straightforward. In the naming task, participants are shown a word on the screen and are asked to name the word as rapidly as possible. The primary measure from this task is the latency between the onset of the stimulus and the onset of acoustic energy. Using the naming task, a number of researchers have shown that orthographic neighborhood density facilitates responding (Andrews, 1989, 1992; Balota et al., 2004; Carreiras et al., 1997; Grainger, 1990; Peereman & Content, 1995; Sears et al., 1995). Likewise, the research seems to indicate that orthographic neighborhood frequency also facilitates naming (Grainger, 1990; Sears et al., 1995, but also see Carreiras et al., 1997).

To be sure, much of the orthographic neighborhood research has been conducted using the lexical decision and naming tasks. However, some have argued that these tasks are not ideal because they do not necessarily require word identification before giving a response, and it would be more appropriate to use a task that requires lexical selection before a response is given (Forster & Shen, 1996). Two such tasks are perceptual identification and semantic categorization. There are a number of different perceptual identification tasks that have been used in orthographic neighborhood research. The common aspect to all of them is that they require the participant to identify the word when it is shown in a degraded form (e.g., masked). In the semantic categorization task, participants are asked to decide if a word belongs to some semantic category (e.g., is it an animal). The results from these tasks are mixed. Using the perceptual identification task, a number of researchers have reported inhibitory effects of neighborhood density and frequency (Carreiras et al., 1997; Grainger, 1990; Grainger & Jacobs, 1996; Snodgrass & Mintzer, 1993), whereas others have reported facilitation (Sears, Lupker, & Hino, 1999; Snodgrass & Mintzer, 1993). For the semantic categorization task, there have been reports of inhibitory (Carreiras et al., 1997), facilitative (Sears, Lupker, & Hino, 1999), and null (Forster & Shen, 1996) effects of orthographic neighbors. As was the case for lexical decision, it is not clear why the results from these various studies are so divergent, but the explanations given above in relation to the lexical decision data may also be relevant in explaining the discrepancy in the perceptual identification and semantic categorization data.

An extension of the original interactive activation model known as the Multiple Read-Out Model (MROM; Grainger & Jacobs, 1996) has been applied extensively to the study of orthographic neighborhood. In the MROM there are multiple ways that a response can be produced. In terms of lexical decisions, one way the model can make a response is when the activation level of an orthographic whole word node reaches a criterion value referred to as the M criterion (Grainger & Jacobs,

1996). The second way that a lexical decision can be made is determined by the Σ criterion. Using this criterion, a response is made based on the total summed orthographic activation. Finally, a nonword response is given if neither the M nor Σ has occurred before a given amount of time has transpired. The amount of time that must elapse before a nonword response is referred to as the T criterion.

In the MROM as the letter nodes receive activation from the feature level they will increase the activation for the whole word orthographic nodes with which they are consistent. The result of this is that the target word's activation at the lexical level will increase. In addition, the target word's orthographic neighbors' nodes will also receive activation due to the shared overlap at the letter level. To give an example, consider the word *drop* that has as one of its neighbors the word *prop*. When the letter nodes for *d, r, o,* and *p* become active they will all increase the activation of the *drop* node at the lexical level. The nodes corresponding to the letters *r, o,* and *p* will also increase the activation for the orthographic neighbor *prop*, but the *d* node will provide inhibition to the *prop* node. An interesting aspect of the MROM model is that it makes very specific predictions about how orthographic neighbors should affect processing. If the Σ criterion is used, the orthographic neighbors should facilitate lexical decisions as the orthographic neighbors would help to increase the amount of summed orthographic activation. On the other hand, if the lexical decision is made based on the M criterion, then orthographic neighbors, particularly those higher in frequency, would slow responding because they would slow the accumulation of activation for the target word through lateral inhibition.

In the MROM, the M criterion is fixed and cannot be adjusted. Conversely the Σ and T criteria are under strategic control. If Σ is set low, then responses will be made based on the summed orthographic activation, but if Σ is set high, responses will be based on the M criterion. This means unique word identification must occur before a response is given. In the lexical decision task, one factor that determines the value of the Σ criterion is the nonword environment. When the nonwords are easy (i.e., they are low in wordlikeness), then the Σ criterion can be set low and unique word identification need not occur to give a response. The reason the Σ criterion can be set low is because nonwords low in wordlikeness will create minimal activation within the orthographic lexicon. Consequently, summed orthographic activation is sufficient for the model to distinguish words and nonwords. On the other hand, if the nonwords are hard (i.e., they are high in wordlikeness), then the Σ criterion will need to be adjusted upward and lexical decisions will rely on the M criterion. In support of these predictions, Grainger and Jacobs (1996) showed that the facilitative effect of orthographic neighborhood size was only evident in the presence of easy nonwords. Interestingly, a similar conclusion was reached by Andrews (1989) who found a significant facilitative effect of orthographic neighborhood density by items only in the presence of easy nonwords. In terms of neighborhood frequency, Grainger and Jacobs (1996) showed that the MROM model could successfully simulate both the inhibitory effect reported by Grainger and Segui (1990) and the facilitative effect reported by Sears et al. (1995). This lead Grainger and Jacobs to conclude that the neighborhood frequency effect can range from inhibition to facilitation and what determines the nature of the effect is how low the Σ criterion is set.

The MROM has been fairly successful in explaining orthographic neighborhood effects in the lexical decision task, and it is clear that the ability to adjust the Σ criterion is responsible for the model's success. However, in other tasks where only the M criterion can be used, the model has had difficulty. For instance, in perceptual identification and semantic categorization tasks it is assumed that unique word identification must occur. For the MROM, this means a response can only be given once an orthographic word node exceeds the M criterion. The prediction from the MROM in this case is straightforward. Orthographic neighbors should slow responding because they will inhibit the accumulation of activation for the target word. Unfortunately, this has not always been the case. As mentioned above, there have been reports of facilitative effects of orthographic neighborhood density and orthographic neighborhood frequency in both perceptual identification and semantic categorization tasks, and this has led some to claim that the MROM overestimates the impact of inhibition on visual word recognition (Sears, Campbell, & Lupker, 2006; Siakaluk, Sears, & Lupker, 2002). Others have noted that it is possible for models with an interactive activation framework, such as the MROM, to simulate facilitative effects of orthographic neighbors by increasing the facilitation between the letter and word levels to offset the lateral inhibition within the word level (Andrews, 1997). Increasing the facilitation between the two levels means that as the neighbors became active they also increase the activation of their constituent letters through feedback activation to the letter level. As these letters are also shared with the target word, the letters in the target word increase in activation. This leads to an increase in activation at the word level for the target word node, allowing it to be identified more rapidly. Thus, it is possible to simulate either inhibitory or facilitative effects of orthographic neighbors as a function of the tradeoff between within level inhibition and between level excitation, and as result, it can be argued that these types of models are too powerful (Andrews, 1992).

Another model that should be discussed in relation to orthographic neighborhood effects on visual word recognition is the dual-route cascaded (DRC) model of Coltheart and colleagues (Coltheart, Rastle, Perry, Langdon, & Ziegler, 2001). The DRC model has primarily been applied to simulating data from the naming task. According to the model, there are two ways that a word can be named. One way is through a sublexical pathway that involves mapping letters to phonemes according to a set of rules. The other pathway is a lexical pathway that incorporates the assumptions of IAC. Both pathways pass activation to a shared phoneme system that consists of a series of phoneme units. A word is said to have been named once a phoneme unit within each of the positions in the phoneme system have reached some criterion.

In relation to orthographic neighborhoods, the lexical pathway of the DRC model has received the most attention, so it is worth describing in more detail. As in the original interactive activation model (McClelland & Rumelhart, 1981), the first part of the lexical pathway of the DRC model consists of a set of visual feature units that are connected to a letter level, which in turn is connected to an orthographic whole word lexicon. Additionally, the orthographic lexicon is attached to a phonological lexicon that consists of whole word phonological units. Finally, the phonological lexicon passes activation to the shared phoneme system. Thus, as a node in the orthographic lexicon becomes activated, it increases the activation of its corresponding phonological node in the phonological lexicon, which in turn increases the activation level of its constituent phonemes. Using the standard parameter set from Coltheart et al. (2001), the DRC model was unable to simulate the facilitative effect of orthographic neighbors on naming, but Coltheart et al. did show that the DRC model could simulate the effect when the within level inhibition was turned off in the orthographic and phonological lexicons and the letter to word inhibition was reduced. Unfortunately, using this modified parameter set, the model failed to simulate effects that it had previously been able to simulate, such as nonword reading (Coltheart et al., 2001). Clearly more work is needed to provide a satisfactory account of how orthographic neighborhood affects visual word naming.

ORTHOGRAPHIC NEIGHBORHOOD EFFECTS ON SPOKEN WORD RECOGNITION

Research demonstrating an effect of orthography on spoken word processing is not new. Early work by Seidenberg and Tanenhaus (1979) showed that participants were slower in a rhyme detection task when two words had different orthographic bodies (e.g., *rye* and *tie*) than when they had the same orthographic bodies (e.g., *pie* and *tie*). However, the interest in the role of orthography on spoken word recognition has increased dramatically in the last decade. Leading this surge was a study by Ziegler and Ferrand (1998) showing that feedback consistency affects auditory lexical decisions. Feedback consistency refers to the reliability with which a word's phonological rhyme maps on its orthographic body. A word is considered feedback consistent if its rhyme can only be spelled one way (e.g., /-ɪmp/ is only spelled –imp). If a word's rhyme can be spelled more than one way, then it is said to be feedback inconsistent (e.g., /-eɪt/ can be spelled –ate and –ait). There have now been numerous studies showing words that are feedback inconsistent are responded to more slowly than are words that are feedback consistent (Pattamadilok, Morais, Ventura, & Kolinsky, 2007; Ventura, Morais, & Kolinsky, 2007; Ziegler, Ferrand, & Montant, 2004; Ziegler, Petrova, & Ferrand, 2008). Furthermore, it has been shown that the feedback consistency effect on auditory word recognition is not present for those without sufficient reading experience (Ventura et al., 2007; Ziegler & Muneaux, 2007), suggesting that the effect is truly orthographic in nature.

In terms of orthographic neighbors, the consensus of the few studies that have studied this variable in relation to auditory word recognition indicate that words with large orthographic neighborhoods are responded to more rapidly than are words with small orthographic neighborhoods (Ziegler & Muneaux, 2007; Ziegler, Muneaux, & Grainger, 2003). Using the bimodal interactive activation model (Grainger & Ferrand, 1994, 1996), Ziegler et al. (2003) showed that this effect can be explained as a consistency effect. The bimodal interactive activation model is based on the work of the original interactive activation model (McClelland & Rumelhart, 1981). The model contains two sublexical (one orthographic and one phonological) and two lexical (one orthographic and one phonological) levels. These levels are connected with excitatory connections, and the lexical levels contain lateral inhibitory connections. In more recent forms of the model, there is a central interface that converts orthography to phonology (e.g., letters to phonemes) and phonology to orthography (e.g., phonemes to letters). By having both phonological and orthographic processing systems, the model has the desirable property of making predictions about both spoken and written word recognition, as well as being able to account for cross modality neighborhood effects.

In the bimodal interactive activation model, when a spoken word is presented to the model it will first activate the phonological sublexical units. Next, it will pass activation to the phonological lexicon. Additionally, activation from the sublexical phonological units will activate their corresponding orthographic sublexical units, leading to an increase in activation within the orthographic lexicon for the target word even though the input is phonological. Importantly, not only will the target word's node become active within the orthographic lexicon, but the word's orthographic neighbors will also receive activation as they share all but one letter with the target word. Thus, in the bimodal interactive activation model, when the input is auditory, both the orthographic and phonological neighbors receive activation. The same is true when the input is visual.

On the face of it, it would seem that the bimodal interactive activation would have trouble explaining a facilitative effect of orthographic neighborhood as the within level inhibition in the orthographic lexicon would lead to inhibition for the target word from its orthographic neighbors. However, Ziegler et al. (2003) state that the effect is being driven by sublexical consistency and not lexical processing. They argue that words with few orthographic neighbors have an atypical orthographic pattern, and as a result, the link between phonology and orthography is weak for these words. For words with many orthographic neighbors, the link between phonology and orthography is stronger. Consequently, words with few orthographic neighbors will take longer to process due to the increased phonological-orthographic inconsistency. There are two findings that lend credence to this account. First, as previously mentioned, there have been numerous studies indicating that feedback consistency affects auditory word recognition. Second, when consistency was regressed out, the effect of orthographic neighborhood was no longer significant (Ziegler et al., 2003). This indicates that it is not the neighborhood size that matters, but rather feedback consistency is what is important.

Regardless of whether the orthographic neighborhood effects arises from neighbors or feedback consistency, the important point is that the effect provides strong support for the assertion that orthography influences auditory word recognition. As virtually all models of auditory word recognition do not include orthographic representations, the finding of orthographic effects on auditory word recognition represents one of the most difficult challenges for these models (Ziegler et al., 2008). Exactly how these models will answer this challenge is unclear at this time.

PHONOLOGICAL NEIGHBORHOOD

Phonological neighborhood research began in the area of auditory word recognition and later was extended to visual word recognition. As will be discussed below, the effect of phonological neighborhood is relatively consistent within the two modalities, although the direction of the effect reverses as a function of input modality. It should be noted that there have been different ways of defining phonological neighbors. In auditory word recognition research, neighbors are typically defined as words differing by one phoneme substitution, deletion, or addition, whereas in visual word recognition research, neighbors are defined as words that differ by one phoneme substitution. The reason for defining neighbors this way in visual word recognition is to make the measure congruent with past research on orthographic neighborhood. The two ways of defining neighbors are obviously highly correlated and should lead to similar measures of neighborhood structure.

PHONOLOGICAL NEIGHBORHOOD EFFECTS ON AUDITORY WORD RECOGNITION

There have been many studies of how phonological neighbors influence spoken word recognition and the data clearly indicate that phonological neighborhood density and phonological neighborhood frequency inhibit auditory word recognition (Goldinger, 1989; Goldinger, Luce, & Pisoni, 1989; Luce, 1986; Luce & Pisoni, 1998; Luce, Pisoni, & Goldinger, 1990; Vitevitch & Luce, 1998, 1999). Furthermore, this inhibitory effect has been found using a number of different tasks including lexical decision, perceptual identification, and auditory naming. In line with the finding that phonological neighbors slow auditory word processing, essentially all models of spoken word recognition assume that neighbors compete for activation in some manner.

One of the first IAC models of spoken word recognition was the TRACE model (McClelland, 1991; McClelland & Elman, 1986). In similar fashion to the interactive activation model of visual word recognition, the TRACE model contains three hierarchical levels. The first is a phonetic feature level that is directly connected to a phoneme level that is in turn connected to a level containing whole word phonological nodes. There are excitatory connections between levels, and within the phoneme and word level there are inhibitory connections. In addition, as auditory word recognition naturally has a temporal component, each unit at the three levels is repeated across multiple time slices. This temporal component means that the between level excitatory connections only extend to units that are in the same or neighboring time slices. Likewise, the inhibitory connections between units will be strongest when they overlap closely in time and nonexistent if there is no temporal overlap.

When a word is first presented to the model, the feature detectors in the first time slice will become active and propagate activation to the phoneme level and then to the word level. As more of the utterance becomes available, activation for subsequent time slices will be computed based on the input pattern at that point in time as well as activation resulting from previous time slices. Word recognition is assumed to occur based on readout from the word level (McClelland & Elman, 1986).

In terms of phonological neighborhood, it is the within level inhibitory connections that account for the effect. As the model is presented with a word, the initial phoneme of the target word will become active via bottom-up activation from the feature level. This phoneme will likewise begin to pass activation to every word with which it is congruent. This means that every word beginning with this phoneme will receive activation early in processing. As more of the utterance becomes available, words that do not match the input will be inhibited by words that do. For words that have many phonological neighbors, there will be increased inhibition from the neighborhood, resulting in slower processing for these words.

The account given by TRACE is not the only account for the neighborhood effect. Indeed, virtually all models of spoken word recognition hold that similar sounding words interfere with recognition, although in very different ways. Therefore, it is worth considering another way of explaining the neighborhood effect. One model that is particularly relevant to neighborhood effects is the neighborhood activation model (NAM; Luce & Pisoni, 1998).

According to NAM, when a word is encountered it will activate a pattern of acoustic-phonetic information. This acoustic-phonetic information then activates a set of word decision units that are congruent with the acoustic-phonetic activation. Once activated, a word decision unit monitors not only the acoustic-phonetic information with which it corresponds but also higher level lexical information (e.g., frequency) that pertains to the particular word it represents. Furthermore, the word decision units monitor the overall level of activation in the word decision system. Word recognition occurs when one of the word decision units reaches a recognition criterion. During word processing, the word decision units compute decision values based on a decision rule where decision values decrease as neighborhood size increases. Because of this, NAM correctly predicts that phonological neighbors should hinder target word processing. It is important to note that both TRACE and NAM predict inhibitory effects of phonological neighbors, but for very different reasons. In TRACE, the inhibitory effect exists because neighbors actively inhibit one another. In NAM, on the other hand, the inhibitory effect arises because neighbors raise the overall level of activity within the decision system, and this has the end result of lowering the decision values, which slows responding.

One related effect that has proven difficult for NAM to explain is the effect of phonotactic probability. Phonotactic probability refers to the frequency of the phonetic segments in a word, and is positively correlated with neighborhood density. Research has shown that *nonwords* that are high density/high phonotactic probability are processed more rapidly than are nonwords that are low density/ low phonotactic probability. The opposite is true for words (Vitevitch & Luce, 1998, 1999). Vitevitch and Luce (1998) argue that when nonwords are processed there is no lexical representation for the stimuli, and as a result, sublexical processing dominates, leading to a facilitative effect. However, when the stimuli are words any sublexical facilitation is squelched by the competition at the lexical level, leading to an inhibitory effect. It is the facilitative effect for nonwords that is problematic for NAM as it predicts that stimuli with large neighborhoods should be processed more slowly (Vitevitch & Luce, 1999). Additionally, NAM suffers from the fact that it does not include a sublexical level, and therefore, cannot accommodate the effect of phonotactic probability. The architecture of the TRACE model is more in agreement with the data in that it contains lexical and sublexical levels. However, there have been no formal simulations of the effect, and it is not clear that the model could simulate the data given that Vitevitch and Luce (1999) have argued that sublexical and lexical processing need to be independent to explain the effects.

Because of the limitations with models such as NAM and TRACE, Vitevitch and Luce (1999) chose to discuss their results in terms of Grossberg's adaptive resonance theory (ART) of speech perception (Grossberg, 1986; Grossberg, Boardman, & Cohen, 1997; Grossberg & Myers, 2000). Within the ART framework, there are two levels of processing. In the first level, the incoming phonetic signal is mapped onto phoneme items in working memory. The second level is a short-term memory that consists of list chunks of different sizes (e.g., phonemes, syllables, whole word, etc.) representing different combinations of the items in working memory. The items in working memory are connected with bidirectional excitatory links to the list chunks in short-term memory. Within short-term memory, list chunks equal in size are connected with inhibitory connections (i.e., all words are connected, all syllables are connected, etc.). Also, larger list chunks in short-term memory can inhibit smaller list chunks (a process referred to as masking). For example, words mask syllables and syllables mask phonemes. When presented with a word, the items in working memory excite the list chunks that contain them. In turn, the active list chunks then send feedback to the items in working memory. As processing continues a resonance emerges between the list chunks and the items that support them. It is this resonance that gives rise to perception.

In terms of phonological neighborhood density, when a word chunk gets activated it will receive inhibition from its phonological neighbors. It will take longer for the chunks of words with many neighbors to overcome this inhibition and establish a resonance with the items in working memory. Furthermore, for word processing, the largest chunks that will be activated are the word chunks, and these will mask all smaller chunks, removing any effect of phonotactic probability. However, when nonwords are processed, the largest chunks that will become active are smaller than the word chunks. Consequently, the resonance between the chunks in short-term memory and the items in working memory are driven by phonotactic probability and not density (Vitevitch & Luce, 1999). Thus, the ART framework seems capable of explaining the opposite effects of phonological neighborhood density and phonotactic probability, and the key to its ability to do so is that processing is driven by the properties of the longest chunks that become strongly activated. Although Vitevitch and Luce (1999) only discuss their effects in terms of a verbal description of ART, recent work has shown that ARTphone, a computational model based on the ART framework, can simulate the Vitevitch and Luce data (Pitt, Myung, & Altteri, 2007).

Phonological Neighborhood Effects on Visual Word Recognition

As detailed in the preceding section, there is a rich history on the effect of phonological neighborhood on auditory word recognition, but in terms of visual word recognition, phonological neighborhood has only recently begun to receive attention. Interestingly, one of the first studies failed to find an effect of phonological neighborhood density on nonword naming (Peereman & Content, 1997). However, later research has shown that phonological neighborhood density facilitates visual word recognition in the lexical decision, naming, and semantic categorization tasks (Mulatti et al., 2006; Yates, 2005; Yates et al., 2004). There has been one report indicating that phonological neighbors may inhibit processing. Grainger, Muneaux, Farioli, and Ziegler (2005) crossed orthographic and phonological neighborhood density in a factorial design. Their results indicated that for words with few orthographic neighbors phonological neighborhood had an inhibitory effect, but for words with large orthographic neighborhoods, the effect of phonological neighborhood was facilitative. They explained this interaction in terms of cross code consistency within the bimodal interactive activation model. Cross code consistency refers to whether activation within the phonological and orthographic systems is in agreement. Any inconsistency between these systems will slow processing. For example, the word *bait* has some phonological neighbors that are not orthographic neighbors (e.g., *gate, hate,* and *bake*). Thus, the activation of these words within the phonological system will be inconsistent with activation in the orthographic system. Grainger et al. argued that words with orthographic and phonological neighborhoods that are similar in size (e.g., both large or both small) should be more cross code consistent while words where one neighborhood is large and the other small should be more cross code inconsistent. This means for words with small orthographic neighborhoods as the phonological neighborhood size *increases* so does the cross code inconsistency. The result is slower responses to words with many phonological neighbors. For words with large orthographic neighborhoods, increasing the number of phonological neighbors *decreases* the cross code inconsistency, leading to faster responses to words with many phonological neighbors.

The cross code consistency account is intriguing, but it does not seem capable of explaining some of the facilitative effects seen in other studies. For example, using words controlled on measures of cross code consistency (i.e., feedback and feedforward consistency), both Yates (2005) and Mulatti et al. (2006) found that phonological neighbors facilitated word recognition. One potential difference between these studies is that Grainger et al. (2005) used French words and Yates and Mulatti et al. used English words. It is also worth noting that Peereman and Content's (1997) study that failed to find an effect of phonological neighborhood on word naming consisted of French stimuli. It is not clear why (or if) language is a determining factor in the nature of the phonological neighborhood effect. Only future research will be able to address this issue.

In terms of the facilitative effect of phonological neighborhood density on English word naming, Yates (2005) argued that phonological neighbors increase the activation levels of the target word's phonemes through interactive activation between the lexical and sublexical levels. More recently it has been shown that what is important is not the number of neighbors per se but instead it is the number of neighbors for the least supported phoneme (LSP) that matters (Yates, Friend, & Ploetz, 2008). The LSP is defined as the phoneme within a word that receives the least amount of support from the word's phonological neighbors. For example, the word *geese* has the following words as neighbors: *cease, lease, niece, piece, gas, goose,* and *guess.* For the word *geese* the first phoneme /g/ is the LSP as it overlaps with the fewest phonological neighbors. As the LSP receives the least support, it should take longer to reach threshold than the other phonemes in the word that benefits from additional neighbor overlap. In word naming, it is assumed that the pronunciation for a word cannot be initiated until the complete phonological code has been determined (Rastle, Harrington, Coltheart, & Palethorpe, 2000). This means that the pronunciation of a word can only be as fast as the amount of time it takes the slowest phoneme (i.e., the LSP) to reach threshold. Yates et al. showed that words with large phonological neighborhoods tended to have more neighbors for their LSP than did words with small phonological neighborhoods. Moreover, they showed that the data from the naming experiments of Yates (2005) and Mulatti et al. (2006) could be explained in terms of the LSP and argued that the important variable was not the overall neighborhood density but was instead the number of neighbors for the LSP. Words with many neighbors overlapping with their LSP are named more rapidly than are words with few neighbors overlapping with their LSP.

SUMMARY AND CONCLUSIONS

As detailed throughout this chapter there is a rich history of studying how similarity among representations stored in memory affects word recognition. One of the most common ways of explaining these effects is in terms of IAC models. However, from the beginning, some of the research on similarity has proven difficult for these models to handle. Most notably are the facilitative effects of neighbors as most IAC models would, on the surface, seem to predict inhibition due to lateral inhibition from their neighbors. Nevertheless, researchers have shown that it is possible for models that employ interactive activation to produce facilitative effects by either reducing the influence of inhibitory connections and/ or increasing the influence of facilitatory connections (Andrews, 1997; Mulatti et al., 2006; Yates et al., 2008). Unfortunately, when the models are modified in this manner they lose the ability to explain other word recognition effects such as nonword naming (Coltheart et al., 2001). A future goal of research will be to see if these models can simulate neighborhood effects while continuing to explain the effects of other variables. Also from a model standpoint, the study of neighborhoods has also brought to light a serious problem that is present in nearly all models of spoken word recognition. Specifically, they do not contain orthographic representations. The finding that orthographic neighbors, or more specifically feedback consistency, affect auditory word recognition poses a serious challenge for these models (Ziegler et al., 2008). Any model that claims to be a complete account of spoken word processing will need to include orthographic representations, just as models of visual word recognition include phonological representations.

Finally, throughout this chapter I have defined similarity in terms of neighbors. Historically this has been the most common way of defining similarity. Nevertheless, this is not the only or necessarily the best way to do so. For instance, research has shown that visual word recognition is influenced by words that share transposed letters (e.g., salt/slat; Andrews, 1996) and neighbors that are formed by deleting a letter (e.g., tablet/table; Davis & Taft, 2005). Although these words are clearly similar, they would not be considered neighbors using the conventions of Coltheart et al. (1977). Additionally, recent work has shown that defining orthographic similarity in terms of Levenshtein distance provides a better account of lexical decision and naming data (Yarkoni, Balota, & Yap, 2008). Clearly there is still much work to be done in determining the best way(s) to define similarity, and as this research progresses, it should prove invaluable in helping to further refine our understanding of the role of orthography and phonology on word recognition.

REFERENCES

Andrews, S. (1989). Frequency and neighborhood effects on lexical access: Activation or search? *Journal of Experimental Psychology: Learning, Memory, and Cognition, 15,* 802–814.

Andrews, S. (1992). Frequency and neighborhood effects on lexical access: Lexical similarity or orthographic redundancy? *Journal of Experimental Psychology: Learning, Memory, and Cognition, 18,* 234–254.

Andrews, S. (1996). Lexical retrieval and selection processes: Effects of transposed-letter confusability. *Journal of Memory and Language, 35,* 775–800.

Andrews, S. (1997). The effect of orthographic similarity on lexical retrieval: Resolving neighborhood conflicts. *Psychonomic Bulletin and Review, 4,* 439–461.

Balota, D. A., Cortese, M. J., Sergent-Marshall, S. D., Spieler, D. H., & Yap, M. (2004). Visual word recognition of single-syllable words. *Journal of Experimental Psychology: General, 133,* 283–316.

Carreiras, M., Perea, M., & Grainger, J. (1997). Effects of the orthographic neighborhood in visual word recognition: Cross-task comparisons. *Journal of Experimental Psychology: Learning, Memory, and Cognition, 23,* 857–871.

Coltheart, M., Davelaar, E., Jonasson, J., & Besner, D. (1977). Access to the internal lexicon. In S. Dornic (Ed.), *Attention and performance VI* (pp. 535–555). Hillsdale, NJ: Erlbaum.

Coltheart, M., Rastle, K., Perry, C., Langdon, R., & Ziegler, J. (2001). DRC: A dual route cascaded model of visual word recognition and reading aloud. *Psychological Review, 108,* 204–256.

Davis, C. J., & Taft, M. (2005). More words in the neighborhood: Interference in lexical decision due to deletion neighbors. *Psychonomic Bulletin & Review, 12,* 904–910.

Forster, K. I., & Shen, D. (1996). No enemies in the neighborhood: Absence of inhibitory neighborhood effects in lexical decision and semantic categorization. *Journal of Experimental Psychology: Learning, Memory, and Cognition, 22,* 696–713.

Goldinger, S. D. (1989). Neighborhood density effect for high frequency words: Evidence for activation-based models of word recognition. *Research on Speech Perception Progress Report, 16*, 163–186.

Goldinger, S. D., Luce, P. A., & Pisoni, D. B. (1989). Priming lexical neighbors of spoken words: Effects of competition and inhibition. *Journal of Memory and Language, 28*, 501–518.

Grainger, J. (1990). Word frequency and neighborhood frequency effects in lexical decision and naming. *Journal of Memory and Language, 29*, 228–244.

Grainger, J., & Ferrand, L. (1994). Phonology and orthography in visual word recognition: Effects of masked homophone primes. *Journal of Memory and Language, 33*, 218–233.

Grainger, J., & Ferrand, L. (1996). Masked orthographic and phonological priming in visual word recognition and naming: Cross-task comparisons. *Journal of Memory and Language, 35*, 623–647.

Grainger, J., & Jacobs, A. M. (1996). Orthographic processing in visual word recognition: A multiple read-out model. *Psychological Review, 103*, 518–565.

Grainger, J., Muneaux, M., Farioli, F., & Ziegler, J. C. (2005). Effects of phonological and orthographic neighbourhood density interact in visual word recognition. *Quarterly Journal of Experimental Psychology A: Human Experimental Psychology, 58*, 981–998.

Grainger, J., O'Regan, J. K., Jacobs, A. M., & Segui, J. (1989). On the role of competing word units in visual word recognition: The neighborhood frequency effect. *Perception and Psychophysics, 45*, 189–195.

Grainger, J., O'Regan, J. K., Jacobs, A. M., & Segui, J. (1992). Neighborhood frequency effects and letter visibility in visual word recognition. *Perception and Psychophysics, 51*, 49–56.

Grainger, J., & Segui, J. (1990). Neighborhood frequency effects in visual word recognition: A comparison of lexical decision and masked identification latencies. *Perception and Psychophysics, 47*, 191–198.

Grossberg, S. (1986). The adaptive self-organization of serial order in behavior: Speech, language, and motor control. In E. C. Schwab & H. C. Nusbaum (Eds.), *Pattern recognition by humans and machines: Vol. 1 Speech perception* (pp. 187–294). New York, NY: Academic Press.

Grossberg, S., Boardman, I., & Cohen, M. (1997). Neural dynamics of variable-rate speech categorization. *Journal of Experimental Psychology: Human Perception and Performance, 23*, 481–503.

Grossberg, S., & Myers, C. W. (2000). The resonant dynamics of speech perception: Interword integration and duration-dependent backward effects. *Psychological Review, 107*, 735–767.

Harm, M. W., & Seidenberg, M. S. (2004). Computing the meanings of words in reading: Cooperative division of labor between visual and phonological processes. *Psychological Review, 111*, 662–720.

Huntsman, L. A., & Lima, S. D. (1996). Orthographic neighborhood structure and lexical access. *Journal of Psycholinguistic Research, 25*, 417–429.

Huntsman, L. A., & Lima, S. D. (2002). Orthographic neighbors and visual word recognition. *Journal of Psycholinguistic Research, 31*, 289–306.

Johnson, N. F., & Pugh, K. R. (1994). A cohort model of visual word recognition. *Cognitive Psychology, 26*, 240–346.

Landauer, T. K., & Streeter, L. A. (1973). Structural differences between common and rare words: Failure of equivalence assumptions for theories of word recognition. *Journal of Verbal Learning and Verbal Behavior, 12*, 119–131.

Luce, P. A. (1986). *Neighborhoods of words in the mental lexicon*. Research on speech perception technical report (No. 6). Bloomington, IN: Speech Research Laboratory, Psychology Department, Indiana University.

Luce, P. A., & Pisoni, D. B. (1998). Recognizing spoken words: The neighborhood activation model. *Ear and Hearing, 19*, 1–36.

Luce, P. A., Pisoni, D. B., & Goldinger, S. D. (1990). Similarity neighborhoods of spoken words. In G. T. M. Altmann (Ed.), *Cognitive models of speech processing: Psycholinguistic and computational perspectives* (pp. 122–147). Cambridge, MA: The MIT Press.

McClelland, J. L. (1991). Stochastic interactive processes and the effect of context on perception. *Cognitive Psychology, 23*, 1–44.

McClelland, J. L., & Elman, J. L. (1986). The TRACE model of speech perception. *Cognitive Psychology, 18*, 1–86.

McClelland, J. L., & Rumelhart, D. E. (1981). An interactive activation model of context effects in letter perception: I. An account of basic findings. *Psychological Review, 88*, 375–407.

Mulatti, C., Reynolds, M. G., & Besner, D. (2006). Neighborhood effects in reading aloud: New findings and new challenges for computational models. *Journal of Experimental Psychology: Human Perception and Performance, 32*, 799–810.

Pattamadilok, C., Morais, J., Ventura, P., & Kolinsky, R. G. (2007). The locus of the orthographic consistency effect in auditory word recognition: Further evidence from French. *Language and Cognitive Processes, 22*, 700–726.

Peereman, R., & Content, A. (1995). Neighborhood size effect in naming: Lexical activation or sublexical correspondences? *Journal of Experimental Psychology: Learning, Memory, and Cognition, 21*, 409–421.

Peereman, R., & Content, A. (1997). Orthographic and phonological neighborhoods in naming: Not all neighbors are equally influential in orthographic space. *Journal of Memory and Language, 37*, 382–410.

Perea, M., & Pollatsek, A. (1998). The effects of neighborhood frequency in reading and lexical decision. *Journal of Experimental Psychology: Human Perception and Performance, 24*, 767–779.

Pitt, M. A., Myung, J. I., & Altteri, N. (2007). Modeling the word recognition data of Vitevitch and Luce (1998): Is it ARTful? *Psychonomic Bulletin & Review, 14*, 442–448.

Plaut, D. C., McClelland, J. L., Seidenberg, M. S., & Patterson, K. (1996). Understanding normal and impaired word reading: Computational principles in quasi-regular domains. *Psychological Review, 103*, 56–115.

Rastle, K., Harrington, J., Coltheart, M., & Palethorpe, S. (2000). Reading aloud begins when the computation of phonology is complete. *Journal of Experimental Psychology: Human Perception and Performance, 26*, 1178–1191.

Reicher, G. M. (1969). Perceptual recognition as a function of meaningfulness of stimulus material. *Journal of Experimental Psychology, 81*, 275–280.

Rumelhart, D. E., & McClelland, J. L. (1982). An interactive activation model of context effects in letter perception: II. The contextual enhancement effect and some tests and extensions of the model. *Psychological Review, 89*, 60–94.

Sears, C. R., Campbell, C. R., & Lupker, S. J. (2006). Is there a neighborhood frequency effect in English? Evidence from reading and lexical decision. *Journal of Experimental Psychology: Human Perception and Performance, 32*, 1040–1062.

Sears, C., Hino, Y., & Lupker, S. J. (1995). Neighborhood size and neighborhood frequency effects in word recognition. *Journal of Experimental Psychology: Human Perception and Performance, 21*, 876–900.

Sears, C., Lupker, S. J., & Hino, Y. (1999). Orthographic neighborhood effects in perceptual identification and semantic categorization tasks: A test of the multiple read-out model. *Perception and Psychophysics, 61,* 1537–1554.

Seidenberg, M. S., & McClelland, J. L. (1989). A distributed, developmental model of word recognition and naming. *Psychological Review, 96,* 523–568.

Seidenberg, M. S., & Tanenhaus, M. K. (1979). Orthographic effects on rhyme monitoring. *Journal of Experimental Psychology: Human Learning and Memory, 5,* 546–554.

Siakaluk, P. D., Sears, C. R., & Lupker, S. J. (2002). Orthographic neighborhood effects in lexical decision: The effects of nonword orthographic neighborhood size. *Journal of Experimental Psychology: Human Perception and Performance, 28,* 661–681.

Snodgrass, J. G., & Mintzer, M. (1993). Neighborhood effects in visual word recognition: Facilitatory or inhibitory? *Memory & Cognition, 21,* 247–266.

Ventura, P., Morais, J., & Kolinsky, R. G. (2007). The development of the orthographic consistency effect in speech recognition: From sublexical to lexical involvement. *Cognition, 105,* 547–576.

Vitevitch, M. S., & Luce, P. A. (1998). When words compete: Levels of processing in perception of spoken words. *Psychological Science, 9,* 325–329.

Vitevitch, M. S., & Luce, P. A. (1999). Probabilistic phonotactics and neighborhood activation in spoken word recognition. *Journal of Memory and Language, 40,* 374–408.

Wheeler, D. D. (1970). Processes in word recognition. *Cognitive Psychology, 1,* 59–85.

Yarkoni, T., Balota, D., & Yap, M. (2008). Moving beyond Coltheart's N: A new measure of orthographic similarity. *Psychonomic Bulletin & Review,15,* 971–979.

Yates, M. (2005). Phonological neighbors speed visual word processing: Evidence from multiple tasks. *Journal of Experimental Psychology: Learning, Memory, and Cognition, 31,* 1385–1397.

Yates, M., Friend, J., & Ploetz, D. M. (2008). Phonological neighbors influence word naming through the least supported phoneme. *Journal of Experimental Psychology: Human Perception and Performance, 34,* 1599–1608.

Yates, M., Locker, L. J., & Simpson, G. B. (2004). The influence of phonological neighborhood on visual word perception. *Psychonomic Bulletin & Review, 11,* 452–457.

Ziegler, J. C., & Ferrand, L. (1998). Orthography shapes the perception of speech: The consistency effect in auditory word recognition. *Psychonomic Bulletin & Review, 5,* 683–689.

Ziegler, J. C., Ferrand, L., & Montant, M. (2004). Visual phonology: The effects of orthographic consistency on different auditory word recognition tasks. *Memory & Cognition, 32,* 732–741.

Ziegler, J. C., & Muneaux, M. (2007). Orthographic facilitation and phonological inhibition in spoken word recognition: A developmental study. *Psychonomic Bulletin & Review, 14,* 75–80.

Ziegler, J. C., Muneaux, M., & Grainger, J. (2003). Neighborhood effects in auditory word recognition: Phonological competition and orthographic facilitation. *Journal of Memory and Language, 48,* 779–793.

Ziegler, J. C., & Perry, C. (1998). No more problems in Coltheart's neighborhood: Resolving neighborhood conflicts in the lexical decision task. *Cognition, 68,* B53–B62.

Ziegler, J. C., Petrova, A., & Ferrand, L. (2008). Feedback consistency effects in visual and auditory word recognition: Where do we stand after more than a decade? *Journal of Experimental Psychology: Learning, Memory, and Cognition, 34,* 643–661.

14 Two Theories of Speech Production and Perception

Mark Tatham and Katherine Morton

INTRODUCTION

In this chapter we focus on two speech theories: Classical Phonetics and Cognitive Phonetics. Classical phonetics forms the basis of all modern research in speech, whereas cognitive phonetics is contemporary.

Classical phonetics (Abercrombie, 1967; Cruttenden, 2001) gave to mental representations of speech a central position in the theory, making it a cognitively based model. Relatively informal inspection of articulation enabled phoneticians to correlate the mental representation with vocal tract shapes for various speech sounds. Together with a symbol system—the International Phonetic Alphabet—the approach often enabled large scale comparisons between representations in many different languages.

There were two key problems with classical phonetics: it failed to tackle the difference between cognitive representation and physical instantiation, believing that because cognitively we tend to proceed in a symbolic categorical way the same must be true of the physical instantiation. In the 1960s, when it was pointed out that the cognitive representations are all about discrete segments and that the physical signals are all about continuousness, the model was restated by Coarticulation Theory (MacNeilage & De Clerk, 1969), which attempted to explain how discrete segments "become" continuous.

The inherent confusions in classical phonetics and its failure to explain more and more empirical observations as instrumentation developed from the 1950s onward led to several developments. Description of the data as the goal of the theory gave way to the more usual scientific goal of *explanation* of the data. Linear representations of speech gave way to nonlinear hierarchical representations. Researchers began to look behind the simple configurations of the vocal tract observed by eye and the audio signal registered by ear. Suggestions for integrated models of speech production and perception began to appear. Action Theory (Fowler, 1980) led the way, suggesting a layered model linking cognitively based speech processing (in linguistics: phonology) and physically based speech processing (phonetics), considerably downgrading the role of mental representation and processing that had been the central consideration of classical phonetics and linguistics.

Cognitive phonetics (Tatham, 1984, 1990) rested on the same basic ideas as action theory, but focused on developing ideas about cognition in speech, particularly concentrating on computationally adequate dynamic modeling of utterances from their phonological representations and on to the perceived soundwave (Tatham & Morton, 2002). Cognitive phonetics embodied a model of the perceiver in the speaker and a model of the speaker in the perceiver. Speech production and perception became essentially relatively simple processes compared with the earlier complex extensions to classical phonetics made by coarticulation theory. In the new model the surface complexity was explained by using the principle of supervision continuously controlling and therefore varying a basic and relatively uncomplicated articulation (Tatham, 1995). The simple *categorical* suggestions of classical phonetics gave way to explanation of the *continuousness* of speech production, but more importantly to a systematic explanation of the continuously *varying* nature of speech.

CLASSICAL PHONETICS (1900+)

Developed from the late 19th century onward, classical phonetics was the first true attempt at a scientific theory of speech. The focus of the theory is the segmental object, strings of which form speech. Experimental techniques as we know them today were not available to early phoneticians who relied on strict training in listening to give them the ability to perceive nuances in the acoustic signal and to introspect on how vocal tract shapes were set up to produce individual sounds. Classical phonetics developed symbolic representations for speech sounds and for some prosodic effects spanning groups of individual sounds.

Classical phonetics is a descriptive theory that does not extend to an explanatory level. Its subjective methodology for investigating speech asserted that speech is a concatenation of individually manipulable sounds. It relied on perception and limited observation of how the articulators produce speech to assign segment labels. Questions such as the shape of the vocal tract and neuromuscular control had to wait until the 1960s when techniques were developed such as electromyography, air pressure measurement, and video x-ray, allowing correlations between shapes and the acoustic wave. The new techniques generated many new questions:

a. What aerodynamic properties of the general vocal tract are used in speaking?
   In general, speech is carried by an egressive air stream; that is, air flows out from the lungs, through the vocal tract, and exits *via* the mouth and/or nose. Some languages employ ingressive sounds, and it is possible to create localized aerodynamic effects (and hence sounds) within the vocal tract, such as clicks, and so on. Researchers have noted that airflow and the dynamic response to its impedance contribute to certain coarticulatory effects such as aspiration.

   b. How are the vocal shapes specified? Various proposals (Baer, Gore, Gracco, & Nye, 1991; Rubin & Vatikiotis-Bateson, 1998) are made in terms of
      1. The overall shape (the projected final shape within which the aerodynamics takes place)
      2. The configuration of the individual organs (a parametric representation)
      3. Parametrically in terms of the individual muscles
      4. Parametrically in terms of muscle groupings (coordinative structures)
   c. What are the constraints (particularly temporal) on the mechanics of the vocal tract in a dynamic mode, rather than static single segment mode? We need to distinguish between constraints in moving in zero time from one static position to another and those constraints associated with dynamic movement (where the emphasis is on the movement rather than the underlying vocal tract shapes).
   d. Are these constraints fixed or can they deliberately be manipulated to the limits of the physical system? For example, manipulation can potentially have a considerable influence on constraints governed by time: it is possible to decide to speak fast or slow, but the constraint, even in slow speech, remains at the "boundaries," though with more time during the segment to render the target specification more accurately.

In general, classical phonetics made no attempt to address such questions, which by the 1970s were becoming center stage in speech production research.

COARTICULATION THEORY (FROM AROUND 1965)

From the 1940s onward, developments in instrumentation enabled researchers to examine directly the nature of the speech soundwave. It became obvious that it is rarely possible to find separate speech sounds within the signal. Work began to investigate how the discontinuity of the cognitive representation of speech (classical phonetics' segments) becomes continuous in the soundwave, and how the perceiver reconstructs the discontinuity when listening to the soundwave. We would not today consider that discrete objects *become* continuous, or that discrete objects are *reconstructed* from the soundwave. The kinds of questions being addressed at that time included:

   a. What is the precise nature of the acoustic signal of speech?
      The acoustic signal of speech has been studied extensively since the 1950s (Fant, 1960). The signal is modeled as the result of a filtered source, where the source can be either periodic, aperiodic, or mixed, originating with vocal cord vibration or due to some constriction-based impedance at some point(s) within the vocal tract. The vocal tract forms a resonance cavity responsible for the filtering of the source signal; the nasal cavity

constitutes an additional resonance cavity that can be shunted into the system at will.

The size and shape of the vocal tract cavities determine some aspects of the resultant waveform's spectral properties, with the resonance energized by characteristically shaped source signals.

Recognition of unclear boundaries and so-called blurred effects across approximate boundaries led to coarticulation theory. A range of summarizing articles can be found in the collection edited by Hardcastle and Hewlett (1999). This model proposed that although a string of speech segments is *intended* by the speaker, the inertial properties of the various stages of production (in the motor control system, mechanics of muscle and articulator movement and the aerodynamics) introduce a smoothing, or overlap effect producing the observed continuousness of the final signal (MacNeilage, 1970). This smoothing is *time dependent*: a landmark change in speech production theory, since for the first time we have a truly dynamic and explanatory perspective on speech, which contrasted strikingly with the static and atemporal descriptive perspective of classical phonetics.

b. What is encoded in the signal?
Initially it was thought that the temporal rendering of the intended speech plan for a sequence of words directly encoded the basic meaning of the string of *syntactic* objects, and it was then up to *phonological processing* and *phonetic rendering* to determine what acoustic features can be assigned to prosody (intonation, stress, rhythm). There was no clear correlation in the sense that it is still unclear, for example, how the prosody of a particular sentence on a particular occasion will turn out in terms of the timing, frequency, and amplitude parameters of the acoustic signal (Matthies, Perrier, Perkell, & Zandipour, 2001).

c. Are there specific aerodynamic coarticulatory constraints? Observations were made, for example, on vocal cord movement.
   1. Intended vocal cord vibration from the start of the rendering of a vowel nucleus segment following a syllable initial voiceless plosive (as in a word like *pat, /pæ.../*, for example), is delayed because of instability in the air pressure and flow above the larynx following the release of the built-up air pressure. There is an oscillatory settling of the pressure, but until the necessary ratio between supra- and subglottal pressures and vocal cord tension is reestablished vibration will not begin. This delay is called voice onset time (VOT; Lisker & Abramson, 1964) and varies across languages.
   2. Vocal cord vibration for a phonologically voiced stop cannot be continued indefinitely if the air flow is stopped above the larynx. Again the build up of supraglottal air pressure behind the stop eventually destroys the required ratio—as in a sequence like /ada/ in English (Higgins, Netsell, & Schulte, 1998).

The general case of coarticulation resulting from a pressure ratio disturbance during stops specified as [+ voice] phonologically involves curtailment of vibration if the air flow is impeded above the larynx. Specific cases are progressive vocal cord vibration attenuation with *partial* impedance (in, say, a voiced fricative in a word like *measure* in English) and vibration failure with *full* impedance (in, say, a voiced stop in a word like *adder*) to air flow through the vocal tract. Deliberate curtailment of vocal cord vibration occurs when tension in the vocal cords (the third parameter in the equation) is too great or the vocal cords are held too stiffly, as in whispered vowels.

COGNITIVE PHONETICS (FROM AROUND 1980)

THE BASIC THEORY

Although coarticulation theory (MacNeilage & De Clerk, 1969) appeared to explain time governed dynamic effects in speech production and was able to use these to throw light on the mismatch between the segmentally oriented focus of classical phonetics and the more recent detailed observations of the acoustic signal, there remained some unexplained phenomena. Cognitive phonetics (Tatham, 1984) was devised to explain a class of observations that coarticulation theory failed to explain.

The idea that the continuousness of the soundwave results from the inertial properties of the production system implies that coarticulation is universal. Closer inspection reveals however that coarticulatory effects vary from language to language, even from accent to accent within a language and even within the speech of a single person on different occasions. Two explanations are possible: either there are no truly universal properties of coarticulation or the concept needs refining to account for these apparent discrepancies.

Cognitive phonetics took the second view, proposing that coarticulation is indeed a truly universal phenomenon since it is determined by the way nonlinguistic universal physical factors that are mechanical or aerodynamic in origin constrain the linguistic *use* of speech production processes. But at the same time linguistically (and therefore cognitively) sourced considerations determine the *extent* of coarticulatory phenomena. In other words, coarticulation is a two-stage process.

1. There are universal physically determined constraints.
2. These constraints are manipulable (Tatham, 1971).

The concept of cognitive intervention in somatic behavior here is different from usage of the term in education and therapy. Here intervention means disturbance or modification of an otherwise automatic or universal process. The source of the intervention is cognitive and relies on tacit knowledge of the coarticulatory process and knowledge of the speaker's phonological intentions. Intervention is rarely a consciously aware process and is performed by the Cognitive Phonetic

Agent (CPA; Tatham, 1995). The concept of the agent is adapted from Artificial Intelligence (Garland & Alterman, 2004).

In phonetics it is impossible to isolate cognitive considerations from physical considerations. In fact, much of the theorizing in phonetics over the past half century has explicitly addressed the relationship between the cognitive processes of phonology and the physical processes of speech production. We feel there must be a relationship, but what that relationship is still defeats theorists: at the most we are able to characterize a rather loose correlative association between the two.

Speech production models usually propose that the cognitive processing underlying speech is handled along with all of language as a symbolic system that ultimately terminates in an output: a symbolic representation that specifies the linguistically significant properties of what is to be spoken. We have called this the *utterance plan* (Figure 14.1).

However this representation as it stands cannot be input directly to physical processing, whether considered statically in terms of its potential, or as a dynamic system characterizing particular utterances. The most usual method of bridging the cognitive/physical gap is to assume some kind of rerepresentation of the cognitive plan in physical terms that lead directly into a physical model of speech production. Along these lines, questions asked by researchers include:

1. What is the nature of the input to physical rendering of the cognitively derived utterance plan? The physical input to the premotor control system needs to be initiated by a cognitive representation of the intended plan. This plan is derived by cognitive processes (the language's phonology) and is currently expressed as a string of extrinsic allophonic objects

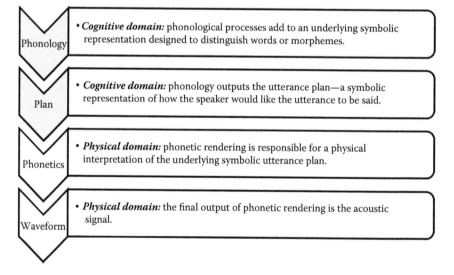

FIGURE 14.1   The relationship between cognitive phonology and physical phonetics.

appropriately wrapped; that is, embedded in a prosody and a framework of expression (Tatham & Morton, 2006), see Figure 14.2.

2. Are there physical units or objects matching the cognitive objects of the plan? It would seem so. We have a clear idea of the psychological reality of the basic objects contained in the plan—we call them extrinsic allophones (as opposed to the phonetic *intrinsic* allophones that are unintended variants resulting from coarticulation (Tatham, 1971). Also, it does seem to be the case that movement results from a system input in terms of a sequence of physical target representations (MacNeilage, 1970). It is possible that at both the cognitive and physical levels the units are organized: in the case of the cognitive plan, in terms of hierarchically structured syllable objects sequenced appropriately; and in terms of the physical plan, as functionally similar physical structures. It is easier to show the structure of the cognitive plan than the physical plan, but the hypothesis has proved productive.

There remain a number of questions about what the physical representation looks like. Is it, for example, in terms of hierarchically organized whole objects or it is parametric? Are the sequenced objects wrapped in the sense that they are contained within a broader domain of prosodic features and, even higher, expressive features?

3. What constraints are there in the equivalence of cognitive and physical plans? The physical plan needs to render all extrinsic allophonic features—these are all linguistically significant (or, by definition, they would not be there). In converting from a cognitive plan to a physical plan the system may find it useful to flag certain known problems further down the line—for example, predicted coarticulatory errors (perhaps hierarchically organized in terms of probability in this context, etc.). Any such flagging could be used to feedback to the cognitive level warning of future stabilization or supervision requirements. So for example the /s/

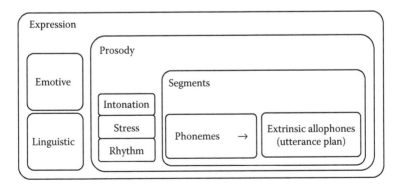

FIGURE 14.2   The wrapper format: expressions wraps prosody, which in turn wraps segmental processing.

and /ʃ/ (*sea vs. she*) proximity in both production and perceptual spaces could be flagged to alert a possible need for supervision or increased precision of articulation.

Cognitive phonetics requires a way of dynamically operating within the physical limits of the articulatory system. The CPA conducts a systematic supervisory intervention in physical processes based on tacit knowledge the speaker has of the production process. Thus coarticulatory effects are characterized in cognitive phonetics as varying along a vector from maximal constraint to maximal enhancement. A speaker may constrain a universal coarticulatory effect or may enhance the effect. A pivot point of no intervention lets the inertial constraint find its own level.

scale of CPA control from fully enhanced through neutral to fully constrained

$$[\text{enhanced}] \quad 1 \quad \leftarrow \quad 0 \quad \rightarrow \quad 1 \quad [\text{constrained}]$$

THE MECHANISMS AVAILABLE TO THE CPA

The basic unit involved in motor control is the coordinative structure first put forward in speech by Action Theory (Fowler, 1980). Coordinative structures are hierarchically nested groupings of the musculature, and are characterized by their internal ability to allow low level messaging between muscles in the group without reference to higher control. The coordinative structure is able to learn certain configurations of its member muscles and the messaging that determines their temporal behavior. Equations of constraint determine the interplay between muscles that, via the messaging system, maintains stability of gestures (coordinated movement in time) and improves their robustness in the face of external constraints.

Control of a coordinative structure is initiated centrally, but expanded locally by the knowledge embodied in the structure's equations of constraint. Knowledge beyond some basic biological behavior has to be acquired as the child learns language such that much of the detail of the behavior of the vocal tract for utterances is derived at this low level. As learning continues gradually acquired low level specifications take over from complete central specification. This approach contrasts sharply with simple coarticulation theory, which postulated that target specifications for a string of speech sounds were worked out cognitively and then issued to the musculature as a set of commands every time the segment was required. Not only would such a system be very complex, it would also fail to show how speakers readily adapt to environmental constraints like the changing direction of the gravitational force as the head is tilted during an utterance, or a sudden increase in background noise, or the need to speak faster or slower.

Central to the working of coordinative structures is the low level gamma loop feedback system (Matthews, 1964), and it is the gamma circuits that stabilize movement. Efferent signals originating in the motor cortex are available to the gamma system and are used effectively to set the bias of particular behavior—it is this property of the motor control system that enables CPA supervision in the way postulated by cognitive phonetics. Action theory used gamma efferent signals to tune the system, but cognitive phonetics employs this tuning mechanism on a dynamic on-going basis to continuously adjust for coarticulatory effects, constraining or enhancing them as needed.

THE UTTERANCE PLAN AND ITS REPRESENTATION

As the concept of the utterance plan is central to cognitive phonetics, we now ask, aside from the generalizations used on static models of speaking, whether there is a cognitively based plan for an *instance* of speech. And if so, how is this plan represented?

The plan is the output representation of the set of phonological processes. This set of processes is modeled in a *static* phonology that simultaneously characterizes *all* the possibilities for a language, and in a *dynamic* phonology as a subset detailing the processes underlying the instantiation of a particular utterance. As such, the plan's representation reflects phonology in the sense that it consists of a string of phonological objects appropriately wrapped with prosodic and expressive layers. The final derived objects in phonology are extrinsic allophones: these represent potential sound or articulatory targets and embody all the information required for a successful rendering of the plan into sound and its subsequent decoding in the listener. The information is linguistic and may reflect contrastive requirements (e.g., this vowel vs. that vowel) derived from underlying modeling of morpheme structure (basic phonemes) or idiosyncratic noncontrastive requirements (two different /l/ targets, for example, in English in words like *leaf* vs. *feel*).

The CPA intervention can optimize or extend the inventory of cognitive objects available for use in a language.

1. The inventory of a language's extrinsic allophonic objects (objects used to specify the utterance plan) must by definition exclude objects unable to be physically rendered under ideal conditions. That is, the inventory consists of extrinsic allophones able to be rendered with some or minimal supervision.
2. The system that sets up the inventory must have access to a model able to predict extrinsic allophones and the degree of supervision they will need when rendered. So, for example, knowing about the aerodynamics of controlling sudden air outflow following a plosive release enables the system to postulate several possible allophones of a plosive by noting that stable objects can be created from the coarticulatory process by CPA intervention. So, we can have prevoiced [b] (the vocal cords start way before the [b] is released), or somewhat prevoiced [b] (the vocal cords start a little before [b] release), or regular [b] (the vocal cords start just after [b] release), or somewhat aspirated [p] or "normally" (minimally

supervised) aspirated [p], or [p] with enhanced aspiration, or [p] with very enhanced aspiration. These are stable at normal rates of delivery and at a useful range of rates from slow to very fast and within a useful range of loudness or overall airflow. Once the perceptual thresholds for these various objects are known (the predictive perceptual model) unusable objects can be filtered out to leave the useful ones. In this way a language builds up additional segments to include phonological objects not possible without CPA intervention.

SUPERVISION

Supervision uses CPA intervention as its mechanism for controlling the precision of utterances. Ongoing adjustment of articulation at the muscular and coordinative structure levels is crucial to cognitive phonetics.

Speech gestures are produced in response to an utterance plan, specifying how an utterance is *intended* to be. As such, it derives from high level abstract "sound" objects designed to keep words separate to avoid confusion of meaning (called phonemes in classical phonetics) and lower level abstract sound objects that reflect phonological pressures such as assimilation (the cognitively based tendency for one of these abstract objects to succumb to contextual effects from its neighbors), idiosyncratic pressures due to pronunciation niceties specific to the language (such as the use of two different /l/ sounds in English)—*all designed to facilitate perception*. These variants are the extrinsic allophones to be used in utterance instantiation.

Coarticulatory constraints occurring after the plan has been assembled and environmental constraints, such as noise levels impinging on the acoustic signal, or even physical effects detracting from ideal articulation, such as a sore throat, tend to degrade the acoustic signal—ultimately making it, if severe enough, unintelligible to the listener. Listeners regularly repair some damage to the signal, but the effect is limited. However, observations of the acoustic signal show that it varies continuously with respect to its *precision* (Charles-Luce, Dressler, & Ragonese, 1999; Tatham & Morton, 1980). Precision is the degree to which the signal, for a specific period of time, matches some idealized physical signal corresponding to the abstract plan. Moreover this variation in precision is systematic: it correlates well with listeners' perceptual difficulties, which themselves vary continuously.

Thus, coarticulation is universal, but its extent or degree on many occasions is not universal. We can vary the degree of coarticulation by limiting or enhancing the effect. Constraint and enhancement has been found to be systematic and stable enough that "new" sounds can be created for use by a language's phonology.

Examples:

1. Unconstrained, an alveolar fricative might take an average tongue position varying broadly around [s] and [ʃ], and this works for a phonology requiring just one fricative in this area (e.g.. Greek, Spanish), but not for

one requiring two (e.g., French, English) in the *same* area. Here, precision of articulation must be tightened, or its variability constrained, to ensure that perceptual confusion is minimized.

2. An example of coarticulation enhancement occurs in languages that manipulate the aerodynamic coarticulatory effect of VOT for the purposes of increasing the phonological inventory to include more plosive consonants. Such a language is Hindi (Ladefoged & Maddieson, 1996).

3. An example of constraining the same VOT aerodynamic coarticulatory effect occurs in a number of languages that need to specify the *supervision* of vocal cord vibration in voiced stops that would otherwise "lose" their target voiced specification; English is an example since VOT occurs only in a constrained way following /b, d, g/. Constraint is necessary to avoid perceptual confusion with /p, t, k/. French extends this supervision to minimise VOT in voiceless stops and preserve vocal cord vibration more fully in voiced stops and fricatives. Loss of target voice specification is enhanced in German and Russian where we find, respectively, *bund* with final /t/, and *хлеб* (transliterated as *khljeb*) with final /p/; examples of a coarticulatory effect so consistently able to be supervised as to attain full phonological status of planned extrinsic allophone (Morton & Tatham, 1980), rather than unplanned intrinsic (coarticulated) allophones in other languages.

PRODUCTION FOR PERCEPTION

Cognitive Phonetics introduces the idea that speech production is a managed process; it is supervised toward a particular goal—that of *optimal perception* (Nooteboom, 1983; Tatham, 1970). Optimal perception does not mean perfect perception; it means perception that works satisfactorily for both speaker and listener. Supervision involves CPA intervention to achieve better precision when the speaker predicts potential failure of the perceptual repair mechanism in dealing with signal error. Actual dynamic speech production is not driven solely by what a speaker wants to say and how they want to say it (speaker plans of utterances and expressive content for those utterances), but also by how well it is *predicted* the overall communication system will behave *at any one moment*. Speech production in this theory incorporates a running predictive model of the environment and its constraints and also of the perceptual process and its constraints.

CPA INTERVENTION

For CPA supervision of the articulatory rendering of the utterance plan the mechanism of cognitive intervention requires:

1. a predictive model of production robustness and sources of error; and
2. a predictive model of perception robustness and sources of error.

Both of these models need to be static to capture the overall general case of supervision, and dynamic to capture the current rendering within a continuously varying context of constraints external to the utterance plan (Tatham & Morton, 2006). The principle of supervision goes beyond any simple mechanism of intervention because it is organized in the *context* of speech production, and is itself continuously variable. Supervision depends on the current situation, and the actual degree of intervention necessary cannot be wholly determined in advance since every utterance instantiation is different. A set of continuously varying parameters interact in an ever changing way to determine locally the current instantiation and how it is constrained.

For example, in pulling in information on the current physical performance of the production process, supervision employs all three major possibilities for feedback (slow auditory, medium speed tactile and fast intramuscular). Locally, coordinative structures are able to be set or tuned to tighten or relax the behavioral precision of an entire group or nested group of muscles in the structure. It is in this way that supervision allows rapid response to changes in mood during conversation, and so on.

Perception

The theory of speech perception addresses the general question: What cognitive processing is involved in interpreting the soundwave the listener is hearing (Pardo & Remez, 2006)?

It is widely felt that once the analyzed physical auditory signals cross to the cognitive domain a number of processes are involved in their interpretation. What must be remembered is that the "meaning" of the utterance is not directly encoded in the acoustic signal: it is pointless to attempt to find linguistic/cognitive objects like phonemes in the signal. They could not exist *in* an acoustic waveform because, of course, they are abstractions. Phonemes and all linguistic units are symbolic objects existing in the linguist's model and, it is hypothesized, perhaps have some psychological reality in the speaker/listener.

The task of perceptual interpretation of the incoming signal is to *assign* to it (not *find* within it) a symbolic representation that will ultimately enable the listener to be aware of the speaker's intended utterance. Various proposals have been made as to how this might be done. These include identification of the incoming signal by consulting a dictionary memory of signals heard in the past, so that the signal can be found and identified.

All such lookup table procedures fail partly because of the theoretically infinite possibilities of the acoustic signal in representing *any* utterance (so the template knowledge base would have to be vast or categorized in some way, and a means of data reduction would have to be found that did not label each incoming signal as unique), and partly because of the near certainty that the incoming acoustic has been degraded in some way. It is easily observed that the signal can be *repaired* by the listener to some meaningful and less degraded version, and that the repair of *identical* signals is often different for different languages or even accents of the same language.

The data that needs to be explained by a theory of perception includes the listener's ability to repair damaged signals, and recover, by assignment, a symbolic representation associated with the speaker's intentions. The recovered symbolic representation matches the speaker's utterance plan, and is an idealized or error free representation of the original intention. In addition, listeners usually realize when they have made an assignment error, then go back and reinterpret a buffered version of the original signal (Hartsuiker, Pickering, & deJong, 2005).

The listener is in effect not interpreting the original signal but a version of that signal recovered from memory—as such the recovered version has no error, is stable, and has no variability. Prosodic and expressive interpretation proceeds along the same lines. This is why listeners are unaware of variants below the extrinsic allophonic level—*they are no longer there: the listener is perceiving their own* reconstructed *version of the signal.*

THEORIES OF PERCEPTION

Theories of perception within the domain of speech production/perception fall basically into two major types: passive and active.

1. Passive theories involve no, or very little, interpretation. The hypothesis here is that there is sufficient information within the signal to enable perception to proceed without active addition of information by the listener. The general theory is called Direct Perception (Gibson, 1954), and the main theory within speech is called Direct Realism (Fowler, 1986).

   The main argument against passive theories is their inability to explain the contextually dependent variation in meaning of identical signals even within a single language.
2. Active theories involve varying degrees of interpretation of the signal. To do this the listener must include:
   a. knowledge of the special nature of the speech signal required [explains the ability to affirm: *I know this is human speech*];
   b. a model of how speech is produced [explains: The *speaker said 'X'*].

Minimally active theories include the Motor Theory of Speech Perception (Cooper, 1966) and the Revised Motor Theory (Liberman & Mattingly, 1985), and the Analysis by Synthesis Theory (Stevens & Halle, 1967).

Fully active theories must include:

a. A means of hypothesising that a production or transmission error has occurred [explains: *His speech is not coming out right or There's too much noise, I can't quite hear*].
b. A means of recovery and reconstruction of the intended signal underlying any degraded version reaching the listeners ears [explains: *He must have meant "X"*].

c. A means of accessing a stored idealized signal to replace the actual heard signal, thereby removing errors [explains: *I know he said "X,"*] when analysis of the acoustic signals shows that X is not exactly what it looks like.

d. A means of buffering and reiterating the error repair process to cope with realization that a repair error has occurred.

Among the more active theories able to detect and repair errors of production or transmission degradation is the Associative Store Theory (incorporated within cognitive phonetics), which proposes a mechanism for dynamic matching of a defective incoming signal with the inventory of symbolic representations (Tatham & Morton, 2006).

QUESTIONS FOR THE MODEL OF PERCEPTION

Contemporary models of speech perception need to address a number of critical questions.

1. Is perception a mirror image of production? Perception seems to depend on the listener's having reference to some model of speech production to be able to anticipate what the speaker is doing. For us, it seems clear that to linguistically interpret the representation assigned to a cognitive version of the incoming acoustic signal, the listener must have reference to a static phonological model capable in principle of characterizing all possible utterances in the language at all the segmental and prosodic/ expressive levels.

2. Is the recovered signal represented as a reconstruction of the speaker's plan—a plan the perceiver could have if they were the speaker? This would make an active mirroring of the speaker an essential part of the general perceptual process.

3. What is the role of the perceiver's own production phonology in this reconstruction? Evidence from mis-hearing, say, of a foreign accent: *If I myself had made this sound I would be trying to make "X."*

4. What is the precise nature of the representation in the listener's mind?
   a. Is the representation expressed in phonological terms; that is, does it match the production phonology?
   b. Is the representation segmental rather than continuous? At an abstract cognitive level the representation only makes sense if it is segmental. A continuous representation would have all representations different, technically, an infinity of representations would be possible. The representation must take a "reduced" symbolic form, a form devoid of nonlinguistic variability.
   c. Cognitive phonetics suggests a continuity between segment and prosody. Standard models *add* prosody, whereas cognitive phonetics *wraps* the segment string in a hierarchical arrangement:

    i   the plan's prosodic environment—wraps the segmental plan;

    ii   the plan's expressive environment—wraps the prosody.

For a full explanation of the wrapper format for the model that relates the components formally, see Morton & Tatham, 2006.

    d.   The representation is wrapped in much the same way as the production process(es).

        i.   Is there a recovery hierarchy mirroring the production wrapper layers?

        ii.   The perceptual system actively assigns expression, prosody, and segmental elements. If these form a wrapped package, then we presume that the unwrapping would show a hierarchical perceptual strategy—expression first (because tone of voice can sometimes be perceived before the actual words), segments last because they are perceived within the expression (and production-wise are the most wrapped, least deep, elements).

The wrapper format for the *dynamic* model is diagrammed in Figure 14.2.

VARIABILITY

In any theory of speech it is necessary to account for variability in production and how it is dealt with in perception. Some variability occurs deliberately, as with essential variant phonemes to distinguish words (e.g., *cat* /kæt/ vs. *cap* /kæp/), some occurs deliberately, as with nonessential extrinsic variant allophones (e.g., *leaf* /ljif/ vs. *feel* /filw/, palatalized and velarized /l/s, respectively), and some occur mostly involuntarily (e.g., *lad* /læd°/, devoiced /d/), symbolically, intrinsic allophones.

Types of Variability

Early researchers working with classical phonetic recognized variability in speech. They were particularly concerned with allophonic variants of phonemes and their descriptions often noted contextual variations due to assimilation. Variation arises under the influence of linearly juxtaposed phonemes in their model. The picture was confused however until two types of allophonic variability were modeled:

    1.   *extrinsic allophones,* which are derived deliberately in cognitively based phonological processing for inclusion in the utterance plan; and

    2.   *intrinsic allophones,* which are derived largely involuntarily during physical phonetic rendering of the plan (Tatham, 1971; Wang & Fillmore, 1961).

The plan's extrinsic allophones can become, according to coarticulation theory, seriously degraded as a result of time constraints on mechanical and aerodynamic processes, and perhaps also on some neurophysiological processes. Even the mood of speakers can distort their physiology to cause changes in the acoustic signal; this occurs for example in the tenseness associated with extreme anger.

Expressive features, both emotive and linguistic, dominate the rendering of the intended segmental pattern of the utterance as set out in the utterance plan (see the diagram above). These features are said to wrap the utterance and influence it prosodically for the most part using variations in timing or rhythm, intonation and stress.

A final type of variability is quite simply randomness, noise or jitter in the physical system. The degree of variability here can be quite wide, but within certain limits does not interfere with the perceptual system's recovery procedures too badly. By definition the idealized abstract cognitive objects of phonology in either production or perception cannot exhibit random variability: variability of this type belongs strictly to the physical world.

It is important to note that speakers and listeners are only aware in any linguistic sense of the symbolic representations in terms of extrinsic allophones and phonemes. The system pivots on the speaker's extrinsic allophonic utterance plan and on the perceiver's recovered interpretation. Neither speakers nor listeners are aware of intrinsic allophones (unless enhanced or constrained—in which case they have achieved extrinsic allophonic status), nor of any variability due to jitter in the system. The listener's recovery process, within its limitations, is so robust and efficient that it almost completely negates any awareness of error, unless it is gross.

CONTROL OF VARIABILITY

Variability in rendering the utterance plan is principally controlled by manipulating precision (Charles-Luce et al., 1999; Tatham & Morton, 1980). Clearly people can control the precision of their articulations, and do so often without knowing that anything has altered. Regularly what is involved is a change in delivery tempo: a decrease eases degradation due to time constrained coarticulatory effects. Tightening up on target specifications further attempts to deliver near ideal articulations. Supervision of articulation control is intensified based on local fast intramuscular feedback and reference to the original intended target (see Figure 14.3).

The required degree of precision can clearly vary. Many factors including local phonological contrast (Did you say "sea" or "she"?), environmental constraints such as a noisy channel (a bad phone circuit or high ambient noise), social constraints (the feeling that we need to speak more carefully to nonnative speakers or listeners perceived to be less intelligent than ourselves). Thus variation of precision can have an effect on a whole conversation and can change from syllable to syllable.

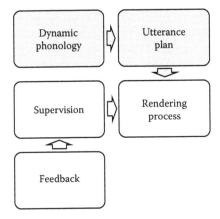

FIGURE 14.3 Diagram showing how feedback from production is one input to supervision of the rendering process. Supervision also benefits from access to the underlying utterance plan.

APPLICATIONS MODELING

Applications models can be thought of as models that can be put to practical use in addressing particular problems. They are derived from more general underlying theories and models in the relevant disciplines, and arise in response to the need to solve problems in special instances. No underlying comprehensive *integrated* speech production/perception model has been developed (Fowler & Galantucci, 2005; Tatham & Morton, 2006). Practitioners are therefore faced with the necessity to develop sections of an incomplete but idealized integrated speech production/perception model.

Language production and perception (including the subset of speech production/perception) is described according to principles operating in two different domains: cognitive and physical (Tatham & Morton, 2006). Applications models can draw on research in these two domains, the cognitive including linguistics (semantics, syntax, phonology) and cognitive psychology, and the physical including physiology (neuromuscular movement, the hearing system) and the anatomically oriented parts of classical phonetics. In addition, some models cross domain boundaries: cognitive phonetics, auditory scene analysis (Bregman, 1990) and some phonology/phonetic modeling.

The *medium of transmission of* ideas and feelings—the speech waveform—is relevant to language/speech disorders since it is the physical event associated with the end product of speaking. The waveform provides the acoustic features that trigger perceptual interpretation.

PRODUCTION AND PERCEPTION

We speak in order to be listened to and understood. It is therefore reasonable to expect that an awareness of the listener is important to the speaker (see p. 303,

Production for Perception). Applications models might include such a concept to take account of some variability in disordered speech that might be because of modifying what can be produced to take account of the listener. Here some variability may be introduced by the emotive stance of the speaker and their attitude toward the person they are speaking to, or to what that person has to say—part of the general social context. Speaking to a friend may result in different characteristics from speaking to a therapist. The range of variability allowed is limited (see p. 307, Variability), and the model builder should ideally take this into account.

Much applications work is not explicitly theory bound, but based on empirically derived hypotheses. In such cases feedback from observation, together with formal empirical procedures, can provide evidence for claims made by the underlying disciplines (see Tatham & Morton, 2006).

CLASSICAL PHONETICS AND APPLICATIONS

Phonetic descriptions based on classical phonetics:

- provide linear descriptions of someone's speech, usually based on the IPA transcription system in combination with the subjective interpretation of the labeller; idealization in the subjective approach confines this to static modeling—dynamic variability is seldom considered;
- enable inferences about the listener's phonological perceptions; and
- allow annotation of departures from expected norms of speech— suggesting possible disorders.

We have suggested a possible format for applications models based on classical phonetics (Tatham & Morton, 2006).

COGNITIVE PHONETICS AND APPLICATIONS

In addition to the descriptions provided by classical phonetics, cognitive phonetics addresses

- The requirement for linking underlying linguistic events (the phonology, including the prosodic features of rhythm, intonation and stress) to descriptions of the waveform. It puts speech processes into a larger language framework, incorporating the derived utterance plan—the intended linguistic shape for the final utterance prior to phonetic rendering.
- The relationship between cognitive and physical phenomena in an active way within a dynamic model through the pivotal mechanism of the utterance plan.
- Variability as a cognitive influence on the waveform, taking into account expressive and emotive effects.

- A focus for the model based on the listener through the principle of "production for perception."
- The listener's ability to reduce variability to meaningful categories by a process of assignment of idealized representations to analyzed waveforms, and by procedures that can repair damage to the intended waveform.
- The need for an integrated speech production and perception model in which errors can be more precisely specified than they can using the classical phonetics model's surface and linear descriptions.

CONCLUSION

In this chapter we have contrasted two distinct theories of speech: classical phonetics and cognitive phonetics. Classical phonetics remains useful as a means of describing subjective observations about articulation and listeners' reactions to the resultant soundwave. Classical phonetics also brought us a comprehensive symbolic representation to record these observations in alphabetic form. Classical phonetics is, however, a strictly linear approach to what we now understand to be a highly complex hierarchically organized system. Consequently it fails to explain the surface observations it seeks to characterize.

Cognitive phonetics is typical of a more rigorous contemporary approach to speech production and perception as exemplified by Keating (1990, 2006). It recognizes the hierarchical structure of language and attempts to model the relationship between cognitive and physical processes in speech production and perception. This model also relates earlier attempts to characterize language in a static way to capture generalizations optimally and a more dynamic modeling that can relate individual instantiations to the underlying generality. This last property seems to increase the usefulness of the model in applications, but also in attempting to answer interdisciplinary questions.

The rigorous computational format of cognitive phonetics (Tatham & Morton, 2005) draws out gaps in the theory leading straight to hypotheses for guiding future thought and experimental work.

REFERENCES

Abercrombie, D. (1967). *Elements of general phonetics*. Edinburgh, Scotland: Edinburgh University Press.

Baer, T., Gore, J. C., Gracco, L. C., & Nye, P. W. (1991). Analysis of vocal tract shape and dimensions using magnetic resonance imaging: Vowels. *Journal of the Acoustical Society of America, 90,* 799–828.

Bregman, A. S. (1990). *Auditory scene analysis*. Cambridge, MA: MIT Press.

Charles-Luce, J., Dressler, K., & Ragonese, E. (1999). Effect of semantic predictability on children's preservation of a phonemic contrast. *Journal of Child Language, 26,* 505–530.

Cooper, F. (1966). Describing the speech process in motor command terms. *Status reports on speech research*. Haskins Laboratories, SR 515, 2.1–2.7.

Cruttenden, A. (2001). *Gimson's pronunciation of English*. London, UK: Hodder Arnold.

Fant, G. (1960). *Acoustic theory of speech production*. The Hague, The Netherlands: Mouton.

Fowler, C. (1980). Coarticulation and theories of extrinsic timing. *Journal of Phonetics, 8*, 113–133.

Fowler, C. (1986). An event approach to the study of speech perception from a direct-realist perspective. *Journal of Phonetics, 14*, 3–28.

Fowler, C., & Galantucci, B. (2005). The relation of speech perception and production. In D. B. Pisoni & R. Remez (Eds.), *The handbook of speech perception* (pp. 633–652). Oxford, UK: Blackwell.

Garland, A., & Alterman, R. (2004). Autonomous agents that learn to better coordinate. *Autonomous Agents and Multi-Agent Systems, 8*(3), 267–301.

Gibson, J. (1954). A theory of pictorial perception. *Audio Visual Communication Review, 1*, 3–23.

Hardcastle, W., & Hewlett, N. (Eds.). (1999). *Coarticulation: Theory, data, and techniques*. Cambridge, UK: Cambridge University Press.

Hartsuiker, R., Pickering, M., & deJong, N. (2005). Semantic and phonological context effects in speech error repair. *Journal of Experimental Psychology: Learning, Memory and Cognition, 31*(5), 921–932.

Higgins, M., Netsell, R., & Schulte, L. (1998). Vowel-related differences in laryngeal articulatory and phonatory function. *Journal of Speech, Language and Hearing Research, 41*, 712–724.

Keating, P. (1990). The window model of coarticulation: Articulatory evidence. In J. Kingston & M. Beckman (Eds.), *Papers in laboratory phonology I* (pp. 451–470). Cambridge, UK: Cambridge University Press.

Keating, P. (2006). Phonetic encoding of prosodic structure. In J. Harrington & M. Tabain (Eds.), *Speech production: Models, phonetic processes, and techniques* (pp. 167–186). Macquarie Monographs in Cognitive Science. New York, NY and Hove, UK: Psychology Press.

Ladefoged, P., & Maddieson, I. (1996). *Sounds of the world's languages*. Oxford, UK: Blackwell.

Liberman, A., & Mattingly, I. (1985). The motor theory of speech perception revised. *Cognition, 21*, 1–36.

Lisker, L., & Abramson, A. (1964). A cross-language study of voicing in initial stops: Acoustical measurements. *Word, 20*, 384–422.

MacNeilage, P. (1970). Motor control of serial ordering of speech. *Psychological Review, 77*, 182–196.

MacNeilage, P., & De Clerk, J. (1969). On the motor control of coarticulation in CVC monosyllables. *Journal of the Acoustical Society of America, 45*, 1217–1233.

Matthews, P. (1964). Muscle spindles and their motor control. *Physiological Review, 44*, 219–288.

Matthies, M., Perrier, P., Perkell, J., & Zandipour, M. (2001). Variation in coarticulation with changes in clarity and rate. *Journal of Speech, Language and Hearing Research, 44*, 552–563.

Morton, K., & Tatham, M. (1980). Production instructions. *Occasional papers 23* (pp. 14–16). Colchester, UK: University of Essex.

Nooteboom, S. (1983). Is speech production controlled by speech perception? In M. van den Broecke, V. van Heuven, & W. Zonneveld (Eds.), *Studies for Antonie Cohen. Sound structures* (pp. 183–194). Dordrecht, The Netherlands: Foris Publications.

Pardo, J. S., & Remez, R. E. (2006). The perception of speech. In M. Traxler & M. A. Gernsbacher (Eds.), *Handbook of psycholinguistics* (2nd ed., pp. 201–248). New York, NY: Academic Press.

Rubin, P., & Vatkiotis-Bateson, E. (1998). Measuring and modelling speech production. In S. L. Hopp, M. J. Owren, & C. S. Evans (Eds.), *Animal acoustic communication* (pp. 251–290). New York, NY: Springer-Verlag.

Stevens, K., & Halle, M. (1967). Remarks on analysis by synthesis and distinctive features. In W. Wathen-Dunn (Ed.), *Models for the perception of speech and visual form* (pp. 88–102). Cambridge, MA: MIT Press.

Tatham, M. (1970). Coarticulation and phonetic competence. *Occasional papers 8.* Colchester, UK: University of Essex.

Tatham, M. (1971). Classifying allophones. *Language and Speech, 14,* 140–145.

Tatham, M. (1984). Towards a cognitive phonetics. *Journal of Phonetics, 12*(11), 37–47.

Tatham, M. (1990). Cognitive phonetics. In W. Ainsworth (Ed.), *Advances in speech, hearing and language processing 1* (pp. 193–218). London, UK: JAI Press.

Tatham, M. (1995). The supervision of speech production. In C. Sorin, J. Mariani, H. Meloni, & J. Schoentgen (Eds.), *Levels in speech communication: Relations and interactions* (pp. 115–125). Amsterdam, The Netherlands: Elsevier.

Tatham, M., & Morton K. (1980). Precision. *Occasional papers 23* (pp. 104–113). Colchester, UK: University of Essex.

Tatham, M., & Morton, K. (2002). Computational modelling of speech production: English rhythm. In A. Braun & H. Masthoff (Eds.), *Phonetics and its applications: Festschrift for Jens-Peter Köster on the occasion of his 60th birthday* (pp. 383–405). Stuttgart, Germany: Franz Steiner Verlag.

Tatham, M., & Morton, K. (2005). *Developments in speech synthesis.* Chichester, UK: Wiley & Sons.

Tatham, M., & Morton, K. (2006). *Speech production and perception.* Basingstoke, UK: Palgrave Macmillan.

Wang, W., & Fillmore, C. (1961). Intrinsic cues and consonant perception. *Journal of Speech and Hearing Research, 4,* 130–136.

15 Psycholinguistic Validity and Phonological Representation

Ben Rutter and Martin J. Ball

INTRODUCTION

Psycholinguistic theories have had a number of important insights for speech–language pathologists. Models of speech production and perception have added to the ways in which researchers and clinicians can conceptualize, analyze, and treat a multitude of speech and language disorders. Linguistic models rationalized using psychological or cognitive principles, often based on experimental findings, are appealing because they offer the potential for both explanatory as well as descriptive adequacy (Stackhouse & Wells, 1997). On the other hand, the application of theoretical ideas from strictly descriptive linguistic theories has not always been able to claim such explanatory power. Rather, theories from generative approaches to syntax or phonology, for example, have often provided new and interesting ways to visualize and label clinical data, but any explanation is often heavily couched in theory internal principles.

In this chapter we explore the concept of abstract phonological representations, the kind discussed in most mainstream phonological theories ranging from the seminal work in generative grammar (Chomsky & Halle, 1968), autosegmental phonology (Goldsmith, 1976, 1990), and more recent generative phonology (Kenstowicz, 1994). We consider the justification for positing highly abstract, single-entry mental representations for lexical items and evaluate the extent to which they have any potential explanatory power for the analysis of disordered speech. We suggest that, like many imports from purely descriptive linguistic theories, abstract phonological representations should not be conflated with genuine attempts to model speech processing and performance. While they are no doubt useful tools for analyzing clinical linguistic data, and perhaps uncovering sound patterns that lie within, their explanatory power for the clinician may in fact be extremely weak. We speculate that the reason lies in the fact that mainstream phonological theories have long concerned themselves purely with linguistic competence, whereas clinical linguists and speech–language pathologists are interested first and foremost in speech performance. What's more, many of the concepts found in phonological theories often take on a slightly different meaning when applied in speech pathology. Our conclusion, however, looks

313

to the possibilities for the future and the development of a more far reaching application of multiple entry, phonetically rich mental representations of lexical items, as suggested by exemplar theory, and the work of Bybee (2001). We predict that, like Ball (2003) and Sosa and Bybee (2007), clinical applications of such a phonological theory may have much to offer the clinical arena.

The structure of the chapter is as follows. We begin with a brief outline of clinical phonology, focusing on its aims as a discipline. We argue that if clinical phonology is to be anything more than an exercise in describing clinical data using a set of terms, labels, and diagrams borrowed from mainstream phonology, it must offer the clinician at least some objective explanatory power and some insight into remediation. With this in mind, the third section provides a brief tour of the various definitions of a phonological representation, in both descriptive linguistics and speech pathology. We then trace the gradual evolution of the phonological representation, including the conception of the phoneme, distinctive feature, and the autosegment and then outline a more recent approach to phonological representations, that of usage-based phonology. In the fifth section, we suggest that the adoption of usage-based phonology might offer clinical phonology a great deal and we conclude by summarizing our position and looking to the future of clinical phonology.

THE AIM OF CLINICAL PHONOLOGY

Clinical phonology (see, for example, Ball & Kent, 1998; Ball, Müller, & Rutter, 2009; Grunwell, 1987) arose from the revolution of applying linguistic theories, usually reserved for the formulation of grammars based on the analysis of normal speakers alone, to clinical data. As with clinical linguistics in general, clinical phonology is usually cited as having two main aims (see, for example, the preface of Ball et al., 2009). Firstly, informing the assessment and treatment techniques of the clinician, and, secondly, the testing of the linguistic theories themselves using novel and challenging types of data (so called talking back to theory). Therefore, clinical phonology, as opposed to many branches of purely descriptive phonology, primarily takes as its aim the analysis of the speech *performance* of individuals. Descriptive phonology, on the other hand, is the business of analyzing the various systems and patterns of sounds found in specific languages. While these two pursuits clearly have similarities, not least the fact that a speech disorder is defined according to the characteristics of a specific language, their differences should not be overlooked (Ball & Müller, 2002). For example, clinical linguists are typically interested in describing, and then possibly accounting for, the difference between a client's speech output and the expected speech output of a normal speaker. Descriptive linguists are, on the whole, concerned with the description of entire languages. A consequence of this disparity is that many of the concepts found in descriptive theories have taken on a double meaning in clinical phonology. Kent sums this up particularly well:

> The discipline of linguistics is concerned primarily with the structure of language. The disciplines of psychology and speech pathology are concerned primarily with the processing of language—with its formulation and its reception. The linguistic

study of language structure has influenced the study of language processing, and, to some degree, the reverse is true as well. Descriptions of language processing often use terms, such as syntax, semantics, phonology, and phonetics, that denote traditional areas of linguistic study. These terms have come to have a dual usage, one referring to structure another to processing. (1998, p. 3)

If the above is true, we should always be careful that the concepts we borrow from descriptive linguistics are truly appropriate for the study of speech performance. It might be the case that, in the domain of phonology for instance, techniques devised for the description of data are not necessarily appropriate for describing what speakers actually do. A useful comparison can be drawn with sociolinguistics, which, we would argue, has experienced a similar such tension. Sociolinguists are generally concerned with the variability observed in speech when individuals engage in functional communication. This variability is often related to factors other than lexical meaning; social variables such as age, class, and gender, for example. Because phonology is concerned solely with lexically significant details, many of the theoretical ideas that abound in mainstream phonology are inapplicable to the study of sociolinguistic variation. Unsurprisingly, sociolinguists have not always found the theoretical ideas of descriptive linguistics to be particularly revealing for their interests, and Kerswell and Shockey (2007) describe the phonology–sociolinguistics interface specifically as an "uneasy coexistence" (p. 52).

Unless clinical linguists are to occupy themselves with purely lexically contrastive material in the speech signal, they too must consider whether abstractionist phonological theories are suitable for describing disordered speech data. Our aim in this chapter is to explore this issue by asking whether abstract, single-entry phonological representations can be considered a psycholinguistically valid concept. More specifically, we propose the following questions: what do the abstract phonological representations of traditional (i.e., generative) theories of phonology denote? Put simply, what are phonological representations? And, likewise, do they represent the same thing in the parlance of descriptive linguistics as in clinical phonology?

The extent to which these questions are answered by researchers is often limited, particularly in applied fields such as child language acquisition and speech pathology, where the phonemic principle* is often taken as a given. However, we will argue that researchers and speech–language pathologists must take seriously the possibility that the foundations on which many of the assumptions we make about speech disorders are based not on psychological reality but in fact on early attempts to simplify transcription methods.

WHAT ARE PHONOLOGICAL REPRESENTATIONS? WHAT DO THEY REPRESENT?

The phonetics–phonology distinction is perhaps the most widely discussed of the linguistic interfaces and is a division that is far from fixed. Defining the distinction

---

* At its simplest, the notion that two distinct levels of representation can be identified, one being concrete or phonetic, the other being abstract or phonological.

is no easy task, but it seems generally agreed upon that a characterization using the notion of levels is essential. This is routinely adopted in textbook definitions of the distinction. Giegerich (1992, p. 31) provides a particularly good definition of the classical phonetics–phonology interface when he states that "[A] phonological analysis entails two levels of representation—a concrete (phonetic) one and an abstract (underlying) one—as well as statements on how the units on one level are connected with corresponding units on the other level."

While this definition is not a comprehensive one, and such a definition would be impossible to find, it is successful in identifying the two critical characteristics of the phonetics–phonology distinction; levels and abstraction.* The notion of levels, and importantly of abstraction, is likely to feature in most, if not all, definitions of the interface. The need for abstraction is argued by citing the vast phonetic variability observable in speech performance. With the same lexeme exhibiting the potential to be produced in multiple ways, it is often suggested that an abstract level of representation is needed to avoid encoding a potentially infinite degree of variability in storage. Therefore, phonological representations employ a finite number of phonological primes with which the lexical representations of words can be written out. The primes are symbolic, as they "stand for" a set of (potentially) infinite phonetic realizations along a continuum.

Therefore, phonology recognizes abstract categories that comprise phonetically distinct but functionally equivalent places along a phonetic continuum. Cohn (2006) uses this as the basis for a schema of the phonetics–phonology distinction (see Figure 15.1).

The notion of levels, of a hierarchical ordering, of representations very much suggests a relationship between this distinction and some physical correlate, be it cognitive or neurological. The history of such a distinction, however, does not have its roots in attempts at psycholinguistic validity or even models of articulatory planning. Rather, the phonetics–phonology distinction can, and probably should, be seen as originating from different approaches to the transcription of speech. This is suggested in the *Handbook of the International Phonetic Association* (1999) itself:

> The International Phonetic Association has aimed to provide "a separate sign for each distinctive sound; that is, for each sound which, being used instead of another, in the same language, can change the meaning of a word." This notion of a "distinctive sound" is what became widely known in the twentieth century as the phoneme. (p. 27)

The phoneme, then, arose from early attempts to reduce the amount of detail needed in phonetic transcriptions that were only intended to convey the differences between words. Phonetic variation that did not contribute to word meaning was not a desirable feature of such transcriptions. Consequently, two forms of representation speech arose, a phonetic (also called allophonic or narrow)

---

* A third possible element could be added to this list in the form of segmentation and the idea that at the phonological level at least, it is possible to represent speech as a series of discrete segments.

Phonology	=	discrete, categorical
≠		
Phonetics	=	continuous, gradient

FIGURE 15.1   A schema of the phonetics/phonology distinction (Adapted from Cohn, A., *Gradience in grammar: Generative perspectives,* Oxford, UK, Oxford University Press, 25–44, 2006.)

representation, and a phonological (also called phonemic or broad) representation. It was this distinction that led to the phonetics–phonology distinction and to the notion of a phonological representation.

> Historically, the IPA has its roots in a tradition of phonology in which the notions of the phoneme, as a contrastive sound unit, and of allophones, as its variant phonetic realizations, are primary; and in which utterances are seen as the concatenation of the realization of phonemes. The use of an alphabetic notation underlines the conceptualization of speech as a sequence of sounds. (International Phonetic Association, 1999, p. 37)

It has been suggested elsewhere that the concept of a phonological representation not only stems from early transcription practices, but that it has been unduly influenced by the conventions of written language (see Coleman, 1998, p. 47; Linell, 2005). Regardless, it is very much apparent that phonological representations were initially ways of representing speech on paper and were not intended as mental objects. However, in many circles they seem to have come to mean just that.

THE MENTAL STATUS OF PHONOLOGICAL REPRESENTATIONS

Querying the mental status of phonological representation is at both a challenging and important endeavor. Are phonological representations intended to be mental objects, perhaps templates or scripts for speech organization and production? Are they perceptual targets, strings of abstract units onto which highly variable incoming speech forms are mapped? Or are they merely graphical images that appear on paper in order to help us better understand sets of data? Coleman (1998, p. 11) discusses the relationship between linguistic representations and cognitive representations, and suggests that generative phonological representations can constitute a number of possible things. These include articulatory scripts, mental scripts, or purely theoretical objects; convenient but fictitious.

Perhaps more important for our endeavor is the intended value of phonological representations in speech pathology, and it seems that for speech pathologists the phonological representation denotes something quite different still. It is not uncommon to come across the suggestion that (underlying) phonological representations are in fact something approaching the target, or adult, form of the word a child is attempting to say. For example, Grunwell (1987, p. 171) notes that in a generative approach to disordered phonology "adult pronunciations … form the 'input' to the phonological rules; the 'output' is the child's pronunciation." This is radically different to what underlying representations are in standard generative phonology (Kenstowicz, 1994). Most importantly, underlying forms in generative phonology are abstract whereas surface forms are concrete. Presumably, both underlying and surface forms in Grunwell's model are concrete, differing only in the extent to which they map onto one another. Moreover, if the input to phonological rules in clinical generative phonology are akin to adult forms, then they must be sociolinguistically accurate and include fine phonetic detail. That is, they must exhibit the phonetic detail that the child is being exposed to and attempting to learn, with sociolinguistic variables such as geographical region and socioeconomic status taken into account. As a result, they must be written out in the same way the output is; in allophones. However, because clinical generative phonology adopts the machinery of standard generative phonology the input is written out in phonemes and the output in allophones. Hence, there exists a clear disconnect between the intended usage of rules and representations and their adoption in the clinical realm.

PHONOLOGICAL REPRESENTATIONS IN THE TWENTIETH CENTURY

The evolution of the notion of phonological representation over the last three quarters of a century is worth tracing for a number of reasons. Firstly, it demonstrates the somewhat uneasy relationship between phonology and phonetics, and the trend for phonological representations to be firmed up, tying them more closely to something pronounceable. Secondly, it reflects the changing approaches to the study of speech disorders in clinical phonology. As new theoretical approaches have emerged in mainstream phonology, so too has their application in clinical settings.

We start first with the splitting of the phoneme into its composite distinctive features and then discuss the autosegmental revolution of the 1970s.

DISTINCTIVE FEATURES

Chomsky and Halle's seminal work *The Sound Pattern of English* (1968) introduced a number of concepts into the mainstream of phonological theory. Referred to as SPE, the book adopted the two way phonetics–phonology distinction outlined above, but divided phonological segments into so-called distinctive features. These were the properties of the segments that were responsible for differentiating them from other segments. Because distinctive features were based on those properties of a sound that distinguish lexical oppositions, which themselves are based on binary opposition, distinctive features were binary in nature. In terms of lexical distinctiveness, a sound is either voiced or voiceless, for example, in the same way that a word is either "pin" or "bin"; there is no middle ground. Therefore, for a given feature [X] a segment would be specified as either [+ X] or [–X], often displayed as [± X].

Distinctive feature analysis has been adopted in speech pathology, primarily as a means of quantifying speech errors (see discussion and exemplification in Ball et al., 2009). However, there are problems using this approach (see also Grunwell, 1987). For example, errors that seem phonetically closely linked to the target may show a larger number of feature errors than other less closely related due to the limits of a binary, phonological system. Also, there is now a way of showing that a change in features in one direction (e.g., /s/ to [t]) is a frequently occurring error, whereas the opposite (/t/ to [s]) is an unusual error, without resorting to a theory of markedness added on to distinctive feature theory. (Even then markedness conventions may not always reflect patterns found in disordered speech as it is predicated on normal).

AUTOSEGMENTAL REPRESENTATIONS

While the distinctive feature approach to phonological representations reduced the size of the unit of analysis to below the level of the segment, the theory of autosegmental phonology (Goldsmith, 1976) tackled the problem of the "absolute slicing hypothesis;" The notion that, at the phonological level at least, speech should be represented as a series of serially ordered segments. Goldsmith's motivations were initially the treatment of tone languages, but autosegmental analysis was soon expanded to incorporate features such as [nasal] and place features.

Importantly, the approach of using autosegmental *graphs* as a means of phonological representation, be it for normal or disordered speech, leads to a radically different idea as to what constitutes a phonological segment. In autosegmental representations, segments are simply the minimal unit of organization on their respective tiers, and behave *autonomously* (hence the name *auto*segment). What emerges is a picture of phonology quite different to that found in SPE. One with several simultaneous tiers of segments, related to each other through association lines, but ordered independently.

Several researchers have applied the insights from this nonlinear approach to phonology to the analysis of disordered speech [see, for example, Bernhardt (1992a, 1992b), Bernhardt & Gilbert (1992), Dinnsen (1997)]. However, as with classical SPE phonology, it is not clear whether devices such as autosegments and different layers of representation, are simply convenient analytic tools, or are intended to have some kind of psycholinguistic or physical (see Goldsmith's 1976 comment referred to above) reality. Further, studies such as Bernhardt (1992b), demonstrate that it is not straightforward to transfer the nonlinear analysis of a disordered speaker into nonlinear means of therapeutic intervention: the therapy recommended still has to deal with individual sounds or sound classes, it cannot target an abstract nonpronounceable autosegment.

GOVERNMENT PHONOLOGY

A move toward a more phonetically concrete phonology, yet still within the broad bounds of generative linguistics, can be found in Government Phonology (Harris, 1990, 1994; Harris & Lindsey, 1995; Kaye, Lowenstamm, & Vergnaud, 1985, 1990). Government phonology eschews the abstractness of underspecification in generative phonology (e.g., Archangeli, 1988), and requires that its phonological primes, called "elements" (unary and privative rather than the binary, equipollent distinctive features we referred to earlier) all be phonetically realizable (i.e., each element has an actual pronunciation; though it is hard to work out how the laryngeal elements are supposed to be pronounced). The theory allows different governing relations between elements, and these combinations can account for the range of segmental units in a language. Changes in governing relations can illustrate diachronic or synchronic sound changes. For example, lenition can be characterized as the gradual removal of different elements and/or changes in governing relations between elements from one sound to the next lenited sound (e.g., /t/ to /s/; /s/ to /h/, etc.).

In the same way, disordered speech can be characterized as changes in the relations between elements, or changes in the actual elements between the target and the realization. Harris, Watson, and Bates (1999) and Ball (2002) both apply government phonology to disordered vowels systems. For example, a pattern reported with vowel errors (see Ball & Gibbon, 2002) involves the lowering of mid back vowels. This can be seen as a progression from [ɔ] to [ɒ] to [ɑ]. Using government phonology, the first step is characterized as a change in government from **[U]** governing **[A]** to **[A]** governing **[U]**. The final step sees the removal of the **[U]** element altogether, leaving just **[A]** (the pronunciation of which is [ɑ]). (See Ball et al., 2009, for full details of these elements.)

Government phonology is, then, a step away from the abstractness often associated with generative phonology. However, in terms of direct input into remediation, we still have to test the status of the claimed basic elements, and consider how therapy could deal with combining elements into specific governing relations. We also need to recall that this model retains a derivational process from underlying to surface forms—an assumption that has been challenged in recent "cognitive" models of phonology (see below).

OPTIMALITY THEORY

Still within the tradition of generative phonology, recent work on theoretical phonology has centered on constraint-based approaches to phonological description (see Archangeli & Langendoen, 1997; Prince & Smolensky, 1993) within a model of language termed Optimality Theory.

Constraint-based phonology, as the name suggests, has constraints only, and is overtly nonrule-based. By this last point we mean that phonological descriptions do not set out to derive a surface realization from an underlying general phonological description through a set of rules, but rather the relation between the input and the output of the phonology is mediated by the ranking of a set of constraints. The set of phonological constraints is deemed universal, their ranking (and possible violability) is language specific.

Optimality theory operates as follows. GEN, short for generator, takes some underlying form, called the input, and generates a set of possible candidates for its surface form. The candidate set is then evaluated, by EVAL, according to which constraints of the language each candidate violates. Candidates are then ranked according to *relative harmony*. That is, the more higher ranked constraints they violate, the least harmonic they are. The optimal candidate is hence at the top of the relative harmonic ranking, and is said to best fit the constraint ranking of the language in question.

As applied to disordered speech (e.g., Dinnsen & Gierut, 2008), constraints can be reordered to account for the client's differences from the target phonology. The candidate set is presumably held to be the same, but the differences in constraint rankings yield a different optimal candidate. It is unclear whether those working with the clinical applications of OT believe that the input is the same as it would be for a normal speaker of English, and that the difference in constraint ranking yields the different output form; or whether the input for a client is the target form; that is, the output for normal speakers. Dinnsen and Gierut (2008) seem to suggest the latter, but this would be completely altering the way OT is claimed to work.

Again, we are left with the question of whether or not this approach is attempting to model psycholinguistic activities. A leading researcher in the field has answered this question. In addressing the requirement that the GEN component of OT generates an infinite number of possible inputs to the EVAL component, which would seem to disqualify the theory as an actual attempt to model speech production, McCarthy (2002) states clearly that OT does not aim to model the performance of speech production. Therefore, OT does not appear to get us closer to an explanatory model.

GESTURAL PHONOLOGY

Gestural, or articulatory, phonology addresses the problem of phonological organization from a phonetic perspective, and proposes the notion that "phonology is a set of relations among physically real events" (Browman & Goldstein, 1992, p. 156). These real events are called "gestures" in articulatory phonology and constitute the prime of the theory. They are neither feature not segment, but represent "the formation and release of constrictions in the vocal tract" (p. 156). The gesture is distinct from the feature in a number of ways, and yields quite a different approach to phonological analysis from traditional feature-based theories.

Broadly speaking, a gesture is the formation of some degree of constriction at some place in the vocal tract. In this sense, the gesture is substantiated through articulatory activity. Distinctive features, on the other hand, are properties of a segment that are responsible for phonological contrast. They are atemporal and are defined in a "present or absent" manner. Gestural phonology defines gestures according to a series of tract variables. A tract variable defines one element of the formation of a constriction in the vocal tract. The tract variables (lip protrusion, lip aperture, etc.) and the articulators that are involved in conducting them (upper and lower lips, jaw, tongue tip, etc.) are described in Browman and Goldstein (1992, p. 157).

A crucial difference between gestural phonology and feature-based systems is the fact that gestures have internal duration. This allows gestures to vary in how they co-occur. Crucially, it means gestures can overlap not at all, partly, or indeed completely. Gestures will not always align with each other in an absolute fashion and may well overlap. In application to disordered speech (see, for example, Ball, Rutter, & Code, 2008), we can use this facility to show how gestures may be uncoupled from one another (e.g., to show loss of aspiration in stops), gestures can be removed altogether (denasalization), or how one gesture can be removed and a remaining one realigned (e.g., the loss of a nasal stop with concomitant nasalization of the vowel).

Clearly, this approach to phonology is extremely concrete, and should prove useful to clinicians wishing to describe the nature of speech disorders. It does not attempt to provide insights into cognitive processes underlying the disorder, but if coupled with a cognitive approach to phonology it would seem to be potentially of considerable worth.

USAGE-BASED PHONOLOGY

Following the work of Goldinger (1997), Johnson (1997), and Bybee (2001), a model of phonology that can loosely be described as *usage-based* is gradually emerging. Based on the principle that (a) both language use and experience play a significant role in shaping a speaker's knowledge of phonology, and that (b) all experiences of lexical items are stored whole, the theory is very much influenced by, and compatible with, an exemplar account of lexical storage (see Pierrehumbert, 2001). Bybee's book *Phonology and Language Use* (2001) drew together many of the concepts, and subsequent applications have been forthcoming. Bybee's (2001) model claims that mental representations of linguistic objects have the same properties as mental representations of other objects. That is, every instance of a speaker's experience with a word is stored as a fully concrete object, along with the contextual information that came with it. This is radically different from the abstractionist theories above, which are based on single, abstract entries for each lexical item, with only the distinctive information contained in them. In usage-based phonology, the problem of explaining phonetic variability, the original motivation for positing an abstract level of representation, is dealt with through a system of organized storage. Words are stored in a fully specified form, with both fine and coarse phonetic detail, and are associated with the context in which they were encountered.

The application of exemplar theory and "cognitive phonology" to clinical data is still developing, however both Ball (2003) and Sosa and Bybee (2007) have speculated as to what insights this approach to phonological description might have in the clinical arena, and Ball et al. (2009) introduce the basic apparatus of the theory from a clinical perspective adopting Bybee's suggestion of using the formalism of gestural phonology (see above).

CONCLUSION

As discussed in the second section, clinical phonology is a subdiscipline of clinical linguistics that takes as its aim the explanation of speech sound disturbances in such a way as to inform both treatment and linguistic theory. As the developments in phonological theory that are discussed above have come about, their application to clinical data has generally followed. Ball et al. (2009) summarize the application of both generative and nongenerative phonological theories to clinical data and demonstrate the far reaching possibilities for modeling the organization of sound patterns.

By far the most influential phonological model in speech pathology has been generative phonology and a very strict phonetics–phonology separation. This has influenced the study of speech disorders in two important ways. Firstly, it has led to the distinction between a phonetic (or articulatory) disorder and a phonological (or underlying) disorder. A decision as to which of these two problems should be diagnosed is based on analysis of the client's productions. In other words, if a client uses the wrong phonological unit, be it an entire phoneme or some distinctive feature of that phoneme, from the target language, this is deemed to be a phonological error, whereas if a wrong variant of the unit is used, or if a sound from outside the language altogether is employed, this is deemed to be an articulatory (or phonetic) error.

The second major sense in which phonological representations have influenced the description of phonological disorders is through the use of the many theories of phonology in describing various symptoms of, for example, child language production. As suggested above, such accounts run the risk of leading to an explanation of the *cause* of the disorder not being due to any physical—be it motoric or neurological—factor but stemming directly from the principles of the theory. As an example, the use of autosegmental representations to explain, for example, consonant harmony, can lead to an analysis that is driven by the constraints on the graphs of the theory rather than any physiological reason. The cause of the symptom, harmonizing word endings with word beginnings, for example, is explained through positing a violation of the no-crossing constraint rather than a problem with the speech production mechanism.

It is perhaps for this reason that the import of theoretical constructs from descriptive linguistics, often via clinical linguistics, into speech–language pathology has not always brought about any real explanatory success. In phonology specifically, the state of the art has often been used to cast speech disorders in new and interesting ways, explaining them using constraints as opposed to rules, for example, but the real benefit for the therapist has not always been clear. This is summarized well by Locke, when discussing the role of articulation disorders in clinical phonology:

> In Speech-Language Pathology we have a tradition of borrowing from other fields, and I am afraid we also have borrowed this tendency to label instead of explain, and to take our labels as explanations" (Locke, 1983, p. 341).

We do not intend this chapter to be an assault on the enterprise of clinical phonology, for it has offered much to speech–language pathology. However, we think it is important that the concept of a phonological representation of speech, as it is used in a clinical setting, be reviewed and possibly revised. For one, the mental status of phonological representations is questionable to begin with. It is not clear whether they constitute scripts for articulation, targets for incoming percepts, or purely theoretical objects. It seems certain, though, the notion of a phonological representation of speech has its roots in the transcription practices of the early twentieth century, and not any attempt to model motor execution or speech perception. Secondly, phonological representations are often used in clinical phonology to mean something quite different from standard generative phonology; something approaching an adult, or target, form. This would presumably have to be specific in terms of sociophonetic detail, however the underlying representations in clinical phonology are still written in phonemes and in slant brackets, not in fine phonetic detail and in square brackets.

Considering recent developments in nongenerative phonology, it might well be the case that the lexicon comprises multiple phonetic entries for a single lexicon item, with the phonological representation of a word functioning essentially like a lexeme. As exposure to the more phonetic variability increases, a speaker's ability to map incoming forms onto the correct item increases. This is very much the model proposed by exemplar theory (Johnson, 1997) and probabilistic approaches to phonology (Pierrehumbert, 2003). The result would be that the phonological representation of a word is merely the sum of the experienced surface forms. In terms of production, speakers are likely to adapt their own production to something approximating the trace with the highest frequency of occurrence. This would succinctly explain how speakers' productions of words can change over time, both during acquisition, and as part of ongoing language change. It would also account for the gradience observed in language change (Bybee, 2001).

Such a model of phonology has quite radical but very exciting implications for the way in which we might regard a disorder of speech production. It would be more heavily grounded in phonetic, or articulatory, evidence and rely less on abstract segments. It would also involve the role of experience, and the extent to which a child is capable of storing instances of language use, and then generalizing across them, coming to the forefront of research, assessment, and remediation. Hopefully, this may well represent a step forward for research as well as practice.

REFERENCES

Archangeli, D. (1988). Aspects of underspecification theory. *Phonology, 5,* 183–208.

Archangeli, D., & Langendoen, T. (1997) *Optimality theory. An overview.* Oxford, UK: Blackwell.

Ball, M. J. (2002). Clinical phonology of vowel disorders. In M. J. Ball and F. Gibbon (Eds.), *Vowel disorders* (pp. 187–216). London: Butterworth-Heinemann.

Ball, M. J. (2003). Clinical applications of a cognitive phonology. *Phoniatrics, Logopedics, Vocology, 28,* 63–69.

Ball, M. J., & Gibbon, F. (Eds.). (2002). *Vowel disorders.* Woburn, MA: Butterworth-Heinemann.

Ball, M. J., & Kent, R. D. (Eds.). (1998). *The new phonologies.* San Diego, CA: Singular.

Ball, M. J., & Müller, N. (2002). The use of the terms phonetics and phonology in the description of disordered speech. *Advances in Speech-Language Pathology, 4,* 95–108.

Ball, M. J., Müller, N., & Rutter, B. (2009). *Phonology for communicative disorders.* Mahwah, NJ: Lawrence Erlbaum.

Ball, M. J., Rutter, B., & Code, C. (2008). Phonological analyses of a case of progressive speech degeneration. *Asia-Pacific Journal of Speech, Language and Hearing, 11,* 305–312.

Bernhardt, B. (1992a). Developmental implications of nonlinear phonological theory. *Clinical Linguistics and Phonetics, 6,* 259–281.

Bernhardt, B. (1992b). The application of nonlinear phonological theory to intervention with one phonologically disordered child. *Clinical Linguistics and Phonetics, 6,* 283–316.

Bernhardt, B., & Gilbert, J. (1992). Applying linguistic theory to speech-language pathology: The case for non-linear phonology. *Clinical Linguistics and Phonetics, 6,* 123–145.

Browman, C., & Goldstein, L. (1992). Articulatory phonology: An overview. *Phonetica, 49,* 155–180.

Bybee, J. (2001). *Phonology and language use.* Cambridge, UK: Cambridge University Press.

Chomsky, N., & Halle, M. (1968). *The sound pattern of English.* New York, NY: Harper & Row.

Cohn, A. (2006). Is there gradient phonology? In G. Fanselow, C. Fery, R. Vogel, & M. Schlesewsky (Eds.), *Gradience in grammar: Generative perspectives* (pp. 25–44). Oxford, UK: Oxford University Press.

Coleman, J. (1998). *Phonological representations: Their names, forms and powers.* Cambridge, UK: Cambridge University Press.

Dinnsen, D. (1997). Nonsegmental phonologies. In M. J. Ball & R. D. Kent (Eds.), *The new phonologies* (pp. 77–125). San Diego, CA: Singular.

Dinnsen, D., & Gierut, J. (2008). Optimality theory: A clinical perspective. In M. J. Ball, M. Perkins, N. Müller, & S. Howard (Eds.), *Handbook of clinical linguistics* (pp. 439–451). Oxford, UK: Blackwell.

Giegerich, H. J. (1992). *English phonology.* Cambridge, UK: Cambridge University Press.

Goldinger, S. D. (1997). Echoes of echoes? An episodic theory of lexical access. *Psychological Review, 105,* 251–279.

Goldsmith, J. (1976). *Autosegmental phonology.* Unpublished PhD dissertation, MIT.

Goldsmith, J. (1990). *Autosegmental and metrical phonology.* Oxford, UK: Blackwell.

Grunwell, P. (1987). *Clinical phonology* (2nd ed.). London, UK: Chapman & Hall.

Harris, J. (1990). Segmental complexity and phonological government. *Phonology, 7,* 255–300.

Harris, J. (1994). *English sound structure.* Oxford, UK: Blackwell.

Harris, J., & Lindsey, G. (1995). The elements of phonological representation. In J. Durand & F. Katamba (Eds.), *Frontiers of phonology* (pp. 34–79). London, UK: Longmans.

Harris, J., Watson, J., & Bates, S. (1999). Prosody and melody in vowel disorder. *Journal of Linguistics, 35,* 489–525.

International Phonetic Association. (1999). *Handbook of the International Phonetic Association: A guide to the use of the International Phonetic Alphabet.* Cambridge, UK: Cambridge University Press.

Johnson, K. (1997). Speech perception without speaker normalization: An exemplar model. In K. Johnson & J. W. Mullennix (Eds.), *Talker variability in speech processing* (pp. 145–165). San Diego, CA and London, UK: Academic Press.

Kaye, J., Lowenstamm, J., & Vergnaud, J.-R. (1985). The internal structure of phonological elements: A theory of charm and government. *Phonology Yearbook, 2,* 305–328.

Kaye, J., Lowenstamm, J., & Vergnaud, J.-R. (1990). Constituent structure and government in phonology. *Phonology, 7,* 193–232.

Kenstowicz, M. (1994). *Phonology in generative grammar.* Cambridge, MA: Blackwell.

Kent, R. D. (1998). Normal aspects of articulation. In J. E. Bernthal and N. W. Bankson (Eds.), *Articulation and phonological disorders* (pp. 1–59). Boston, MA: Allyn & Bacon.

Kerswell, P., & Shockey, L. (2007). The production and acquisition of variable phonological patterns: Phonology and sociolinguistics. In M. Pennington (Ed.), *Phonology in context* (pp. 51–75). Basingstore, UK: Pelgrave Macmillan.

Linell, P. (2005). *The written language bias in linguistics: Its nature, origins and transformations.* London, UK and New York, NY: Routledge.

Locke, J. (1983). Clinical phonology: The explanation and treatment of speech sound disorders. *Journal of Speech and Hearing Disorders, 48,* 339–341.

McCarthy, J. (2002). *A thematic guide to optimality theory.* Cambridge, MA: Cambridge University Press.

Pierrehumbert, J. (2001). Exemplar dynamics: Word frequency, lenition, and contrast. In J. Bybee & P. Hopper (Eds.), *Frequency effects and the emergence of lexical structure* (pp. 137–157). Amsterdam, The Netherlands: John Benjamins.

Pierrehumbert, J. (2003). Probabilistic phonology: Discrimination and robustness. In R. Bod, J. Hay, & S. Jannedy (Eds.), *Probabilistic linguistics* (pp. 177–228). Cambridge, MA: MIT Press.

Prince, A., & Smolensky, P. (1993). *Optimality theory: Constraint interaction in generative grammar.* RuCCs Technical Report #2. Piscataway, NJ: Rutgers University Center for Cognitive Science.

Sosa, A. V., & Bybee, J. (2007). A cognitive approach to clinical phonology. In M. J. Ball, M. Perkins, N. Müller, & S. Howard (Eds.), *Handbook of clinical linguistics.* Oxford, UK: Blackwell.

Stackhouse, J., & Wells, B. (1997). *Children's speech and literacy difficulties: A psycholinguistic framework.* London, UK: Whurr.

16 From Phonology to Articulation: A Neurophonetic View

Wolfram Ziegler, Hermann Ackermann, and Juliane Kappes

INTRODUCTION

In this chapter we present a neurophonetic perspective on how phonological representations transform into speech movements during verbal communication. Our "neurophonetic view" approaches speech production from its bottom end, not from the top, and the empirical evidence presented here will predominantly relate to neurologic conditions and brain imaging work. As a consequence, we consider phonological and phonetic processes to be constrained by the properties of the vocal tract motor system, on the one hand, and the auditory system, on the other. We start out by describing some crucial elements of a tripartite model of normal and impaired spoken language production, and then sketch the representations operating at each processing stage. In the last section of this chapter, we will delineate the neuroanatomic basis of speech production, from motor execution processes up to the level of cortical auditory-somatosensory-motor integration, with a focus on properties fundamental to the emergence of phonological structure.

A TRIPARTITE ARCHITECTURE OF SPEECH PRODUCTION

PHONOLOGICAL IMPAIRMENT, APRAXIA OF SPEECH, DYSARTHRIA

Neurolinguistic and neurophonetic investigations of phonetic–phonological operations and speech motor processes are centered around the observation that brain lesions may compromise verbal communication at different levels of the speech production chain. A fundamental distinction has been made—at least since the work by Pierre Marie—between "language" and "motor" deficits of spoken language. Within the clinical domain, this classical demarcation line separates the two syndromes of *phonological paraphasia* as a linguistic impairment and *dysarthria* as a plain motor disorder. The term *phonological* (better: *phonemic*) *paraphasia* refers to a class of symptoms characterized by the substitution, omission, addition, or metathesis of one or several phonemes of a word. As an example, a patient suffering from acquired brain damage might say [da:bel] instead of [ga:bel] (English: *fork*) with perfectly fluent and clear articulation of each segment of the produced nonword. A popular and straightforward symbolic interpretation of such a paraphasic error is that during the encoding of the target word the patient has mis-selected a [d] for a [g] (e.g., Alexander & Hillis, 2008). The units implicated in this encoding failure could equally well represent syllables ([da:] for [ga:]), distinctive phonetic features ([ALVEOLAR] for [VELAR]) or even articulatory gestures (tongue tip for tongue back). Connectionist theories would ascribe such errors to an inefficient transmission of activation across the nodes of a neural network or to reduced decay rates (Dell, Schwartz, Martin, Saffran, & Gagnon, 1997). "Dual-origin" models of phonological impairment postulate these errors of spoken language to arise either at the level of lexical representation or during postlexical processing steps (Schwartz, Wilshire, Gagnon, & Polansky, 2004). Irrespective of any details, these models assume subsequent speech motor control processes to be uncompromised. As a consequence, the speaker produced a well-articulated but phonemically inaccurate sound category.

By contrast, the term *dysarthria* refers to a class of disorders characterized, at the bottom end of the speech production chain, by impaired movement execution due to paresis, ataxia, akinesia, tremor, or any other pathological condition of motor control mechanisms (Duffy, 2005). The word [ga:bel] produced by a dysarthric speaker comes out—depending on the specific variant of this syndrome—with overall imprecise consonant articulation, reduced or increased mouth opening, rough, strained, or breathy voice quality, hypernasality, and so on. Nevertheless, a preserved phonemic structure still can be recognized behind these motor implementation problems.

Since Broca's time, a third kind of speech disorder has emerged between these two syndromes. Broca had assumed damage to the posterior component of the left inferior frontal gyrus, a region now bearing his name, to give rise to a distinct variant of speechlessness ("aphemia"): These patients were not "paralyzed" (in our terms: not dysarthric), but appear to have lost the "memory of the procedures that must be followed in the articulation of words" (Broca, 1861). More specifically, he envisaged an impairment of the *faculty of speaking* (i.e., a loss of the overlearned motor routines pertaining to a speech motor memory). Liepmann, a German neurologist who worked on apraxic disorders of limb movements, later characterized aphemia, which was then called "motor aphasia" or "Broca's aphasia," as an "apraxia of the language muscles" (Liepmann, 1900), suggesting that aphemic patients have "a correct concept of what they ought to do" (here: to say), "but cannot transform the image of the intended action into appropriate motor commands" (Liepmann, 1907). This characterization of aphemia has almost literally entered modern descriptions of a syndrome that is now—following a proposal by Darley (1968)—called "apraxia of speech" (e.g., Hillis et al., 2004, p. 1479). A patient with mild or moderate apraxia of speech, confronted with the task of producing [ga:bel], would typically display problems initiating this word, grope for the initial [g] and eventually produce some sound in between [g] and [d] or [g] and [k] or often even a plain phonemic substitution, try a new start, and finally articulate the word in a disfluent manner, with varying misarticulations, phonemic errors, and repeated self-corrections. By contrast to dysarthria syndromes, none of the pathomechanisms known from neurological movement disorders (such as paresis, ataxia, tremor, etc.) are recognizable behind the behavioral pattern of apraxia of speech. Furthermore, even moderately impaired apraxic speakers may at times produce stretches of unimpaired speech, a phenomenon that cannot be explained within the framework of dysarthric impairments. Unlike phonological disorders, on the other hand, apraxic speech is not well-articulated and shows a markedly nonfluent character, phenomena that led clinicians and researchers to allocate this constellation to the motor domain.

PHONOLOGICAL ENCODING, PHONETIC PLANNING, ARTICULATION

The classification of neurogenic speech impairments into *phonological impairment*, *apraxia of speech*, and *dysarthria* largely parallels the architecture of psycholinguistic information processing models of spoken language production, especially of the model proposed by Levelt, Roelofs, and Meyer (1999). In this model, the words stored in a speaker's mental lexicon are considered to be composed of a serially ordered set of phonemes. During production of a lexical item, the respective phonemes are read out in their correct order and, in Levelt's theory, are syllabified according to universal syllabification rules. In interactive activation theories of word production (e.g., Dell et al., 1997), the sequence of phonemes of a lexical item is generated by forward and backward activation flows within a network of nodes representing words, syllables, syllable constituents, and phonemes. The two approaches referred to have in common that the phonological stage of word production ends up with an ordered set of discrete phonemes (Dell) or phonological syllables (Levelt), providing the input to the phonetic encoding stage or the motor component of speech production.

How do these strings of phonological units translate into movements? In Levelt's theory, the phonological syllables of a word activate motor programs stored in a repository of syllable-sized "phonetic plans." At this point, a motor learning concept enters the scene, since the entries of a speaker's "mental syllabary" are considered to represent crystallized speech motor routines, acquired through extensive exercise during language learning (Levelt et al., 1999). This suggestion is reminiscent of Broca's idea of a "memory" of speech motor procedures (see above). The retrieved phonetic plans encompass the "gestural scores" that specify the articulatory movements required for the production of the syllables of a word.

The theoretical accounts mentioned so far consider phonemes the smallest units of word form encoding. However, this basic assumption of phoneme-based approaches is obviously incompatible with the surface characteristics of speech movements and acoustic speech signals. As a fundamentally different approach, *articulatory phonology* postulates that the word forms housed in a speaker's mental lexicon consist of abstract *gestures* rather than segments. Gestures are defined as goal-directed vocal tract actions of the speech organs (i.e., lips, tongue tip, tongue body, velum, and glottis). They have a temporal extension and are characterized by the type and location of vocal tract constrictions underlying the formation of speech sounds. Furthermore, the gestures of a word are organized across parallel tiers, with different "bonding strengths" between them. The coherence between two gestures is expressed by their relative timing, technically, by the phase relationship that governs the coupling of two moving masses. Unlike phoneme-based theories, articulatory phonology makes no distinction between a phonological and a phonetic encoding level (Goldstein, Byrd, & Saltzman, 2006). As a consequence, this theory would not propose a fundamental difference between aphasic phonological impairment and apraxia of speech, but rather explain the well-articulated phonemic errors of aphasic patients and the sound distortions of apraxic speakers by similar mechanisms of impaired selection or coupling of articulatory gestures.

All the theoretical accounts mentioned so far assume the final stage of spoken language production to encompass the mechanisms of speech *motor execution*. These processes, however, are not further specified beyond the suggestion that the commands conveyed to the articulators to move in a phonetically meaningful are prescribed, for instance, by the syllabic gestural scores created by Levelt's phonetic encoder, by the segmental phonetic features activated at the bottom level of connectionist-type models, or by the abstract phonetic gestures that constitute a word in articulatory phonology. More specifically, it is not known how detailed the motor signals sent to the "vocal apparatus" must be in order to allow for accurate and smooth movement sequences. Among others, theories of the motor execution component of speech production should delineate the interplay between sensory-afferent and motor-efferent functions and also account for the adjustment of speech movement parameters to faster or louder speaking modes. Current computational theories of speech motor control are based on feedforward and feedback mechanisms involving orosensory and auditory afferent information, emerging from an extensive adaptive entrainment during a babbling period of language learning (e.g., Guenther & Perkell, 2004). On these grounds, impaired motor execution in dysarthria would reflect a downscaling of movement parameters (paretic or hypokinetic syndromes), intermittent derailments of scaling parameters (hyperkinetic or dyskinetic variants), or a misadaptation of motor commands to afferent sensory information (ataxic dysarthria).

THE NATURE OF PHONOLOGICAL, PHONETIC, AND MOTOR REPRESENTATIONS

Classical aphasiology considers the linguistic and the motor domains of speech production as entirely disjunct or mutually "irrelevant" processing stages (e.g., Alexander & Hillis, 2008). Within this traditional account, phonological impairment pertains to the *linguistic* realm and, therefore, must be assigned—like agrammatism or semantic disorders—to the aphasic syndrome complex. On the other hand, speech motor deficits, including apraxia of speech, are considered part of the nonlinguistic world, relating to a peripheral *instrument* rather than language proper. This strict dichotomy of linguistic versus motor disorders of spoken language is grounded in implicit assumptions concerning the computational structure (representations, operations) of the phonological, phonetic, and motor levels of speech production, especially the view of an impermeable demarcation between a symbolic-phonological and a physical-motor domain. The following paragraphs discuss some of the properties that must be ascribed to data structures of each of the three stages of speech production.

THE DISCRETE NATURE OF PHONOLOGICAL REPRESENTATIONS

The observation that phonemic paraphasias are *discrete* phenomena has been invoked as an argument for a symbolic nature of the substitution-, deletion-, or addition-mechanisms underlying aphasic phonological impairments. Discreteness of word forms is an indispensable requirement since words refer to—concrete or abstract—discrete objects in our environment (e.g., to knives or forks), hence our vocal motor apparatus must be capable of generating discrete and separable acoustic signals referring to these concepts. As an example, [ga:bel] (fork) must be sufficiently distinct from [ka:bel] (cable) to serve its referential function, and therefore the onsets of these two similar sounding words must differ by at least one discrete feature. Phonological theories congruently assume that words consist of discrete sub-lexical "atoms," though they may differ in their assumptions on the nature and size of these entities (e.g., Goldstein et al., 2006). This *particulation* of word forms constitutes the basis of our ability to create a potentially infinite number of verbal messages from a small number of primitives (Levelt, 1998).

An important question arising at this point is how discreteness of phonological form can emerge from continuous physical processes such as muscle contractions, mass movements, or aerodynamic events. The ancient dictum *natura non facit saltus* (i.e., nature does not change in leaps) would suggest that a fundamental dualism must exist between discrete phonology, on the one hand, and gradual movements, on the other, and would force us to postulate a purely symbolic nature of phonological representations.

Yet, nature *does* behave discontinuously and does make leaps. As a first fundamental source of discreteness, speech motor activity involves distinct articulatory organs (i.e., the lips, tongue, velum, etc.). Hence, vocal tract movements inject discreteness into speech production and, reciprocally, we perceive the contributions of discrete articulators when listening to speech. A parallel can be found in general action theory, especially in accounts of how we perceive and imitate actions of the upper extremities (e.g., the hand). Some authors assume action perception to be in general mediated by a *body part coding* mechanism, supporting the recognition or imitation of the motor actions of other organisms (Goldenberg, in press).

Notwithstanding the fractionation of motor behavior into contributions of separate body parts, even the trajectories of single moving organs are considered to demonstrate—for purely mechanical reasons—instabilities or attractor states, respectively. These biomechanical properties surface into discrete behavioral patterns. Dynamic field theories or coupled oscillator accounts of biological motion provide the theoretical framework for a description of these phenomena, assuming, for example, movement planning models to be based on nonsymbolic representations that by virtue of their nonlinear physical properties exhibit discontinuous behaviors (Erlhagen & Schöner, 2002).

Further sources of emergent discreteness can be found in the aerodynamic processes associated with spoken language. For instance, a small gradual change in transglottal airflow rate may give rise to a discrete bifurcation between oscillating and nonoscillating vocal folds, hence, between voiced and voiceless consonants. Or an equally small gradual step may turn a turbulent into a laminar airflow (i.e., a fricative into an approximant). Finally, our auditory-perceptual system imposes a great deal of discreteness by fine-tuning its acuity to language-specific, discriminative features of the acoustic signal.

Taken together, there is no sufficient reason to maintain a strict dualism between the discreteness of phonological units and the gradedness of speech movement parameters. The movement-to-sound transformations that underlie human speech embrace a variety of mechanisms that generate discreteness within the domains of motor behavior and sound production, providing a basis for particulation in phonology. As a consequence, discreteness of the units implicated in phonemic paraphasia is by far not incompatible with the view that paraphasic errors arise at some abstract level of speech motor control.

PHONETIC REPRESENTATIONS: FROM GESTURES TO RHYTHMS

Given that phonological primitives are discrete entities, how are they combined in order to specify the input to the speech motor execution system? Psycholinguistic theories converge on the notion that the phonetic plans for speaking are linear strings of phonetic primitives; that is, syllables (in Levelt's model) or phonemes (in connectionist accounts such as Dell's proposal). As a consequence, the unfolding speech movements operate on information chopped into linearly ordered fragments. In Levelt's model, for instance, articulation of the word [ga:bel] is based on two motor programs, one for each syllable, which are implemented one-by-one in a serial fashion by the motor execution system. As concerns Dell's account, the phonological network would generate five phonemes for [ga:bel], each specified by its distinctive features, which are then fed into the neural motor apparatus of spoken language.

This architecture leaves a large part of the "articulation work" unspecified, delegating it to lower level mechanisms of motor execution. Levelt's syllable-based phonetic plans, for example, do not contain any information concerning the concatenation of two or more syllables to form a word, or any suprasyllabic information concerning its rhythmical structure. These shortcomings loom even larger in case of phoneme-based motor programs, in which all coarticulation processes and any prosodic modulation is left to the motor implementation component.

From the perspective of speech motor planning impairment (i.e., apraxia of speech), linear concatenation models of phonetic planning make very clear predictions: if all motor programming work were encapsulated in the syllables or the phonemes of a word, the number of speech errors of a patient in an utterance would depend solely on the number of phonetic units the utterance contains, but would not be influenced by structural properties from above or below the supposed phonetic unit. If, for instance, Levelt's view is adopted and phonetic representations are conceived of as strings of syllables, the pattern of apraxic errors occurring in a stretch of speech should depend on the number of syllables, but not on their subsyllabic architectures or their metrical parsing (Ziegler, Thelen, Staiger, & Liepold, 2008).

Yet, empirical data are at variance with this prediction. When we count apraxic errors, we find that their frequency in fact depends on syllable number, but also on the complexity of syllable structure (more errors on complex than on simple syllables) and on the grouping of syllables into metrical feet (more errors on two stressed syllables than on a trochee). This implies that phonetic representations (or motor plans) of speech utterances have a complex, hierarchical architecture (Ziegler et al., 2008).

The probability of phonetic encoding to fail in patients with apraxia of speech can be modeled rather efficiently by metrical tree structures of phonological words, with "phonetic gestures" at the bottom level and metrical feet at the top level (Figure 16.1).

The structure in Figure 16.1 is reminiscent of the connectionist network postulated in Dell's phonological encoding model (Dell et al., 1997), with the difference

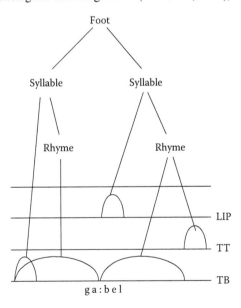

FIGURE 16.1 Gestural and metrical structure of the word [ga:bel] (engl.: fork), as a model of the non-linear architecture of its phonetic plan.

that it extends to the level of phonetic gestures and that it is designed to describe the makeup of motor programs, as inferred from the behaviors of patients with speech motor programming disorders. The model depicted in Figure 16.1 also borrows from articulatory phonology in that it uses vocal tract gestures as its primitives and parameterizes the bonding strengths between them (cf. Goldstein et al., 2006). It thereby creates phonetic representations that integrate the signature of the evolving movement sequence from the gestural to the rhythmical level.

By such a model we were able to predict the errors of a large sample of apraxic speakers on a large variety of word forms (Ziegler, 2009). The prediction was by far better than predictions based on linear string models. The coefficients of the resulting nonlinear model indicated that consonantal gestures in the onset of a syllable or multiple consonants within a syllable constituent impose a high load on phonetic encoding, whereas the consonants in a syllabic rhyme and the syllables in a trochaic foot are less vulnerable than one would predict on purely combinatorial grounds (Ziegler, 2005, 2009). These results suggest that low "bonding strengths" exist between the phonetic gestures at syllable onset and within consonant clusters, and that syllabic rhymes and trochaic feet are highly integrated motor patterns. Hence, if an apraxic patient substitutes [d] for [g] in the onset of [ga:bel], which is not an unlikely event, this may be due to a weak coupling of the velar gesture to the syllabic rhyme of the first syllable.

Overall, the model depicted in Figure 16.1 gives credit to the suggestion that phonetic gestures are basic units of speech motor planning, and it also recognizes that the coupling of these units to form increasingly larger motor patterns, up to the level of metrical feet, must be part of the phonetic information that is finally handed down to the speech motor execution apparatus.

To What Extent is Speech Motor Control Nonlinguistic?

At the bottom end of the speech production cascade, the vocal tract movements generating the sounds of a word unfold in space and time. According to conventional theories, the neural machinery controlling the speech motor apparatus is prepared to execute all kinds of movement specifications in the same, universal manner. Therefore, lesions to this system are expected to cause motor impairments (e.g., ataxia, paresis, apraxia, etc.), irrespective of the specific motor act to be performed (Ballard, Granier, & Robin, 2000).

Yet, from a clinical perspective this hypothesis must be rejected. It is true that impairments of speech and nonspeech vocal tract movements often co-occur, but numerous clinical reports have also documented instances of brain lesions that compromised speech production, but left other oral motor functions unimpaired. Vice versa, neurologic disorder may interfere with motor activities like swallowing, smiling, tongue protrusion, and so on, sparing spoken language however. Such clinical dissociations suggest a task-specific perspective on vocal tract motor control, which postulates different neural organizations for autonomous metabolic motor functions (breathing, swallowing), emotional expression (laughter, smiling, sobbing, crying, etc.), nonspeech voluntary motor activities (imitation of mouth movements, visuomotor tracking, etc.), and speech (Bunton, 2008; Ziegler, 2003).

The clinical dissociation between voluntary vocal tract movements, on the one hand, and emotionally expressive facial or laryngeal movements, on the other, has a clear neural basis that will be sketched in a later section. The control of vegetative-autonomous motor functions like breathing or swallowing by distinct neural "pattern generators" in the brainstem is also relatively well understood. Yet, dissociations obviously also exist between different types of voluntary vocal tract actions, on the one hand, and speaking, on the other (Connor & Abbs, 1991; McAuliffe, Ward, Murdoch, & Farrell, 2005; Ziegler, 2002). One of the core arguments for a specific neural organization of speech as compared to nonspeech voluntary vocal tract movements implies that verbal communication is based on a lifelong motor learning process that, through mechanisms of experience-dependent neural plasticity, creates a motor network specifically tuned to the control of speech (see below). As a result, the motor processes at the bottom end of the speech production chain are not at all exclusively nonlinguistic phenomena. They are patterned in a way unique to speech, integrate respiratory, laryngeal, and articulatory muscles in a characteristic manner that is not seen in any other motor activity, are tuned toward the goal of producing sounds, and are entrained over many years, through extensive daily exercise, to subserve this specific goal. Motor control of spoken language must, therefore, be considered an extension of the human language faculty into the periphery of its vocal execution apparatus (Ziegler, 2006).

FROM ARTICULATION TO PHONOLOGY: NEURAL CORRELATES

As outlined above, one of the most salient properties that distinguish human spoken language from vocal communication in subhuman primates is the generative nature of the speech code. Macaques or squirrel monkeys produce calls of a holistic and largely invariant acoustic structure, highly contingent upon specific stimulus constellations and rigidly bound to distinct social functions. As a consequence, monkeys and apes show very limited vocal learning capabilities (Fitch, 2000). In contrast, human verbal communication is based upon patterned signals: The lexical signs of human speech consist of separable and recombinable units, which is fundamental to our capacity to expand our lexicon by learning or creating new words for new concepts (Levelt, 1998). In the following paragraphs, we briefly sketch the neural basis of this capacity, with a particular emphasis on some of the functional properties that distinguish human speech from primate vocal signaling.

MOTOR EXECUTION

A Dual-Route System of Vocal Communication in Humans

Vocal behavior of monkeys and apes, on the one hand, and human speech, on the other, are mediated by largely different neural networks. The monkey vocal motor system is based on a *limbic-mesencephalic-bulbar* pathway, which plays only a subordinate role in human communication. Vice versa, human speech is supported by a *neocortical-bulbar* motor system, extended by two subcortical pathways, which also exists in subhuman primates, but is "silent" in these species.

The primate vocal motor system has been investigated most extensively in the squirrel monkey model (Jürgens, 2002). Spontaneous calls of these animals arise from neuronal activity in the anterior cingulate gyrus, a cortical structure on the mesial surface of the frontal lobes. The anterior cingulate gyrus is part of the limbic system and is considered to be associated with motivational and affective aspects of behavior. The primate vocal pathways descend from this structure via the midbrain periaqueductal grey to the reticular formation and the vocal tract motor nuclei in the brainstem, eliciting, ultimately, vocalization-related contractions of the laryngeal and supralaryngeal muscles. This system also exists in humans, where it is considered to mediate intrinsic vocalizations like laughter or crying (Ackermann & Ziegler, 2010).

However, the neural pathway conveying volitional vocal tract motor control in humans is almost entirely separate from the limbic vocalization pathway of subhuman primates. It originates from rolandic motor cortex on the anterior bank of the central sulcus and the precentral gyrus, from where it descends to the brainstem motor nuclei. The various vocal tract muscles are represented within the lower third of the lateral precentral motor strip. As a consequence, intraoperative electrical stimulation of this cortical area has been found to elicit vocalizations and facial movements. Bilateral lesions to the face, mouth, and larynx region of primary motor cortex or the descending cortico-bulbar fiber tracts yield a severe dysarthric syndrome, eventually even complete aphonia and anarthria, indicating that this neural pathway plays a crucial role in human speech. In monkeys, on the contrary, complete bilateral destruction of lower sensorimotor cortex does not compromise vocal behavior, although it renders the animals unable to chew, lick, and swallow.

Remarkably, patients who are severely dysarthric or entirely mute after bilateral corticobulbar lesions often display preserved or even exaggerated facial and laryngeal motor patterns in emotionally expressive behavior such as laughter or crying (Ackermann & Ziegler, 2010). Moreover, unilateral lesions of motor cortical pathways projecting on the facial nucleus yield a similar dissociation of emotional and volitional motor behavior. The patients are unable to abduct the contralesional side of their mouth when instructed to volitionally spread their lips, whereas emotional stimuli may elicit an entirely symmetrical spontaneous smile (*volitional* facial paresis). The reverse pattern of a unilateral *emotional* facial paresis has also been described. This syndrome is characterized by a preserved volitional abduction of the mouth on the contralesional side, but an asymmetric spontaneous smile (Hopf, Müller-Forell, & Hopf, 1992). As a conclusion, these clinical observations demonstrate that human volitional and emotional vocal motor functions are mediated by distinct neural pathways. As will be outlined below, the specific properties of the neocortical, volitional vocal motor pathway are fundamental to the emergence of a communication system based on particulated vocal signals.

Fractionation and Dexterity of the Corticobulbar Motor System

The vocal motor responses elicited through electrical stimulation of inferior precentral gyrus in humans are not speech-like or well-articulated. This system conveys only fractionated gestural elements of sounds or syllables rather than phonologically structured information. More generally, primary motor cortex activity is considered to be implicated in controlling gestural fractions of complex motor acts rather than holistic actions, which is considered an important basis of the fractionated architecture of skilled motor activity (Brooks, 1986). As we have seen, gestural fractionation is also a salient feature of phonological structure, especially from the perspective of articulatory phonology, in which words are considered to be composed of co-ordinated vocal tract gestures (Goldstein et al., 2006).

Importantly, the human vocal motor pathway contains *direct, monosynaptic* fibers projecting onto the vocal tract motor nuclei of the brainstem, including the laryngeal motor nucleus (nucleus ambiguus). The nucleus ambiguus is remarkable, because in monkeys and apes this nucleus lacks a direct, monosynaptic connection with cortical motor cells (Kuypers, 1958). In humans, this direct projection entails that the human laryngeal muscles, like the muscles of the face and mouth, can be addressed directly by cortical signals and may therefore be implicated in versatile vocal motor activity. This allows for a laryngeal contribution to articulated speech, for example, through rapid ad- and abductions of the vocal folds for the distinction between voiced and voiceless consonants, or through a fine-tuning of vocal fold stiffness in the control of pitch for the expression of accent and intonation.

Plasticity of the Vocal Tract Motor System

Unlike the limbic motor system of intrinsic vocalizations, the motor network involved in human speech motor control is characterized by a high functional and structural plasticity. Studies in monkeys and humans have shown that motor exercise of the extremities leads to a structural and functional reorganization at the level of the primary motor cortex. The mechanisms of motor cortical plasticity are mainly characterized by a restructuring of connections between motor cortical neurons and a modulation of synaptic processes. These mechanisms can be triggered by motor learning and motor exercise. The dynamic architecture of primary motor cortex and its resulting functional plasticity are viewed as an important prerequisite of behavioral flexibility and adaptivity (Sanes & Donoghue, 2000). Practice-related plasticity is not confined to the hand area of the motor strip, but in humans has also been shown for cortical vocal tract muscle representations, especially the tongue (Svensson, Romaniello, Wang, Arendt-Nielsen, & Sessle, 2006). Therefore, the cortical maps for the control of speech movements in adults must be viewed as the result of a long-lasting vocal motor learning process, with the consequence that vocal tract movements for speaking have their own specific motor cortical representation.

Learning-induced plasticity extends beyond primary sensorimotor cortex and also encompasses the two subcortical motor loops subserving volitional movement control (i.e., the basal ganglia and the cerebellar loop). The basal ganglia and cerebellum are even considered to play an important active role in the acquisition of motor skills, and their contribution to movement control itself is continuously modulated throughout the motor learning process (Ungerleider, Doyon, & Karni, 2002). Again, this knowledge comes from investigations of manual functions, but there is no reason to assume that the results of these studies not also apply to vocal tract movements.

As a conclusion, the plasticity of the human vocal tract motor system entails that over the many years of language acquisition motor execution for the production of speech attains a high degree of linguistic specificity. The acquired routines lend themselves to the emergence of phonological representations for the control of speech movements.

Motor Planning

As mentioned above, the corticobulbar pathways—in cooperation with cerebellar and striatal motor loops—operate as a *speech motor execution* system. Bilateral functional organization represents one of the salient features of this neural circuitry. Besides this network, a further cerebral system has been identified that is lateralized to the language-dominant hemisphere and is assumed to subserve speech motor *planning* processes. Based on observations in patients with severe speech production deficits after damage to the "foot of the third frontal convolution" of the left hemisphere, Broca proposed this area to represent the seat of the "faculty of spoken language" (Broca, 1861, 1865). Since Broca's time, both the status of the disorder we now call apraxia of speech as well as the location of the respective lesions have been disputed passionately. Besides Broca's area, dysfunctions of the white matter underlying left anterior inferior frontal gyrus, of the left anterior insular cortex, and of the oral-facial region of the left primary motor strip have been reported to give rise to apraxia of speech (Ziegler, 2008). Despite the many controversies revolving around this syndrome, one finding has stood the test-of-time: Apraxia of speech is bound to a lesion of the left hemisphere, more specifically, of the anterior peri- and/or subsylvian regions of the language-dominant cortex.

Brain imaging studies have repeatedly identified left anterior insular cortex and ipsilateral inferior frontal gyrus as components of the cerebral network of motor aspects of speech production (for an overview see Riecker, Brendel, Ziegler, Erb, & Ackermann, 2008). Their role within the hierarchical organization of the speech production process was specified in an fMRI-study by Riecker et al. (2005), who identified left dorsolateral premotor and left anterior insular cortex as part of a "premotor" network whose activation precedes activation of the motor execution pathways mentioned above and is considered to be responsible for higher-order motor planning processes. In Broca's understanding, left posterior inferior frontal cortex houses the implicit memories for the motor procedures constituting the faculty of spoken language (see above), in Levelt's theory this region would be considered as the neural substrate of a store of syllabic motor plans, still others have used the terms *planning*, *programming*, or *orchestration of articulation* to describe its role. More specifically, Broca's area has been assumed to participate in hierarchical sequential processing (Fiebach & Schubotz, 2006), functions crucially engaged in motor planning processes, as described in Figure 16.1. Furthermore, ventral premotor cortex and Broca's area play a key role as target areas in the mapping of sensory onto motor representations (see below).

Although the Broca-homologue of macaque monkeys seems to take part in the control of orofacial and jaw muscles (Petrides, Cadoret, & Mackey, 2005), electrical stimulation of this region does neither evoke nor interrupt vocalizations in subhuman primates, but reliably interferes with speaking in humans. Therefore, the contribution of this region distinguishes human speech from vocal communication behaviors of subhuman species. Existence of this network lends support to the notion of a phonetic planning component in speech production, which is distinct from the bilaterally organized motor execution system.

AUDITORY-MOTOR INTEGRATION

While limb movements navigate us through visual space, speaking unfolds in acoustic space. When we learn to speak, we learn to steer our vocal tract organs in a way that they produce intelligible and natural speech sound sequences. This is not a trivial task, since spoken language requires mastery of a complex tool for the generation of air pressure, regulation of airflow, control of resonances, and creation of noises. There is high flexibility and adaptivity of this system, in the sense that a great variety of different patterns of muscle contractions can be used to bring about the same sound under different circumstances (Guenther, Hampson, & Johnson, 1998). Development and maintenance of such a system requires a high degree of integration of motor and auditory processes, since speech movements are exclusively tuned to the generation of sound sequences.

The guidance of movement through perceptual goals has been a major topic in theories of visuomotor action control. Skillful limb motor activity is considered to involve a "dorsal stream" system, by which visual mental images of a movement are transformed into actual movements. This concept goes back to Liepmann, who identified the "idea" of a movement with an internally generated "movement formula" in terms of some abstract visual image of the movement. Liepmann's concept was taken up and refined in modern neuropsychology, with the persistent view that the left inferior parietal lobe plays a crucial role as an interface between occipital visual and frontal motor areas. In these theories, the parietal lobe is assumed to house mental representations of intended motor actions (for a critical discussion see Goldenberg, 2009).

Hickok and Poeppel (2004) transferred the dorsal stream concept into the motor domain of speech production by postulating the existence of a bidirectional "dorsal" pathway involved in the mapping of sound to movement. This concept is reminiscent of a long-standing connectionist tradition, tracing back to Wernicke, based upon the existence of a fiber tract system (i.e., the arcuate fascicle), which projects from posterior superior temporal gyrus toward inferior parietal and dorsolateral inferior frontal cortex. The dorsal stream system of the left hemisphere plays an obvious role in tasks like word repetition, where the acoustic signal must be transformed into a speaker's own movements (Peschke, Ziegler, Kappes, & Baumgärtner, 2009), but appears to be engaged in various other modalities of speech production as well. For example, overlapping hemodynamic activation of left inferior frontal and posterior temporal regions has been found in brain imaging studies both during perceptual and expressive tasks, an observation that highlights the perceptual-motor integrative role of this system. According to a more refined analysis of the dorsal stream, the posterior superior temporal plane of the left temporal lobe is characterized as a device that matches the speech signal with stored auditory templates, in order to disambiguate the incoming acoustic signal and to extract a sequence of speech-specific auditory representations. These data are then mapped onto motor representations, constrained by the auditory input, and further onto the speech motor plans stored within inferior frontal cortex (Warren, Wise, & Warren, 2005).

A dorsal "do-system" based on auditory information appears also to be present in nonhuman primates and, thus, is not restricted to speech production. Yet, the auditory dorsal stream used in producing and perceiving speech has several specific properties that may explain its key role in the development of a phonological communication system in humans. One is that the lateralization of this network to the dominant hemisphere begins early in childhood. This may indicate its specification as a basis for auditory-vocal learning in human infants. Second, its subcomponents, including the auditory and the motor component, are shaped by mechanisms of experience-dependent plasticity, which is fundamental to the generative properties of the phonological architecture of speech. Third, the system also encompasses left inferior parietal regions that may be considered, in analogy to the visual motor system, to make an important contribution to the mapping of auditory "images" of sounds, syllables, or words onto representations of intended movements. Taken together, this neural architecture can be expected to house an embodiment of the sound generating "tool" of the vocal tract with its rather abstract physical relationships between movement and sound. The representations generated by this system acquire a strong potential of being utilized, beyond speaking and listening, in cognitive operations of many other kinds, such as mental imagery of speech, verbal working memory, or alphabetic script.

SUMMARY AND CONCLUSION

The path from phonology to articulation during verbal communication was characterized here as a processing chain, unfolding from abstract representations of intended motor acts via hierarchical motor plans to motor executive functions. Despite the tripartite fragmentation of this process in psycholinguistic models, our knowledge about the exact specification of motor information at each stage is still limited, and there is still considerable disagreement about the separation of phonological from phonetic encoding or of phonetic planning from motor execution stages, respectively. The transitions between the three processing levels distinguished here are continuous, and the motor nature of the information is visible on even the highest stage. We emphasized the functional coherence of the phonology-to-articulation interface by highlighting that phonological representations specify motor information at the upper end of the processing chain, and the motor processes are shaped by linguistic form at its bottom end.

The neural substrate of the phonology-to-articulation system has its origin in a left peri-sylvian cortical auditory-motor integration network, which is at the core of human vocal communicative behavior. This dorsal stream system targets a lateralized premotor system, considered to store acquired "motor knowledge" about the makeup of speech movements for words and phrases. As a subsequent step of speech production, a bilaterally organized system subserving voluntary control of vocal tract movements is activated. All components of this system are characterized by a high potential for experience-related plasticity, fundamental to the generative potential of particulation in phonology. The connectivity of the components of this system is well established, which makes the whole network identifiable as the basis of human auditory-vocal linguistic behavior. In the light of the coherent architecture of this system, there is no room for a strict demarcation between linguistic and motor speech processing, or between aphasic phonological and nonaphasic speech impairments.

FURTHER READING

Ackermann, H., & Ziegler, W. (in press). A birdsong perspective on human speech. In J. J. Bolhuis & M. Everaert (Eds.), *Birdsong, speech, and language. Converging views.* Boston, MA: MIT Press.

Ziegler, W. (2002a). Psycholinguistic and motor theories of apraxia of speech. *Seminars in Speech and Language, 23,* 231–243.

Ziegler, W., Staiger, A., & Aichert, I. (2009). Apraxia of speech: What the deconstruction of phonetic plans tells us about the construction of articulate language. In B. Maassen & P. H. H. M. van Lieshout (Eds.), *Speech motor control: New developments in basic and applied research.* Oxford, UK: Oxford University Press.

REFERENCES

Ackermann, H., & Ziegler, W. (2009). Brain mechanisms underlying speech. In W. J. Hardcastle (Ed.), *The handbook of phonetic sciences* (2nd ed.). Oxford, UK: Blackwell.

Alexander, M. P., & Hillis, A. E. (2008). Aphasia. In G. Goldenberg & B. Miller (Eds.), *Handbook of clinical neurology* (pp. 287–309). London, UK: Elsevier.

Ballard, K. J., Granier, J. P., & Robin, D. A. (2000). Understanding the nature of apraxia of speech: Theory, analysis, and treatment. *Aphasiology, 14,* 969–995.

Broca, P. (1861). Remarks on the seat of the faculty of articulate language; followed by an observation of aphemia. *Bulletins de la Societé d'Anatomie, 36,* 330–357.

Broca, P. (1865). On the seat of the faculty of articulate language in the left hemisphere of the brain. *Bulletins de la Societé d'Anthropologie, 6,* 377–393.

Brooks, V. B. (1986). *The neural basis of motor control.* New York, NY: Oxford University Press.

Bunton, K. (2008). Speech versus nonspeech: Different tasks, Different neural organization. *Seminars in Speech and Language, 29,* 267–275.

Connor, N. P., & Abbs, J. H. (1991). Task-dependent variations in Parkinsonian motor impairments. *Brain, 114,* 321–332.

Darley, F. L. (1968). Apraxia of speech: 107 years of terminological confusion. Paper presented at the Annual Convention of the ASHA.

Dell, G. S., Schwartz, M. F., Martin, N., Saffran, E. M., & Gagnon, D. A. (1997). Lexical access in aphasic and nonaphasic speakers. *Psychological Review, 104,* 801–838.

Duffy, J. R. (2005). *Motor speech disorders: Substrates, differential diagnosis, and management* (2nd ed.). St. Louis, MO: Elsevier Mosby.

Erlhagen, W., & Schöner, G. (2002). Dynamic field theory of movement preparation. *Psychological Review, 109,* 545–572.

Fiebach, C. J., & Schubotz, R. I. (2006). Dynamic anticipatory processing of hierarchical sequential events: A common role for Broca's area and ventral premotor cortex across domains? *Cortex, 42,* 502.

Fitch, W. T. (2000). The evolution of speech: A comparative review. *Trends in Cognitive Sciences, 4,* 258–267.

Goldenberg, G. (2009). Apraxia and the parietal lobes. *Neuropsychologia, 47,* 1449–1459.

Goldstein, L., Byrd, D., & Saltzman, E. (2006). The role of vocal tract gestural action units in understanding the evolution of phonology. In M. A. Arbib (Ed.), *Action to language via the mirror neuron system* (pp. 215). Cambridge, UK: Cambridge University Press.

Guenther, F. H., Hampson, M., & Johnson, D. (1998). A theoretical investigation of reference frames for the planning of speech movements. *Psychological Review, 105,* 611–633.

Guenther, F. H., & Perkell, J. S. (2004). A neural model of speech production and its application to studies of the role of auditory feedback in speech. In B. Maassen, R. Kent, H. Peters, P. van Lieshout, & W. Hulstijn (Eds.), *Speech motor control in normal and disordered speech* (pp. 29–49). Oxford, UK and New York, NY: Oxford University Press.

Hickok, G., & Poeppel, D. (2004). Dorsal and ventral streams: A framework for understanding aspects of the functional anatomy of language. *Cognition, 92,* 67–99.

Hillis, A. E., Work, M., Barker, P. B., Jacobs, M. A., Breese, E. L., & Maurer, K. (2004). Re-examining the brain regions crucial for orchestrating speech articulation. *Brain, 127,* 1479–1487.

Hopf, H. C., Müller-Forell, W., & Hopf, N. J. (1992). Localization of emotional and volitional facial paresis. *Neurology, 42,* 1918–1923.

Jürgens, U. (2002). Neural pathways underlying vocal control. *Neuroscience & Biobehavioral Reviews, 26,* 235–258.

Kuypers, H. G. J. M. (1958). Some projections from the peri-central cortex to the pons and lower brainstem in monkey and chimpanzee. *Journal of Comparative Neurology, 110,* 221–255.

Levelt, W. J. M. (1998). The genetic perspective in psycholinguistics or where do spoken words come from. *Journal of Psycholinguistic Research, 27,* 167–180.

Levelt, W. J. M., Roelofs, A., & Meyer, A. S. (1999). A theory of lexical access in speech production. *Behavioral and Brain Sciences, 22,* 1–38.

Liepmann, H. (1900). The clinical pattern of apraxia („motor asymbolia"), based on a case of unilateral apraxia (I). *Monatsschrift für Psychiatrie und Neurologie, VIII,* 15–41.

Liepmann, H. (1907). Two cases of destruction of the lower left frontal convolution. *Journal für Psychologie und Neurologie, IX,* 279–289.

McAuliffe, M. J., Ward, E. C., Murdoch, B. E., & Farrell, A. M. (2005). A nonspeech investigation of tongue function in Parkinson's disease. *The Journals of Gerontology, 60A,* 667–674.

Peschke, C., Ziegler, W., Kappes, J., & Baumgärtner, A. (2009). Auditory-motor integration during fast repetition: The neuronal correlates of shadowing. *Neuroimage, 47,* 392–402.

Petrides, M., Cadoret, G., & Mackey, S. (2005). Orofacial somatomotor responses in the macaque monkey homologue of Broca's area. *Nature, 435,* 1235–1238.

Riecker, A., Brendel, B., Ziegler, W., Erb, M., & Ackermann, H. (2008). The influence of syllable onset complexity and syllable frequency on speech motor control. *Brain and Language, 107,* 102–113.

Riecker, A., Mathiak, K., Wildgruber, D., Erb, M., Hertrich, I., Grodd, W., & Ackermann, H. (2005). fMRI reveals two distinct cerebral networks subserving speech motor control. *Neurology, 64,* 700–706.

Sanes, J. N., & Donoghue, J. P. (2000). Plasticity and primary motor cortex. *Annual Review of Neuroscience, 23,* 393–415.

Schwartz, M. F., Wilshire, C. E., Gagnon, D. A., & Polansky, M. (2004). Origins of nonword phonological errors in aphasic picture naming. *Cognitive Neuropsychology, 21,* 159–186.

Svensson, P., Romaniello, A., Wang, K., Arendt-Nielsen, L., & Sessle, B. J. (2006). One hour of tongue-task training is associated with plasticity in corticomotor control of the human tongue musculature. *Experimental Brain Research, 173,* 165–173.

Ungerleider, L. G., Doyon, J., & Karni, A. (2002). Imaging brain plasticity during motor skill learning. *Neurobiology of Learning and Memory, 78,* 553–564.

Warren, J. E., Wise, R. J., & Warren, J. D. (2005). Sounds do-able: Auditory-motor transformations and the posterior temporal plane. *Trends in Neuroscience, 28,* 636–643.

Ziegler, W. (2002). Task-related factors in oral motor control: Speech and oral diadochokinesis in dysarthria and apraxia of speech. *Brain and Language, 80,* 556–575.

Ziegler, W. (2003). Speech motor control is task-specific. Evidence from dysarthria and apraxia of speech. *Aphasiology, 17,* 3–36.

Ziegler, W. (2005). A nonlinear model of word length effects in apraxia of speech. *Cognitive Neuropsychology, 22,* 603–623.

Ziegler, W. (2006). Distinctions between speech and nonspeech motor control. A neurophonetic view. In M. Tabain & J. Harrington (Eds.), *Speech production: Models, phonetic processes, and techniques* (pp. 41–54). New York, NY: Psychology Press.

Ziegler, W. (2008). Apraxia of speech. In G. Goldenberg & B. Miller (Eds.), *Handbook of clinical neurology* (pp. 269–285). London, UK: Elsevier.

Ziegler, W. (2009). Modelling the architecture of phonetic plans: Evidence from apraxia of speech. *Language and Cognitive Processes, 24*(5), 631–661.

Ziegler, W., Thelen, A.-K., Staiger, A., & Liepold, M. (2008). The domain of phonetic encoding in apraxia of speech: Which sub-lexical units count? *Aphasiology, 22,* 1230–1247.

Section II

Developmental Disorders

17 (Central) Auditory Processing Disorders: Current Conceptualizations

Terri Shive and Teri James Bellis

INTRODUCTION

Professionals in audiology and related fields have demonstrated an interest in auditory processing for more than 50 years. Myklebust (1954) highlighted the need to evaluate central auditory function in children suspected of communication disorders. However, it was not until 1977, when the first conference to focus entirely on (Central) Auditory Processing Disorders ((C)APD) in children was held that research with this population began to increase dramatically (Keith, 1977). Since that time, myriad studies have been conducted that have focused on the relationship between performance on both behavioral and electrophysiologic measures of central auditory dysfunction and auditory, communication, and related difficulties in both children and adults. Through the use of tests that have been documented to demonstrate sensitivity and efficiency for the diagnosis of central auditory nervous system (CANS) dysfunction, we have come to a better understanding of the nature of (C)APD. In addition, our knowledge of the physiology of the central auditory system has increased significantly over the last half century, enabling more accurate diagnosis of and appropriate intervention for the disorder. This chapter will provide an overview of the current conceptualizations of (C)APD, methods of diagnosing and treating the disorder, and the relationship between (C)APD and functional language, learning and communicative sequelae.

CURRENT DEFINITION AND CONCEPTUALIZATION OF (C)APD

The information that guides our conceptualization of (C)APD is drawn from studies in a variety of disciplines, including but not limited to auditory and cognitive neuroscience, cognitive psychology, neuropsychology, psycholinguistics, and others. As such, several definitions and theories of (C)APD have been proposed throughout the years, with the result that a great deal of controversy has existed regarding the nature of the disorder, methods of appropriate diagnosis and intervention, and even whether the disorder exists as a distinct diagnostic entity at all (e.g., Cacace & McFarland, 2005; McFarland & Cacace, 1995). In 1996, The American Speech-Language-Hearing Association (ASHA) convened a consensus conference to elucidate these issues (ASHA, 1996). This effort was followed by other, similar conferences (e.g., Jerger & Musiek, 2000). Finally, in 2005, a technical report and position statement were set forth that form the bases for our current conceptualization of the disorder in accordance with the available evidence to date (ASHA, 2005a, 2005b).

ASHA (2005a, 2005b) defines (C)APD as a deficit in the perceptual processing of auditory stimuli and its underlying neurobiological activity in the CANS. A key element of this definition is the focus on the underlying CANS dysfunction at the neurobiological level. Support for a neurobiological basis to (C)APD has been evidenced by a plethora of studies demonstrating abnormal neurophysiologic representation of speech as well as nonspeech signals, atypical interhemispheric transfer, inefficient timing in the auditory system, and atypical hemispheric asymmetries in children and adults with the disorder (see Musiek, Bellis, & Chermak, 2005 for a review). This definition holds significant implications for the diagnosis of (C)APD in that, in order to identify the presence of a central auditory disorder, it must be shown that a deficit exists in the CANS using test tools that have been documented to demonstrate validity for the detection of CANS dysfunction (ASHA, 2005a).

Another key element of the current conceptualization of (C)APD is that, although (C)APD may lead to, or be associated with, functional difficulties in higher order language, learning, and communication, it cannot be attributed to higher order language, cognitive, or related confounds. That is, the term central auditory processing is not synonymous with the terms phonological processing, language processing, or cognitive processing, even though the overt behaviors may be similar. Therefore, application of the diagnostic label of (C)APD to the listening difficulties exhibited by children and adults with higher order, global, or pansensory deficits [e.g., attention deficit/hyperactivity disorder (ADHD), limited cognitive capacity, autism, language disorder] is not appropriate without the demonstration of a coexisting CANS deficit using test tools designed for that purpose. The interactive nature of brain organization underlies the comorbidity of (C)APD with other disorders that rely on shared neuroanatomical substrates, but (C)APD is not the result of dysfunction in other modalities (ASHA, 2005a; Bellis, 2003).

Behavioral Manifestations of (C)APD

Central auditory processing deficits can impact negatively the underlying perceptual and neural processes for localization and lateralization of sound, auditory discrimination of speech and nonspeech signals, auditory pattern recognition, temporal processing, and performance with competing and/or degraded acoustic signals (ASHA, 1996, 2005a; Bellis, 2003; Chermak & Musiek, 1997). Subsequently, persons suspected of (C)APD often present with difficulty understanding spoken language in less than ideal circumstances. For these people, challenging situations may include listening in the presence of background noise, reverberation, or competing messages. This may result in inconsistent or inappropriate responses; frequent requests for repetition, often saying "huh?" and "what?"; needing more time to respond to oral communication; difficulty following complex auditory directions or commands; inability to localize sounds; difficulty interpreting tone-of-voice and other prosodic cues; poor musical skills; and associated reading, spelling, and learning difficulties (see Bellis, 2002a, 2003 for a review). By far, this list is not exhaustive and these behaviors certainly are not exclusive to (C)APD. Individuals with learning and language disorders, ADHD, Asperger's Syndrome, and others may exhibit similar behavioral characteristics, rendering the need for accurate differential diagnosis even more critical so that appropriate, deficit-specific intervention can be undertaken.

MODALITY-SPECIFICITY OF (C)APD

One particular area of controversy concerning (C)APD has focused on the degree to which the disorder can be expected to be specific to the auditory modality. Currently, there are two primary viewpoints regarding the issue of modality-specificity as a criterion for diagnosing (C)APD. Cacace and McFarland (2005; McFarland & Cacace, 1995) have postulated that, because (C)APD is defined as an auditory perceptual dysfunction and because perceptual dysfunctions are modality-specific, (C)APD should manifest itself as an auditory-specific disorder. Further, the authors suggest that, unless modality specificity can be demonstrated, the clinical utility of a diagnosis of (C)APD is questionable. According to this viewpoint, the cortex is traditionally divided into sensory, associative, and motor areas. As such, the sensory systems are fundamentally modular, although polysensory areas are located at the borders of the modality-specific areas. It follows then that auditory-modality-specific effects can and should be expected in (C)APD.

Because any psychophysical test can be influenced by a variety of factors including language, attention, and memory, the authors suggest the need for the use of multimodal analogs of central auditory tests to verify the presence of an auditory-specific deficit in individuals suspected of (C)APD. To accomplish this goal, it is necessary to vary systematically the nature of the stimulus, while holding all other variables constant, to determine whether observed deficits are truly due to the nature of the stimulus. To diagnose (C)APD accurately, deficits in the auditory modality should be greater than those seen in other sensory modalities. The test results then may offer three possible findings: (1) "Pure" (C)APD, in which deficits are seen only in the auditory modality; (2) comorbid dysfunction, with a mixed pattern of deficits; or (3) global dysfunction, with difficulties exhibited regardless of modality. To differentiate among these possible findings, multimodal testing is critical. The authors conclude that multimodal analogs of central auditory tests are required to validate specific measures of central auditory dysfunction and, further, the clinical utility of a (C)APD diagnosis is questionable until this is done.

Logical as these assertions may seem, the ecological validity of this viewpoint has been called into question in recent years (e.g., ASHA, 2005a; Bellis, 2002b, 2003; Bellis, Billiet, & Ross, 2008; Musiek et al., 2005). There is substantial neurobiological evidence to indicate that there are few, if any, entirely compartmentalized areas of the brain responsible for a single sensory modality (e.g., Poremba et al., 2003; Salvi et al., 2002). Even in those areas of the brain previously considered to be auditory-specific, multisensory neurons exist that may respond primarily, but not solely, to auditory stimuli. Further, the close proximity of rare modality-specific neurons to polysensory areas limits the likelihood of a pure modality-specific dysfunction. In addition, studies have shown that multimodal influences can affect even the most basic of neural coding and manipulation of sensory stimuli (e.g., Calvert et al., 1997; Musacchia, Sams, Nicol, & Kraus, 2006; Sams et al., 1991). Therefore, processing of sensory data is interdependent and integrated, and supported by cognitive domains and language representations (see Musiek et al., 2005 for a review). For these reasons, ASHA (2005a) concluded that the expectation of complete modality-specificity of (C)APD is neurophysiologically untenable as it does not represent the manner in which auditory processing occurs in the human brain. Nonetheless, (C)APD certainly should manifest itself primarily in the auditory modality.

This viewpoint supports the diagnosis of (C)APD when dysfunction is primarily manifested in the auditory modality as confirmed by valid tests of central auditory function. However, because of the organizational structure of the brain, this position also acknowledges that (C)APD may coexist with other disorders that have shared or adjacent neuroanatomical substrates. Use of norm-referenced criteria is important for diagnosis; however, because nonauditory factors can influence performance on psychophysical tests of central auditory function, comparison against age-specific normative values is insufficient for differential diagnosis. Instead, test results should be analyzed for inter- and intratest patterns that are consistent with dysfunction in specific CANS regions to rule out global, supramodal, or pansensory influences. Therefore, while it is essential that the diagnosis of (C)APD relies upon tests of auditory function, multidisciplinary assessment is necessary for accurate differential diagnosis (ASHA, 2005a; Bellis, 2002a, 2002b, 2003; Musiek et al., 2005).

These two viewpoints are not entirely contradictory. Both agree that (C)APD should manifest primarily in the auditory modality, although they disagree on the issue of whether the expectation of *complete* modality specificity is consistent with the available neuroscience literature. Further, both agree that accurate differential diagnosis through a multimodal/multidisciplinary approach is imperative for the diagnosis to be meaningful. However, the two views differ on the issue of the nature of the multimodal testing that should be performed, with Cacace and McFarland (2005) suggesting the use of direct multimodal analogs and Musiek et al. (2005) and ASHA (2005a) questioning the construct validity of analog tests and advocating, instead, for the use of a multidisciplinary approach in which other modalities are assessed via test tools designed for those purposes. More recently, findings have cast further doubt on the clinical utility of multimodal analogs of central auditory function for differential diagnostic purposes, demonstrating that the use of valid central auditory tests alone can differentiate among normal listeners, listeners with (C)APD, and listeners with pansensory dysfunction such as ADHD when interpreted appropriately (Bellis, 2008; Bellis et al., 2008).

In summary, (C)APD is conceptualized as a deficit in neurobiological CANS activity that manifests itself in auditory and related symptoms. The label of (C)APD is applicable only when a specific CANS deficit can be demonstrated through the use of valid tests of central auditory function. Finally, although (C)APD typically manifests itself primarily in the auditory modality, the organization of the brain supports comorbidity of disorders. Therefore, a multidisciplinary approach to the assessment of the child or adult suspected of (C)APD is critical for differential diagnosis as well as to elucidate the relative contribution of the central auditory dysfunction to the individual's overall presenting complaints so as to direct intervention efforts.

DIAGNOSIS OF (C)APD

Because (C)APD is an auditory disorder and because diagnosis of (C)APD requires the administration of acoustically controlled and valid psychophysical and/or electrophysiologic tests of central auditory function, audiologists are the professionals uniquely qualified to make the diagnosis (ASHA, 2002, 2004). That being said, to arrive at an accurate differential diagnosis, information from a variety of sources also must be considered. Such sources may include, but are not limited to, the speech–language pathologist, educational psychologist, neuropsychologist, teacher, physician, parent or other family member, and the patients themselves. Several screening measures have been developed to aid nonaudiologists in screening for (C)APD and to facilitate diagnostic evaluation for those deemed to be at risk. Screening measures may include simple questionnaires or checklists, comprehensive multidisciplinary records review, speech-language and related measures of phonological processing and listening/auditory comprehension skills, and/or specific central auditory screening test protocols (Bellis, 2003; Jerger & Musiek, 2000; Keith, 1994, 2000b; Richard & Ferre, 2006). At this time, no one screening method has been universally accepted and, in fact, often several measures are used in combination. Unfortunately, because of the overly common and imprecise use of the term "auditory processing," several of the tools in the speech–language pathologist's or psychologist's armamentarium have been offered as diagnostic tests of (C)APD when, in fact, they are functional measures of listening and related abilities that may or may not be related to CANS integrity. It is important to note that screening tools cannot be used for diagnostic purposes, but can only indicate whether a given child or adult may require further comprehensive central auditory diagnostic testing by an audiologist.

A test battery approach is necessary to assess central auditory processes comprehensively (ASHA, 2005a; Bellis, 2003; Chermak & Musiek, 1997). Several tests are available but not all tests may be appropriate for every individual; therefore, the test battery should be developed on a case-by-case basis, depending on presenting symptoms and supplemental preassessment information. It is critical that tests selected are both sensitive (i.e., detect the presence of a disorder when it truly exists) and specific (i.e., do not identify a disorder when one is not present) for disorders of the central auditory pathways. It is equally important to recognize that results on nonaudiological tests (e.g., phonological awareness, phonemic synthesis, auditory comprehension, language) cannot be used to diagnose the presence of (C)APD; however, they may be quite useful to delineate the cognitive/communicative and related speech–language difficulties that may be associated with (C)APD (ASHA, 2005a; Bellis, 2003; Chermak & Musiek, 1997).

Both behavioral and electrophysiological auditory tests may be used to diagnose (C)APD. Electrophysiological tests aid in the objective demonstration of abnormal neurophysiologic representation of sound in the central auditory system; however, these tests may be normal in many cases of (C)APD (Bellis, 2003). Further, even when abnormal, the information obtained from these tests may provide little direction for intervention, as they do not illuminate functional difficulties. Finally, although it has been proposed that electrophysiologic tests be included as part of a standard test battery for (C)APD (e.g., Jerger & Musiek, 2000), the equipment may not be available at many sites that offer (C)APD assessment. Therefore, behavioral tests of central auditory function currently provide the best means of delineating deficient auditory processes and diagnosing (C)APD in most cases.

Several factors may affect individual performance on behavioral central auditory processing tests and need to be considered when determining appropriateness of referral, test selection, and interpretation. Factors such as chronological and developmental age, language age and experience, cognitive function, attention and memory, medications, motivation, peripheral hearing status, and other abilities all may impact results obtained on diagnostic tests (ASHA, 2005a). For example, formal behavioral diagnostic tests of central auditory function may not be warranted if a child is already known to exhibit significant cognitive impairment or if he or she is younger than approximately 7 or 8 years of age. Testing should be performed in the child's primary language; therefore, children who use English as a second language and exhibit nonnative proficiency may require limited evaluation using only nonspeech stimuli. Significant attention concerns or peripheral hearing loss likewise may preclude diagnostic central auditory testing. In short, all efforts must be made to ensure that performance deficits observed on tests of central auditory function are due to (C)APD and not to other, nonauditory-related factors.

To arrive at a diagnosis of (C)APD, performance that is more than two standard deviations below the mean must be identified on two or more central auditory tests (ASHA, 2005a; Chermak & Musiek, 1997). In addition, a pattern of test findings consistent with dysfunction in specific brain regions must be present. It is important to rule out poor performance as a result of nonauditory factors (e.g., attention, cognitive, or language issues). When inconsistency or a lack of pattern consistent with underlying neuroscience tenets is observed across the test battery, the diagnosis of (C)APD should be suspect. If performance is poor on all central tests, and other mitigating factors have been ruled out, it is most likely that a higher-level more global problem exists and the diagnostic label of (C)APD is not appropriate (ASHA, 2005a; Bellis, 2003).

INTERVENTION FOR (C)APD

Once (C)APD diagnosis is confirmed, a comprehensive intervention plan that is individualized should be implemented. Treatment and management goals should be based on the unique needs of the individual while focusing on those interventions that are most likely to have a significant impact on daily function. Selection of "high impact" recommendations that are more likely to promote compliance is essential.

A comprehensive tripod model of intervention for (C)APD has been proposed (ASHA, 2005a; Bellis, 1996, 2002a, 2002c, 2003; Bellis & Ferre, 1999). The primary components include: (1) modifications to the communication environment, especially at home, work, or school; (2) teaching of compensatory strategies that utilize higher order skills; and (3) direct remediation of skills to improve deficit skills.

Environmental (bottom-up) modifications should be used to help improve clarity and access to auditory information. In many cases, use of personal or sound field amplification systems may be warranted; however this should not be a blanket recommendation for everyone identified with (C)APD. For example, if clarity of the acoustic signal is not the main problem, use of amplification would not be warranted. If amplification is used, pre- and postassessments are necessary to determine benefit. Use of amplification should not be global. That is, it is not necessary to use the technology in nonacademic or nonwork environments. Overuse can lead to exacerbation of listening problems when technology is not available.

Compensatory strategies should be used to facilitate compensation for auditory deficits. Activities for strengthening higher order top-down skills are designed to compensate for deficient auditory skills. If less energy is expended deciphering the incoming signal, higher order resources can better support processing of auditory information and improve listening, learning, and communicative success. Compensatory strategies generally fall within two categories: cognitive/metacognitive and linguistic/metalinguistic strategies. Cognitive strategies promote self-regulation and monitoring of one's own listening to strengthen the ability to attend to auditory stimuli, enhance memory skills, and improve related cognitive resources (Chermak & Musiek, 1997). These strategies help with the development of problem-solving and self-monitoring techniques that facilitate understanding of the auditory message. Further, development of these skills encourages individuals with (C)APD to take ownership of their auditory problem.

Direct remediation activities are focused primarily on improving, to the greatest extent possible, the auditory deficit through the use of targeted auditory training activities. Such activities have been shown to result in brain reorganization and functional improvement in auditory skills (Russo, Nicol, Zecker, Hayes, & Kraus, 2005; see Musiek, Shinn, & Hare 2002; Musiek et al., 2005 for reviews).

Specific activities must be based on the functional deficit profile of the individual and be appropriate to developmental level. Further, activities should be intense, frequent, and sufficiently challenging (Chermak & Musiek, 2002). Activities may be formal (i.e., using acoustically controlled stimuli) or informal.

CENTRAL AUDITORY PROCESSING AND LANGUAGE, LEARNING, AND COMMUNICATION

Chermak and Musiek (1997) estimated that as many as half of all children identified with a learning disorder (i.e., 2–5% of the school-age population) exhibit (C)APD. Research on the older adult population has yielded substantial variation (e.g., 2–76%), largely related to differing criteria used for subject inclusion in the studies (e.g., Cooper & Gates, 1991; Golding, Carter, Mitchell, & Hood, 2004; see Bellis, 2007a for a review). Of primary interest to clinicians, educators, and others are the functional sequelae associated with (C)APD. As indicated in the previous section, (C)APD may lead to or be associated with difficulties that span language, learning, and communicative domains. However, because of the heterogeneous nature of (C)APD, along with the heterogeneity observed in language, learning, and related disorders, a direct one-to-one correlation between fundamental auditory processes and language/learning outcomes is difficult to demonstrate in large groups of subjects (ASHA, 2005a). Moreover, not every (C)APD is associated with learning, language, or related disorders and, conversely, not every learning or related difficulty can be attributed to an underlying (C)APD, even if the behavioral manifestations are similar. Nonetheless, recent research has highlighted relationships among (C)APD and specific language impairment, reading difficulties, ADHD, learning disability, speech production disorders, and others (e.g., Bellis, 2002a, 2003; Bellis & Ferre, 1999; Moncrieff & Musiek, 2002; Tillery, Katz, & Keller, 2000).

In the previous section, the importance of inter- and intratest pattern analysis of performance on central auditory tests for diagnosis of (C)APD was emphasized. In recent years, these patterns have been analyzed and developed into functional deficit profiling models (Bellis, 2002a, 2003; Bellis & Ferre, 1999; Katz, 1992). Bellis (2007b) identified three caveats when using functional deficit profiling methods. First, the profiles must be consistent with the underlying neuroscience. Therefore, they must be iterative in nature, evolving as additional information is gleaned from the auditory neuroscience and related literature. Second, profiling methods should not be used as "cookbook" approaches to diagnosing or treating processing disorders. Rarely, if ever, will a child or adult fit every symptom and finding possible in a given subprofile, and individualization of both the diagnosis and the intervention is critical. Third, causality should not be assumed when comorbidity of functional deficits is observed. In some cases, evidence does support a causal relationship between deficient auditory processes and higher order language-learning or related difficulties. In these situations, intervention for the auditory deficit may be expected to facilitate improvement in these higher order functions. However, in others, comorbidity may be a reflection of shared neuroanatomical

substrates and the interactive nature of brain organization. In these cases, differential intervention for each of the co-presenting disorders is indicated.

Drawing from the vast body of literature investigating brain-behavior relationships across functional domains, Bellis and Ferre (1999) have proposed a functional deficit profiling model of (C)APD that relates specific CANS dysfunction and associated central auditory test findings with language, learning, and communicative sequelae. First offered by Bellis (1996), this model has undergone substantial revisions in recent years in accordance with new findings in the auditory neuroscience, neuropsychology, cognitive science, and related literature. At present, the Bellis/Ferre Model consists of three primary subprofiles, representing dysfunction in left-, right-, and interhemispheric brain regions. A brief overview of each of these profiles follows. Readers are referred to Bellis (2002a, 2003) for a comprehensive treatment of this topic.

LEFT-HEMISPHERE (PRIMARY AUDITORY CORTEX) DYSFUNCTION

Speech sounds, especially those with very rapidly changing spectrotemporal acoustic features such as stop consonants, as well as linguistic content are processed primarily in the dominant (usually left) hemisphere. Specifically, the primary auditory cortex is highly specialized to represent temporal (timing-related) aspects of speech sounds and to facilitate auditory closure, or the ability to fill in missing components of a message. Individuals with dysfunction in this region often present with the hallmark symptom of difficulty listening in noise due to poor phonemic representation and auditory closure abilities. They may request repetitions and may "mis-hear" words, often substituting similar sounding phonemes. For example, some sounds/words may be easily confused such as *dime* and *time*, or *shop* and *shock*. Central auditory dysfunction involving the primary auditory cortex of the left hemisphere has been termed Auditory Decoding Deficit in the Bellis/Ferre model.

Associated symptoms may include reading and spelling difficulties primarily focused on word-attack abilities, or the "sound" portion of sound–symbol association. A phonics approach often is used to teach children to spell and read. If sounds are not processed correctly, it becomes a challenge to acquire adequate spelling and reading skills. The phonics approach assumes the child can hear the fine acoustic differences between speech sounds and apply them to sound–symbol relationships. Children with left-hemisphere central auditory dysfunction may struggle with sounding out new words, generating "invented spelling" samples, and other aspects of reading and spelling associated with phonological representation. These same children may, likewise, exhibit difficulties with speech production, particularly of speech sounds with very similar acoustic features, and may exhibit substitutions of similar sounding phonemes (e.g., /d/ for /g/), deletions of weak or final phonemes, and other hallmarks of a "hearing loss," despite normal peripheral hearing sensitivity.

Other language and vocabulary concerns may be apparent as well, as is often seen with peripheral hearing loss. However, as (C)APD is conceptualized as an input disorder, receptive skills typically are poorer than (or commensurate with) expressive skills. In addition, these individuals may exhibit better nonverbal cognitive abilities as compared to verbal, and likely perform best with visual or multimodal augmentations.

Behavioral central auditory diagnostic testing in children and adults with this type of (C)APD reveals a clear pattern of deficits that points to primary auditory cortical dysfunction, poor auditory discrimination of speech sounds involving rapid spectrotemporal acoustic change, and poor temporal resolution abilities. In addition, if electrophysiologic evaluation is conducted, responses often are attenuated over left-hemisphere electrode sites, suggesting inefficient neurophysiologic representation of acoustic signals, especially speech stimuli.

Because the associated sequelae in the areas of reading–spelling, speech production, and other areas are presumed to be causally related to inefficient speech sound representation in the auditory cortex in Auditory Decoding Deficit, auditory interventions for the (C)APD are critical to the overall intervention plan, and often can facilitate improvement in these other, higher order functional areas.

RIGHT-HEMISPHERE DYSFUNCTION

Right-hemisphere dysfunction, or Prosodic Deficit in the Bellis/Ferre model, is associated with deficits in processing rhythm, stress, intonation, and other prosodic elements of speech. Because the nondominant (usually right) hemisphere is implicated in nonspeech processing, especially that related to music, linguistic, and speech-sound processing typically is spared in children and adults with Prosodic Deficit. Instead, individuals with right-hemisphere (C)APD often exhibit difficulties with comprehending the *intent*, rather than the *content*, of a communication. This may lead to communicative misunderstandings related to misreading tone-of-voice cues. Associated communicative symptoms may include difficulty sequencing auditory events, extracting key words from a message, part-to-whole synthesis required for understanding the main idea of a communication, and comprehending abstract language forms.

The right hemisphere also has been implicated in a variety of other functions, including but not limited to visual–spatial abilities, part-to-whole Gestalt processing, mathematics calculation, the ability to disengage and re-engage attention, and others. Therefore, (C)APD involving the right hemisphere may be accompanied by difficulties in these areas as well. Further, nonverbal cognitive capacity may be lower than verbal capacity, and music and art skills may be described as weak or nonexistent. Reading and spelling difficulties may occur; however, these differ in nature from those associated with Auditory Decoding Deficit. In children with Prosodic Deficit, the "symbol" portion of sound–symbol association is more likely to be impacted, leading to poor sight-word (or automatic) reading and spelling abilities, but spared phonological decoding (word attack) abilities.

Behavioral central auditory testing reveals a clear pattern of deficit consistent with right-hemisphere dysfunction, including difficulty perceiving nonverbal tonal patterns and difficulty with nonspeech discrimination. Electrophysiologic testing may indicate reduced responses over right-hemisphere electrode sites to nonspeech stimuli.

It is important to note that the nonauditory sequelae that may accompany Prosodic Deficit likely arise due to shared neuroanatomical resources in the affected hemisphere and, thus, are not likely to be causally related to the auditory deficit. Thus, while auditory interventions are indicated to address the functional listening and communicative complaints, presenting symptoms in visuospatial processing, reading–spelling, mathematics calculation, and other areas, if present, likely will require deficit-specific intervention.

Interhemispheric (Corpus Callosum) Dysfunction

Dysfunction of the interhemispheric pathways via the corpus callosum may result in difficulties with any task, auditory or not, in which both sides of the brain need to work in coordination. This, the most common form of (C)APD, has been termed Integration Deficit in the Bellis/Ferre model.

The hallmark, and often the primary symptom, of Integration Deficit is significant difficulty hearing in noise. The corpus callosum is critical to localization and tracking of a sound source across the midline and, as such, dysfunction in these pathways will disrupt speech-in-noise abilities. Associated symptoms vary widely, and may include difficulty with bimanual/bipedal skills, difficulty playing musical instruments such as the piano, dislike of video games requiring rapid bimanual movements, and others. Inability to link prosodic and linguistic elements of speech, such as that required for the appreciation of sarcasm, may be impacted, as well, as may reading and spelling abilities reliant upon the "association" element of sound–symbol association. That is, word-attack and sight-word abilities typically are intact when assessed independently of one another, but rapid switching between the two strategies such as is required for fluent reading may be difficult, thus leading to reduced reading fluency. Despite the presence of these associated symptoms in corpus callosum dysfunction, it is critical to note that the auditory symptoms are paramount, and these other difficulties typically are subtle and not consistent with global dysfunction such as that seen in sensory integration disorder.

Behavioral central auditory findings reveal a classic pattern of deficit consistent with corpus callosum dysfunction; however, electrophysiologic testing often is normal in cases of Integration Deficit. Nonetheless, atypical hemispheric asymmetries in response amplitudes to speech stimuli may be observed in some cases (Bellis, Nicol, & Kraus, 2000).

Auditory intervention for Integration Deficit typically focuses on improving binaural separation abilities (the ability to attend to one stimulus in the presence of a competing signal). Interestingly, any activity that requires the two hemispheres of the brain to work cooperatively can have a beneficial impact on the auditory and related symptoms of this disorder, including video games and piano lessons. The multimodal nature of the corpus callosum lends itself to a variety of intervention techniques.

In summary, the Bellis/Ferre model of (C)APD provides a guide for clinicians to recognize the auditory neuroscience findings and related functional multi-modal sequelae that may be associated with dysfunction in left-, right-, and inter-hemispheric cortical regions. It is not intended to be a catch-all, cookie-cutter approach to (C)APD diagnosis and intervention and, indeed, a great deal of individual variability exists within each of these functional deficit profiles. Neither is it intended to suggest that all forms of (C)APD are represented in the model. Indeed, recent research indicates that a substantial portion of children with reading-related disorders may exhibit abnormal brainstem timing for speech as measured by the Biological Marker of Auditory Processing (BioMARK) elec-trophysiologic tool (Johnson, Nicol, & Kraus, 2005) These same children have been shown to respond favorably to auditory training (Russo et al., 2005). Most interestingly, it appears that the children with abnormal brainstem timing may not meet current diagnostic criteria for (C)APD based upon behavioral tests of central auditory function and, as such, would be missed and likely would not receive a recommendation for auditory intervention (Billiet, 2008). These emerging findings suggest that consideration of additional functional deficit pro-files, especially ones that take into account brainstem-level processing of speech signals, is indicated.

SUMMARY AND CONCLUSIONS

(Central) auditory processing disorder is considered a perceptual disorder that is primarily related to processing of auditory stimuli and the neurobiological activity underlying that processing. The (C)APD may coexist with other language and learning disorders due to shared neuroanatomical substrates in the brain. Although the diagnosis of (C)APD is made by the audiologist, it is imperative that a multidisciplinary approach be utilized to facilitate accurate diagnosis and effective comprehensive intervention.

REFERENCES

American Speech-Language-Hearing Association. (1996). Central auditory processing: Current status of research and implications for clinical practice. *American Journal of Audiology, 5*(2), 41–54.

American Speech-Language-Hearing Association. (2002). *Guidelines for audiology service provision in and for the schools.* Rockville, MD: American Speech-Language-Hearing Association.

American Speech-Language-Hearing Association (2004). *Scope of practice in audiology.* Rockville, MD: American Speech-Language-Hearing Association.

American Speech-Language-Hearing Association. (2005a). (Central) Auditory Processing Disorders. Available at http://www.asha.org/members/deskref-journals/deskref/default

American Speech-Language-Hearing Association. (2005b). (Central) Auditory Processing Disorders—The role of the audiologist [Position statement]. Available at http://www.asha.org/members/deskref-journals/deskref/default

Bellis, T. J. (1996). *Assessment and management of central auditory processing disorders in the educational setting: From science to practice.* San Diego, CA: Singular Publishing.

Bellis, T. (2002a). *When the brain can't hear: Unraveling the mystery of auditory processing disorder.* New York, NY: Pocket Books.

Bellis, T. J. (2002b). Considerations in diagnosing auditory processing disorders in children. *American Speech-Language-Hearing Association Special Interest Division 9 (Hearing and Hearing Disorders in Children), 12,* 3–9.

Bellis, T. (2002c). Developing deficit-specific intervention plans for individuals with auditory processing disorders. *Seminars in Hearing, 23*(4), 287–295.

Bellis, T. (2003). *Assessment and management of central auditory processing disorders in the educational setting: From science to practice* (2nd ed.). Clifton Park, NY: Thomson Learning.

Bellis, T. J. (2007a). Differential diagnosis of (C)APD in older listeners. In G. D. Chermak & F. E. Musiek (Eds.), *Handbook of central auditory processing disorder: Volume 1: Diagnosis.* San Diego, CA: Plural Publishing.

Bellis, T. (2007b). Historical foundations and the nature of (C)APD. In F. Musiek, & G. Chermak (Eds.), *Handbook of (central) auditory processing disorder: Auditory neuroscience and diagnosis volume I* (pp. 128–129). San Diego, CA: Plural Publishing.

Bellis, T. J. (2008, November). *Defining and diagnosing (C)APD: A question of modality specificity.* Paper presented at the American Speech-Language-Hearing Association Annual meeting, Chicago, IL.

Bellis, T. J., Billiet, C., & Ross, J. (2008). Hemispheric lateralization of bilaterally presented homologous visual and auditory stimuli in normal adults, normal children, and children with central auditory dysfunction. *Brain and Cognition, 66,* 280–289.

Bellis, T., & Ferre, J. (1999). Multidimensional approach to the differential diagnosis of central auditory processing disorders in children. *Journal of the American Academy of Audiology, 10,* 319–328.

Bellis, T. J., Nicol, T., & Kraus, N. (2000). Aging affects hemispheric asymmetry in the neural representation of speech sounds. *Journal of Neuroscience, 20,* 791–797.

Billiet, C. R. (2008). *Relationship between brainstem temporal processing and performance on tests of central auditory function in children with reading disorders.* Unpublished audiology capstone, University of South Dakota.

Cacace, A. T., & McFarland, D. J. (2005). The importance of modality specificity in diagnosing central auditory processing disorder. *American Journal of Audiology, 14,* 112–123.

Calvert, G. A., Bullmore, E. T., Brammer, M. J., Campbell, R., Williams, S. C. R., McGuire, P. K., … David, A. S. (1997). Activation of auditory cortex during silent lipreading. *Science, 276,* 593–596.

Chermak, G., & Musiek, F. (1997). *Central auditory processing disorders: New perspectives.* San Diego, CA: Singular Publishing Group.

Chermak, G., & Musiek, F. (2002). Auditory training: Principles and approaches for remediating and managing auditory processing disorders. *Seminars in Hearing, 23*(4), 297–308.

Cooper, J., & Gates, G. (1991). Hearing in the elderly: The Framingham cohort, 1983–1985. Part II. Prevalence of central auditory processing disorders. *Ear and Hearing, 12,* 304–311.

Golding, M., Carter, N., Mitchell, P., & Hood, L. (2004). Prevalence of central auditory processing (CAP) abnormality in an older australian population: The Blue Mountains hearing study. *Journal of the American Academy of Audiology, 15,* 633–642.

Jerger, J., & Musiek, F. (2000). Report of the consensus conference on the diagnosis of auditory processing disoders in school-aged children. *Journal of the American Academy of Audiology, 11,* 467–474.

Johnson, K. L., Nicol, T., & Kraus, N. (2005, review). The brainstem response to speech: A biological marker. *Ear and Hearing, 26*(5), 424–433.

Katz, J. (1992). Classification of auditory processing disorders. In J. Katz (Ed.), *Central auditory processing: A transdisciplinary view* (pp. 81–91). St. Louis, MO: Mosby Year Book.

Keith, R. (1977). *Central auditory dysfunction.* New York, NY: Grune & Stratton.

Keith, R. (1994). *SCAN-A: A test for auditory processing disorders in adolescents and adults.* San Antonio, TX: Psychological Corporation.

Keith, R. (2000a). *Random gap detection test.* St. Louis, MO: Auditec.

Keith, R. (2000b). *SCAN-C: Test for auditory processing disorders in children-revised.* San Antonio, TX: The Psychological Corporation.

McFarland, D. J., & Cacace, A. T. (1995). Modality specificity as a criterion for diagnosing central auditory processing disorders. *American Journal of Audiology, 4*(3), 36–48.

Moncrieff, D., & Musiek, F. (2002). Interaural asymmetries revealed by dichotic listening tests in normal and dyslexic children. *Journal of the American Academy of Audiology, 13,* 428–437.

Musacchia G. E., Sams, M., Nicol, T. G., & Kraus, N. (2006). Seeing speech affects acoustic information processing in the human brainstem. *Experimental Brain Research, 16,* 1–10. Also at http://www.soc.northwestern.edu/brainvolts/documents/MusacchiaetalExpBrainRes2005.pdf

Musiek, F., Bellis, T., & Chermak, G. (2005). Nonmodularity of the central auditory nervoussystem: Implications for (central) auditory processing disorder. *American Journal of Audiology, 14,* 128–138.

Musiek, F. E., Shinn, J., & Hare, C. (2002). Plasticity, auditory training, and auditory processing disorders. *Seminars in Hearing, 23*(4), 263–275.

Myklebust, H. (1954). *Auditory disorders in children.* New York, NY: Grune & Stratton.

Poremba, A., Saunders, R., Crane, A., Cook, M., Sokoloff, L., & Mishkin, M. (2003). Functional mapping of the primate auditory system. *Science, 299,* 568–571.

Richard, G. J., & Ferre, J. M. (2006). *Differential screening test for processing.* East Moline, IL: LinguiSystems, Inc.

Russo, N., Nicol, T., Zecker, S., Hayes, E., & Kraus, N. (2005). Auditory training improves neural timing in the human brainstem. *Behavioural Brain Research, 156,* 95–103. Also at www.soc.northwestern.edu/brainvolts/projects/documents/Russoetal2005BehavBrainRes.pdf

Salvi, R., Lockwood, A., Frisina, R., Coad, M., Wack, D., & Frisina, D. (2002). PET imaging of the normal human auditory system: Responses to speech in quiet and background noise. *Hearing Research, 170,* 96–106.

Sams, M., Aulanko, R., Hamalainen, M., Hari, R., Lounasmaa, O. V., Lu, S. T., & Simola, J. (1991). Seeing speech: Visual information from lip movements modifies activity in the human auditory cortex. *Neuroscience Letters, 127,* 141–145.

Tillery, K., Katz, J., & Keller, W. (2000). Effects of methylphenidate (Ritalin) on auditory performance in children with attention and auditory processing disorders. *Journal of Speech, Language, and Hearing Research, 43,* 893–901.

18 Temporal Processing in Children With Language Disorders

Martha Burns

Scientists have attempted to understand the seemingly effortless process of language acquisition in infants for decades. Despite the acoustic complexity of speech input and apparent limited neurological processing resources of an immature neonatal brain, most infants master their native language in a few years. To accomplish this, the infant must extract from the continuous auditory signals in the environment meaningful segments that constitute phonemes, syllables, and words and determine how they combine into meaningful strings (Dehaene-Lambertz et al., 2006). The process proceeds predictably and effortlessly despite variability in language exposure or culture (Kuhl, 2000). This ease with which children acquire language and the uniformity across languages led Noam Chomsky in 1986 to propose that human infants must possess an innate neurological capacity to acquire language (Chomsky, 1986). The exact nature of this "language acquisition device" has been debated and researched ever since. Yet, as Patricia Kuhl states in a thorough review of the research on language acquisition mechanisms, "cracking the speech code is child's play for human infants but [remains] an unsolved problem for adult theorists and our machines" (Kuhl, 2004). Even more perplexing, perhaps, is why a small proportion (6–7%) of children, without sensory, motor, or nonverbal cognitive deficits, fail to develop normal language skills despite exposure to their native language (Tomblin, Records, & Zhang, 1996).

HISTORICAL PERSPECTIVE ON ISSUES OF CAUSATION IN LANGUAGE DISORDERS

Although the cause(s) of problems learning language might seem an important issue for those scientific disciplines that study normal language acquisition as well as those that treat language disorders, the issue of causation has been mired in controversy and led to divisions within and between those scientific disciplines for over 40 years. In the 1960s, the relatively new fields of speech pathology and audiology began to back away from "etiologic" approaches to classification of communicative disorders in general in an abandonment of the "medical model" that biased research and training toward finding and curing disease (Irwin, 1964). Marge, in a chapter in one of the early books on language disorders written in the early 1970s, further elaborated on the need to deemphasize etiology in under-standing language disorders, citing a primary reason that it implies that there might be a single cause that, if identified, could be corrected and the disability eliminated (1972). But perhaps a greater influence on attempts to find and treat causes of language disorders came from the impact of two scientific disciplines that dramatically influenced language research in the late 1950s and continue to influence research on language pathology to this day. The first was behavioral psychology, B. F. Skinner's reaction to Gestalt psychology, which predominated discussions of language learning beginning in the late 1950s. He attributed lan-guage learning to stimulus-response contingencies, and advocated for measure-ment (and by implication treatment) of only observable phenomenon (Skinner, 1957). The second, which stood in opposition to Skinner's behaviorist explana-tions of language development, was linguistics, where Noam Chomsky's seminal theories of generative grammar (1959) revolutionized the study of language as a solely human capacity and focused on the study of language structure (1957). As he developed his theory, Chomskyís underlying assumption was that although language performance may not be error free, humans possess an innate capacity to learn and use language, a "language competence" that consists of a set of finite computational "rules" that allow children to acquire language quickly, easily, and effortlessly and allow for infinite and creative use of language to express complex ideas (1964).

Chomsky's theories revolutionized not only the field of linguistics, but also cog-nitive psychology and speech pathology. The study of language acquisition changed from attempts to "measure language skill" milestones (such as Templin's norms for specific speech sound use or vocabulary counts) to specifying the hierarchy for how word order and grammatical form are acquired (Brown, 1973). Instead of relying on vague quantitative measures to gauge language development, one could analyze phrase structure, average length of utterance, and acquisition of specific gram-matical and morphological forms (Lee, 1974). Transformational grammar, and the developmental studies that applied it, also provided a framework for systematically analyzing language disorders and treating the presumed underlying hierarchical linguistic deficits using a developmental model. The availability of a developmen-tal model and tests that provided objective measures of syntactical comprehension and use reduced the concern over identification of etiology. Chomsky's theories ultimately led to the emergence of a new scientific discipline, psycholinguistics (Boden, 2006), which focused the fields of cognitive science and psychology on the importance of language to human cognition. This in turn, provided an enor-mous boost to the field of speech pathology by emphasizing the need for identifica-tion and remediation of language problems in children; ultimately leading in 1978 to the addition of Language in the name of the professional organization ASHA (from the American Speech and Hearing Association to the American Speech-Language-Hearing Association), and resulting in an approximate fivefold increase in certified ASHA members during the same time period (www.asha.com).

However, despite the decreased interest in and emphasis on causation in lin-guistics and speech–language pathology, others scientific disciplines continued to seek causative explanations for language disorders in children. The field of learning disabilities, for example, was initially rooted in neurological explanations for language disorders (Johnson & Myklebust, 1967). Similarly, some cognitive psychology researchers continued to seek causal explanations for language disorders. Tallal and Piercy were among the most influential researchers in the field of psychology to explore nonverbal auditory processing disturbances that might underlie problems learning language (1973). Yet, because of the profound influence of Chomsky during the period when their original research was published and the prevailing viewpoint that language was an innate human capacity, many psycholinguists originally dismissed their findings, maintaining that nonverbal processing could not play a significant part in a neurological faculty innately derived through a "language acquisition device" (Burns, 2007). Today, although some controversy persists regarding the importance of auditory processing in language acquisition (Bishop, Carlyon, Deeks, & Bishop, 1999), the prevalence of interdisciplinary research involving developmental psycholinguistics, clinicians and neuroscientists has led to a resurgence of interest in causal mechanisms of language disturbance and recognition of the importance of timing and synchrony in neurological cognitive systems (Boden, 2006).

In this regard, what is now often referred to as the "temporal processing hypothesis," stemming from the research of Tallal and Piercy in the 1970s, has been refined and studied extensively in recent years. Essentially the hypothesis asserts that some language impaired children have difficulty processing rapidly changing acoustic details, which interferes with their ability to adequately parse incoming language signals into phonemes and thereby have an increased risk of developing speech, language, and/or reading problems (Tallal & Piercy, 1974; Tallal & Stark, 1981). This explanation essentially views the capacity to process rapidly changing sensory inputs as a probable core neurological component of phonological processing. How this core capacity is understood by neuroscience and the role it may play in language acquisition is an unfolding scientific inquiry. This chapter will attempt to review and clarify the current state of neuroscience research that led to and supports the temporal processing hypothesis and will review research on assessment and the remediation value to auditory training of temporal processing skills. However, the viewpoint of this chapter is that the consideration of the role of temporal processing in language learning does not necessitate rejecting Chomsky or the vast accumulation of psycholinguistic research on language learning and language disorders. Rather, it is the perspective of this author, that understanding temporal processing adds to what some might consider the top-down influence of language and conceptual knowledge on learning by specifying co-occurring bottom-up processes that influence language learning as well.

ORIGINS OF THE TEMPORAL PROCESSING HYPOTHESIS

All scientific disciplines begin with a set of underlying principles that define the science. Margaret Boden, a preeminent archivist of historical perspectives in cognitive science, has recently likened the child learning language to the scientist, who, "formulates theories and hypotheses which suggest what to look for, and where to look for it" (Boden, 2006, p. 647). As speech–language pathologists, audiologists, and psychologists, our science is based in behavior. We tend to study the observable behavioral outcomes to controlled stimuli. In general, we attempt to conduct group research studies where we test hypotheses about factors we theorize may lead to specific behavioral outcomes. Neuroscience is a relatively new scientific discipline that is an outgrowth of medicine (neurology), cognitive science, psychology, and computational studies of neurophysiology that blends all disciplines in an attempt to understand brain function (Bishop, Carlyon, Deeks, & Bishop, 1999). Cognitive neuroscience, for example, uses physical data from brain imaging of various types to attempt to understand the brain processes that underlie specific behaviors. The Temporal Processing Hypothesis is an outgrowth cognitive neuroscience research that seeks to identify neurological processing characteristics that may define and underlie cognitive development. To that end, cognitive neuroscientists distinguish bottom-up from top-down neurological factors in neurological information processing, and seek to define those processes that seem critical to acquisition of any cognitive skill.

TOP-DOWN VERSUS BOTTOM-UP ATTENTIONAL AND PERCEPTUAL PROCESSES

Imagine you are on a bus in a foreign country for the first time and you hear a stream of dialogue in a foreign tongue that you have never experienced before. At the same time you are aware that the speakers, sitting just across from you are having a very animated discussion about what appears to be a minor accident in the street. Chances are, as an adult with a well-developed knowledge of how language is organized and years of experience using nonverbal pragmatic cues to guide comprehension, you would begin to use context, gestures, intonation, and facial expression to figure out some of the content of the conversation. You could, for example, probably very easily discern whether the speakers are happy, angry, or sad; in agreement or disagreement; friends or strangers; and so on. If they are pointing or looking at the scene outside the bus, you may also be able to extract meaning from some of their spoken words, especially if spoken with expression and if they resemble words of your own language. That ability to use past knowledge and experience to extract meaning from a sensory event is referred to in neuroscience as "top-down" processing. It has been described and researched thoroughly in the visual processing neuroscience literature (Corbetta & Schulman, 2002) and applied to conceptualization and research on auditory processing disorders in children (Chermak & Musiek, 1998). If on the other hand you wanted to say or repeat words or phrases that were spoken by the foreign speakers, with no prior experience with that language, you would need to attend to different aspects of the conversation. As an adult you would struggle to attend to the internal details of the words. As linguists we could describe that task as determining the phonological composition of the words. As acousticians we might describe the process as identifying and discriminating the relevant temporal or spatial acoustic events that signal differences in meaning. Cognitive neuroscientists and audiologists refer to that, "data driven" analysis of incoming sensory events as "bottom-up" processing (Chermak & Musiek, 1998).

In most human sensory processing, both top-down and bottom-up processing is thought to occur simultaneously, through distributed neuronal networks that allow application of past knowledge and experience to the task of attending to and learning from novel sensory information. Fortunately, through advances in neuroimaging technology, scientists can now observe these processing systems at work by carefully controlling sensory events and responses and documenting how the brain changes its strategy to handle top-down versus bottom-up tasks (Cabeza, Ciaramelli, Olson, & Moscovitch, 2008). One component of bottom-up processing of auditory information gleaned from neuroscience research that appears to be essential for learning language is the ability to process rapidly changing sensory inputs (Tallal, 2004). To understand how this relates to language acquisition a discussion of neurological processing of sensory information is helpful.

HOW THE BRAIN PROCESSES SENSORY INFORMATION

To explain neuroscience exploration of perception, one has to review a few principles of neurological processing. First, although a neuron essentially has only two ways to respond to a stimulus, fire or not fire, the firing rate of serial spikes is likely the mechanisms neurons use to convey information. This is often referred to in systems neuroscience as the "neural code" (Van Vreeswijk, 2006). Therefore single neurons probably do not convey much information in isolation, but rather form networks by connecting to other neuron groups that work together to fire in patterns (Mesulam, 2000). Just as a single instrument in a symphony orchestra might not play a recognizable melody by itself, the combined contribution of all of the instruments yields a recognizable composition (Kenet, Arieli, Tsodyks, & Grinvald, 2006). Following that analogy, neurons fire in patterns that must combine to convey information. But what are these patterns?

Neuroscientists have discovered through several different methods of studying neuronal firing patterns that neurons, similar to musical instruments in a band or orchestra, seem to convey information by their firing rate and rhythm. Rate and rhythm are temporal (timed) aspects of a signal. If a person claps out the rhythm of "Happy Birthday," without humming the melody or singing the words, most people who know the song can identify it just from the rhythm. But if the rhythm gets distorted by clapping some of the measures too quickly in relation to the others, omitting some of the claps, or inserting pauses or extra claps where they do not belong, then the rhythm becomes unidentifiable. It is no accident that the temporal lobe of the brain is responsible for perception of sound; perception of sound requires analysis of the temporal aspects of the acoustic signal that are referred to as temporal acoustic cues. When one observes the brain at work, processing speech for example, there are regions of the left frontal lobe that appear to be essential when decoding requires handling rapidly changing temporal events (Temple et al., 2000). There is recent evidence that abnormal processing in that area correlates with reading disability (Nagarian et al., 1999), and, of perhaps greater importance, is remediable (Merzenich et al., 1996), and when remediated, improves language (Tallal et al., 1996) and reading skills (Gaab, Gabrieli, Deutsch, Tallal, & Temple, 2007). This research points to the importance of understanding this neurological capacity to process information in a temporal array, and how that contributes to bottom-up processing required for language acquisition and reading skill.

TEMPORAL PROCESSING AND LANGUAGE ACQUISITION

Speech is, of course, a flow of rapidly changing acoustic events. As stated above, "temporal processing" refers to the ability to process rapidly changing temporal events, both in a stream of speech and also in nonspeech acoustic events. From a neurological perspective, rapid changes are those that occur in tens of milliseconds. In speech, acoustic cues that we use to discriminate phonemes, like voice onset time and place of articulation, for example, are signaled by such rapidly occurring changes in the acoustic signal. Neuroscientists have found that those rapid changes in the physical properties of sound are represented by rapid neurological firing patterns in the primary auditory cortex that can be directly measured through various psychophysical and physiological methods. These cortical representations have been shown to differ in adults with reading problems when compared to those with no history of reading problems (Nagarijan et al., 1999) as well as infants as young as three months old who have immediate family members with language problems (Benasich et al., 2006).

Tallal and Piercy's finding that problems processing rapidly successive auditory changes are correlated with language problems does not by itself support the contention that language acquisition is dependent on the fidelity of this processing system. Some authors over the past two decades have questioned the possibility of a causative relationship between temporal processing and language acquisition because most individuals with reading problems, especially, ultimately develop adequate phonological production and do not appear to have altered aural speech recognition abilities (Bishop et al., 1999) and that studies of children with language problems suggest that the auditory processing issues may be the result of immature patterns that resolve naturally over time (Bishop & McArthur, 2004). These authors and others believe that the failure to master language and/or reading is more likely due to problems with top-down ability to segment words into sounds and syllables (phonological awareness) or other deficits in higher-level aspects of language learning, perhaps affected by working memory or other cognitive constraints (Snowling, 1990; Swan & Goswami, 1997). But interdisciplinary cognitive scientists and developmental psychologists are asserting that, given the abundance of research supporting both scientific contentions, both bottom-up and top-down processing are necessary for normal language acquisition (Thomas & Karmiloff-Smith, 2003).

ASSESSMENT OF TEMPORAL PROCESSING DISORDERS

Fortunately, audiologists who specialize in diagnosing auditory processing disorders (APD) have developed a battery of tests that can be used to diagnose temporal processing. The original research of Tallal and Piercy, used a two-tone temporal sequencing task to measure temporal processing in children with language disorders (see Figure 18.1). The test, later named the Tallal Repetition Test, involved asking children to sequence two tones in which the interstimulus interval (the period of time between the two tones) decreased from slightly over 4 seconds between tones (4062 ms) to less than a 100th of a second (8 ms). This is the task that has been consistently shown to distinguish children with language problems from those developing language normally.

Rawool has recently provided an excellent summary of tasks used by audiologists to assess temporal processing (2007). The tests include gap detection, backward masking, temporally degraded speech, masking level differences, and many others. It is beyond the scope of this chapter to describe the tests that are used by audiologists to diagnosis differing temporal processing disorders and it is not known which of those tests are best at identifying the temporal processing difficulties that distinguish children with language problems from those with normal language. However, it is recommended that children with speech language or literacy problems for whom speech discrimination, phonic decoding, phonological awareness, or auditory working memory are present receive a thorough auditory processing evaluation by a qualified audiologist to determine the degree to which temporal processing problems may be contributing to the difficulties.

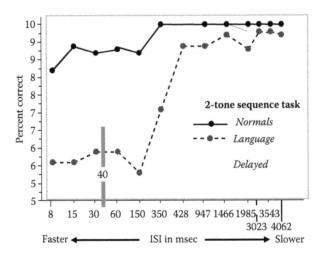

FIGURE 18.1   Normal vs. language impaired seven year old's % correct on a two tone sequencing task as interstimulus interval decreases (right to left) from just over 4 seconds to 8 ms.

TEMPORAL PROCESSING AND REMEDIATION
OF LANGUAGE PROBLEMS

The final issue to be addressed with respect to the Temporal Processing Hypothesis and language disorders is twofold: Can temporal processing problems be remediated and if so, what is the effect on language skills? The first controlled research studies that demonstrated the value of temporal processing intervention with language impaired children was published in 1996. The first study reported by Merzenich et al., was conducted with seven children, ages 5.9–9.1 with language learning impairments who participated in two 20-minute temporal processing exercises (one very similar to the two-tone sequencing task of Tallal and Piercy, the other a phonetic element recognition exercise) 5 days a week for 4 weeks. At the conclusion of the training the children showed significant gains in temporal processing as measured by the Tallal Repetition Test as well as significant gains in speech discrimination as well as averaging 1.5 years gain in measures of language development (Merzenich et al., 1996; Tallal, et al., 1996).

A second study was then conducted using a larger sample of 22 language impaired children who were divided into two groups matched for nonverbal intelligence and receptive speech and language skills. Four exercises were used for training the experimental group, the initial two exercises that had been improved for ability to maintain the childrenís attention and two other exercises that stressed categorical perception of sounds in syllables and the other, a minimal pairs forced choice task. The control group played video games. Both groups received language intervention, but the experimental group had exposure to speech that had been digitally modified to enhance rapid temporal elements and the control group had the same exercises without the acoustic enhancement. Both groups showed benefit from the language intervention, but the experimental group showed significantly greater improvement in language and temporal processing skills (Merzenich et al., 1996; Tallal, et al., 1996). Taken together these two studies provided further evidence that temporal processing deficits were a factor in language disorders and that remediation of temporal processing could be achieved through practice with temporal processing tasks and speech sound discrimination activities. But of great import was the finding of the second study showing that when temporal processing tasks and acoustically modified speech are included in a treatment protocol it enhances the therapeutic outcomes significantly.

Several studies have been conducted since the original 1996 research that have reported positive effects of the intervention protocol developed by Merzenich, Tallal, and colleagues subsequently published as Fast ForWord and later Fast ForWord Language, with children who have cochlear implants (Schopmeyer, Mellon, Dobaj, Grant, & Nipapko, 2000), adults with aphasia (Dronkers et al., 1999), adults with dyslexia (Temple et al., 2003), and children with dyslexia (Gaab, et al., 2007; Temple, et al., 2003). There has been a study reported where Fast ForWord Language was not shown to be more effective than computerized remediation without the temporal processing components of acoustically modified speech (Cohen et al., 2005), and another with a small group of reading impaired children with half from impoverished socioeconomic environments (Pokorni, Worthington, & Jamison, 2004).

Recently, Ron Gillam and associates reported on a 3-year randomized controlled trial comparing Fast ForWord Language with other interventions including one-on-one language therapy, other computerized language interventions with language impaired children showing that all the interventions, when administered in an intensive 2 hour per day, 5 day a week protocol during 8 week summer sessions resulted in significant language improvements with no significant differences between the groups. In addition, using backward masking as a measure of temporal processing the authors reported that all the groups showed improvements in the backward masking measures as well (Gillam et al., 2008). When combined, the research conducted to this date support the view that both top-down and bottom-up approaches to language intervention, when conducted using an intensive treatment protocol 5 days a week for several consecutive weeks have a significant impact on language skills, and perhaps temporal processing skills as well.

SUMMARY AND CONCLUSIONS

Temporal processing is a bottom-up component of neurolinguistic processing that is impaired in many children with language disorders. The degree to which it is a predisposing factor in language disorders is still being debated, but the research to date is persuasive that temporal processing disorders do increase the risk of problems with language development for some children.

The intensive treatment approaches that include remediation of temporal processing deficits, have been shown through replicated random controlled studies, to result in significant improvements in language skills and temporal processing skills in a short period of time. However, it is clear that other intensive interventions that work directly on language structure and function (top-down approaches) are also effective when used intensively. Future research is needed that will begin to differentiate those patterns of language impairment and temporal processing impairment that benefit preferentially from top-down versus bottom-up approaches or a combination of both. In the meantime, the research overwhelmingly supports the value of intensive language interventions that combine bottom-up (perceptual and temporal processing exercises) and top-down (language structure, function, and use) for children with language disorders.

REFERENCES

American Speech-Language-Hearing Association Web site, www.asha.org

Benasich, A., Choudbury, N., Friedman, J., Realpe-Bonilla, T., Chojnowska, C., & Gou, Z. (2006). The infant as a prelinguistic model for language learning impairments: Predicting event-related potentials to behavior. *Neuropsychologia, 44*(3), 396–411.

Bishop, D. V. M., Carlyon, R. P., Deeks, J. M., & Bishop, S. J. (1999). Auditory temporal processing impairment: Neither necessary nor sufficient for causing language impairment in children. *Journal of Speech & Hearing Research, 42*, 1295–1310.

Bishop, D. V. M., & McArthur, M. (2004). Immature cortical responses to auditory stimuli in specific language impairment: Evidence from ERPs to rapid tone sequences. *Developmental Science, 7*, 11–18.

Boden, M. (2006). Transforming linguistics. *The mind as machine: A history of cognitive science*. Oxford, UK: Oxford University Press.

Brown, R. A. (1973). *First language: The early stages*. Cambridge, MA: Harvard University Press.

Burns, M. (2007). Auditory processing disorders and literacy. In D. Geffner & D. Ross-Swain (Eds.), *Auditory processing disorders: Assessment, management and treatment* (p. 973). San Diego, CA: Plural.

Cabeza, R., Ciaramelli, E., Olson, I., & Moscovitch, M. (2008). The parietal cortex and episodic memory: An attentional account. *Nature Reviews Neuroscience, 9*(8), 613–625.

Chermak, G., & Musiek, F. (1998). *Central auditory processing disorders: New perspectives*. New York, NY: Singular.

Chomsky, N. (1957). *Aspects of language*. The Hague, The Netherlands: Mouton.

Chomksy, A. N. (1959). Review of B. F. Skinner, Verbal behavior, *Language, 35*, 26–58.

Chomsky, A. N. (1964). *Aspects of the theory of syntax*. Cambridge, MA: MIT Press.

Chomsky, N. (1986). *Knowledge of language: Its nature, origin and use*. New York, NY: Praeger Publishers.

Cohen, W., Hodson, A., OíHare, A., Boyle, J., Durrani, T., McCartney, E., . . . Watson, J. (2005). Effects of computer-based intervention through acoustically modified speech (Fast ForWord) in severe mixed receptive–expressive language impairment: Outcomes from a randomized controlled trial. *Journal of Speech, Language, and Hearing Research, 48*, 715–729.

Corbetta, M., & Schulman, G. (2002). Control of goal-directed and stimulus-driven attention in the brain. *Nature Reviews Neuroscience, 3*(3), 201–215.

Dehaene-Lambertz, G., Hertz-Pannier, L., Dubois, J., Mériaux, S., Roche, A., Sigman, M., & Dehaene, S. (2006). Functional organization of perisylvian activation during presentation of sentences in preverbal infants. *Proceedings of the National Academy of Sciences, 103*(38), 14240–14245.

Dronkers, N., Husted, D., Deutsch, G., Taylor, K., Saunders, G., & Merzenich, M. (1999). Lesion site as a predictor of improvement after "Fast ForWord" treatment in adult aphasic patients. *Brain and Language, 69*, 450–452.

Gaab, N., Gabrieli, J., Deutsch, G., Tallal, P., & Temple, E. (2007). Neural correlates of rapid auditory processing are disrupted in children with developmental dyslexia and ameliorated with training: An fMRI study. *Restorative Neurology and Neuroscience, 25*, 295–310.

Gillam, R., Loeb, D., Hoffman, L., Bohman, B., Champlin, C., Thibodeau, L., . . . Friel-Patti, S. (2008). The efficacy of Fast ForWord language intervention in school-age children with language impairment: A randomized controlled trial. *Journal of Speech and Hearing Research, 51*, 57–119.

Irwin, J. (1964). Comments. In A. House (Ed.), *Proceedings of the conference on communicating by language: The speech process*. Bethesda, MA: National Institute of Child Health and Human Development, NIH.

Johnson, D. J., and Myklebust, H. R. (1967). *Learning disabilities: Educational principles and practices*. New York, NY: Grune and Stratton.

Kenet, T., Arieli, A., Tsodyks, M., & Grinvald, A. (2006). Are single cortical neurons soloists or are they obedient members of a huge orchestra? In J. L. van Hemmen & T. J. Sejnowski (Eds.), *23 Problems in systems neuroscience* (pp. 160–181). Oxford, UK: Oxford University Press.

Kuhl, P. K. (2000). A new view of language acquisition. *Proceedings of the National Academy of Sciences, 97*, 11850–11857.

Kuhl, P. (2004). Early language acquisition: Cracking the speech code. *Nature Reviews Neuroscience, 5*(11), 831.

Lee, L. (1974). *Developmental sentence analysis.* Evanston, IL: Northwestern University Press.

Marge, M. (1972). The general problem of language disabilities in children. In J. Irwin & M. Marge (Eds.), *Principles of childhood language disabilities* (pp. 75–98). New York, NY: Appleton-Century-Crofts.

Merzenich, M., Jenkins, W., Johnston, P., Schreiner, C., Miller, S., & Tallal, P. (1996). Temporal processing deficits of language-learning impaired children ameliorated by training. *Science, 271*, 77–81.

Mesulam, M.-M. (2000). *Principles of behavioral neurology.* Oxford, UK: Oxford University Press.

Nagarian, S., Mahncke, H., Salz, T., Tallal, P., Roberts, T., & Merzenich, M. (1999). Cortical auditory signal processing in poor readers. *Proceedings of the National Academy of Sciences, 96*, 6483–6488.

Pokorni, J. L., Worthington, C. K., & Jamison, P. J. (2004). Phonological awareness intervention: Comparison of Fast ForWord, Earobics, and LiPS. *Journal of Educational Research, 97*, 147–157.

Rawool, V. (2007). Temporal processing in the auditory system. In D. Geffner & D. Ross-Swain (Eds.), *Auditory processing disorders: Assessment, management and treatment* (pp. 117–138). San Diego, CA: Plural.

Schopmeyer, B., Mellon, N., Dobaj, H., Grant, G., & Nipapko, J. (2000). Use of Fast ForWord to enhance language development in children with cochlear implants. *Annals of Otology, Rhinology, and Laryngology*, Suppl. 85, 96–98.

Skinner, B. F. (1957). *Verbal behavior.* New York, NY: Appleton-Century-Crofts.

Snowling, M. (1990). *Dyslexia: A cognitive developmental perspective.* Oxford, UK: Blackwell.

Swan, D., & Goswami, U. (1997). Phonological awareness deficits in developmental dyslexia and the phonological representations hypothesis. *Journal of Experimental Child Psychology, 66*, 18–41.

Tallal, P. (2004). Improving language and literacy is a matter of time. *Nature Reviews Neuroscience, 5*(9), 721–728.

Tallal, P., Miller, S., Bedi, G., Byma, G., Wang, X., Srikantan, S., . . . Merzenich, M. (1996). Language comprehension in language-learning impaired children improved with acoustically modified speech. *Science, 271*, 81–84.

Tallal, P., & Piercy, M. (1973). Deficits of non-verbal auditory perception in children with developmental aphasia. *Nature, 241*, 468–469.

Tallal, P., & Piercy, M. (1974). Developmental aphasia: Rate of auditory processing and selective impairment of consonant perception. *Neuropsychologia, 12*(1), 83–93.

Tallal, P., & Stark, R. E. (1981). Speech acoustic-cue discrimination abilities of normally developing and language-impaired children. *Journal of the Acoustic Society of America, 69*(2), 568–574.

Temple, E., Deutsch, G., Poldrack, R., Miller, S., Tallal, P., & Merzenich, M. (2003). Neural deficits in children with dyslexia ameliorated by behavioral remediation: Evidence from functional MRI. *Proceedings of the National Academy of Sciences, 100*(5), 2860–2865.

Temple, E., Poldrack, R., Protopapas, A., Nagarajan, S., Salz, T., & Tallal, P. (2000). Disruption of the neural response to rapid acoustic stimuli in dyslexia: Evidence from functional MRI. *Proceedings of the National Academy of Sciences, 97*(25), 13907–13912.

Thomas, M., & Karmiloff-Smith, A. (2003). Connectionistic models of development, developmental disorders, and individual differences. In R. J. Sternberg, J. Lautrey, & T. I. Lubart (Eds.), *Models of intelligence: International perspectives* (pp. 133–150). Washington, DC: American Psychological Association.

Tomblin, J. B., Records, N. L., & Zhang, X. (1996). A system for the diagnosis of specific language impairment in kindergarten children. *Journal of Speech and Hearing Research, 39,* 1284–1294.

Van Vreeswijk, C. (2006). What is the neural code? In J. L. van Hemmen & T. J. Sejnowski (Eds.), *23 problems in systems neuroscience* (pp. 143–159). Oxford, UK: Oxford University Press.

19 Language Processing in Children With Language Impairment

Bernard Grela, Beverly Collisson,
and Dana Arthur

INTRODUCTION

It is estimated that approximately 7% of the general population has a syndrome known as specific language impairment (Tomblin et al., 1997). The term specific language impairment (SLI) is used to identify children who have difficulty with the acquisition and use of language. When compared to their typically developing peers, these children's scores on standardized measures of language development fall greater than one standard deviation below the mean, yet their cognitive abilities are within normal limits, they have normal hearing acuity, no frank neurological impairment, and no social-emotional problems (Leonard, 1998; Stark & Tallal, 1981). The acquisition and use of grammatical morphology appears to be the aspect of language most severely affected in children with SLI and they often produce grammatical markers less frequently than younger, typically developing children matched for mean length of utterance (MLU; e.g., Leonard, 1998; Rice & Wexler, 1996). The morphemes that appear to be most problematic for children with SLI include inflectional markers (e.g., third person singular: s, regular past tense: ed, contractible copula and auxiliary forms of *to be*) and functional words (e.g., uncontractible copula and auxiliary forms of *to be*). These morphemes may be completely absent or produced inconsistently across utterances (Leonard, Eyer, Bedore, & Grela, 1997; Miller & Leonard, 1998). When errors do occur, children with SLI are more likely to make omission rather than commission errors (Leonard et al., 1997; Rice & Wexler, 1996). Furthermore, they often have problems with other aspects of language such as phonology, vocabulary, and syntax (e.g., Leonard, 1998; Rice, 2004). Recent studies of language intervention have shown that while these children do show progress in their acquisition of language as a result of intervention, they are resistant to mastery of language in a timely manner (Bishop, Adams, & Rosen, 2006; Ebbels, van der Lely, & Dockrell, 2007; Leonard, Camarata, Pawlowska, Brown, & Camarata, 2008; Rice & Wexler, 1996). This difficulty with language may persist into adulthood (van der Lely, 1997, 2005).

While numerous studies have identified the language characteristics of children with SLI, relatively little is known about the underlying cause of this impairment. This has been complicated by the findings that children with SLI comprise a heterogeneous group (Bishop, Bright, James, Bishop, & van der Lely, 2000; Leonard, 1998; van der Lely, 2005). Furthermore, the symptoms associated with the disorder may have different underlying causes, or a combination of factors (Bishop, 2002; McArthur & Bishop, 2004). This provides a challenge for researchers and clinicians who strive to find the best assessment and intervention practices for children with SLI. Our goals as language interventionists are to identify measures that are highly sensitive in isolating the cause of the disorder and to develop intervention techniques that are effective in ameliorating the symptoms associated with the disorder. These assessment and intervention procedures will be most effective if we can identify the underlying cause, or causes, of the disorder. The focus of this chapter is to review evidence that children with SLI have a limitation in processing linguistic information. In addition, the implications for assessment and intervention will be discussed.

THEORIES OF SLI

Several theories have been proposed that attempt to explain the cause of SLI. The theories can be divided into two opposing perspectives with each consisting of several related but distinct theories of SLI. The first perspective assumes that children with SLI have a problem with the innate structures of grammar that prevents the application of productive morphosyntactic rules or leads to erroneous parameter settings for a language (e.g., Crago & Gopnik, 1994; Rice & Wexler, 1996; van der Lely, 1994). This faulty linguistic system inhibits the children from determining the linguistic parameters that are appropriate for the language they are learning. When grammatical morphemes are produced correctly, it is assumed that the children have either memorized a specific linguistic form (Crago & Gopnik, 1994) or set a tense optional grammar when tense is obligatory (Rice & Wexler, 1996). The commonality of this set of theories is that children with SLI are exposed to acceptable examples of linguistic input from their caregivers, but they are unable to correctly hypothesize the linguistic rules of their ambient language because of a faulty underlying grammar.

The second perspective proposes that children with SLI have an intact underlying grammatical structure, but processing systems (e.g., working memory, attention, general processing) that are essential for the acquisition of language function less than optimally (Bishop, 1994; Johnston, 1991; Kail, 1994; Leonard et al., 1997). These systems are affected by a processing capacity limitation, which prevents children with SLI from acquiring grammatical rules as efficiently and rapidly as their typically developing peers. During the process of acquisition, children with SLI may develop weak representations of grammatical structures that result in within individual variation in the use of these structures at any one point in development (Leonard et al., 1997; Miller & Leonard, 1998). Therefore, a child may produce a grammatical morpheme in one situation (e.g., The dog's running), but omit it in another (e.g., *The dog chasing the cat). Therefore, grammatical structures may be used productively, but not in every situation where they are required. This differs from a deficit in linguistic knowledge perspective, which proposes that children with SLI use grammatical markers because they memorize them in particular contexts.

ASSUMPTIONS OF PROCESSING CAPACITY LIMITATIONS

It is well recognized that the human brain functions as a system that processes and organizes incoming sensory information to make sense of the world. However, it is also known that the brain has a limited capacity for processing incoming information and so it can perform only a limited amount of work within a specific period of time (Johnston, 1991, 1994). When the processing system is taxed, information is lost because of an inability to cope with an overwhelming amount of information. This would be similar to composing an e-mail while conversing on the phone. These tasks are difficult to accomplish simultaneously and often lead to frustration on the part of the person to whom we are talking. We may be able to switch from one task to the other rapidly, but we have difficulty processing several sources of information at the same time. In this scenario, our processing system is receiving and encoding more information than our brain is capable of managing, resulting in a loss of information.

There are several factors that must be considered when taking into account the amount of information that the brain is capable of processing within a given period of time. These include the familiarity of the information, the attentional resources required for processing, and the type of processing that will be necessary (Bishop, 2000). When a new skill is being learned, controlled processing is required. Controlled processing consumes a large percentage of available attentional resources and makes the completion of a task difficult and effortful. As a result, few attentional resources are available to perform other tasks. On the other hand, automatic processing occurs after a skill has been mastered through practice. This mastered skill consumes few attentional resources and can be completed automatically. Automatic processing frees up the processing resources so that other tasks can be performed simultaneously.

In addition, the operational resources available for processing information efficiently are thought to be dependent on at least three other factors: speed of processing, space available for processing, and energy available to drive the processing system (Leonard, 1998; Leonard et al., 2007). These factors have been divided into functional- (speed of processing) and structural-based (space and energy) systems of processing (Montgomery & Windsor, 2007). According to the functional-based perspectives, if information is presented too rapidly, our ability to process the information is compromised (Hayiou-Thomas, Bishop, & Plunkett, 2004). It would follow that if the processing system is abnormally slow, then information will be lost when it is presented at a normal rate (Kail, 1991). In contrast, structural-based systems emphasize the amount of space allocated for processing (Daneman & Carpenter, 1983). It seems logical that a large volume processor should be capable of handling more information within a specific period of time than a small volume processor. Furthermore, a small volume processor may be overwhelmed if too much information is presented within a particular time frame in comparison to a large volume processor. A final way of thinking about information processing is to consider the amount of energy that is required to complete a task (Lapointe, 1985). This perspective assumes that a processing system requires energy in order to complete a task or several tasks simultaneously. If there is insufficient energy to complete the task, only a portion of it will be accomplished. If this involves information processing, a portion of that information will be missing because the energy source required to finish the task will be depleted.

The three factors listed above may contribute to a processing capacity limitation. They may occur in isolation, but are more likely to be codependent factors (Ellis Weismer et al., 2000; Lahey, Edwards, & Munson, 2001). For example, a small volume processor will take longer to process large volumes of information. A combination of reduced space and speed will have an impact on the amount of information that can be processed within a given timeframe. Finally, a large volume of information may take more energy than is available to complete a task. Therefore, any of these factors combined may contribute to a processing capacity limitation.

A major assumption of the processing capacity limitation perspectives for children with SLI is that these children have an intact grammatical structure. An intact grammatical structure has the potential for learning the linguistic rules of a child's ambient language. However, it needs an appropriate flow of linguistic information in order to acquire these rules. If this flow of information is incomplete, degraded, or interrupted due to an improperly functioning processing system, then it will take children with SLI a longer time to acquire language.

There are several reasons to suspect that children with SLI have difficulty processing linguistic information. Physiologically-based studies have used functional magnetic resonance imaging (fMRI; e.g., Ellis Weismer, Plante, Jones, & Tomblin, 2005; Hugdahl et al., 2004) and event related potentials (ERPs; e.g., Bishop & McArthur, 2005; McArthur & Bishop, 2004) to examine brain function in children with SLI. The fMRI studies found less activation in the areas of the cortex critical for language processing in children with SLI (Ellis Weismer et al., 2005; Hugdahl et al., 2004). These included the parietal regions, the precentral gyrus, and inferior frontal gyrus. The ERP studies examined processing at a lower level of processing in the auditory cortex (Bishop & McArthur, 2005; McArthur & Bishop, 2005). These authors argue that children with SLI have immature processing systems. However, the auditory system eventually matures and processes information as efficiently as typically developing children.

The advantage of the physiological studies is that they do not require behavioral responses from the children and may be more sensitive in identifying differences between children with SLI and their typically developing peers. However, the disadvantages are that these procedures are expensive and in many cases can only be used on older disordered populations. Therefore, a large percentage of studies on children with SLI have used behavioral observations including reaction times, comprehension tasks, and production tasks. The next section describes these studies and the different hypotheses suggesting the underlying cause of SLI. Some of the theories assume a general processing capacity limitation for language, while others identify specific systems that result in degraded linguistic input to the grammatical system. The general consensus behind these theories is that the brain has a limited processing capability and when the processing system is taxed, information is lost. These processing limitations have a significant impact on children's abilities to acquire the grammar of their ambient language.

SPECIFIC THEORIES OF PROCESSING CAPACITY LIMITATION IN CHILDREN WITH SLI

GENERALIZED SLOWING HYPOTHESIS

According to the generalized slowing hypothesis (Kail, 1994), the amount of work that can be accomplished within a given period of time is determined by speed. It then follows that individuals who perform a task slowly complete less work within a specified period of time than individuals who perform a task rapidly. Using a meta-analysis procedure, Kail (1994) found that children with SLI took longer to complete a variety of linguistic (e.g., object naming) and nonlinguistic (e.g., judging picture similarity) tasks when compared to typically developing peers. Furthermore, the response times of the children with SLI increased linearly in comparison to the response times of the typically developing children. Kail concluded that the slower response times of the children with SLI was not specific to any particular task, but more general across both linguistic and nonlinguistic domains. Thus, children with SLI were slower at a variety of tasks including the comprehension and production of language. Kail believes that this reduced speed of processing accounts for the delayed acquisition of language.

Several recent studies have attempted to replicate Kail's results (Hayiou-Thomas et al., 2004; Miller, Kail, Leonard, & Tomblin, 2001; Miller et al., 2006). Miller and colleagues (2001) examined the response times of third grade children with SLI across a variety of linguistic and nonlinguistic tasks. The linguistic tasks included lexical decision making, grammaticality judgment, and phonological awareness. The nonlinguistic tasks included motor response, visual scan, and mental rotation. The results of this study were consistent with Kail's (1994) findings that children with SLI responded more slowly than their typically developing peers across all task domains. They argued that the slower reaction times by the children with SLI provided evidence for a general processing deficit in comparison to their typically developing peers. Several years following the Miller et al. (2001) study, the same tasks were administered to a group of 14-year-old children with SLI (Leonard et al., 2007; Miller et al., 2006). Again, a strong relationship between performance on language tasks and speed of processing was found. They concluded that children with SLI continue to lag behind their typically developing peers in speed of performance as they age. Other studies have reported similar findings for other areas of nonlinguistic processing such as slower visual processing, attentional orientation, and motor responses on the part of children with SLI (Schul, Stiles, Wulfeck, & Townsend, 2004; Windsor & Hwang, 1999). Therefore, there is evidence to suggest that speed of processing is correlated with the language difficulties of children with SLI.

SURFACE HYPOTHESIS

The surface hypothesis as described by Leonard and colleagues (Leonard & Bortolini, 1998; Leonard et al., 1997; Leonard, McGregor, & Allen, 1992) assumes that children with SLI have a general processing capacity limitation. Therefore, they process information at a slower rate than their typically developing peers. In addition, the theory emphasizes the physical properties of language in that morphemes of low phonetic substance are vulnerable to decay when the processing system is taxed. Leonard (1998) defines low phonetic substance as grammatical morphemes that are brief in duration. These include grammatical morphemes consisting of single consonants or weak syllables that occur in sentence positions where they are less likely to be lengthened. When these morphemes are encountered in an utterance, children must perceive them and then hypothesize their grammatical function while subsequent auditory and linguistic information continues to be heard and processed. In children with SLI, some verbal input will be lost because they cannot process the information quickly enough to store it in long-term memory. The information likely to be lost includes forms consisting of low phonetic substance. As a result, it is likely that the information contained within these grammatical morphemes decays from memory before it can be completely processed. Thus, it will take children with SLI longer to determine the function of these grammatical markers and they are less likely to build a productive rule for their use in comparison to their peers.

Studies examining children's ability to perceive grammatical morphemes have lent support to the surface hypothesis (Montgomery & Leonard, 1998, 2006). Montgomery and Leonard (1998) found that children with SLI showed sensitivity to morphemes of high phonetic substance but not to morphemes of low phonetic substance. Their typically developing peers matched either for age or receptive language showed sensitivity to both high and low phonetic substance morphemes. A later study (Montgomery & Leonard, 2006) included a condition where morphemes of low phonetic substance were manipulated by increasing the duration and intensity of these morphemes. The results of this study showed that the children with SLI performed as well on the enhanced morphemes as they did on the morphemes of high phonetic substance. The results of these two studies suggest that the children with SLI have more difficulty processing morphemes of low phonetic substance and provide support for the surface hypothesis.

DEFICIT IN TEMPORAL PROCESSING

Comprehending language involves the perception of complex and rapidly changing acoustic information. According to Tallal and colleagues (Tallal, 1980;

Tallal & Piercy, 1974, 1975), children with developmental language disorders (such as SLI) cannot respond to rapidly changing acoustic events as are found in consonant to vowel transitions in speech. This inability results in difficulty with speech perception that in turn has a significant impact on language acquisition. To test this hypothesis, Tallal and colleagues (Tallal, 2004; Tallal, Miller, & Fitch, 1993; Tallal, Sainburg, & Jernigan, 1991; Tallal, Stark, & Mellits, 1985) described several tasks where children with SLI were asked to detect the difference between two tones presented with either short interstimulus intervals (ISI) or with tones of short duration. The children with SLI had difficulty detecting differences between the tones when the ISIs were short and when the tones were of brief duration. However, they performed as well as their typically developing peers when the ISI between tones and the length of tones were increased. Similar results were found when the children were presented with verbal stimuli that included consonant-vowel (CV) syllables (i.e., /ba/ vs. /da/; Burlingame, Sussman, Gillam, & Hay, 2005; Tallal & Piercy, 1974, 1975). The children with SLI had difficulty identifying the CV pairs when the formant transitions were presented at a normal rate, but improved when the formant transitions were lengthened. Tallal and colleagues argued that this showed evidence of a temporal processing disorder on the part of the children with SLI.

WORKING MEMORY LIMITATIONS

Montgomery (2003) provides a comprehensive description of two models of working memory and how they relate to children with SLI. The first model of working memory has been referred to as phonological working memory (PWM; Baddeley, 1986). PWM consists of a central executive and a phonological loop. The central executive functions to regulate the flow of information, the retrieval of information from other memory systems, and the processing and storage of information. The phonological loop consists of a capacity limited system that subvocally rehearses auditory information for a short period of time while information is processed in the central executive. It is thought that the phonological loop is problematic for children with SLI (Adams & Gathercole, 1995; Archibald & Gathercole, 2006b; Gathercole & Baddeley, 1995; Gathercole, Willis, Baddeley, & Emslie, 1994). Therefore, they are not able to rehearse and maintain information in the phonological loop long enough for information to be stored in long-term memory. As a result, it will take children with SLI longer to learn vocabulary, grammatical morphology, and other grammatical forms. Evidence for a problem with the phonological loop has been found in various nonword repetition tasks (Adams & Gathercole, 1995; Archibald & Gathercole, 2006a, b; Archibald & Gathercole, 2007; Dollaghan & Campbell, 1998; Ellis Weismer et al., 2000; Gathercole et al., 1994). In nonword repetition tasks, children are required to repeat nonsense words ranging from one to four syllables in length. These studies have found that children with SLI both tend to make more errors overall and make more errors as the number of syllables per word increases in comparison to their typically developing peers (Dollaghan & Campbell, 1998; Gathercole et al., 1994; Roy & Chiat,

2004). This may be because words with more syllables take longer to rehearse in the phonological loop.

The second model of working memory has been referred to as functional working memory (FWM). This model assumes that information must be held in memory while other processing operations take place (Just & Carpenter, 1992). FWM is similar to PWM, except that the existence of a phonological loop is deemphasized while the relationship between the storage and processing of information is emphasized. In this model, the central executive has a limited capacity and the tasks of storing and processing information must share a limited pool of resources. When the working memory system is taxed, there is a trade-off between attentional resources required for storage and those required for retrieval. To assess the dual function of working memory, Daneman and Carpenter (1983) devised a task where adult participants were asked to answer questions about sentences while remembering the last word of each sentence. This task was modified and used as a measure of working memory in school age children (Gaulin & Campbell, 1994). This procedure was adopted for use in children with SLI to assess their ability to process and store information simultaneously (Ellis Weismer, Evans, & Hesketh, 1999). Ellis Weismer et al. (1999) found that children with SLI responded to questions about the sentences as well as typically developing children matched for age, but were unable to recall as many sentence final words as their peers. This experimental design was later used to assess adolescent children with SLI using both behavioral and fMRI data (Ellis Weismer et al., 2005). The results of this study supported previous findings (Ellis Weismer et al., 1999) that children with SLI recalled fewer words than their typically developing peers. In addition, the fMRI results indicated that the children with SLI had lower levels of activation in areas of the brain responsible for attentional, memory, and language processing. The results of these studies were used to support the argument that children with SLI have structural deficits in verbal working memory that affect their acquisition and use of language.

PHONOLOGICAL DEFICIT HYPOTHESIS

It has been suggested that the general processing capacity limitations of children with SLI result in an impairment in the processing of speech that has a significant impact on the development of good phonological representations. These degraded phonological representations are thought to be the central cause of delayed acquisition of morphology and syntax because children with SLI have difficulty translating the auditory forms of words and morphemes into a phonological code necessary for learning these forms (Criddle & Durkin, 2001; Joanisse, 2004; Joanisse & Seidenberg, 2003). This may be the case as children with SLI often have phonological impairments as well as problems with syntax and morphology (e.g., Leonard, 1998; Leonard et al., 1997; Rice, 2004). Adopting a connectionist model, Joanisse (Joanisse, 2004; Joanisse & Seidenberg, 2003) suggested that the phonological form of grammatical morphemes is degraded during exposure and as a result the productive rules for use of inflectional markers take longer to learn. Therefore, the deficit in inflectional morphology is secondary to a phonological impairment. One of the assumptions of connectionist modeling is that knowledge is a distributed and inter-active system. So if there is an impairment in one aspect of the system other aspects within the system are also be affected. Joanisse (2004) created a network model to simulate degraded phonological representations. The network acquired some of the knowledge for use of inflections so occasionally they were produced. His results were remarkably similar to the language profiles of children with SLI where omission errors are more frequent than commission errors. Therefore, a general processing capacity limitation resulting in poor phonological representations may have a significant impact on the acquisition and use of grammatical morphology.

LINGUISTIC COMPLEXITY

Linguistic complexity can be thought of as the amount of linguistic information bundled within a particular linguistic structure. More complex structures consist of more linguistic features and require a greater number of mental computations to encode or produce an utterance (e.g., Grela, 2003b; Grela, Snyder, & Hiramatsu, 2005). Therefore, if children with SLI have limited processing capabilities for language, then linguistic structures that have higher levels of complexity should be problematic for these children. This may be due to limited space available for mental computations of these structures or limited energy to complete the computations. Several studies have examined linguistic complexity as a contributing factor to comprehension problems and production errors characteristic of children with SLI (Dick, Wulfeck, Krupa-Kwiatkowski, & Bates, 2004; Grela, 2003a; Grela & Leonard, 2000; Grela et al., 2005; Marton, Schwartz, Farkas, & Katsnelson, 2006). Some of the complex linguistic structures that have been examined include argument structure (Grela, 2003a; Grela & Leonard, 2000), novel root compounds (Grela et al., 2005), verb particles (Juhasz & Grela, 2008; Watkins & Rice, 1991), number of propositions per utterance (Johnston & Kamhi, 1984), and clausal imbedding (Dick et al., 2004). In general, these studies have found that children with SLI tend to make more errors or use fewer linguistic features than their typically developing peers as complexity levels increase.

Johnston and Kamhi (1984) found that children with SLI produced fewer propositions per utterance in comparison to typically developing children matched for MLU. Therefore, even when sentence length was a controlled factor, the children with SLI produced fewer idea units, suggesting that they were limited in the amount of information that could be contained within each utterance. More recently, a study examining use of grammatical morphology associated with phonological mean length of utterance (PMLU), as opposed to MLU in morphemes, found that children with SLI used fewer grammatical structures in comparison to children matched for PMLU (Polite & Leonard, 2006). In other words, when children with SLI attempt to produce utterances of similar length, or of increasing length, they make more grammatical errors than their typically developing peers (Marton et al., 2006). This provides evidence of a grammatical system that reaches its limits at relatively lower levels of linguistic complexity in comparison to typically developing children.

When linguistic complexity has been manipulated, children with SLI have been found to have difficulty comprehending and producing grammatical sentences (Dick et al., 2004; Grela, 2003b; Grela & Leonard, 2000; Grela et al., 2005). These studies have shown that children with SLI make more grammatical errors as argument structure complexity increases (Grela, 2003a, 2003b; Grela & Leonard, 1997, 2000). For example, Grela and Leonard (2000) found that children with SLI omitted more auxiliary verbs when attempting ditransitive sentences (e.g., The boy is giving the ball to the witch) than when producing intransitive (e.g., The boy is jumping) or transitive (e.g., The boy is pushing the car) sentences. Similar results were found for the omission of subject arguments of sentences (Grela, 2003a, 2003b). A study of French-speaking children with SLI found that they were likelier to omit grammatical morphemes in obligatory contexts as more complex argument structures were attempted (Pizzioli & Schelstraete, 2008). In addition, children with SLI were found to have difficulty interpreting the meaning of sentences when clausal imbedding was used to add complexity to sentences (Dick et al., 2004).

Linguistic complexity may have a significant impact on the mechanisms involved in the comprehension (e.g., working memory) and production of linguistic structures. The arguments have been that if children with SLI are presented with too much information while learning, the processing mechanisms are overwhelmed and information is compromised resulting in a slower rate of learning (Ellis Weismer et al., 1999; Gathercole et al., 1994; Johnston, 1994; Montgomery, 2000). It is also possible that during production, children with SLI may reach their processing limitations earlier than typically developing children. This is thought to be true when children with SLI have weak representations of grammatical structures (Grela & Leonard, 2000; Leonard, 1998; Leonard et al., 1997, 2000; Miller & Leonard, 1998). More specifically, the information that needs to be retrieved for sentence production may overwhelm the children's production "buffer" resulting in more grammatical errors as the demands associated with linguistic complexity increases (Grela, 2003a, 2003b; Grela & Leonard, 2000). To support this hypothesis, Leonard and colleagues (2000) devised an experiment where children with SLI were primed for the production of a targeted morpheme. The children with SLI produced more grammatical morphemes when the prime and the target sentence contained the same syntactic frame and prosodic structure (Prime: The birds are building the nest, Target: The horse is kicking the cow) than when they differed (Prime: The doctor smiled, Target: The horse is driving the car). They suggested that the matching prime and target reduced the processing load associated with the retrieval of the syntactic structure and grammatical morphemes required for sentence production. Therefore, linguistic complexity may have a significant impact on the learning and use of grammatical structures.

IMPLICATIONS FOR ASSESSMENT

Clearly there is evidence to support processing capacity limitations for at least some children with SLI. Therefore, thoughtful evaluation of processing capacity should become an integral part of any assessment battery for children with

SLI. Furthermore, these measures should have sufficient sensitivity to identify an existing language impairment and, ideally, have some evidence of construct validity for assessing processing capacity limitations (Hutchinson, 1996; McCauley & Swisher, 1984; Plante & Vance, 1994; Spaulding, Plante, & Farinella, 2006). It is also important that clinicians and researchers use guidelines to help differentiate children with SLI from other types of language impairments (Leonard, 1998; Stark & Tallal, 1981).

This being said, assessment of processing ability in children can present particular challenges to clinicians and researchers. Few standardized measures of processing capacity are available (Montgomery, 2003), and not every purported test of processing or memory is created equally. In fact, many tasks labeled as working memory measures tap other memory systems as well (Dehn, 2008). Conversely, tasks designed to evaluate language can tax any and all of the facets of processing discussed above. For example, a test requiring children to imitate sentences of increasing length and/or complexity may place a strain on working memory, while a timed test may indirectly measure processing speed. To evaluate the nature and severity of processing capacity limitations in children with SLI—a crucial step toward creating an intervention plan—an effort must first be made to understand the strengths and limitations of the assessment tools available (Hutchinson, 1996; Spaulding et al., 2006). Therefore, it is critical that clinicians and researchers carefully read test manuals to determine if the test items are indeed assessing processing capacity or some other aspect of language.

TESTS OF PROCESSING CAPACITY

Even though few standardized measures of processing capacity exist, some specific tasks have emerged in the literature as assessments of processing capacity and short-term memory. Some can be found as subtests of larger language assessment batteries, such as the nonword repetition subtest of the Comprehensive Test of Phonological Processing (CTOPP; Wagner, Torgeson, & Rashotte, 1999), or Gaulin and Campbell's Competing Language Processing Test (CLEP; Gaulin & Campbell, 1994), which may be adapted as an informal measure of processing ability.

NONWORD REPETITION TESTS

One of the more promising measures for identifying SLI is the nonword repetition task (also known as CNRep or NRT; Dollaghan & Campbell, 1998; Gathercole et al., 1994). Children with SLI have significant difficulties with nonword repetition compared to their typically developing peers (e.g., Archibald & Gathercole, 2007; Dollaghan & Campbell, 1998; Ellis Weismer et al., 2000). Even compared to younger children matched for language level, children with SLI perform significantly worse on this task (Ellis Weismer et al., 2000). Furthermore, Montgomery and Windsor (2007) found that performance on the NRT predicted significant unique variance on the Clinical Evaluation of Language Fundamentals (CELF-R;

Semel, Wiig, & Secord, 1987), suggesting a strong relationship between verbal working memory and direct tests of language ability. When dealing with non-words, children cannot rely on long-term representations or vocabulary knowledge. Therefore, the task of recalling and repeating each item falls primarily on the child's working memory. Children with SLI, working at a reduced processing capacity, are unable to keep up with the demands of the task.

Despite its seeming utility in detecting processing capacity limitations in children with SLI, some researchers caution against its use as a primary determiner of such limitations (Conti-Ramsden, Botting, & Faragher, 2001; Gathercole et al., 1994). One such caution centers around the shared nonword repetition deficit between children with SLI, children at risk for dyslexia, and children with poor working memory abilities, but appropriate oral and written language (Bishop, 2002; Conti-Ramsden et al., 2001). Therefore the ability of nonword repetition tasks to differentially identify SLI from children who are at risk for language problems comes into question.

A second caution centers on the skills assessed by the nonword repetition task itself. Phonological working memory, while it may loom large as an underlying skill contributing to nonword repetition, is not the only skill brought to bear on this task. Long-term lexical knowledge, according to some researchers (Archibald & Gathercole, 2006a, b; Gathercole et al., 1994), is also at work in nonword repetition despite the seeming unfamiliarity of the nonword items. Specifically, when presented with a nonword item, subjects may draw on their semantic knowledge as well as their working memory in order to repeat it. This may be particularly true when a nonword is similar in phonological structure to a familiar word (Gathercole et al., 1994). If a nonword item is too similar to a real word, children may be able to draw on their long-term representation of the real word to mitigate the strain on working memory. To support this argument, Estes, Evans, and Else-Quest (2007) found significant variability among nonword repetition tasks and cited word likeness as a contributing factor to this variability. With these cautions in mind, nonword repetition cannot be viewed as a strictly nonverbal task, purely assessing children's processing abilities. Clinically, nonword repetition may be a task best utilized as a screening tool and not as the primary assessment of processing limitations.

SENTENCE REPETITION TASKS

How are we to fill the gaps in assessment left by nonword repetition tasks? Another type of repetition task, sentence repetition, shows promise as an assessment tool for processing capacity limitations and identification of SLI. The Recalling Sentences subtest of the CELF-R (Semel, Wiig, & Secord, 1987) presents children with sentences that increase in length and complexity. The child's task is to repeat the sentences verbatim. Children with processing capacity limitations, such as SLI, should perform poorly as the complexity of the sentences increases. Conti-Ramsden and colleagues (2001) compared several assessment tasks, including nonword repetition and sentence repetition in terms of their potential as phenotypic markers of SLI. Sentence repetition was found to be the most accurate measure studied, showing both high accuracy and predictive value.

COMPLEX SPAN TASKS

Gaulin and Campbell's (1994) Competing Language Processing Task (CLPT) was designed specifically to assess processing trade-offs in children as young as 6 years of age. The CLPT presents the child with groups of short sentences and requires a truth-value response to each. At the same time, the child must recall the final word of each sentence. This requires concurrent processing of meaning and retention of words in working memory, thus forcing the central executive to compete for processing resources involved in storage and processing. Ellis Weismer et al. (1999) revealed that the CLPT was far more taxing for children with SLI than for their typically developing peers.

PROCESSING INVOLVEMENT IN OTHER LANGUAGE TASKS

Despite the critical role that processing capacity is thought to play as the underlying cause of SLI, assessment of these limitations should in no way be viewed as a complete assessment of SLI. Direct measures of language ability remain necessary, particularly given the heterogeneous nature of the SLI population. Tasks like nonword repetition, or the CLPT, can reveal the presence of limitations on processing, but only broader testing can show how these limitations are manifested in a child's linguistic system.

The need for additional language testing is far from a burden. In fact, it can be considered a remedy for the relative dearth of standardized processing assessment measures. Tasks in formal language testing usually draw on some aspect of processing, and each can tax the capacity of the child's system in different ways. By analyzing the tasks of a standardized assessment battery, the clinician–researcher can observe how a child's processing capacity affects overall language performance. For example, the *Token Test for Children* (Revised; DiSimoni, Ehrler, & McGhee, 2007), was originally designed to assess comprehension of verbal commands. However, as those commands become increasingly long and complex, it is easy to see the influence that limited processing capacity has on a child's performance. Processing can play more subtle roles as well. Rapid naming tests, popular for assessing expressive vocabulary, can demonstrate weaknesses in the child's processing speed, as can any timed assessment. In the end, nearly any task employed by formal testing has a processing component. By examining each task carefully, standard language batteries can provide useful information about a child's processing capacity limitations.

THE DYNAMIC ASSESSMENT PARADIGM

The most effective method of evaluating processing capacity in children with SLI may lie not with the specific measure used, but with the overall assessment paradigm employed. Dynamic assessment (DA) moves the focus of the evaluation from the answer that the child provides to the process the child uses to reach that answer. Instead of determining the level at which the child can perform a task without help, this paradigm interactively assesses what the child can do given strategic adult assistance (e.g., Gutierrez-Clellen & Peña, 2001; Hasson & Joffe, 2007; Peña & Gillam, 2000; Peña, Iglesias, & Lidz, 2001; Peña, Quinn, & Iglesias, 1992). By focusing on the process children with SLI use to approach evaluation tasks, the DA paradigm can provide specific information about how their processing ability differs from their typically developing peers. Thus, a DA approach can fill in the gaps that may be left by formal testing. Further, DA provides insight into a child's stimulability and potential for positive change (e.g., Gutierrez-Clellen & Peña, 2001; Hasson & Joffe, 2007). Dynamic assessment provides us with the opportunity to carefully employ various intervention strategies during testing, in order to determine what will provide the most benefit to the child.

IMPLICATIONS FOR INTERVENTION

In this chapter, we have explored SLI from a processing limitation perspective. This perspective provides the framework from which intervention approaches will be discussed. Within the language domain itself, children and adolescents with SLI may experience difficulty with one or more of the various aspects of spoken and written language: phonology, semantics, grammatical morphology, syntax, and pragmatics (Leonard, 1998). Further, evidence suggests that factors in the related areas of speed of processing (Kail, 1994), working memory (Gathercole et al., 1994; Montgomery, 2003), phonological quality (Joanisse, 2004), executive functioning and attentional capacity (Im-Bolter, Johnson, & Pascual-Leone, 2006) contribute to poor language learning.

A critical component of selecting an intervention program is to consider the theoretical construct underpinning the intervention procedure to ensure that it is consistent with the hypothesized underlying cause of the language impairment. Second, the intervention program chosen should demonstrate evidence of effectiveness and efficacy in ameliorating the characteristics of the language problem in the population with which it is being used (Dollaghan, 2007; Gillam & Gillam, 2006). Finally, the intervention approach should focus on the content, form, and use of language within pragmatically appropriate contexts (Fey, Long, & Finestack, 2003). For children with processing capacity limitations, the interventionist strives to make the acoustic signal more salient and to decrease processing demands placed on children with SLI. These are key elements for children who demonstrate deficits in their ability to store and process information. For example, teaching new forms in old contexts allows the clinician to control the amount of new information to the child's existing level of prior knowledge (Fey, 1986), this in turn allows for increased storage and better coordination of executive processes. Reducing processing demands may free cognitive resources necessary for new skill acquisition.

Based on their results that both verbal processing speed and working memory are differentially implicated in language impairment and the important role that nonlinguistic/nonverbal factors take, Leonard et al. (2007) suggested that clinicians develop intervention goals for children with SLI that not only target the desired linguistic forms, but encompass nonlinguistic targets as well. Activities that promote both linguistic goals and the organization/regulation of material previously attained serve to promote the relationship between information processing and language learning. Ultimately, the goal in intervention for children with SLI is to simultaneously enhance language performance and the efficiency of information processing. Therefore, an intervention program will endeavor to decrease the amount of controlled processing that occurs and increase the automatic processing in children with SLI. This should free up attentional resources and allow the children to learn new information more efficiently. The following intervention practices are meant to serve as illustrations of a broad range of language treatment methods that serve to make the language signal more salient, to decrease processing demands, or to compensate for these processing limitations by training meta cognitive strategies.

Decreasing Processing Demands and Making the Signal Salient

If children with SLI have difficulty processing the speech signal, the signal must be made more salient. One way to deliver more salient input is to alter the manner in which it is presented. The supersegmental features of a language can be altered by modifying intonation, stress, pause time, or rate of delivery (Montgomery, 2005; Montgomery & Leonard, 2006). Montgomery and Leonard (2006) found that children with SLI were more sensitive to morphemes of low phonetic substance when the intensity and duration of these morphemes was increased. Clinicians may use auditory trainers to increase the intensity of the acoustic signal and reduce background noise for children with SLI. This may function to enhance morphemes of low phonetic substance.

Ellis Weismer and Hesketh (1993, 1996, 1998) conducted a number of investigations to identify the linguistic variables that had an influence on children's language learning. One study examined the influence of varying speaking rate on novel word learning (Ellis Weismer & Hesketh, 1996). Children with SLI and typically developing children were taught two sets of novel words under three speaking rates: a slow rate, a normal rate, and a fast rate. It was found that children with SLI were able to produce fewer of the target words that had been introduced in the fast rate than at the normal rate, however, presentation of the target words at the slow rate did not assist the children with SLI learn the novel words. The authors concluded that fast rates of presentation for children with SLI be avoided. Further they suggested that a slower speaking rate may be beneficial to some children with SLI, however, they were not able to make this claim for the entire group of children with SLI in their investigation. The role of speaking rate, as in other manipulations of input, may demonstrate differential effects on the divergent group of children with SLI. It is important to carefully examine the influence of these modifications on each child individually.

Using the same experimental paradigm as their other investigations of linguistic input modification, Ellis Weismer and Hesketh (1998) examined the role of emphatic stress in word learning. Both typically developing children and children with SLI were exposed to single syllabic words produced with either neutral or emphatic stress. Both groups appeared to benefit from marking the novel lexical term with emphatic stress when tested for production ability. Coupling these findings with other investigations Ellis Weismer (1997) conjectured that emphatic stress does play a role in promoting language learning and this practice can be extended to real words in a clinical setting.

FOCUSED STIMULATION

Focused stimulation refers to the technique in which a target linguistic form is made highly salient to a child by modeling it at a high frequency rate in a natural context. The child is not required to repeat the form, however, opportunities to produce the target are provided by carefully arranging the environment to promote it in an expected context (Fey, 1986; Fey, Cleave, Long, & Hughes, 1993). A number of treatment studies delivered by both clinicians and parents (e.g., Cleave & Fey, 1997; Girolametto, Pearce, & Weitzman, 1996) that promote both lexical and grammatical targets have demonstrated the effectiveness of this treatment approach with delayed language learners.

CONVERSATIONAL RECASTS

A recast is a response to a child's inaccurate or immature utterance that both corrects the utterance and includes additional phonological, semantic, and/or grammatical information (Camarata & Nelson, 2006). An example of a recast would be, "The baby is sleeping" in response to a child's observation, "Baby sleep." While making the input more salient, the adult tailors his response directly to the child's production. Experimental investigations comparing the relative effectiveness of the conversational recast technique with the direct imitation technique have demonstrated the effectiveness of conversational recasts to develop both absent and partially mastered grammatical structures in the language of children with SLI (Camarata, Nelson, & Camarata, 1994; Nelson, Camarata, Welsh, & Butkovsky, 1996). The investigators in these treatment studies hypothesized that the conversational recast technique allowed the children with SLI to exploit the meaningfulness of the discourse to aid in the processing of the target structure.

SELF-TALK AND PARALLEL TALK

Self-talk and parallel talk are both techniques that fall under the umbrella of child-centered approaches (Fey, 1986). Typically clinicians and parents facilitate general linguistic development while engaged with a child in play. These techniques may be extended to other contexts in which caregivers find themselves at any time of the day. A linguistic target is not selected for directed reinforcement, rather the conversational partner bases his comments on his or the child's particular activity in that moment in time. Self-talk describes the clinician's or parent's enthusiastic comments on or description of what the parent is engaged in while playing with a child. This serves as a language model for the child. Parallel talk shifts the focus of the adult's comments to what the child is engaged in. Parallel talk was one of several child-centered techniques used in a treatment study successfully targeting the linguistic and social skills of toddlers with delayed language development (Robertson & Weismer, 1999). Toddlers who were not yet using words were provided with a verbal description of their actions (e.g., "Hug the bear"), which in combination with a number of additional child-oriented techniques successfully moved the toddlers forward both linguistically and socially.

ELICITED IMITATION

Elicited imitation is an intervention technique that directs a child's attention to a target form by highlighting it in contrast to another syntactic target form (Cleave & Fey, 1997; Connell, 1987; Connell & Stone, 1992). This serves to make the target more salient by focusing the child's attention to the target, providing opportunity for the child to produce the features of the target and illuminating the grammatical function of the target (Fey, Long, & Finestack, 2003). To promote success with this technique, the target form should be contrasted with a competing grammatical target in a pragmatically appropriate context (Cleave & Fey, 1997). This technique has been used to successfully promote new language forms by children with SLI (Connell, 1987; Connell & Stone, 1992) and as a beneficial component of a treatment study that facilitated the acquisition of grammatical forms in children with language impairments (Fey et al., 1993).

MODIFYING THE SPEECH INPUT

Computer modification of the speech signal provides a way to make the signal perceptually more salient for children with SLI. Tallal, Miller, Bedi, Wang, and Nagarajan (1996) introduced modified speech that temporally prolonged the signal and amplified the phonetic contrasts in the ongoing speech signal in order to assist children with language impairment to enhance speech discrimination and overall language comprehension abilities. Half of the children in this study were exposed to prerecorded acoustically modified speech using computer games, audio tapes, and CD-ROMS designed for this study for approximately 5 hours each day over a 4-week period. The other half of the children received the same training, however, the speech input was not modified. The authors concluded that training children with a temporally prolonged and emphasized speech signal lead to significant improvement in measures of speech discrimination, language processing, and grammatical comprehension. Further, testing at 6 weeks postintervention revealed that the gains the children made during the intervention were maintained. Based on the positive results of this study, a number of the modified speech computer games introduced by Tallal et al. (1996) were packaged as a commercially available software program called Fast ForWord® Language (FFW-L; Scientific Learning Corporation, 1998).

A number of researchers have closely examined the success of intervention in children with SLI when modifications have been made to the speech signal. Cohen et al. (2005) evaluated the efficacy of adding the FFW-L software to the treatment programs of children with severe mixed receptive expressive SLI in a randomized controlled trial. The children who participated in this study received either: (a) FFW-L intervention delivered at home by each child's parents, (b) a number of language learning computer programs that did not contain modified speech delivered at home by each child's parents, and (c) a control group who received no additional home intervention. During the study, all of the children continued to receive their regular speech and language intervention programs at school. The children made significant gains in language outcome measures, but did not demonstrate any significant benefit among any of the three groups. The authors concluded that the inclusion of a modified speech signal into an existing intervention regime did not offer additional benefit.

Bishop, Adams, and Rosen (2006) examined the efficacy of computer training with and without modified speech on the grammatical comprehension abilities of children with receptive language impairments. The children participated in one of three possible intervention groups aimed at enhancing grammatical comprehension of constructs already known to the children: (a) grammatical training using slow speech developed by inserting pauses before critical words, (b) grammatical training using both slow speech and modified speech based on an algorithm used in FFW-L, and (c) an untrained control group. The children in the two intervention groups received anywhere from 6 to 29 sessions consisting of 15-minute training blocks. The results of this intervention study revealed that none of the children in any of the groups demonstrated improved proficiency of the grammatical constructions targeted. The authors were not able to demonstrate any benefit of delivering the stimuli using modified speech.

Gillam and colleagues (2008) conducted a randomized controlled study of the efficacy of FFW-L that included 216 children over a span of 3 years. In this trial, the authors compared the language and auditory processing outcomes of children with language impairments assigned to one of four treatment groups. The interventions included: (a) the FFW-L computer program using modified speech designed to develop temporal processing abilities (Scientific Learning Corporation, 1998), (b) a language learning computer program designed to promote the same skills targeted by FFW-L without a modified speech signal, (c) a series of academic enrichment computer games not designed to improve language or auditory processing skills, and (d) a clinician delivered language intervention program. Following a summer program of intervention in one of the four conditions, all the children with language impairments demonstrated a significant improvement in both the language and the auditory processing measures from pre- to posttest and follow up testing at both 3 and 6 months later. The children who received FFW-L intervention and a similar computer program without a modified speech signal performed better on a subtest of phonological performance than did the children in the other two treatment conditions. The authors suggest that children should demonstrate improvement in language and auditory processing skills when they receive a time intensive intervention that requires that they focus on and immediately respond to verbal input, coupled with feedback from attentive adults and interactions with peers. In a comprehensive review of intervention practices, Cirrin and Gillam (2008) concluded that use of modified speech to improve language processing abilities is not superior to other forms of intervention including computer software programs without modified speech or clinician-based treatment.

TEACHING MEMORY STRATEGIES

It is accepted that the role of memory in intervention is compensatory in nature. Thus rather than trying to increase memory capacity, intervention serves to improve performance through enhancing the efficiency of memory resources (Dehn, 2008). It is difficult to separate memory intervention from language intervention (Gillam, 1997). Children with SLI require strategies that allow them to remember information long enough to use it for learning or for academic demands (Gill, Klecan-Aker, Roberts, & Fredenburg, 2003). Gill et al. (2003) compared three memory strategies in their intervention study that employed 30 school aged children with SLI. Each child was seen twice weekly for a 30-minute period that was divided between 15 minutes of expressive language activities and 15 minutes of following directions. During the following directions components, children received instruction that included: (a) traditional direction following instruction that included teaching prepositional phrases and vocabulary, as well as commercially available worksheet exercises, (b) imposed rehearsal where the children were instructed to repeat the clinician's instructions aloud (i.e., "copy me" or "say what I say" before the child performed the direction), or (c) both rehearse the direction (as above) as well as visualize the instruction (i.e., "see it happen" or "imagine the task finished"). Following 5 weeks of intervention, the children who received either imposed rehearsal or imposed rehearsal and visualization performed significantly better on a posttreatment measure of following directions than children who received traditional following directions instructions. Eight months following the treatment study, however, only children who received imposed rehearsal and visualization intervention maintained a significant difference from the traditional direction instruction suggesting that this intervention was superior to imposed instruction alone at maintaining the ability to follow directions after the period of direct instruction ended. Importantly, this intervention study demonstrated that children with SLI are able to successfully learn and apply a strategy of rehearsal.

Adolescents with language learning disabilities (LLD) can improve their learning performance after being taught metacognitive strategies (Wynn-Dancy & Gillam, 1997). Dehn (2008) identifies key aspects of metacognitive instruction including teaching skills such as: awareness of processing deficits and strengths, accurate selection of appropriate strategies to match the situation or task, self-monitoring and self-evaluation, and ability to revise or change strategies when necessary. Wynn-Dancy and Gillam (1997) describe two metacognitive strategies (ARROW and BRIDGE). However, they caution that adolescents with LLD not only require direction strategy instruction, but also need to be taught how to act strategically in applying these learning strategies.

SUMMARY AND CONCLUSIONS

The original classification of SLI was developed to help differentiate this population from children with other language related problems such as intellectual disability (Stark & Tallal, 1981). However, as we learn more about children with SLI it has become obvious that they comprise a heterogeneous group with potentially different underlying causes of the language disorder. One possible subgroup of children with SLI displays strong evidence of a processing capacity limitation that contributes to their language learning problem. There are several different processing theories about SLI, but they have at least one factor in common. That is that children with SLI have an intact underlying grammatical structure, but the systems involved in the processing of language prevent these children from acquiring language as efficiently as their typically developing peers. Some theories emphasize a functional problem associated with slow speed of processing while others support a structural disorder that emphasizes reduced space for processing or insufficient energy for processing. The general, or specific, systems responsible for processing acoustic and linguistic information are unable to respond to the rate or volume of information as rapidly as the systems of their typically developing peers. As a result, language development is impaired in children with SLI.

Continued research within this population is essential to help shed light on the causal factors of processing limitations and how they influence language development. Identification of the underlying cause of language impairments is critical for developing sensitive assessment measures and effective intervention procedures for children with SLI. Assessment of processing capacity (such as nonword repetition and CLPT tasks) will assist in identifying children with, or at risk for, SLI. These types of assessment procedures are relatively short in duration and easy to administer. It is unlikely that they identify those components of language that are affected or qualify children for intervention services. However, they will help determine why language learning is affected in this population. This information can be used to help establish what intervention procedures are most likely to be appropriate for children with processing problems, how to use appropriate compensatory strategies, or provide ideas of how to modify the communication environment so that the children receive the maximum benefit from language intervention. There is still much more research that needs to be completed on this population. Recent technological advances (e.g., ERP, fMRI, genetic mapping) are likely to drive research endeavors into areas that were not possible in the past.

Indeed, more advanced research designs will continue to enlighten our knowledge of this group of children with language problems. For a comprehensive overview of specific language impairment, *Specific Language Impairment* by Leonard (1998) is a recommended reading for anyone interested in this population.

REFERENCES

Adams, A. M., & Gathercole, S. E. (1995). Phonological working memory and speech production in preschool children. *Journal of Speech and Hearing Research, 38*, 403–414.

Archibald, L. M., & Gathercole, S. E. (2006a). Nonword repetition: A comparison of tests. *Journal of Speech, Language, and Hearing Research, 49*(5), 970–983.

Archibald, L. M. D., & Gathercole, S. E. (2006b). Short-term and working memory in specific language impairment. *International Journal of Language and Communication Disorders, 41*, 675–693.

Archibald, L. M. D., & Gathercole, S. E. (2007). Nonword repetition in specific language impairment: More than a phonological short-term memory deficit. *Psychonomic Bulletin and Review, 14*(5), 919–924.

Baddeley, A. (1986). *Working memory*. New York, NY: Clarendon Press/Oxford University Press.

Bishop, D. (1994). Grammatical errors in specific language impairment: Competence or performance limitations? *Applied Psycholinguistics, 15*, 507–550.

Bishop, D. V. M. (2000). How does the brain learn language? Insights from the study of children with and without language impairment. *Developmental Medicine & Child Neurology, 42*(2), 133–142.

Bishop, D. V. M. (2002). The role of genes in the etiology of specific language impairment. *Journal of Communication Disorders, 35*(4), 311–328.

Bishop, D. V. M., Adams, C. V., & Rosen, S. (2006). Resistance of grammatical impairment to computerized comprehension training in children with specific and non-specific language impairments. *International Journal of Language and Communication Disorders, 41*, 19–40.

Bishop, D. V. M., Bright, P., James, C., Bishop, S. J., & van der Lely, H. K. J. (2000). Grammatical SLI: A distinct subtype of developmental language impairment? *Applied Psycholinguistics, 21*(2), 159–181.

Bishop, D. V. M., & McArthur, G. M. (2005). Individual differences in auditory processing in specific language impairment: A follow-up study using event-related potentials and behavioural thresholds. *Cortex, 41*(3), 327–341.

Burlingame, E., Sussman, H. M., Gillam, R. B., & Hay, J. F. (2005). An investigation of speech perception in children with specific language impairment on a continuum of formant transition duration. *Journal of Speech, Language, and Hearing Research, 48*(4), 805–816.

Camarata, S. M., & Nelson, K. E. (2006). Conversational recast intervention with preschool and older children. In R. J. McCauley & M. E. Fey (Eds.), *Treatment of language disorders in children* (pp. 237–264). Baltimore, MD: Paul H Brookes Publishing.

Camarata, S. M., Nelson, K. E., & Camarata, M. N. (1994). Comparison of conversational-recasting and imitative procedures for training grammatical structures in children with specific language impairment. *Journal of Speech & Hearing Research, 37*(6), 1414–1423.

Cirrin, F. M., & Gillam, R. B. (2008). Language intervention practices for school-age children with spoken language disorders: A systematic review. *Language, Speech, and Hearing Services in Schools, 39*(1), 110–137.

Cleave, P. L., & Fey, M. E. (1997). Two approaches to the facilitation of grammar in children with language impairments: Rationale and description. *American Journal of Speech-Language Pathology, 6*(1), 22–32.

Cohen, W., Hodson, A., O'Hare, A., Boyle, J., Durrani, T., McCartney, E., . . . Watson, J. (2005). Effects of computer-based intervention through acoustically modified speech (Fast ForWord) in severe mixed receptive-expressive language impairment: Outcomes from a randomized controlled trial. *Journal of Speech, Language, and Hearing Research, 48*(3), 715–729.

Connell, P. J. (1987). An effect of modeling and imitation teaching procedures on children with and without specific language impairment. *Journal of Speech & Hearing Research, 30*(1), 105–113.

Connell, P. J., & Stone, C. A. (1992). Morpheme learning of children with specific language impairment under controlled instructional conditions. *Journal of Speech & Hearing Research, 35*(4), 844–852.

Conti-Ramsden, G., Botting, N., & Faragher, B. (2001). Psycholinguistic markers for specific language impairment (SLI). *Journal of Child Psychology and Psychiatry, 42*(6), 741–748.

Crago, M. B., & Gopnik, M. (1994). From families to phenotypes: Theoretical and clinical implications of research into the genetic basis of specific language impairment. In R. V. Watkins & M. L. Rice (Eds.), *Specific language impairments in children* (pp. 35–51). Baltimore, MD: Paul H Brookes Publishing.

Criddle, M. J., & Durkin, K. (2001). Phonological representation of novel morphemes in children with SLI and typically developing children. *Applied Psycholinguistics, 22*(3), 363–382.

Daneman, M., & Carpenter, P. A. (1983). Individual differences in integrating information between and within sentences. *Journal of Experimental Psychology: Learning, Memory, and Cognition, 9*(4), 561–584.

Dehn, M. (2008). *Working memory and academic learning: Assessment and intervention* (1st ed.). Hoboken, NJ: John Wiley & Sons.

Dick, F., Wulfeck, B., Krupa-Kwiatkowski, M., & Bates, E. (2004). The development of complex sentence interpretation in typically developing children compared with children with specific language impairments or early unilateral focal lesions. *Developmental Science, 7*(3), 360–377.

DiSimoni, F., Ehrler, D. J., & McGhee, R. L. (2007). *Token test for children* (Rev.). Greenville, SC: Super Duper Publications.

Dollaghan, C. A. (2007). *The handbook for evidence-based practice in communication disorders*. Baltimore, MD: Paul H Brookes Publishing.

Dollaghan, C., & Campbell, T. F. (1998). Nonword repetition and child language impairment. *Journal of Speech, Language, and Hearing Research, 41*(5), 1136–1146.

Ebbels, S. H., van der Lely, H. K. J., & Dockrell, J. E. (2007). Intervention for verb argument structure in children with persistent SLI: A randomized control trial. *Journal of Speech, Language, and Hearing Research, 50*, 1330–1349.

Ellis Weismer, S. E. (1997). The role of stress in language processing and intervention. *Topics in Language Disorders, 17*(4), 41–52.

Ellis Weismer, S., Evans, J. L., & Hesketh, L. J. (1999). An examination of verbal working memory capacity in children with specific language impairment. *Journal of Speech, Language, and Hearing Research, 42*, 1249–1260.

Ellis Weismer, S. E., & Hesketh, L. J. (1993). The influence of prosodic and gestural cues on novel word acquisition by children with specific language impairment. *Journal of Speech & Hearing Research, 36*(5), 1013–1025.

Ellis Weismer, S. E., & Hesketh, L. J. (1996). Lexical learning by children with specific language impairment: Effects of linguistic input presented at varying speaking rates. *Journal of Speech & Hearing Research, 39*(1), 177–190.

Ellis Weismer, S., & Hesketh, L. J. (1998). The impact of emphatic stress on novel word learning by children with specific language impairment. *Journal of Speech, Language, and Hearing Research, 41*, 1444–1458.

Ellis Weismer, S. E., Plante, E., Jones, M., & Tomblin, J. B. (2005). A functional magnetic resonance imagining investigation of verbal working memory in adolescents with specific language impairment. *Journal of Speech, Language, and Hearing Research, 48*, 405–425.

Ellis Weismer, S., Tomblin, J. B., Zhang, X., Buckwalter, P., Chynoweth, J. G., & Jones, M. (2000). Nonword repetition performance in school-age children with and without language impairment. *Journal of Speech, Language, and Hearing Research, 43*, 865–878.

Estes, K. G., Evans, J. L., & Else-Quest, N. M. (2007). Differences in the nonword repetition performance of children with and without specific language impairment: A meta-analysis. *Journal of Speech, Language, and Hearing Research, 50*, 177–195.

Fey, M. E. (1986). *Language intervention with young children.* San Diego, CA: College-Hill Press.

Fey, M. E., Cleave, P. L., Long, S. H., & Hughes, D. L. (1993). Two approaches to the facilitation of grammar in children with language impairment: An experimental evaluation. *Journal of Speech & Hearing Research, 36*(1), 141–157.

Fey, M. E., Long, S. H., & Finestack, L. H. (2003). Ten principles of grammar facilitation for children with specific language impairments. *American Journal of Speech-Language Pathology, 12*(1), 3–15.

Gathercole, S. E., & Baddeley, A. D. (1995). Short-term memory may yet be deficient in children with language impairments: A comment on van der Lely & Howard (1993). *Journal of Speech & Hearing Research, 38*(2), 463–466.

Gathercole, S. E., Willis, C. S., Baddeley, A. D., & Emslie, H. (1994). The children's test of nonword repetition: A test of phonological working memory. *Memory, 2*(2), 103–127.

Gaulin, C. A., & Campbell, T. F. (1994). Procedure for assessing verbal working memory in normal school-age children: Some preliminary data. *Perceptual and Motor Skills, 79*, 55–64.

Gill, C. B., Klecan-Aker, J., Roberts, T., & Fredenburg, K. A. (2003). Following directions: Rehearsal and visualization strategies for children with specific language impairment. *Child Language Teaching & Therapy, 19*(1), 85–101.

Gillam, R. B. (1997). Putting memory to work in language intervention: Implications for practitioners. *Topics in Language Disorders, 18*(1), 72–79.

Gillam, R. B., Loeb, D. F., Hoffman, L. M., Bohman, T., Champlin, C. A., Thibodeau, L., . . . Friel-Patti. S. (2008). The efficacy of Fast ForWord language intervention in school-age children with language impairment: A randomized controlled trial. *Journal of Speech, Language, and Hearing Research, 51*(1), 97–119.

Gillam, S. L., & Gillam, R. B. (2006). Making evidence-based decisions about child language intervention in schools. *Language, Speech, and Hearing Services in Schools, 37*(4), 304–315.

Girolametto, L., Pearce, P. S., & Weitzman, E. (1996). Interactive focused stimulation for toddlers with expressive vocabulary delays. *Journal of Speech & Hearing Research, 39*(6), 1274–1283.

Grela, B. G. (2003a). The omission of subject arguments in children with specific language impairment. *Clinical Linguistics and Phonetics, 17*, 153–169.

Grela, B. G. (2003b). Production based theories may account for subject omission in normal children and children with SLI. *Journal of Speech-Language Pathology and Audiology, 27,* 221–228.

Grela, B. G., & Leonard, L. B. (1997). The use of subject arguments by children with specific language impairment. *Clinical Linguistics and Phonetics, 11*(6), 443–453.

Grela, B. G., & Leonard, L. B. (2000). The influence of argument-structure complexity on the use of auxiliary verbs by children with SLI. *Journal of Speech, Language, and Hearing Research, 43*(5), 1115–1125.

Grela, B. G., Snyder, W., & Hiramatsu, K. (2005). The production of novel root compounds in children with specific language impairment. *Clinical Linguistics and Phonetics, 19,* 701–715.

Gutierrez-Clellen, V. F., & Peña, E. (2001). Dynamic assessment of diverse children: A tutorial. *Language, 32*(4), 212–224.

Hasson, N., & Joffe, V. (2007). The case for dynamic assessment in speech and language therapy. *Child Language Teaching and Therapy, 23*(1), 9–25.

Hayiou-Thomas, M. E., Bishop, D. V. M., & Plunkett, K. (2004). Simulating SLI: General cognitive processing stressors can produce a specific linguistic profile. *Journal of Speech, Language, and Hearing Research, 47*(6), 1347–1362.

Hugdahl, K., Gundersen, H., Brekke, C., Thomsen, T., Rimol, L. M., Ersland, L., & Niemi, J. (2004). fMRI brain activation in a Finnish family with specific language impairment compared with a normal control group. *Journal of Speech, Language, and Hearing Research, 47*(1), 162–172.

Hutchinson, T. A. (1996). What to look for in the technical manual: Twenty questions for users. *Language, Speech, and Hearing Services in Schools, 27*(2), 109–121.

Im-Bolter, N., Johnson, J., & Pascual-Leone, J. (2006). Processing limitations in children with specific language impairment: The role of executive function. *Child Development, 77,* 1822–1841.

Joanisse, M. F. (2004). Specific language impairments in children: Phonology, semantics, and the English past tense. *Current Directions in Psychological Science, 13*(4), 156–160.

Joanisse, M. F., & Seidenberg, M. S. (2003). Phonology and syntax in specific language impairment: Evidence from a connectionist model. *Brain and Language, 86*(1), 40–56.

Johnston, J. R. (1991). Questions about cognition in children with specific language impairment. In J. Miller (Ed.), *Research on child language disorders* (pp. 299–307). Austin, TX: Pro-Ed.

Johnston, J. R. (1994). Cognitive abilities of children with language impairment. In R. Watkins & M. Rice (Eds.), *Specific language impairments in children* (pp. 107–121). Baltimore, MD: Paul H. Brookes Publishing Co., Inc.

Johnston, J. R., & Kamhi, A. G. (1984). Syntactic and semantic aspects of the utterances of language impaired children: The same can be less. *Merrill-Palmer Quarterly, 30*(1), 65–85.

Juhasz, C., & Grela, B. G. (2008). Verb particle errors in preschool children with specific language impairment. *Contemporary Issues in Communication Sciences and Disorders, 35,* 76–83.

Just, M. A., & Carpenter, P. A. (1992). A capacity theory of comprehension: Individual differences in working memory. *Psychological Review, 99,* 122–148.

Kail, R. (1991). Developmental change in speed of processing during childhood and adolescence. *Psychological Bulletin, 109*(3), 490–501.

Kail, R. (1994). A method for studying the generalized slowing hypothesis in children with specific language impairment. *Journal of Speech and Hearing Research, 37,* 418–421.

Lahey, M., Edwards, J., & Munson, B. (2001). Is processing speed related to severity of language impairment? *Journal of Speech, Language, and Hearing Research, 44*(6), 1354–1361.

Lapointe, S. G. (1985). A theory of verb form use in the speech of agrammatic aphasics. *Brain and Language, 24*(1), 100–155.

Leonard, L. B. (1998). *Children with specific language impairment.* Cambridge, MA: MIT Press.

Leonard, L. B., & Bortolini, U. (1998). Grammatical morphology and the role of weak syllables in the speech of Italian-speaking children with specific language impairment. *Journal of Speech, 41*(6), 1363–1374.

Leonard, L. B., Camarata, S. M., Pawlowska, M., Brown, B., & Camarata, M. N. (2008). The acquisition of tense and agreement morphemes by children with specific language impairment during intervention: Phase 3. *Journal of Speech, Language, and Hearing Research, 51*, 120–125.

Leonard, L. B., Eyer, J. A., Bedore, L. M., & Grela, B. G. (1997). Three accounts of the grammatical morpheme difficulties of English-speaking children with specific language impairment. *Journal of Speech, Language, and Hearing Research, 40*(4), 741–753.

Leonard, L. B., McGregor, K. K., & Allen, G. D. (1992). Grammatical morphology and speech perception in children with specific language impairment. *Journal of Speech & Hearing Research, 35*(5), 1076–1085.

Leonard, L. B., Miller, C. A., Grela, B., Holland, A. L., Gerber, E., & Petucci, M. (2000). Production operations contribute to the grammatical morpheme limitations of children with specific language impairment. *Journal of Memory and Language, 43*(2), 362–378.

Leonard, L. B., Weismer, S. E., Miller, C. A., Francis, D. J., Tomblin, J. B., & Kail, R. (2007). Speed of processing, working memory and language impairment in children. *Journal of Speech, Language, and Hearing Research, 50*, 408–428.

Marton, K., Schwartz, R. G., Farkas, L., & Katsnelson, V. (2006). Effect of sentence length and complexity on working memory performance in Hungarian children with specific language impairment (SLI): A cross-linguistic comparison. *International Journal of Language & Communication Disorders, 41*(6), 653–673.

McArthur, G. M., & Bishop, D. V. M. (2004). Which people with specific language impairment have auditory processing deficits? *Cognitive Neuropsychology, 21*(1), 79–94.

McArthur, G. M., & Bishop, D. V. M. (2005). Speech and non-speech processing in people with specific language impairment: A behavioural and electrophysiological study. *Brain and Language, 94*(3), 260–273.

McCauley, R. J., & Swisher, L. (1984). Psychometric review of language and articulation tests for preschool children. *Journal of Speech and Hearing Disorders, 49*, 34–42.

Miller, C. A., Kail, R., Leonard, L. B., & Tomblin, J. B. (2001). Speed of processing in children with specific language impairment. *Journal of Speech, Language, and Hearing Research, 44*, 416–433.

Miller, C. A., & Leonard, L. B. (1998). Deficits in finite verb morphology: Some assumptions in recent accounts of specific language impairment. *Journal of Speech, Language & Hearing Research, 41*(3), 701–707.

Miller, C. A., Leonard, L. B., Kail, R. V., Zhang, X., Tomblin, J. B., & Francis, D. J. (2006). Response time in 14-year-olds with language impairment. *Journal of Speech, Language, and Hearing Research, 49*(4), 712–728.

Montgomery, J. W. (2000). Verbal working memory and sentence comprehension in children with specific language impairment. *Journal of Speech, Language, and Hearing Research, 43*, 293–308.

Montgomery, J. W. (2003). Working memory and comprehension in children with specific language impairment: What we know so far. *Journal of Communication Disorders, 36*, 221–231.

Montgomery, J. W. (2005). Effects of input rate and age on the real-time language processing of children with specific language impairment. *International Journal of Language & Communication Disorders, 40*(2), 171–188.

Montgomery, J. W., & Leonard, L. B. (1998). Real-time inflectional processing by children with specific language impairment: Effects of phonetic substance. *Journal of Speech, Language, and Hearing Research, 41*, 1432–1443.

Montgomery, J. W., & Leonard, L. B. (2006). Effects of acoustic manipulation on the real-time inflectional processing of children with specific language impairment. *Journal of Speech, Language, and Hearing Research, 49*, 1238–1256.

Montgomery, J. W., & Windsor, J. (2007). Examining the language performances of children with and without specific language impairment: Contributions of phonological short-term memory and speed of processing. *Journal of Speech, Language, and Hearing Research, 50*(3), 778–797.

Nelson, K. E., Camarata, S. M., Welsh, J., & Butkovsky, L. (1996). Effects of imitative and conversational recasting treatment on the acquisition of grammar in children with specific language impairment and younger language-normal children. *Journal of Speech & Hearing Research, 39*(4), 850–859.

Peña, E. D., & Gillam, R. B. (2000). Dynamic assessment of children referred for speech and language evaluations. *Advances in Cognition and Educational Practice, 6*, 543–575.

Peña, E., Iglesias, A., & Lidz, C. S. (2001). Reducing test bias through dynamic assessment of children's word learning ability. *American Journal of Speech-Language Pathology, 10*(2), 138–154.

Peña, E., Quinn, R., & Iglesias, A. (1992). The application of dynamic methods to language assessment: A nonbiased procedure. *The Journal of Special Education, 26*(3), 269–280.

Pizzioli, F., & Schelstraete, M.-A. (2008). The argument-structure complexity effect in children with specific language impairment: Evidence from the use of grammatical morphemes in French. *Journal of Speech, Language, and Hearing Research, 51*, 706–721.

Plante, E., & Vance, R. (1994). Selection of preschool language tests: A data-based approach. *Language, 25*(1), 15–24.

Polite, E. J., & Leonard, L. B. (2006). Finite verb morphology and phonological length in the speech of children with specific language impairment. *Clinical Linguistics & Phonetics, 10*, 751–760.

Rice, M. L. (2004). Growth models of developmental language disorders. In M. L. Rice & S. F. Warren (Eds.), *Developmental language disorders: From phenotypes to etiologies* (pp. 207–240). Mahwah, NJ: Lawrence Erlbaum Associates Publishers.

Rice, M. L., & Wexler, K. (1996). Toward tense as a clinical marker of specific language impairment in English-speaking children. *Journal of Speech and Hearing Research, 39*(6), 1239–1257.

Robertson, S. B., & Weismer, S. E. (1999). Effects of treatment on linguistic and social skills in toddlers with delayed language development. *Journal of Speech, Language, and Hearing Research, 42*(5), 1234–1248.

Roy, P., & Chiat, S. (2004). A prosodically controlled word and nonword repetition task for 2- to 4-year-olds: Evidence from typically developing children. *Journal of Speech, Language, and Hearing Research, 47*(1), 223–234.

Schul, R., Stiles, J., Wulfeck, B., & Townsend, J. (2004). How "generalized" is the "slowed processing" in SLI? The case of visuospatial attentional orienting. *Neuropsychologia, 42*(5), 661–671.

Scientific Learning Corporation. (1998). *Fast Forward Language* [Computer Software]. Berkeley, CA: Author.

Semel, E., Wiig, E., & Secord, W. (1987). *Clinical evaluation of language fundamentals-revised.* San Antonio, TX: The Psychological Corporation.

Spaulding, T. J., Plante, E., & Farinella, K. A. (2006). Eligibility criteria for language impairment: Is the low end of normal always appropriate? *Language, 37*(1), 61–72.

Stark, R., & Tallal, P. (1981). Selection of children with specific language deficits. *Journal of Speech and Hearing Disorders, 46,* 114–122.

Tallal, P. (1980). Language disabilities in children: A perceptual or linguistic deficit? *Journal of Pediatric Psychology, 5*(2), 127–140.

Tallal, P. (2004). Improving language and literacy is a matter of time. *Nature Reviews Neuroscience, 5*(9), 721–728.

Tallal, P., Miller, S. L., Bedi, G., Wang, X., & Nagarajan, S. S. (1996). Language comprehension in language-learning impaired children improved with acoustically modified speech. *Science, 271*(5245), 81–84.

Tallal, P., Miller, S., & Fitch, R. H. (1993). Neurobiological basis of speech: A case for the pre-eminence of temporal processing. In P. Tallal, A. M. Galaburda, R. R. Llinás, & C. von Euler (Eds.), *Temporal information processing in the nervous system: Special reference to dyslexia and dysphasia* (pp. 27–47). New York, NY: New York Academy of Sciences.

Tallal, P., & Piercy, M. (1974). Developmental aphasia: Rate of auditory processing and selective impairment of consonant perception. *Neuropsychologia, 12*(1), 83–93.

Tallal, P., & Piercy, M. (1975). Developmental aphasia: The perception of brief vowels and extended stop consonants. *Neuropsychologia, 13*(1), 69–74.

Tallal, P., Sainburg, R. L., & Jernigan, T. (1991). The neuropathology of developmental dysphasia: Behavioral, morphological, and physiological evidence for a pervasive temporal processing disorder. *Reading and Writing, 3*(3), 363–377.

Tallal, P., Stark, R. E., & Mellits, E. D. (1985). Identification of language-impaired children on the basis of rapid perception and production skills. *Brain and Language, 25*(2), 314–322.

Tomblin, J. B., Records, N. L., Buckwalter, P., Zhang, X., Smith, E., & O'Brien, M. (1997). Prevalence of specific language impairment in kindergarten children. *Journal of Speech and Hearing Research, 40*(6), 1245–1260.

van der Lely, H. K. J. (1994). Canonical linking rules: Forward versus reverse linking in normally developing and specifically language-impaired children. *Cognition, 51,* 29–72.

van der Lely, H. K. J. (1997). Language and cognitive development in a grammatical SLI boy: Modularity and innateness. *Journal of Neurolinguistics, 10*(2), 75–107.

van der Lely, H. K. J. (2005). Domain-specific cognitive systems: Insight from grammatical-SLI. *Trends in Cognitive Sciences, 9*(2), 53–59.

Wagner, R., Torgeson, J., & Rashotte, C. (1999). *Comprehensive test of phonological processing (CTOPP)* (1st ed.). Bloomington, MN: Pearson Assessment Group.

Watkins, R. V., & Rice, M. L. (1991). Verb particle and preposition acquisition in language-impaired preschoolers. *Journal of Speech & Hearing Research, 34*(5), 1130–1141.

Windsor, J., & Hwang, M. (1999). Testing the generalized slowing hypothesis specific language impairment. *Journal of Speech, Language, and Hearing Research, 42,* 1205–1210.

Wynn-Dancy, M. L., & Gillam, R. B. (1997). Accessing long-term memory: Metacognitive strategies and strategic action in adolescents. *Topics in Language Disorders, 18*(1), 32–44.

20 Grammatical-Specific Language Impairment: A Window Onto Domain Specificity

Heather van der Lely and Chloë Marshall

INTRODUCTION

There has been much debate as to which aspects of language are specific to language rather than shared with other aspects of cognition, and which aspects of language are specific to humans rather than shared with other groups of animals (Hauser, 2001; Hauser, Chomsky, & Fitch, 2002; Pinker & Jackendoff, 2005). In addition, there continues to be much discussion about how this specialized language system is represented and develops in the brain. New insight into this debate comes from studying people with a developmental language disorder, Specific Language Impairment (SLI), and particularly a subtype of this disorder known as Grammatical (G)-SLI. Such insight is bidirectional: our growing understanding of language and brain-systems enhances and directs our line of enquiry into SLI, furthering our knowledge of the underlying nature of both typical and atypical language development. In turn, this informs our enquiries about language and brain systems.

In this context, our chapter reviews the findings from G-SLI, and aims to contribute to our understanding both of specialized cognitive systems, specifically language, and of the nature of typical and atypical language acquisition. We argue that our data provide evidence that certain aspects of grammar are domain-specific and can be selectively impaired.

THEORETICAL FOUNDATIONS

SLI: What Do We Agree On?

SLI is a disorder of language acquisition in children, in the absence of any obvious language-independent cause, such as hearing loss, low nonverbal IQ, motor difficulties, or neurological damage (Bishop, 1997; Leonard, 1998). Children, teenagers, or even adults with SLI may produce sentences such as "Who Marge saw someone?" (van der Lely & Battell, 2003) or "Yesterday I fall over" (Leonard,

Dromi, Adam, & Zadunaisky-Ehrlich, 2000; Rice, 2003; van der Lely & Ullman, 2001), or may fail to correctly interpret sentences such as "The man was eaten by the fish" (Bishop, 1982; van der Lely, 1996). SLI is one of the most common developmental disorders, affecting around 7% of children in its "pure form" (Tomblin et al., 1997), and the prevalence is even greater when children with co-occurring impairments (e.g., Autism, ADHD) are included.

The disorder heterogeneously affects components of language such as syntax, morphology, phonology and, often to a lesser extent, the lexicon. It has a strong genetic component as shown by familial aggregation studies (for a review see Stromswold, 1998), twin studies (Bishop & Bishop, 1998), and genetic analyses (Fisher, Lai, & Monaco, 2003). The current view is that SLI is likely to have a complex geno-phenotypic profile, with different genetic forms of the disorder causing different phenotypes and possibly even the same genotype resulting in varied phenotypes (Fisher et al., 2003).

SLI: WHAT DON'T WE AGREE ON?

It is perhaps not surprising that, given the heterogeneous nature of SLI, there is disagreement over two areas: a taxonomy of SLI, and its cause at the cognitive level.

The discussion surrounding the taxonomy of SLI concerns the variation and number of component deficits in children who fall under the broad umbrella of "SLI." Broadly speaking, the following disorders and language component deficits are found in the literature. Note that we are focusing on the 7% of children who fall within the "typical definition" of SLI; that is, those who do not have co-occurring problems. It is the particular combination or specification of component deficits that characterizes the various definitions of SLI, some of which are considered SLI subgroups. On the one hand, Bishop and Snowling (2004) reviewed children with SLI who have a double deficit of phonological deficits plus "language impairments." We understand this to mean some or perhaps any other component impairments within the language system. Therefore, we might expect a range of different profiles in the children they study. In contrast to this group of SLI, a highly restrictive subgroup are those called "Syntactic-SLI," characterized by only syntactic and morphosyntactic impairments (Friedmann & Novogrodsky, 2004). The "Grammatical(G)-SLI" subgroup, however, is defined by similar core impairment in syntax and morphology, but in addition the majority suffer from phonological impairment too (Gallon, Harris, & van der Lely, 2007). Even within these component deficits in syntax, morphology and phonology, the deficit is restricted to structures that are hierarchically complex, as we will discuss in due course. Interestingly, the distinction between phonology on the one hand and syntax and morphology on the other appears to be relevant to geno-phenotypic associations. Whereas a locus on Chromosome 16, now identified as CNTNAP2 is associated with children with phonological deficits and/or phonological memory deficits, a locus on Chromosome 19 is associated with expressive grammatical impairments, with no significant overlap between the groups (Bishop, Adams, & Norbury, 2006; Vernes et al., 2008).

In contrast, a subgroup who appear to have relative strengths in the grammatical aspects of language are those with "Pragmatic(P)-SLI," who, as their name implies, have impaired pragmatic abilities (Bishop & Norbury, 2002). There is one subgroup—which we shall refer to as Familial-SLI (of which the most famous is the KE family), which has an identified simple genotype—a mutation of the gene FOXP2 with a simple autosomal, dominant inheritance—but which results in a rather complex phenotype (Fisher et al., 2003). Familial-SLI is characterized by not only impairments in language components, most notably morpho-syntax, morphology, phonology as well as the lexicon, but also outside the language system. Specifically the impaired family members have an oral dyspraxia concerning problems in motor programming of fine articulatory movements for speech sounds (Fisher & DeFries, 2002; Watkins, Dronkers, & Vargha-Khadem, 2002). It is also of note that some members of the KE family have a low IQ; however low IQ doesn't segregate with the language impairment (Fisher & DeFries, 2002). In other children, low IQ is frequently (but not always) associated with a delayed pattern of language development, which we shall call the "delayed language" subgroup (Rice, 2004). Children in this group often exhibit delayed vocabulary acquisition and immature pragmatic development, alongside other language impairments (Rice, 2004).

In addition, many children with a diagnosis of SLI also have Dyslexia, and vice versa. However, these two disorders are not synonymous, and can occur in isolation. For the majority of children with Dyslexia, impairments center around the phonological component, either with the Phonological representations themselves, or with accessing and/or manipulating those representations (Ramus & Szenkovits, 2008; Snowling, 2000). Whether such phonological deficits are identical or different to those found in SLI children is the focus of much current research (de Bree, 2007; Marshall, Harcourt-Brown, Ramus, & van der Lely, 2009; Marshall & van der Lely, 2009 and papers in Messaoud-Galusi & Marshall 2010).

The second area of discussion concerns the cognitive cause of SLI. Given the considerable heterogeneity in the phenotype, it could well be that different cognitive causes and pathways underlie different forms of SLI. But equally, there could be different routes to a particular surface impairment, for example, omission of tense marking. In this context, we now consider the two predominant approaches to the cognitive origins of SLI that can be broadly characterized as the domain-general and domain-specific perspectives.

Domain-General (D-G) deficit proponents identify the primary deficit in general cognitive mechanisms such as temporal discrimination, lower-level sensory processing speed, processing capacity, and short-term memory (Bishop, 1997; Leonard, 1998; Montgomery, 2000; Tallal, 2002). These deficits are considered to impair auditory processing of nonspeech and speech sounds, or alternatively memory and/or general learning. The resulting phonological deficit in turn causes problems in language learning (Joanisse & Seidenberg, 1998). Although the primary source of the domain-general deficit varies across different accounts, they share the common view that the underlying deficit is not in mechanisms specific to grammar, but in lower-level processing or later nongrammatical cognitive processing. Note that whereas temporal deficits alone are proposed by some to be sufficient to cause SLI (Tallal et al., 1996), short-term memory deficits are thought to cause SLI only when found in combination with other impairments (Gathercole, 2006). Within this framework, Joanisse provides perhaps the most clearly specified model starting from an auditory or speech processing deficit, and he describes the resulting developmental trajectory of SLI (Joanisse, 2004; Joanisse, 2007).

Domain-Specific (D-S) deficit proponents, in contrast, claim that in some children the deficit affects the development of neural circuitry underlying the components of grammar (Bishop et al., 2006; Friedmann & Gvion, 2002; Rice, 2003; van der Lely, Rosen, & Adlard, 2004; van der Lely, Rosen, & McClelland, 1998). Thus, although both D-G and D-S mechanisms are likely to contribute to language (Gathercole, 2006; Jakubowicz & Strik, 2008; Marcus, 2004), SLI is thought to be caused by deficits to specialized computational mechanisms underlying grammar processing itself. Although a number of hypotheses have been proposed from this perspective, the Computational Grammatical Complexity (CGC) hypothesis (van der Lely, 2005), provides a framework for our research and investigations of the G-SLI subgroup. Specifically the CGC claims that the deficit is in hierarchical structural knowledge that is core to the computational grammatical system. Our work reveals that many school-aged children and teenagers with G-SLI lack the computations to consistently form hierarchical, structurally complex forms in one or more components of grammar that normally develop between 3 and 6 years of age. This working hypothesis emphasizes the notion that impairments in syntax, morphology, and phonology are functionally autonomous, but cumulative in their effects (Marshall & van der Lely, 2007a, b; van der Lely, 2005)

Figure 20.1 illustrates this model and in the following sections, we will elaborate on the characterization for these three components of grammar and how they affect language. For the purposes of this paper Figure 20.1 only shows the arrows that are key to the discussion below. Based on this component model of language impairment the CGC predicts that there is no causal relation between lower-level auditory abilities or short-term memory abilities and grammatical development, although these abilities, as with typically developing (TD) children, contribute to general language performance. These relations are shown by lines rather than arrows.

We will now consider the CGC in more detail with respect to each of the three impaired grammatical components, syntax, morphology, and phonology, and present evidence that the impairment in the G-SLI subgroup is domain-specific.

SYNTAX

The CGC claims that the deficit in hierarchical structure is characterized by impairment in syntactic dependencies. Specifically, whereas dependences within

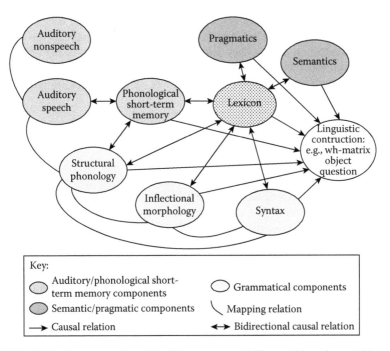

FIGURE 20.1   A component model of language acquisition and impairment. Note for clarity, only lines pertinent to the discussion have been included. There are clearly many more relations between components than depicted.

the phrase are preserved (e.g., agreement), those outside the phrase but within the clause are impaired. Broadly speaking, this can be characterized by what Chomsky terms "movement" or "feature checking"(Chomsky, 1998) or in current terminology "internal merge" (Chomsky, 2004). The impairment affects a large number of structures. For example, tense marking is impaired, resulting in errors such as *"Yesterday I walk to school"* (van der Lely & Ullman, 2001). Such errors have been eloquently described and explored by Wexler and Rice and colleagues and have led them to claim that this "extended optional infinitive" phase is the primary impairment within syntax (Rice, Wexler, & Redmond, 1999). However, the CGC claims that, at least for the G-SLI subgroup, their impairment with syntactic dependencies also affects assignment of theta roles, particularly when more general pragmatic and world knowledge is not available to facilitate interpretation, such as in reversible passive sentences (*The man was eaten by the fish*), or when assigning reference to pronouns or anaphors within sentences (*Mowgli said Baloo was tickling him/himself*; van der Lely, 1994, 1996; van der Lely & Stollwerck, 1997), as well as embedded sentences and relative clauses. The nature of the G-SLI children's syntactic deficits is clearly illustrated in a series of studies of wh-questions. Object matrix and embedded questions are particularly problematic in English because the wh-word has to move from the end of the sentence to the beginning, and "do support" requires checking of tense and question features.

Thus, G-SLI children produce questions such as "Who Joe see someone?" (van der Lely Battell, 2003) and judge such sentences to be grammatical (van der Lely Jones & Marshall, in press). They also make "copying" errors of the wh-word in embedded questions as in (1) (Archonti, 2003). This pattern is sometimes found in young children (Thornton, 1995), suggesting that such structures are syntactically simpler and easier.

(1)   "Who did Joe think who Mary saw?"

Furthermore, using a cross-modal priming paradigm, we found that G-SLI children showed no reactivation at the "gap" [marked by **"t"** in (2)] in preposition object questions in scenarios such as (2), in contrast to age and language matched control groups (Marinis & van der Lely, 2007).

(2)   Balloo gives a long carrot to the rabbit.
      "Who$_i$ did Balloo give the long carrot to t_i at the farm?"

However, we found reactivation for the G-SLI children at the offset of the verb, where subcategorized arguments might be activated, suggesting that, in contrast to their peers, they were using semantic-lexical processing rather than syntactic processing (Marinis & van der Lely, 2007).

Following these findings, our next question was "Is there evidence at the brain level of impaired processing of just these syntactic dependencies, but normal functioning in other language processes?" If this was so, it would provide good evidence for the domain-specificity of this particular syntactic operation. However, the alternative domain-general hypothesis would be supported if brain correlates showed generally slow or abnormal characteristics to all (or most) language and/or auditory processing. To investigate these alternative hypotheses we recorded electrophysiological time-locked, event-related brain potentials (ERPs) in 18 G-SLI participants aged 10–21 years, plus age-matched, language-matched, and adult controls, when they were listening to questions containing a syntactic violation. The particular syntactic violation we were interested in concerns structural syntactic dependencies at the clause level such as those that occur between a question word (*who, what*) and the word, which in declarative sentences follows the verb, but typically is absent in questions. In our particular design, the first possible "wh-word-gap" following the verb was filled. Pretesting of the sentences (see 3a) indicated that, at the critical noun following the verb to which our EEG recordings were time-locked, the listener would perceive the word as a violation. This is because, if the gap is filled, the animacy property of the noun should mismatch that of the wh-word (see 3b). Therefore, an animacy match (3a) was highly unexpected (a syntactic violation), where as the amimacy mismatch (3b) provided the control condition.

(3) a) **Who** did the man push the **clown** into? (violation)
     b) **What** did the man push the **clown** into? (control)

Crucially, the syntactic violation relied on a structural syntactic dependency between two nonadjacent words in the sentence. What is at issue here is not merely to know whether the children noticed the violation/unexpectancy of the noun, but to identify the different functional neural circuitries that are used to detect such a violation/unexpectancy. We found an "Early Left Anterior Negativity" (ELAN),

a language-specific neural correlate associated with structural syntactic violations (Friederici, 2002), in all the control groups but not in the G-SLI children.
The electrophysiological brain responses revealed a selective impairment to only
this neural circuitry that is specific to grammatical processing in G-SLI. The
participants with G-SLI appeared to be partially compensating for their syntactic
deficit by using neural circuitry associated with semantic processing (N400), and
all nongrammar-specific (N400, P600) and low-level auditory neural responses
(N1, P2, P3) were normal (Fonteneau & van der Lely, 2008). Thus, we found
that the G-SLI children did indeed notice the violation, but they were using a
different brain system to do this compared to the control subjects. The findings
indicate that grammatical neural circuitry underlying this aspect of language is
a developmentally unique system in the functional architecture of the brain, and
this complex higher cognitive system can be selectively impaired.

In summary, our syntactic findings from G-SLI show a consistent impairment
in syntactic dependencies outside the phrase but within the clause, which are
manifest across a broad range of structures. The findings from the cross-modal
priming and ERP studies indicated that G-SLI children use semantic mechanisms
to compensate for their syntactic deficits. The use of such a semantic system leads
to the speculation that the optional pattern of performance for syntax that is commonly reported in the literature results from this imprecise form of sentence
processing, rather than an optional functioning of the syntactic mechanism(s).
Such imprecise processing may not sufficiently restrict interpretation or production. Further research is warranted to explore this possibility. Note that children
who do not necessarily fit the G-SLI criterion exhibit syntactic impairments
with similar characteristics in both English speaking children (Bishop, Bright,
James, Bishop, & van der Lely, 2000; Norbury, Bishop, & Briscoe, 2002; O'Hara
& Johnston, 1997) and languages that are typologically different from English,
such as French, Greek, and Hebrew (Friedmann & Novogrodsky, 2004, 2007;
Jakubowicz, Nash, & van der Velde, 1999; Stavrakaki, 2001; Stavrakaki & van
der Lely, 2010). The largely similar characteristics of the component deficit across
different SLI subgroups is also illustrated in morphology and indeed phonology,
which we turn to in the next sections.

MORPHOLOGY

Within the morphology component, the CGC hypothesizes a hierarchical deficit
that impacts on morphologically complex forms. Thus, over and above the syntactic deficits that affect both irregular and regular tense marking, regular forms
are particularly problematic for children with G-SLI. Investigations using both
elicited production (e.g., *Every day I walk to school, Yesterday I . . .*) and grammaticality judgements of correct and incorrect forms reveal a lack of the regularity advantage found in typically developing children (van der Lely & Ullman,
1996, 2001). Furthermore, individuals with G-SLI show an atypical pattern of
frequency effects for both irregular *and* regular past tense forms. The Words and
Rules model of past tense forms (Marcus et al., 1992; Pinker, 1999) provides a

parsimonious explanation for these data: for typically developing children, irregular, morphologically simple forms are stored, which leads to frequency effects, whereas regular, morphologically complex forms are computed online and show no frequency effects. Van der Lely and Ullman (2001) therefore hypothesized that G-SLI children preferentially store regular inflected forms whole, as they do irregular forms. Thus, phonological-to-semantic mapping is key to the learning and processing of both regular and irregular forms.

We report two direct tests of van der Lely and Ullman's hypothesis. The first test explored plural compounds, building on Gorden's study of young children (Gordon, 1985). Gordon showed that 3–5 year olds use irregular plurals inside compounds, such as *mice-eater*, but avoid using regular plurals to create forms such as *rats-eater*. This is because only stored forms can enter the compounding process (Gordon, 1985). Therefore, we hypothesized that if G-SLI children were storing regular plural forms whole, then these would be available to the compounding process, just like irregular plurals. Consistent with our hypothesis, G-SLI children, in contrast to language-matched controls, produced compound forms such as *rats-eater* (van der Lely & Christian, 2000).

The second test of the hypothesis considered the phonotactics of regular past tense marking, and specifically the clusters formed at the verb end when the suffix is added. Some of these clusters also occur in monomorphemic words, for example the cluster at the end of *missed* (*mist*) and *scowled* (*cold*), and we refer to these as "monomorphemically legal clusters." In contrast, some clusters, such as those at the end of *slammed*, *robbed,* and *loved*, only occur in morphologically complex words (past tense or past participles), and we call these "monomorphemically illegal clusters." Because these illegal clusters only occur in inflected words, their frequency is much lower than that of legal clusters. Thus if, as we hypothesized, G-SLI children are storing past tense forms, they should find it harder to inflect verbs when an illegal cluster would be created. On the other hand, if typically developing children are able to compute regular past tense verb forms online, then cluster frequency should have no effect, and they should be equally able to infect the stem whatever the legality of the final cluster.

Reanalysis of the past tense elicitation data collected by van der Lely and Ullman (2001), a new elicitation experiment conducted with a new group of G-SLI children, plus re-analysis of data previously collected by Michael Thomas et al. (2001) confirmed our predictions. Whereas typically developing children from all three studies showed no differences between regular past tense forms containing legal or illegal clusters, the G-SLI children performed consistently worse on verbs containing illegal clusters (Marshall & van der Lely, 2006).

A further investigation of this phenomenon studied past participle forms in online processing of passive sentences, which contained a past participle with either a monomorphemically legal cluster (*kissed*; see 4a) or a monomorphemically illegal cluster (*bathed*; see 4b).

(4) a) I think that the squirrel with the gloves was ki<u>ssed</u> by the tortoise at his house last weekend.

b) I think that the squirrel with the gloves was ba<u>thed</u> by the tortoise at his house last weekend.

We predicted that typically developing children would be able to use the phonotactic cues provided by an illegal cluster to identify the past participle, and therefore interpret the passive sentence more accurately than when this cue was not available; that is, in the forms with legal clusters. G-SLI children, however, were predicted not to be able to use this parsing cue, and therefore show no advantage for sentences where the past participle contained an illegal cluster. Using a self-passed listening task involving a sentence-picture judgement task, this is exactly what we found: typically developing children were significantly more accurate on their judgements for sentences containing the monomorphemically illegal past participle forms. In contrast, G-SLI children did not show a difference between legal and illegal forms, suggesting that the phonotactic cue to the words morphological complexity did not facilitate their parsing of the sentence.

Our investigations into the phonotactics of clusters with respect to morphology is at the interface of morphology and phonology. We now turn to the phonology component itself and our findings from G-SLI children.

PHONOLOGY

Just as the deficit in G-SLI affects hierarchical structures in syntax and morphology, so it affects hierarchical structures in phonology. Phonological constituents such as syllables and prosodic words are grouped into successively higher levels of the prosodic hierarchy (Selkirk, 1978). Certain aspects of phonological structure cause difficulty for children with G-SLI. Children with G-SLI have clear and fluent speech, and are intelligible for known words. Their phonological deficit manifests as a difficulty with forms that are complex at the syllable and foot levels of the prosodic hierarchy (Gallon et al., 2007). In a nonword repetition task, G-SLI children simplify consonant clusters in all word positions, while unfooted syllables are deleted or cause syllabic simplifications and segmental changes elsewhere in the word (Marshall, 2004; Marshall, Ebbels, Harris, & van der Lely, 2002).

For example, in Gallon et al.'s study, *fə. klɛs. tə. lə* (where dots indicate syllable boundaries) was repeated by some children as, *fə. kɛs. tə. lə* with cluster simplification, and by others as *fə. glɛs. tə.,* with erroneous voicing of the velar stop and deletion of the final unfooted syllable (Gallon et al., 2007). Furthermore, systematically increasing the complexity of phonological structure resulted in a systematic increase in errors, regardless of the number of syllables, indicating that it is not just the length of phonological material to be retained in phonological short-term memory that is relevant to repetition accuracy, but the arrangement of that material in the prosodic hierarchy. Even monosyllabic nonwords with two clusters (e.g. *klɛst*) were more difficult for G-SLI children than those with one cluster (e.g., *klɛt*) or no clusters (e.g., *kɛt*), and for disyllabic nonwords, a marked initial weak syllable caused weak-strong forms (e.g., *bə.dremp*) to be more difficult than strong-weak forms (e.g., *drɛm.pə*). This contrasts with previous studies of nonword repetition in children with SLI, which have not shown group differences between SLI and typically developing children when nonwords are only one or two syllables long.

However, it is how these deficits in phonology and other components of language impact on language processing and production that is of ultimate concern to both researcher and clinician.

THE CUMULATIVE EFFECT OF COMPONENT DEFICITS

The CGC model hypothesizes that for children with G-SLI, the deficit is in representing linguistic structural complexity in three components of the computational grammatical system—syntax, morphology, and phonology. Deficits in these components impact on a variety of linguistic constructions as a function of their syntactic, morphological, and phonological complexity. The regular past tense deficit that is found not only in children with G-SLI, but also the vast majority of children with SLI, has been explored most thoroughly. We have already discussed the impact of syntactic and morphological deficits on G-SLI children's realization of tense. Here we complete the picture by considering the effects of phonological complexity. Using an elicitation task we manipulated the phonological complexity of the inflected verb end, and found that, as predicted, phonological complexity impacted on suffixation. G-SLI children were less likely to inflect stems when the suffixed form would end in a consonant cluster, for example *jumped* and *hugged*, compared to when no cluster would result, for example, *weighed*. Furthermore, stems ending in a cluster (*jump*) were less likely to be suffixed than stems ending in a single consonant (*hug*). In contrast, typically developing controls showed no effect of phonological complexity on inflection (Marshall & van der Lely, 2007b).

In another study, we found that morphological and phonological deficits impact even on an aspect of language that is not traditionally noted as being problematic for English-speaking children with SLI—derivational morphology (Marshall & van der Lely, 2007a). We elicited two types of derived forms—adjectives derived from nouns by the addition of *-y* (*sand* → *sandy*, *rocks* → *rocky*), and comparative and superlative adjectives (*happy* → *happier, happiest*). In the former case, the stimulus was either a singular or a regular plural noun, while in the latter the adjectival stem was either one or two syllables long. G-SLI children almost invariably supplied the *-y*, *-er,* and *-est* suffixes, in stark contrast to their high omission of the past tense suffix. Moreover, increasing the morphological or phonological complexity of the stimulus did not trigger suffix omission, but did result in nontarget forms that were uncharacteristic of typically developing children. Some G-SLI children included *-s* inside *-y* when presented with a plural stimulus, producing forms such as *holesy, rocksy,* and *frillsy*, whereas typically developing children very rarely did so (*holey, rocky, frilly*). In forming comparative and superlative adjectives, both G-SLI and typically developing children reduced three-syllable outputs (e.g., *happier, narrowest*) to two-syllable outputs, providing evidence of a maximal word effect on derivation; that is, pressure to limit the output to the size and shape of a trochaic (strong-weak) foot, a constraint that is characteristic of

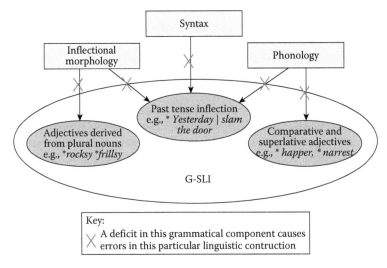

FIGURE 20.2   The computational grammatical complexity model of G-SLI: The impact of component deficits on different linguistic constructions.

young English-speaking children. However, the groups responded differently—G-SLI children's favored strategy was to truncate the stem and retain the suffix (*happer, narrest*), whereas for typically developing children the favored strategy was to omit the suffix and retain the stem-final weak syllable (*happy, narrow*).

The cumulative impact of independent component deficits in the grammatical computational system is illustrated in Figure 20.2.

DO AUDITORY DEFICITS MAINTAIN G-SLI?

One possibility is that an auditory deficit causes and maintains the grammatical impairments found in G-SLI. Evidence of subtle auditory deficits would conflict with domain-specific hypotheses and, instead, support domain-general perspectives. However, neither behavioral nor electrophysiological data have revealed any consistent auditory deficit in individuals with G-SLI that is independent of their language deficit. First, we explored G-SLI children's auditory perception for speech and nonspeech sounds, at varying presentation rates, and controlling for the effects of age and language on performance (van der Lely et al., 2004). For nonspeech formant transitions, 69% of the G-SLI children showed normal auditory processing, whereas for the same acoustic information in speech, only 31% did so. For rapidly presented tones, 46% of the G-SLI children performed normally. Auditory performance with speech and nonspeech sounds differentiated the G-SLI children from their age-matched controls, whereas speed of processing did not. A further set of experiments looked at "backward masking"; that is, their ability to detect a brief tone in quiet, and in the presence of a following noise (Rosen, Adlard, & van der Lely, 2009). Here group analyses showed that mean thresholds for the G-SLI group were never worse than those obtained for the two younger language control groups, but were higher in both backward and simultaneous masking compared to age-matched controls. However, more than half of the G-SLI group (8/14) were within normal limits for all thresholds. Furthermore, the G-SLI children consistently evinced no relationship between their auditory and phonological/grammatical abilities.

A further possibility is that a more sensitive measure might identify an impairment. To test this we explored the neural correlates to auditory processing using event related potential techniques. ERPs can measure brain responses with a millisecond precision, and therefore have the time resolution to detect delayed or deviant brain responses. We recorded Auditory Evoked Potentials (AEPs) of G-SLI and age matched control participants to pure tones in a classical auditory oddball paradigm. Auditory processing elicits early electrophysiological responses known as the N100/P200 (or N1/P2) complex. This complex is associated with perceptual detection of a discrete change in the auditory environment. In addition, they elicit a later P300 component that reflects attentional control processes to detect and categorize a specific event. We discovered that children with G-SLI have age-appropriate waveforms for the N100, P200, and the P300 components (latency, amplitude, distribution on the scalp; Fonteneau & van der Lely, 2008). Our results reveal that G-SLI children have normal auditory processing during the discrimination of pure tones.

These findings, along with those investigating nonverbal cognitive abilities thought to possibly co-occur with, but not cause SLI (or G-SLI; see van der Lely et al., 1998), are consistent with a number of other researchers in the field investigating other SLI subgroups (Bishop et al., 2000; Bishop, Carlyon, Deeks, & Bishop, 1999) and dyslexia (Ramus, 2003). Auditory and nonverbal deficits are more prevalent in the SLI population than in typically developing populations, but no consistent nonverbal deficit has yet been found to co-occur or cause any form of SLI. This of course does not mean that such deficits, when they do co-occur, do not have an impact on language development: it is likely that they do to some extent. We set out in the discussion of our model just why and how we see different components of language affecting performance.

THE CGC MODEL OF LANGUAGE IMPAIRMENT IN THE CONTEXT OF A COMPONENT MODEL OF LANGUAGE ACQUISITION

Our discussion above provides details of the nature of component deficits within the CGC model, and specifically the nature of the hierarchical deficits within each grammatical component. This model has led to clear predictions with respect to precisely those structures in syntax, morphology, and phonology that will be impaired. In addition, the model has enabled us to predict how component deficits would individually impact on processing of linguistic forms, such as wh-questions, and tense marking. The model provides a parsimonious explanation for the pattern of impairments in G-SLI: cumulative effects of component deficits, alongside compensation by components that potentially function normally. Although the CGC model was originally developed to account for G-SLI, the component nature of this model and the detail within the grammatical components enables it to be applied to other forms of SLI, in both English and other languages, and indeed to typical language acquisition. For example, the model predicts that an auditory speech deficit will impact on phonology (specifically at the segmental level) due to mapping relations between the two, and thereby impact on language. It will not, however, directly *cause* the basic mechanisms and representations of phonology to be impaired. The CGC differs from domain-general perspectives in this respect, and this is, of course, an empirical issue. However, the specification of the CGC goes some way to helping understand *how* different components can affect language processing and performance. There is still much to understand about the role of mapping relations between components in normal and impaired acquisition, but we hope that this model will contribute to clarifying these relations.

CONCLUSION

This chapter has focused on the G-SLI subgroup. It has shown the existence of a relatively pure grammatical impairment that affects syntax, morphology, and phonology, but spares other cognitive abilities. More specifically, the deficit affects particular aspects of the grammatical system: complex hierarchical structure. This deficit in the CGC system manifests itself as an impairment in the computation of syntactic dependencies at the level of clause structure, complex morphological words, involving abstract rules, and complex phonological forms involving, for example, clusters and unfooted syllables. All these aspects of language are those learned through development and vary in interesting ways from language to language. Our data challenge views denying that some forms of language impairment are caused by underlying deficits to highly specialized domain-specific mechanisms that normally develop in the young child to facilitate language learning. The fact that other subgroups of SLI show deficits that have similar characteristics in syntax, morphology, and phonology, regardless of any co-occurring problems (Norbury et al., 2002), points to multiple genetic causes impacting on these components, with some genetic causes being more discrete than others.

Finally, the CGC model explains how processing in many different components of language—some within and some outside the grammatical system—in addition to factors pertinent to language such as phonological memory, contributes to language performance. In other words, processing is a reflection of "multiple processing systems." Our model clarifies how each component impacts on language performance in highly predictable ways. Thus, language performance will depend on both the linguistic characteristics of the material with respect to its complexity in each component, and the basic functioning of each component itself. We have shown how G-SLI children appear to use their strengths in certain components to compensate, at least partially, for deficits in others. Thus, for G-SLI children and perhaps other SLI subgroups too, a relative strength in semantic processing could be targeted to help compensate for their syntactic impairment.

In conclusion, our data from the G-SLI subgroup show how some components in grammar can be selectively impaired, supporting a domain-specific view of at least some cognitive systems. These findings provide a valuable window onto the functional architecture of the brain and the development of uniquely human and specialized higher cognitive systems.

ACKNOWLEDGMENTS

We thank the children, parents, schools, and speech and language therapists who have contributed so much to the work reported here. The work was supported by the Wellcome Trust Grant number 063713, the ESRC Grant number RES-000-23-0575, and a Leverhulme Trust Visiting Fellowship to H. van der Lely. Particular thanks are due to the insightful comments and discussion from participants of the Biocomp Workshop on "Specific language impairment and the language faculty" at Harvard University, February 20, 2008 where many of the above issues were discussed.

REFERENCES

Archonti, A. (2003). Wh-Question formation in typically developing children and children with Grammatical SLI. *Human communication science.* London, UK: UCL.

Bishop, D. V. M. (1982). Comprehension of spoken, written and signed sentences in childhood language disorders. *Journal of Child Psychology and Psychiatry, 23*, 1–20.

Bishop, D. V. M. (1997). *Uncommon understanding: Comprehension in specific language impairment.* Hove, UK: Psychology Press.

Bishop, D. V. M., Adams, C. V., & Norbury, C. F. (2006). Distinct genetic influences on grammar and phonological short-term memory deficits: Evidence from 6-year-old twins. *Genes Brain Behavior, 5*(2), 158–169.

Bishop, D. V. M., & Bishop, S. J. (1998). "Twin language": A risk factor for language impairment? *Journal of Speech, Language, and Hearing Research, 41*(1), 150–160.

Bishop, D. V. M., Bright, P., James, C., Bishop, S. J., & van der Lely, H. K. J. (2000). Grammatical SLI: A distinct subtype of developmental language disorder?" *Applied Psycholinguistics, 21*, 159–181.

Bishop, D. V. M., Carlyon, R. P., Deeks, J. M., & Bishop, S. J. (1999). Auditory temporal processing impairment: Neither necessary nor sufficient for causing language impairment in children. *Journal of Speech, Language, and Hearing Research, 42*(6), 1295–1310.

Bishop, D. V. M., & Norbury, C. F. (2002). Exploring the borderlands of autistic disorder and specific language impairment: A study using standardised diagnostic instruments. *Journal of Child Psychology & Psychiatry, 43*(7), 917–929.

Bishop, D. V. M., & Snowling, M. J. (2004). Developmental dyslexia and specific language impairment: Same or different?" *Psychological Bulletin, 130*(6), 858–886.

Chomsky, N. (1998). *Minimalist inquiries: The framework Ms.* Cambridge, MA: MIT Press.

Chomsky, N. (2004). Beyond explanatory adequacy. In A. Belletti (Ed.), *Structures and beyond: The cartography of syntactic structures* (Vol. 3, pp. 104–131). Oxford, UK: Oxford University Press.

de Bree, E. (2007). *Dyslexia and phonology: A study of the phonological abilities of Dutch children at-risk of dyslexia.* University of Utrecht, The Netherlands: LOT.

Fisher, S. E., & DeFries, J. C. (2002). Developmental dyslexia: Genetic dissection of a complex cognitive trait. *Nature Reviews Neuroscience, 3,* 767–780.

Fisher, S. E., Lai, C. S., & Monaco, A. P. (2003). Deciphering the genetic basis of speech and language disorders. *Annual Review Neuroscience, 8,* 8.

Fonteneau, E., & van der Lely, H. K. J. (2008). Electrical brain responses in language-impaired children reveal grammar-specific deficits. *PLoS ONE, 3*(3), e1832.

Friederici, A. D. (2002). Toward a neural basis of auditory sentence processing. *Trends in Cognitive Sciences, 6*(2), 78–84.

Friedmann, N., & Gvion, A. (2002). Modularity in developmental disorders: Evidence from SLI and peripheral dyslexias. *Behavioral and Brain Sciences, 25*(6), 756–757.

Friedmann, N., & Novogrodsky, R. (2004). The acquisition of relative clause comprehension in Hebrew: A study of SLI and normal development. *Journal of Child Language, 31*(3), 661–681.

Friedmann, N., & Novogrodsky, R. (2007). Is the movement deficit in syntactic SLI related to traces or to thematic role transfer?" *Brain & Language, 101*(1), 50–63.

Gallon, N., Harris, J., & van der Lely, H. K. J. (2007). Non-word repetition: An investigation of phonological complexity in children with Grammatical SLI. *Clinical Linguistics & Phonetics, 21*(6), 435–455.

Gathercole, S. (2006). Nonword repetition and word learning: The nature of the relationship. *Applied Psycholinguistics, 27,* 513–543.

Gordon, P. (1985). Level-ordering in lexical development. *Cognition, 21,* 73–93.

Hauser, M. D. (2001). What"s so special about speech? In E. Dupoux (Ed.), *Language, brain and cognitive development: Essays in honor of Jacques Mehler* (pp. 417–433). Cambridge, MA: MIT Press.

Hauser, M. D., Chomsky, N., & Fitch, W. T. (2002). The faculty of language: What is it, who has it, and how did it evolve? *Science, 298*(5598), 1569–1579.

Jakubowicz, C., Nash, L., & van der Velde, M. (1999). *Inflection and past tense morphology in French SLI.* Somerville, MA: BUCLD, Cascadilla Press.

Jakubowicz, C., & Strik, N. (2008). Scope-marking strategies in the acquisition of long-distance wh-questions in French and Dutch. *Language and Speech: On Phonological, Lexical and Syntactic Components of Language Development, 51,* 101–132.

Joanisse, M. (2004). Specific language impairments in children: Phonology, semantics and the English past tense. *Current Directions in Psychological Science, 13,* 156–160.

Joanisse, M. (2007). Phonological deficits and developmental language impairments. In D. Mareschal, S. Sirois, & G. Westermann (Eds.), *Neuroconstructivism, Vol. 2: Perspectives and Prospects.* Oxford, UK: Oxford University Press.

Joanisse, M., & Seidenberg, M. (1998). Specific language impairment: A deficit in grammar or processing? *Trends in Cognitive Sciences, 2,* 240–247.

Leonard, L. (1998). *Children with specific language impairment.* Cambridge, MA: MIT Press.

Leonard, L. B., Dromi, E., Adam, G., & Zadunaisky-Ehrlich, S. (2000). Tense and finiteness in the speech of children with specific language impairment acquiring Hebrew. *International Journal of Language and Communication Disorders, 35*(3), 319–335.

Marcus, G. (2004). *The birth of the mind: How a tiny number of genes creates the complexities of human thought.* New York, NY: Basic Books.

Marcus, G. F., Pinker, S., Ullman, M., Hollander, M., Rosen, T. J., & Xu, F. (1992). *Overregularization in language acquisition. Monographs of the Society for Research in Child Development Series 228,* Chicago, IL: University of Chicago Press.

Marinis, T., & van der Lely, H. K. J. (2007). On-line processing of questions in children with G-SLI and typically developing children. *International Journal of Language and Communication Disorders, 42,* 557–582.

Marshall, C. (2004). *The morpho-phonological interface in specific language impairment.* PhD Thesis; DLDCN Centre. London: University College.

Marshall, C. R., Ebbels, S., Harris, J., & van der Lely, H. (2002). Investigating the impact of prosodic complexity on the speech of children with Specific Language Impairment. In R. Vermeulen & A. Neeleman (Eds.), UCL Working Papers in Linguistics (Vol. 14, pp. 43–68).

Marshall, C. R., Harcourt-Brown, S., Ramus, F., & van der Lely, H. K. J. (2009). The link between prosody and language skills in children with SLI and/or dyslexia. *International Journal of Language & Communication Disorders, 44,* 466–488.

Marshall, C. R., & van der Lely, H. K. J. (2006). A challenge to current models of past tense inflection: The impact of phonotactics. *Cognition, 100,* 302–320.

Marshall, C. R., & van der Lely, H. K. J. (2007a). Derivational morphology in children with grammatical-specific language impairment. *Clinical Linguistics & Phonetics, 21*(2), 71–91.

Marshall, C. R., & van der Lely, H. K. J. (2007b). The impact of phonological complexity on past tense inflection in children with Grammatical-SLI. *Advances in Speech Language Pathology, 9,* 191–203.

Marshall, C. R., & van der Lely, H. K. (2009). Effects of word position and stress on onset cluster production: Evidence from typical development, SLI and dyslexia. *Language, 85,* 39–57.

Messaoud-Galusi, S., & Marshall, C. R. (2010). Introduction to this special issue. Exploring the overlap between dyslexia and SLI: the role of phonology. *Scientific Studies of Reading,* 14, 1–7.

Montgomery, J. W. (2000). Verbal working memory and sentence comprehension in children with specific language impairment. *Journal of Speech Language Hearing Research, 43*(2), 293–308.

Norbury, C. F., Bishop, D. V. M., & Briscoe, J. (2002). Does impaired grammatical comprehension provide evidence for an innate grammar module? *Applied Psycholinguistics, 23,* 247–268.

O'Hara, M., & Johnston, J. (1997). Syntactic bootstrapping in children with specific language impairment. *European Journal of Disorders of Communication, 2,* 189–205.

Pinker, S. (1999). *Words and rules: The ingredients of language.* London, UK: Weidenfeld & Nicolson.

Pinker, S., & Jackendoff, R. (2005). The faculty of language: What's special about it? *Cognition, 95*(2), 201–236.

Ramus, F. (2003). Developmental dyslexia: Specific phonological deficit or general sensorimotor dysfunction? *Current Opinion in Neurobiology, 13*(2), 212–218.

Ramus, F., & Szenkovits, G. (2008). What phonological deficit? *Quarterly Journal of Experimental Psychology, 61*(1), 129–141.

Rice, M. (2003). A unified model of specific and general language delay: Grammatical tense as a clinical marker of unexpected variation. In Y. Levy & J. Schaeffer (Eds.), *Language competence across populations: Toward a definition of Specific Language Impairment* (pp. 63–95). Mahwah, NJ: Lawrence Erlbaum.

Rice, M. (2004). Language growth of children with SLI and unaffected children: Timing mechanisms and linguistic distinctions. In A. Brugos, L. Micciulla, & C. Smith (Eds.), *Proceeding of the 28th Annual Boston University Conference on Language Development* (Vol. 1, pp. 28–49). Somerville, MA: Cascadilla Press.

Rice, M., Wexler, K., & Redmond, S. M. (1999). Grammaticality judgments of an extended optional infinitive grammar: Evidence from English-speaking children with specific language impairment. *Journal of Speech, Language, and Hearing Research, 42*, 943–961.

Rosen, S., Adlard, A., & van der Lely, H. K. J. (2009). Backward and simultaneous masking in children with grammatical specific language impairment: No simple link between auditory and language abilities. *Journal of Speech, Language, and Hearing Research, 52*, 396–411.

Selkirk, E. O. (1978). On prosodic structure and its relation to syntactic structure. In T. Fretheim (Ed.), *Nordic prosody* (Vol. 2, pp. 111–140). Trondheim, The Netherlands: TAPIR.

Snowling, M. (2000). *Dyslexia*, Second Edition. Oxford, UK: Blackwell.

Stavrakaki, S. (2001). Comprehension of reversible relative clauses in specifically language impaired and normally developing Greek children. *Brain and Language, 77*, 419–431.

Stavrakaki, S., & van der Lely, H. (2010). Production and comprehension of pronouns by Greek children with specific language impairment. *British Journal of Developmental Psychology, 28*, 189–216.

Stromswold, K. (1998). Genetics of spoken language disorders. *Human Biology, 70*(2), 297–324.

Tallal, P. (2002). Experimental studies of language learning impairments: From research to remediation. In D. Bishop & L. Leonard (Eds.), *Speech and language impairments in children* (pp. 131–156). East Sussex, UK: Psychological Press..

Tallal, P., Miller, S. L., Bedi, G., Byma, G., Wang, X., Nagarajan, S. S., . . . Merzenich, M. M. (1996). Language comprehension in language-learning impaired children improved with acoustically modified speech. *Science, 271*, 81–83.

Thomas, M. S. C., Grant, J., Barham, Z., Gsödl, M., Laing, E., Lakusta, L., . . . Karmiloff-Smith, A.(2001). Past tense formation in Williams Syndrome. *Language and Cognitive Processes, 16*, 143–176.

Thornton, R. (1995). Referentiality and wh-movement in child English: Juvenile D-Linkuency *Language Acquisition, 1–2*(4), 139–175.

Tomblin, J. B., Records, N. L., Buckwalter, P., Zhang, X., Smith, E., & O'Brien, M. (1997). Prevalence of specific language impairment in kindergarten children. *Journal of Speech Language Hearing Research, 40*(6), 1245–1260.

van der Lely, H. K. J. (1994). Canonical linking rules: Forward versus reverse linking in normally developing and specifically language-impaired children. *Cognition, 51*(1), 29–72.

van der Lely, H. K. J. (1996). Specifically language impaired and normally developing children: Verbal passive vs. adjectival passive sentence interpretation. *Lingua, 98*, 243–272.

van der Lely, H. K. J. (2005). Domain-specific cognitive systems: Insight from grammatical-specific language impairment. *Trends in Cognitive Sciences, 9*, 53–59.

van der Lely, H. K. J., & Battell, J. (2003). Wh-movement in children with grammatical SLI: A test of RDDR Hypothesis. *Language, 79*, 153–181.

van der Lely, H. K. J., & Christian, V. (2000). Lexical word formation in children with grammatical SLI: A grammar-specific versus an input-processing deficit? *Cognition, 75*(1), 33–63.

van der Lely, H. K. J., Jones, M., & Marshall, C. R. (in press). * Who did Buzz see some-one? Grammaticality judgement of wh-questions in typically developing and children and children with Grammatical-SLI. *Lingua.*

van der Lely, H. K. J., Rosen, S., & Adlard, A. (2004). Grammatical language impairment and the specificity of cognitive domains: Relations between auditory and language abilities. *Cognition, 94*(2), 167–183.

van der Lely, H. K. J., Rosen, S., & McClelland, A. (1998). Evidence for a grammar-specific deficit in children. *Current Biology, 8*(23), 1253–1258.

van der Lely, H. K. J., & Stollwerk, L. (1997). Binding theory and grammatical specific language impairment in children. *Cognition, 62,* 245–290.

van der Lely, H. K. J., & Ullman, M. (1996). *The computation and representation of past-tense morphology in normally developing and specifically language impaired children.* The 20th Annual Boston University Conference on Language Development. Vol. 2, Somerville, MA: Cascadilla Press.

van der Lely, H. K. J., & Ullman, M. (2001). Past tense morphology in specifically language impaired children and normally developing children. *Language and Cognitive Processes, 16,* 113–336.

Vernes, S. C., Newbury, D. F., Abrahams, B. S., Winchester, L., Nicod, J., Groszer, M., et al. (2008). A functional genetic link between distinct developmental language disorders. *New England Journal of Medcine,* 359(22), 2337–2345.

Watkins, K. E., Dronkers, N. F., & Vargha-Khadem, F. (2002). Behavioural analysis of an inherited speech and language disorder: Comparison with acquired aphasia. *Brain, 125*(Pt 3), 452–464

21 The Developing Mental Lexicon of Children With Specific Language Impairment

Holly Storkel

INTRODUCTION

The mental lexicon refers to "the collection of words stored in the human mind" (Trask, 1997, p. 140) with each entry "detailing the properties of a single lexical item: its pronunciation, its meaning, its word class, its subcategorization behavior, any grammatical irregularities, and possibly other information" (Trask, 1997, p. 130). This chapter will focus on a subset of the properties of lexical items that are frequently incorporated in adult and child models of spoken language processing, namely phonological, lexical, and semantic representations (Dell, 1988; Gupta & MacWhinney, 1997; Levelt, 1989; Luce, Goldinger, Auer, & Vitevitch, 2000; Magnuson, Tanenhaus, Aslin, & Dahan, 2003; McClelland & Elman, 1986; Norris, 1994). The phonological representation includes information about individual sounds, with models varying in the specific information incorporated (e.g., phonetic features, context-specific allophones, phonemes). For simplicity of illustration, phoneme units will be used to illustrate the phonological representation in this chapter. Thus, the phonological representation of the word "cat" would consist of the individual phonemes /k/, /æ/, and /t/ (i.e., three separate units). The lexical representation includes information about the sound structure of the word as an integrated unit. Continuing the illustration, the lexical representation for "cat" would be /kæt/ (i.e., one unit). Lastly, the semantic representation consists of information about the meaning or referent of the word. Here, the semantic representation for "cat" would include, but not be limited to, information such as "four-legged furry pet that purrs."

For the developing mental lexicon, there are two processes of critical importance. The first process involves the actual creation of the mental lexicon. That is, children are not born knowing the words of their language. Instead, words must be learned through exposure to the language during every day interactions. The second process involves accessing the words in the mental lexicon for language production or comprehension. This is the process that allows children to use the words that they know to communicate. It is critical to understand the potential relationship between these two processes to differentiate different underlying causes of the same behavior. For example, one commonly used paradigm to assess the status of the mental lexicon is to have children name pictures (e.g., Brownell, 2000; Williams, 1997). If a child fails to produce a name for the target picture (i.e., no response is provided), there are at least two possible explanations. The first possible explanation is that the child may not have learned the name for the picture, either because the child has never encountered that item before (i.e., lack of exposure) or because the child has failed to create an appropriate phonological, lexical, and/or semantic representation for the word despite being exposed to the word (i.e., word learning deficit). The second potential explanation is that the child has created an appropriate phonological, lexical, and semantic representation for the word but is having difficulty accessing those representations to produce a correct response within the time constraints of the test format (i.e., retrieval deficit). It should be clear that these two potential underlying causes of the same observed behavior would lead to different diagnostic conclusions and different treatment approaches.

MODELS OF THE LEXICON

One of the difficulties in disentangling learning and access in the developing lexicon is that there are few models that incorporate both processes (but see Magnuson et al., 2003). The tendency is for models of word learning to account for patterns observed in learning new words without accounting for patterns observed in production or recognition of known words (e.g., Gupta & MacWhinney, 1997). Likewise, many models of production or recognition of known words do not account for how those words were acquired (e.g., Dell, 1988; Levelt, 1989; Luce et al., 2000; McClelland & Elman, 1986; Norris, 1994). It is not the case that researchers are disinterested in creating models of the lexicon that learn new words and access known words, but rather that the complexities of both processes make an omnibus model somewhat intractable. Although a complete model or theory does not exist, important components can be garnered from existing models of each process.

One critical component in a model that integrates lexical learning and access is to provide some mechanism to trigger learning. That is, when listening to spoken language, the child must have some way of determining whether a word is novel, and thus new lexical and semantic representations need to be created (i.e., learning), or whether a word is known, and thus existing lexical and semantic representations should be accessed so that the word can be produced or recognized. Some types of models include just such a mechanism. Specifically, adaptive resonance theory, which has been used to model a variety of cognitive processes, involves activation of existing representations whenever novel or known information is encountered (e.g., Carpenter & Grossberg, 1987). However, when the information in the environment sufficiently mismatches the representations in memory, learning is triggered. This allows for the creation of new representations in memory as well as modification to existing representations. Thus, when listening to a word, existing representations will be activated. In the case of a novel word, existing lexical and semantic representations will not sufficiently match the novel word, thereby triggering learning. In the case of a known word, an existing lexical and semantic representation will sufficiently match the known word, thereby triggering production or recognition of the word.

Assuming that word learning is triggered, how does it proceed? Here, models of word learning are useful in outlining the process (e.g., Gupta & MacWhinney, 1997). Figure 21.1 offers a schematic of the learning process when the novel word /goᴜm/ is encountered. Phonological representations of the individual phonemes comprising the novel word will be activated and may aid in maintaining the sound sequence in working memory while a new lexical representation is created. Likewise, a new semantic representation will be created. Various forms of working memory will likely play a role in temporary storage of information while the semantic representation is being created but this will depend on the details of how the referent is presented (e.g., whether there is a visual referent or not). In addition to creating new lexical and semantic representations, a link must be created between the two new representations to support future production and recognition of the word. Finally, links must be created between the new representations and existing representations in the lexicon so that the new representations are integrated with the old. These new representations and links are accessed upon subsequent exposure to the novel word, allowing modification of the representations and links (in the case of incorrectly learned or missing information) as well as strengthening of the representations and links. Thus, word learning is a protracted process with the potential for incorrect or gradient representations prior to mastery (e.g., Capone & McGregor, 2005; Gershkoff-Stowe, 2002; Metsala & Walley, 1998).

For production or recognition, multiple existing representations are activated until one representation is selected. In the case of spoken word production, activation of semantic representations will be initiated first (e.g., Dell, 1988; Levelt, 1989). In the case of spoken word recognition, activation of form based units, namely phonological and lexical representations, will be initiated first (e.g., Luce et al., 2000; McClelland & Elman, 1986; Norris, 1994). Models differ in the amount of interaction between lexical and semantic activation. Some models hypothesize that activation of one type of representation must be completed before activation of the other is initiated (e.g., Levelt, 1989), whereas others assume that activation of one type of representation influences activation of the other (e.g., Dell, 1988). This debate has not fully reached the developmental literature. Thus, the developmental literature does not necessarily favor one type of model over the other.

NORMAL DEVELOPMENT

Past research documents that typically developing children rapidly acquire a lexicon. Following just a single exposure, children are able to associate a novel word form with its referent (Dickinson, 1984; Dollaghan, 1985; Heibeck &

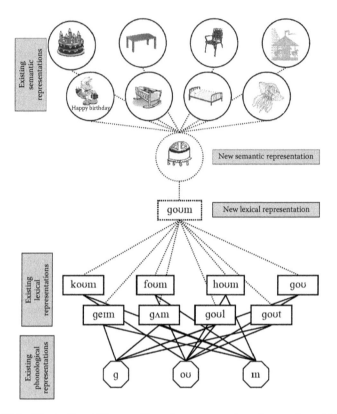

FIGURE 21.1 Illustration of the word learning process when the novel word /goʊm/ is encountered. Existing representations are depicted by solid lines and new representations are depicted with dashed lines. Pictures of known objects are taken from www.freeclipart-now.com (i.e., jellyfish) and www.clker.com (i.e., all pictures except jellyfish). The picture of the novel object is from Kroll and Potter (1984). Semantic neighbors of the novel object are based on the child data from Storkel and Adlof (2009a). Lexical neighbors of the novel words are based on the child calculator described by Storkel and Hoover (2010).

Markman, 1987). This ability has been termed fast mapping (Carey & Bartlett, 1978). It is not assumed that a child has mastered a word following a single exposure but rather has initiated the creation of an initial lexical and semantic representation, which is then refined over time and with repeated exposure to the word. This period of long-term learning is often referred to as extended mapping (Carey & Bartlett, 1978). Typically developing children also are able to create initial lexical and semantic representations of words with relatively few exposures in naturalistic discourse (e.g., television programs), sometimes referred to as quick incidental learning (QUIL; Rice & Woodsmall, 1988). These abilities allow children to rapidly build a lexicon, learning as many as nine words per day by some naturalistic counts (Bloom, 1973; Clark, 1973; K. Nelson, 1973; Templin, 1957).

Additional research on typically developing children has attempted to determine what factors account for this rapid word learning. There is ample research in this area with studies focusing on phonological (Bird & Chapman, 1998; Leonard, Schwartz, Morris, & Chapman, 1981; Schwartz & Leonard, 1982; Storkel, 2001, 2003, 2009; Storkel, Armbruster, & Hogan, 2006; Storkel & Rogers, 2000), prosodic (Cassidy & Kelly, 1991; Cutler & Carter, 1987; Morgan, 1986), lexical (Storkel, 2004a, 2009; Storkel et al., 2006); semantic (Gershkoff-Stowe & Smith, 2004; Grimshaw, 1981; Pinker, 1984; Samuelson & Smith, 1999; Smith, Jones, Landau, Gershkoff Stowe, & Samuelson, 2002; Storkel, 2009; Storkel & Adlof, 2009b), syntactic (Gleitman, 1990; Gleitman & Gleitman, 1992; Landau & Gleitman, 1985), and pragmatic cues (Baldwin, 1993; Baldwin et al., 1996; Sabbagh & Baldwin, 2001; Tomasello, Strosberg, & Akhtar, 1996). Below, some of the research on phonological, lexical, and semantic cues relevant to word learning is highlighted.

One phonological cue that has received recent attention is phonotactic probability. Phonotactic probability is the frequency of occurrence of individual sounds or pairs of sounds such that some legal sound sequences in a language can be identified as common (e.g., /kæt/—"cat") whereas others are classified as rare (e.g., /dɑg/—"dog"). Phonotactic probability appears to be learned early in development with sensitivity emerging around 9 months of age (Jusczyk, Luce, & Charles-Luce, 1994). Phonotactic probability is positively correlated with a lexical cue, namely neighborhood density (Storkel, 2004c; Vitevitch, Luce, Pisoni, & Auer, 1999). Neighborhood density refers to the number of words in a language that are phonologically similar to a given word, such that some words reside in dense neighborhoods (e.g., /kæt/—"cat") with many phonologically similar neighbors (i.e., 27 neighbors for "cat"), whereas others reside in sparse neighborhoods (e.g., /dɑg/—"dog") with few phonologically similar neighbors (i.e., six neighbors for "dog"). The correlation between phonotactic probability and neighborhood density arises because words with common sound sequences tend to reside in dense neighborhoods (e.g., /kæt/—"cat") and words with rare sound sequences tend to reside in sparse neighborhoods (e.g., /dɑl/—"dog"). Note that this correlation is not perfect and that is it possible to identify words with common sound sequences residing in sparse neighborhoods (e.g., /dɑl/—"doll" with nine neighbors) and those with rare sound sequences residing in dense neighborhoods (e.g., /geɪm/— "game" with 18 neighbors).

Word learning studies of correlated phonotactic probability and neighborhood density show that typically developing preschool children learn common/dense novel words more accurately than rare/sparse novel words, when given limited exposure to the novel words (Storkel, 2001, 2003, 2004b; Storkel & Maekawa, 2005). Recently, the individual effects of phonotactic probability and neighborhood density have been disentangled. In experimental studies of adult and child word learning, both phonotactic probability and neighborhood density appear to influence word learning with each variable affecting a different step of the word learning process (Hoover, Storkel, & Hogan, 2010; Storkel et al., 2006). Specifically, phonotactic probability appears to play a role in triggering word learning, such that novel words with rare sound sequences are learned more accurately than novel words with common sound sequences. It was hypothesized that because rare sound sequences are more unique from other known sound sequences, they create larger mismatches, triggering creation of a new representation immediately. In contrast, common sound sequences are deceptively similar to many other known sound sequences, creating smaller mismatches. This potentially impedes the recognition of the word as novel and delays the triggering of word learning. Neighborhood density appeared to play a role in the integration of a new lexical representation with existing lexical representations. Here, novel words from dense neighborhoods were learned more accurately than novel words from sparse neighborhoods. It was hypothesized that forming links with many existing lexical representations served to strengthen the newly created lexical representation, improving retention of the new representation. Similar results were obtained in a corpus analysis of the words known by typically developing infants (Storkel, 2009).

Recent work has examined a semantic variable similar to neighborhood density, namely semantic set size (Storkel & Adlof, 2009a, 2009b). Semantic set size refers to the number of words that are meaningfully related to or frequently associated with a given word, as determined by discrete association norms (D. L. Nelson, McEvoy, & Schreiber, 1998). We collected discrete association data from preschool children and adults for novel objects so that the novel objects could be classified as similar to many other known objects, namely a large semantic set size, or similar to few other known objects, namely a small semantic set size (Storkel & Adlof, 2009a). An experimental word learning study showed that preschool children learned novel words with small and large semantic set sizes equivalently. However, children retained novel words with a small semantic set size better than novel words with a large semantic set size (Storkel & Adlof, 2009b). Note that this finding is counter to the findings for neighborhood density where similarity to many known items facilitated learning. In the case of semantic set size, it was hypothesized that forming links with many existing semantic representations leads to confusion between the newly created semantic representation and existing semantic representations. This likely degraded the newly created representation, impeding retention. Further research is needed to better understand this discrepancy between the influence of lexical versus semantic similarity on word learning; however, one initial hypothesis is that lexical and semantic neighborhoods differ in neighbor diversity and this may impact how these representations influence word learning. Specifically, lexical neighbors always share the majority of phonemes with the new word (i.e., by definition, a neighbor differs by only one sound), whereas semantic neighbors could share few features with the new word and differ by many features, leading to a less focused and cohesive neighborhood.

The studies reviewed to this point have focused primarily on the early stages of learning a word when learning is triggered or when a new representation was recently created or retained over a relatively short delay. There is evidence that these newly created representations may be graded (e.g., Capone & McGregor,

2005; Gershkoff-Stowe, 2002; Metsala & Walley, 1998), such that the representation is incomplete or lacks detail. This hypothesis is supported by empirical study. For example, Storkel (2002) showed that lexical representations of known words from dense neighborhoods were phonologically detailed, whereas lexical representations of known words from sparse neighborhoods were less detailed, particularly for sounds in word final position. Likewise, McGregor and colleagues (McGregor, Friedman, Reilly, & Newman, 2002) showed that semantic representations of known words could be rich and complete or meager and incomplete. Thus, even when a typically developing child knows a word, the underlying lexical and semantic representation may not be as complete and detailed as in the adult lexicon. This, in turn, has consequences for production and recognition. For example, Newman and German (2005) demonstrated that the impact of neighborhood density on spoken word production diminished with development, presumably because the difference in completeness of lexical representations diminishes with development. That is, completeness of lexical representations is hypothesized to vary by neighborhood density in children. In contrast, adults arguably have complete and detailed representations of words in dense as well as sparse neighborhoods. Turning to spoken word recognition, Garlock and colleagues (Garlock, Walley, & Metsala, 2001) showed minimal developmental changes in the recognition of dense words in a gating task but greater developmental changes in the recognition of sparse words. They attribute this developmental pattern to changes in the completeness of lexical representations of words in sparse neighborhoods.

CHILDREN WITH SLI

Children with Specific Language Impairment (SLI) are children who show significant deficits in language acquisition in the absence of any obvious cause (Leonard, 1998). In general, language deficits in children with SLI are noted across all domains of language, although some argue that the most severe deficits occur in morphosyntax (Rice & Wexler, 1996; Rice, Wexler, & Cleave, 1995; Rice, Wexler, & Hershberger, 1998). Prevalence rates for SLI are approximately 7% for kindergarten children (Tomblin et al., 1997). There are a variety of theories about the nature of SLI, with some focusing on limitations in linguistic knowledge and others focusing on general or domain-specific processing deficits (see Leonard, 1998 for review). In terms of the lexicon, children with SLI usually score lower than their age-matched typically developing peers on standardized tests of vocabulary, although their scores may still fall within the normal range (Gray, Plante, Vance, & Henrichsen, 1999). Experimental word learning studies generally show that children with SLI learn fewer words than their same aged typically developing peers, although there is variability across studies and there is evidence of individual differences within the SLI group (specific studies reviewed below). Research by Gray (2004; Kiernan & Gray, 1998) examining individual differences in word learning indicated that approximately 30–73% of children with SLI learned as many words as their typically developing peers. Thus, word learning by 27–70% of children with

SLI fell outside the normal range. These estimates of the percentage of children with SLI who exhibit word learning difficulties should be viewed with caution because they are based on small samples of children with SLI. However, these individual differences should be kept in mind when reviewing the results of group studies (see below).

In terms of fast mapping, deficits in fast mapping have been documented in some studies (Dollaghan, 1987; Gray, 2004) but not others (Gray, 2003, 2004). Across studies, there is no evidence that children with SLI have difficulty associating the novel word with a novel object. When difficulties occur, they appear in later comprehending (Gray, 2004) or producing the novel word (Dollaghan, 1987). Deficits are observed more consistently during extended mapping (Gray, 2003, 2004; Kiernan & Gray, 1998; Oetting, Rice, & Swank, 1995; Rice, Buhr, & Nemeth, 1990), with some studies suggesting that children with SLI may need twice as many exposures to achieve the same comprehension and production accuracy as same aged typically developing children (Gray, 2003).

Where in the word learning process do these deficits occur in children with SLI? Triggering of word learning has received less attention in the literature on word learning by children with SLI. The results of at least some fast mapping studies would hint that triggering word learning may not be problematic for children with SLI (Gray, 2003, 2004). However, this conclusion can only be viewed as tentative, given the paucity of research in this area. In contrast, there is clear and consistent evidence that children with SLI have difficulty creating and retaining mental representations of novel words. Moreover, this difficulty appears to impact both lexical and semantic representations. For example, Alt and colleagues (Alt & Plante, 2006; Alt, Plante, & Creusere, 2004) exposed children to novel words paired with novel objects. After exposure, they examined lexical representations by having the children judge whether a sound sequence was the correct name of the novel object (i.e., the name paired with the object during exposure). Children with SLI recognized fewer names than their typically developing peers, suggesting deficits in the creation and/or retention of lexical representations. In addition, Alt and colleagues examined semantic representations by presenting the novel word and asking children whether its referent had certain semantic features. Children with SLI correctly identified fewer semantic features than their typically developing peers, indicating deficits in the creation and/or retention of semantic representations.

Work by Gray provides a similar conclusion, although suggests that these deficits may be true of only certain children with SLI. Gray (2004) identified children with SLI who performed significantly more poorly on the word learning task than the rest of the group. Approximately 35% of the children with SLI were classified as poor word learners. Gray then examined the word learning profiles of these children to identify potential areas of deficit. For each novel word that the child did not learn, lexical representations were viewed as the area of deficit if the child never learned to produce the novel word during training, whereas semantic representations were viewed as the area of deficit if the child drew a poor picture of referent of the novel word after training. For 79% of the unlearned words, lexical representations were implicated whereas semantic representations were implicated for the remaining 21%. Interestingly, both areas of deficit generally were observed for each child. Moreover, Gray (2005) has shown that providing phonological (e.g., initial sound, initial syllable, rhyming word) or semantic cues (e.g., superordinate category, physical characteristics, action or use) during training improves word learning by children with SLI. Presumably, provision of cues improves the child's ability to create a new lexical or new semantic representation, depending on the cue provided.

Even when children are successful in creating a new lexical or semantic representation, there is evidence that they have difficulty retaining these representations over time. Rice and colleagues (Rice, Oetting, Marquis, Bode, & Pae, 1994) examined the influence of amount of exposure on word learning by children with SLI. With three exposures to the novel words, the children with SLI performed more poorly than the typically developing children on an immediate posttest of comprehension. In contrast, with 10 exposures to the novel words, children with SLI performed similarly to typically developing children in an immediate posttest of comprehension. Thus, immediate learning by the children with SLI was similar to the typically developing children when greater exposure was provided. However, when the posttest was re-administered 1–3 days after the 10 exposures, group differences emerged with the children with SLI performing more poorly than the typically developing children, especially for verbs. This suggests that children with SLI had greater difficulty retaining new representations over time and implicates the integration of newly created representations with existing representations as a potential area of deficit in children with SLI.

These potential word learning deficits have consequences for spoken word production and recognition by children with SLI. Considering first production and semantic representations, McGregor and colleagues (McGregor, Newman, Reilly, & Capone, 2002) provide evidence that naming by children with SLI is affected by the quality of semantic representations. Children were asked to name pictures and their responses were categorized as correct, semantic error, indeterminate error (e.g., "I don't know"), or other error. Children then were asked to draw pictures and define the same items that they had been asked to name. Analyses compared the quality of drawings and definitions for correct versus semantic errors versus indeterminate errors as a means of examining the quality of the semantic representations of the words in each response category. Results showed that children with SLI named fewer pictures correctly than their typically developing peers. For both groups of children, drawings and definitions for correctly named items were richer and more accurate than those for incorrectly named items, with no differences noted between semantic versus indeterminate errors. McGregor and colleagues (2002) also examined the pattern of responses across tasks for each word and determined that approximately one-third of erred responses were attributable to retrieval failure during naming despite adequate semantic representations (i.e., rich drawing, rich definition, and correct comprehension). Approximately another one-third of erred responses were attributable to sparse semantic representations (i.e., poor drawing, or poor definition, or incorrect comprehension). The final one-third of erred responses was attributable to missing lexical or semantic representations (i.e., poor drawing, poor definition, and incorrect comprehension). Taken together, approximately one-third of naming errors were due to retrieval failures, whereas two-thirds of naming errors were attributable to word learning deficits.

Turning to word recognition and lexical representations, Maillart and colleagues (Maillart, Schelstraete, & Hupet, 2004) provide evidence that recognition by children with SLI is affected by the quality of lexical representations. Children completed a lexical decision task where they were asked to identify auditorially presented stimuli as real words or nonwords. Children with SLI were less accurate than typically developing children in this task. Moreover, children with SLI had much greater difficulty rejecting nonwords that differed only slightly (i.e., a phoneme change rather than a syllable change) from a real word. This pattern suggests that children with SLI may have had more holistic lexical representations of real words leading to confusion between slightly modified nonwords and real words.

Finally, research suggests that the quality of lexical and semantic representations has implications for learning to read and write, placing children with SLI at risk for future academic deficits (e.g., Catts, Adolf, Hogan, & Weismer, 2005; Catts, Fey, Tomblin, & Zhang, 2002; Walley, Metsala, & Garlock, 2003).

SUMMARY AND CONCLUSIONS

The theoretical framework outlined at the onset of this chapter provides a means for investigating and understanding differences in the lexicons of children with SLI and their typically developing counterparts. In terms of the different types of representations in the lexicon, children with SLI exhibit deficits in both lexical and semantic representations. The status of phonological representations has received less attention. Most of the research in this area has focused on accessing phonological representations (e.g., Tallal, Stark, & Mellits, 1985), rather than examining the quality of phonological representations. Turning to the process of word learning, children with SLI appear to have deficits in creating, retaining, and/or integrating new representations in their lexicons. Additional research is needed in this area to more fully differentiate the deficits in each process (i.e., creating vs. retaining vs. integrating). Investigation of variables from studies of normal development (e.g., neighborhood density, semantic set size) may be useful in this endeavor. The process of triggering word learning has not been fully investigated, warranting future study. Considering production and recognition of known words, children with SLI show complex deficits in spoken word production and recognition. At least some of their difficulties in this area can be attributed to problems in accessing detailed representations, whereas others can be attributed to holistic or incomplete representations. This pattern highlights the interplay between word learning and production/recognition in the developing mental lexicon.

While much has been learned about the nature of the developing mental lexicon of children with SLI, clinical methods have not yet been fully informed by this knowledge. Specifically, most diagnostic tools take a global approach to assessment by examining the words that a child has already learned. The words a child has already learned, as revealed by this type of test, is a function of the child's exposure to words, the child's ability to learn words, and the child's ability to produce or recognize the words within the format and time constraints of the test. Thus, most diagnostic tools fail to differentiate environment, learning, and access in their examination of the lexicon. Consequently, if a child performs poorly on such a task, the underlying cause of that poor performance cannot be immediately identified. Moreover, a deficit could be missed because strengths in one (or more) of these areas (environment, learning, access) could mask weaknesses in the other areas. Given this situation, it is important to supplement standardized test scores with clinician developed probes that are informed by theory. Probes that examine the quality of representations (lexical vs. semantic), different stages of learning (triggering learning vs. creation of new representations vs. retention/integration of new representations), and differentiate these from access to representations would be the most informative for treatment planning (see Gray, 2004, 2005, for a potentially clinically adaptable example).

FURTHER READING

Bloom, P. (2000). *How children learn the meanings of words*. Cambridge, MA: MIT Press.

Golinkoff, R. M., Hirsh-Pasek, K., Bloom, L., Smith, L. B., Woodward, A., Akhtar, N., et al. (2000). *Becoming a word learner: A debate on lexical acquisition*. Oxford: Oxford University Press.

ACKNOWLEDGMENTS

Preparation of this chapter was supported by NIH grant DC08095. S. M. Adlof, M. S. Bridges, T. P. Hogan, and J. R. Hoover provided valuable comments on an earlier version of this chapter.

REFERENCES

Alt, M., & Plante, E. (2006). Factors that influence lexical and semantic fast mapping of young children with specific language impairment. *Journal of Speech, Language and Hearing Research, 49*(5), 941–954.

Alt, M., Plante, E., & Creusere, M. (2004). Semantic features in fast-mapping: Performance of preschoolers with specific language impairment versus preschoolers with normal language. *Journal of Speech, Language and Hearing Research, 47*(2), 407–420.

Baldwin, D. A. (1993). Infants' ability to consult the speaker for clues to word reference. *Journal of Child Language, 20*, 395–418.

Baldwin, D. A., Markman, E. M., Bill, B., Desjardins, R. N., Irwin, J. M., & Tidball, G. (1996). Infants' reliance on a social criterion for establishing word-object relations. *Child Development, 67*, 3135–3153.

Bird, E. K. R., & Chapman, R. S. (1998). Partial representations and phonological selectivity in the comprehension of 13- to 16-month-olds. *First Language, 18*, 105–127.

Bloom, L. (1973). *One word at a time: The use of single word utterances before syntax*. The Hague, The Netherlands: Mouton.

Brownell, R. (2000). *Expressive one-word picture vocabulary test* (3rd ed.). Novato, CA: Academic Therapy Publications.

Capone, N. C., & McGregor, K. K. (2005). The effect of semantic representation on toddlers' word retrieval. *Journal of Speech, Language and Hearing Research, 48*(6), 1468–1480.

Carey, S., & Bartlett, E. (1978). Acquiring a single new word. *Papers and Reports on Child Language Development, 15*, 17–29.

Carpenter, G. A., & Grossberg, S. (1987). A massively parallel architecture for a self-organizing neural pattern recognition machine. *Computer, Vision, Graphics, and Image Processing, 37*, 54–115.

Cassidy, K. W., & Kelly, M. H. (1991). Phonological information in grammatical category assignments. *Journal of Memory and Language, 30*, 348–369.

Catts, H., Adolf, S. M., Hogan, T. P., & Weismer, S. (2005). Are specific language impairment and dyslexia distinct disorders? *Journal of Speech, Language and Hearing Research, 48*(6), 1378–1396.

Catts, H. W., Fey, M. E., Tomblin, J. B., & Zhang, X. (2002). A longitudinal investigation of reading outcomes in children with language impairments. *Journal of Speech, Language, and Hearing Research, 45*, 1142–1157.

Clark, E. (1973). What's in a word? On the child's acquisition of semantics in his first language. In T. Moore (Ed.), *Cognitive development and the acquisition of language* (pp. 65–110). New York, NY: Academic.

Cutler, A., & Carter, D. (1987). The predominance of strong initial syllables in the English vocabulary. *Computer Speech and Language, 2*, 133–142.

Dell, G. S. (1988). The retrieval of phonological forms in production: Tests of predictions from a connectionist model. *Journal of Memory and Language, 27*, 124–142.

Dickinson, D. K. (1984). First impressions: Children's knowledge of words gained from a single exposure. *Applied Psycholinguistics, 5*, 359–373.

Dollaghan, C. A. (1985). Child meets word: "Fast mapping" in preschool children. *Journal of Speech and Hearing Research, 28*, 449–454.

Dollaghan, C. A. (1987). Fast mapping in normal and language-impaired children. *Journal of Speech and Hearing Disorders, 52*, 218–222.

Garlock, V. M., Walley, A. C., & Metsala, J. L. (2001). Age-of-acquisition, word frequency, and neighborhood density effects on spoken word recognition by children and adults. *Journal of Memory and Language, 45*, 468–492.

Gershkoff-Stowe, L. (2002). Object naming, vocabulary growth, and development of word retrieval abilities. *Journal of Memory and Language, 46*, 665–687.

Gershkoff-Stowe, L., & Smith, L. B. (2004). Shape and the first hundred nouns. *Child Development, 75*(4), 1098–1114.

Gleitman, L. (1990). The structural sources of verb meanings. *Language Acquisition, 1*, 3–55.

Gleitman, L., & Gleitman, J. (1992). A picture is worth a thousand words, but that's the problem: The role of syntax in vocabulary acquisition. *Current Directions in Psychological Science, 1*, 1–5.

Gray, S. (2003). Word-learning by preschoolers with impairment: What predicts success? *Journal of Speech, Language and Hearing Research, 46*(1), 56–67.

Gray, S. (2004). Word learning by preschoolers with specific language impairment: Predictors and poor learners. *Journal of Speech, Language, and Hearing Research, 47*(5), 1117–1132.

Gray, S. (2005). Word learning by preschoolers with specific language impairment effect of phonological or semantic cues. *Journal of Speech, Language and Hearing Research, 48*(6), 1452–1467.

Gray, S., Plante, E., Vance, R., & Henrichsen, M. (1999). The diagnostic accuracy of four vocabulary tests administered to preschool-age children. *Language, Speech, and Hearing Services in Schools, 30*, 196–206.

Grimshaw, J. (1981). Form, function, and the language acquisition device. In C. Baker & J. McCarthy (Eds.), *The logical problem of language acquisition* (pp. 183–210). Cambridge, MA: MIT Press.

Gupta, P., & MacWhinney, B. (1997). Vocabulary acquisition and verbal short-term memory: Computational and neural bases. *Brain and Language, 59*, 267–333.

Heibeck, T. H., & Markman, E. M. (1987). Word learning in children: An examination of fast mapping. *Child Development, 58*, 1021–1034.

Hoover, J. R., Storkel, H. L., & Hogan, T. P. (2010). A cross-sectional comparison of the effects of phonotactic probability and neighborhood density on word learning by preschool children. *Journal of Memory and Language, 63*, 100–116.

Jusczyk, P. W., Luce, P. A., & Charles-Luce, J. (1994). Infants' sensitivity to phonotactic patterns in the native language. *Journal of Memory and Language, 33*, 630–645.

Kiernan, B., & Gray, S. (1998). Word learning in a supported-learning context by preschool children with specific language impairment. *Journal of Speech, Language, and Hearing Research, 41*, 161–171.

Kroll, J. F., & Potter, M. C. (1984). Recognizing words, pictures, and concepts: A comparison of lexical, object, and reality decisions. *Journal of Verbal Learning and Verbal Behavior, 23*, 39–66.

Landau, B., & Gleitman, L. (1985). *Language and experience: Evidence from the blind child.* Cambridge, MA: Harvard University Press.

Leonard, L. B. (1998). *Children with specific language impairment.* Cambridge, MA: The MIT Press.

Leonard, L. B., Schwartz, R. G., Morris, B., & Chapman, K. L. (1981). Factors influencing early lexical acquisition: Lexical orientation and phonological composition. *Child Development, 52*, 882–887.

Levelt, W. J. M. (1989). *Speaking: From intention to articulation.* Cambridge, MA: MIT Press.

Luce, P. A., Goldinger, S. D., Auer, E. T., & Vitevitch, M. S. (2000). Phonetic priming, neighborhood activation, and PARSYN. *Perception & Psychophysics, 62*, 615–625.

Magnuson, J. S., Tanenhaus, M. K., Aslin, R. N., & Dahan, D. (2003). The time course of spoken word learning and recognition: Studies with artificial lexicons. *Journal of Experimental Psychology: General, 132*(2), 202–227.

Maillart, C., Schelstraete, M., & Hupet, M. (2004). Phonological representations in children with SLI: A study of French. *Journal of Speech, Language, and Hearing Research, 47*(1), 187–198.

McClelland, J., & Elman, J. (1986). The TRACE model of speech perception. *Cognitive Psychology, 18*, 1–86.

McGregor, K.K., Friedman, R., Reilly, R., & Newman, R. (2002). Semantic representation and naming in young children. *Journal of Speech, Language and Hearing Research, 45*(2), 332–346.

McGregor, K. K., Newman, R. M., Reilly, R. M., & Capone, N. C. (2002). Semantic representation and naming in children with specific language impairment. *Journal of Speech, Language, and Hearing Research, 45*, 998–1014.

Metsala, J. L., & Walley, A. C. (1998). Spoken vocabulary growth and the segmental restructuring of lexical representations: Precursors to phonemic awareness and early reading ability. In J. L. Metsala & L. C. Ehri (Eds.), *Word recognition in beginning literacy* (pp. 89–120). Mahwah, NJ: Lawrence Erlbaum Associates, Inc.

Morgan, J. (1986). *From simple input to complex grammar.* Cambridge, MA: MIT Press.

Nelson, D. L., McEvoy, C., & Schreiber, T. (1998). The University of South Florida word association, rhyme, and word fragment norms. Retrieved from http://www.usf.edu/FreeAssociation/

Nelson, K. (1973). Concept, word and sentence: Interrelations in acquisition and development. *Psychological Review, 81,* 267–295.

Newman, R. S., & German, D. J. (2005). Life span effects on lexical factors in oral naming. *Language and Speech, 48*(2), 123–156.

Norris, D. (1994). Shortlist: A connectionist model of continuous speech recognition. *Cognition, 52,* 189–234.

Oetting, J. B., Rice, M. L., & Swank, L. K. (1995). Quick incidental learning (QUIL) of words by school-age children with and without SLI. *Journal of Speech and Hearing Research, 38,* 434–445.

Pinker, S. (1984). *Language learnability and language development.* Cambridge, MA: Harvard University Press.

Rice, M. L., Buhr, J. C., & Nemeth, M. (1990). Fast mapping word-learning abilities of language-delayed preschoolers. *Journal of Speech and Hearing Disorders, 55,* 33–42.

Rice, M. L., Oetting, J. B., Marquis, J., Bode, J., & Pae, S. (1994). Frequency of input effects on word comprehension of children with specific language impairment. *Journal of Speech and Hearing Research, 37,* 106–122.

Rice, M. L., & Wexler, K. (1996). Toward tense as a clinical marker of specific language impairment in English-speaking children. *Journal of Speech and Hearing Research, 39*(6), 1239–1257.

Rice, M. L., Wexler, K., & Cleave, P. L. (1995). Specific language impairment as a period of extended optional infinitive. *Journal of Speech and Hearing Research, 38,* 850–863.

Rice, M. L., Wexler, K., & Hershberger, S. (1998). Tense over time: The longitudinal course of tense acquisition in children with specific language impairment. *Journal of Speech, Language, and Hearing Research, 41,* 1412–1431.

Rice, M. L., & Woodsmall, L. (1988). Lessons from television: Children's word learning when viewing. *Child Development, 59,* 420–429.

Sabbagh, M. A., & Baldwin, D. A. (2001). Learning words from knowlegeable versus ignorant speakers: Links between preschoolers' theory of mind and semantic development. *Child Development, 72*(4), 1054–1070.

Samuelson, L. K., & Smith, L. B. (1999). Early noun vocabularies: Do ontology, category structure and syntax correspond? *Cognition, 73,* 1–33.

Schwartz, R. G., & Leonard, L. B. (1982). Do children pick and choose? An examination of phonological selection and avoidance in early lexical acquisition. *Journal of Child Language, 9,* 319–336.

Smith, L. B., Jones, S. S., Landau, B., Gershkoff Stowe, L., & Samuelson, L. (2002). Object name learning provides on-the-job training for attention. *Psychological Science, 13*(1), 13–19.

Storkel, H. L. (2001). Learning new words: Phonotactic probability in language development. *Journal of Speech, Language, and Hearing Research, 44,* 1321–1337.

Storkel, H. L. (2002). Restructuring of similarity neighbourhoods in the developing mental lexicon. *Journal of Child Language, 29*(2), 251–274.

Storkel, H. L. (2003). Learning new words II: Phonotactic probability in verb learning. *Journal of Speech, Language and Hearing Research, 46*(6), 1312–1323.

Storkel, H. L. (2004a). Do children acquire dense neighbourhoods? An investigation of similarity neighbourhoods in lexical acquisition. *Journal of Applied Psycholinguistics, 25*(2), 201–221.

Storkel, H. L. (2004b). The emerging lexicon of children with phonological delays: Phonotactic constraints and probability in acquisition. *Journal of Speech, Language, and Hearing Research, 47*(5), 1194–1212.

Storkel, H. L. (2004c). Methods for minimizing the confounding effects of word length in the analysis of phonotactic probability and neighborhood density. *Journal of Speech, Language and Hearing Research, 47*(6), 1454–1468.

Storkel, H. L. (2009). Developmental differences in the effects of phonological, lexical, and semantic variables on word learning by infants. *Journal of Child Language, 36*, 291–321.

Storkel, H. L. & Adlof, S. M. (2009a). Adult and child semantic neighbors of the Kroll and Potter (1984) nonobjects. *Journal of Speech, Language, and Hearing Research, 52*, 289–305.

Storkel, H. L. & Adlof, S. M. (2009b). The effect of semantic set size on word learning by preschool children. *Journal of Speech, Language, and Hearing Research, 52*, 306–320.

Storkel, H. L., Armbruster, J., & Hogan, T. P. (2006). Differentiating phonotactic probability and neighborhood density in adult word learning. *Journal of Speech, Language, and Hearing Research, 49*(6), 1175–1192.

Storkel, H. L. & Hoover, J. R. (2010). An on-line calculator to compute phonotactic probability and neighborhood density based on child corpora of spoken American English. *Behavior Research Methods, 42*, 497–506.

Storkel, H. L., & Maekawa, J. (2005). A comparison of homonym and novel word learning: The role of phonotactic probability and word frequency. *Journal of Child Language, 32*, 827–853.

Storkel, H. L., & Rogers, M. A. (2000). The effect of probabilistic phonotactics on lexical acquisition. *Clinical Linguistics & Phonetics, 14*, 407–425.

Tallal, P., Stark, R. E., & Mellits, E. D. (1985). Identification of language-impaired children on the basis of rapid perception and production skills. *Brain and Language, 25*, 314–322.

Templin, M. C. (1957). *Certain language skills in children, their development and interrelationships (Institute of Child Welfare, Monograph Series 26).* Minneapolis, MN: University of Minnesota Press.

Tomasello, M., Strosberg, R., & Akhtar, N. (1996). Eighteen-month-old children learn words in non-ostensive contexts. *Journal of Child Language, 23*, 157–176.

Tomblin, J. B., Records, N. L., Buckwalter, P., Zhang, X., Smith, E., & O'Brien, M. (1997). Prevalence of specific language impairment in kindergarten children. *Journal of Speech, Language, and Hearing Research, 40*, 1245–1260.

Trask, R. L. (1997). *A student's dictionary of language and linguistics.* London, UK: Arnold.

Vitevitch, M. S., Luce, P. A., Pisoni, D. B., & Auer, E. T. (1999). Phonotactics, neighborhood activation, and lexical access for spoken words. *Brain and Language, 68*, 306–311.

Walley, A. C., Metsala, J. L., & Garlock, V. M. (2003). Spoken vocabulary growth: Its role in the development of phoneme awareness and early reading ability. *Reading and Writing: An Interdisciplinary Journal, 16*, 5–20.

Williams, K. T. (1997). *Expressive vocabulary test.* Circle Pines, MN: American Guidance Services.

22 Language–Speech Processing in Developmental Fluency Disorders

Peter Howell

INTRODUCTION

This chapter focuses on developmental stuttering, a fluency disorder that is affected by psycholinguistic and speech-motor factors. Stuttered speech has been described as consisting of relatively fluent episodes of speech interspersed with dysfluent events. According to Johnson and associates (1959), the main dysfluent events are: (1) interjections (silent or filled pauses), (2) word repetitions, (3) phrase repetitions, (4) part-word repetitions, (5) prolongations, (6) broken words, (7) incomplete phrases (abandonments), and (8) revisions. Only the first six events are consistent with the ICD-10 definition (World Health Organization, 1992), which maintains that speakers know what they wish to say but are unable to do so. None of these six categories includes an overt speech error. For this reason, our model does not assume fluency problems are linked with speech errors.

The first six event-types tend to be associated with particular linguistic structures. Pauses occur around the onsets of grammatical or prosodic units (according to different theorists), word and phrase repetitions occur (again depending on theoretical position) around onsets of prosodic words (PW) or at points prior to a presumed word error, while part-word repetitions, prolongations, and broken words occur on content words rather than function words* (Howell, 2007a).

All these events occur in fluent speakers' speech, although their incidence is low and their distribution differs relative to speakers who stutter (in particular, fluent speakers have a low proportion of event-types 4–6, Howell, 2007a). The overlap in event-types seen in fluent and stuttered speech makes diagnosis of the disorder difficult. Both fluent children (Clark & Clark, 1977) and children who stutter show a high proportion of word and phrase repetitions, which adds to the problem of differential diagnosis. The incidence of stuttering is at its peak

---

* Function words are pronouns, articles, prepositions, conjunctions, and auxiliary verbs and content words are nouns, main verbs, adverbs, and adjectives (Hartmann & Stork, 1972; Quirk, Greenbaum, Leech, & Svartvik, 1985).

at ages at which language development is maximal. Thus, modal onset ages of 3 and 5 years were reported by Andrews and Harris (1964) and onset around these ages has been confirmed in a number of other studies. In the same work, incidence of the disorder up to 15 years was about 5% and recovery rate was about 80%. Recovery rate declines with age (Andrews and Harris's study reported that no new cases occurred after age 12). The incidence of different dysfluency events change over ages as the proportion of event-types 4–6 is higher in older, compared to younger, speakers who stutter (Howell, Davis, & Williams, 2008). A satisfactory theory should address all these points.

A further observation relevant to theoretical accounts is that the language system operates independently of the motor system. Thus, a particular linguistic representation can be output in several different ways (as speech, in writing, as semaphore, etc.). Speakers can produce nonsense material as if it is speech despite it having no linguistic content. This independence is entrenched in approaches to stuttering where many authors take the stance that stuttering is either a linguistic (Bernstein Ratner & Wijnen, 2007; Kolk & Postma, 1997) or a motor (Max & Caruso, 1997; van Lieshout & Namasivayam, 2010) problem. My team's work suggests that this is misguided. Speakers who stutter have been reported to have various language deficits, but other speakers who have the same deficits do not stutter. This suggests language alone is not causal. Similarly, speakers who stutter have been reported to have motor deficits, but some speakers with these same deficits do not stutter. There has to be something additional that makes a person stutter. There could be something extraneous to language and speech that leads to stuttering (e.g., personality type). Alternatively, the problem could involve the process by which language and speech are coupled. Our work has supported the latter view.

This review starts by examining approaches that promote language processes as the main factor leading to stuttering (including theories that we disagree with and others that we draw on). Problems are highlighted for which our model offers answers. Our model, which involves motor as well as language processes, is then presented.

THEORIES THAT INCLUDE LANGUAGE MONITORING

Our theory contrasts with two proposals about stuttering that draw their inspiration from Levelt's (1989) work on fluent speech control. These are Kolk and Postma's (1997) covert repair hypothesis (CRH) and Bernstein Ratner and Wijnen's (2007) vicious cycle account. The common features of these views are that (1) they all give primacy to language, as it is in this process that errors are made that could lead to stuttering; and (2) speakers monitor their language output to detect and respond to any such errors.

Levelt's Blueprint

Levelt's (1989) model has been influential in many areas of language research. It is singled out for extensive consideration as it includes an explanation of how speech–language processes interface that contrasts with our proposal. Also, the other theories reviewed in this section draw on it to different extents, so it is a convenient vehicle to flag the general problems for these accounts. Figure 22.1, a schematic representation of Levelt's model, shows production and perception as both being involved in speech control. Production (left) starts at conceptualization, then language formulation occurs before speech is output. The formulator performs a hierarchy of linguistic processing steps, the last of which is to generate a phonetic string. This is input to the speech-motor system, after which speech is output. Errors can occur in language formulation. We would define an error as having occurred in an utterance when at least one phone is in the wrong position relative to that intended (so saying "hissed" instead of "missed" would include an initial error). This definition is consistent with Levelt's (1989) use of the term. A speaker does not want to issue a message with errors, so Levelt proposed that these are detected by retrieving the message in one of two ways. First, after speech output, the sound is processed by the auditory and speech perception systems where the linguistic content of the message is retrieved. This information is sent back to the formulator where the monitor resides. The monitor knows the original intention and can use this to determine any erroneous forms that were produced. The monitor determines whether there is a match (i.e., the speaker said what was intended and speech was fluent) or mismatch (i.e., the speaker did not say what was intended and speech was in error) between the two. In the latter case, the message is interrupted, reformulated, and the speaker

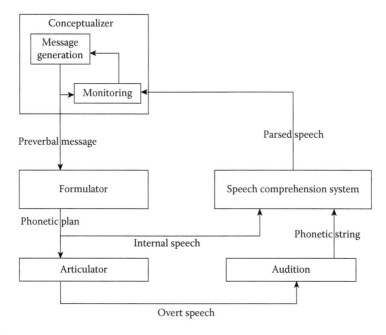

FIGURE 22.1   Levelt's model of the processes involved in speech production. Production is on the left and perception on the right.

tries again (i.e., corrects the error). In this situation there is an overt error that, as already noted, is not usually the case when stuttering occurs. The overall process is called the external loop.

Overt speech repairs such as "to the left of, no, to the right of the curtain" provide support for the *external* loop. The speaker has produced the word "left" when "right" was intended. The Levelt (1983) account assumed that the speaker heard this, interrupted speech (signified by the comma), and repeated some components that are not essential ("to the," called a *retrace*) before the correction was made. Using "left" instead of "right" may not be the result of an error in the linguistic system and, consequently, would have little relevance to the workings of psycholinguistic processes.

Levelt's model has a second way of detecting errors. This involves speech being sent directly from the language formulation process to the speech perception system (before speech is output, so there is no evidence of error). The language error is also detected by the monitor as a mismatch between the intended and current forms. Speech is corrected covertly using the internal loop (language input sent directly through the perceptual system to the monitor). Although there is no overt error, there are signs that an error occurred in the form of hesitation- and repetition-type behavior (features seen in stuttering). Thus, the repair described earlier that was detected over the external loop, might be realized as "to the, to the right of the curtain" over the internal loop. Such structures are called *covert repairs*.

Although the Levelt model was established in the late 1980s, updated versions still rely on the two monitoring routes (Roelofs, 2004). The internal and external loops are feedback routes. It is noteworthy that the loops go from audio or language output right back to the first step in message formulation.

Problems for the Levelt Account

The Levelt model has an autonomous production route, invokes the perceptual system accessed through internal and external loops, and a monitoring process—all of which Levelt used to explain fluent speech control and its breakdown. Each of these components is critically examined.

Production

a. Does the production system supply the speech perception system with error information?

Only around half of overt errors are repaired (Nooteboom, 2005). In addition, the 50% estimate of the correction rate to overt errors is probably higher than that which occurs in normal listening conditions, as these data may reflect a collector's bias, given that these estimates are derived from self-reports (Cutler, 1982). From this, it would appear that production either does not transmit information about all errors or that they are not detected or acted on by subsequent processes. To counter this, Hartsuiker, Kolk, and Martensen (2005) argue that if two loops are operational and both have 50% accuracy, then overall accuracy increases

to 75%. Detection rates of 50–75% indicate that it is not essential for errors to be intercepted during speech control.

There are other grounds for the view that errors are produced without being repaired (even if the speaker can detect them). The output form of children's speech is simpler than that of adults because it is affected by consonant cluster reduction, homogenization of consonants with respect to place, manner, and voicing. These processes would lead children to produce a large number of words that would be characterized as production errors that, perceptually, they are able to detect (Menyuk & Anderson, 1969). It would not make sense for a young child to monitor and correct the errors in these productions, because the child would continue to make the same errors if they are due to cognitive or motor control limitations. This suggests that during phonological development, a child can attempt speech forms and ignore errors that are made.

b. Are the repetitions produced as part of covert errors similar to the retraces in overt errors?

If events associated with the internal and external loop are related, the common constituents (retraces and pauses) should be similar. However, Blackmer and Mitton (1991) argued that phrase repetitions in covert, unlike overt, repairs occur at too rapid a rate to be consistent with the assumption that an internal error underlies these events.

Perception

a. How accurate is the perception mechanism at detecting errors?

No consideration has been given in the monitoring perspective as to whether the perceptual system itself makes errors. As opposed to slips of the tongue, sometimes listeners misperceive, a phenomenon called slips of the ear (Bond, 1999). The perceptual mechanism is reasoned to operate equivalently when used for production or perception (Postma, 2000). Thus, perceptual errors—when a speaker processes his or her own voice—would signal to the monitor that a correction is required, in the same way as a production error (although no production error occurred). Any response the monitor makes on the basis of this incorrect information would create, rather than remove, an error in production (i.e., false alarms that probably surface as repetitions). Thus, the errors made in perception suggest it is _not_ a suitable guide for production.

There is other evidence that different speaker groups either cannot or do not use input over the external loop. Hartsuiker et al. (2005) have modeled the relative contribution of internal and external loops in speakers with aphasia. Following a suggestion by Howell, they were able to show that the speech of speakers with aphasia can be modeled with the external loop making no contribution at all. Adventitiously deafened speakers cannot use the external loop but they do not lose the ability to speak (Borden, 1979), as would be the case if this loop was essential for controlling speech. An alternative possibility is that loss of the external loop would lead to speech that contains many errors, as the speaker has no way of monitoring whether output is correct or not. However, there is no empirical evidence that supports the view that postlingually deafened speakers produce more errors than hearing controls. On the other hand, perceptual errors, such as those involving judgments of place of articulation, are ubiquitous in profound hearing loss and would occur when listening to self-produced speech. The listening errors would be expected to trigger many false alarms, which would surface as repairs to correct utterances, which should introduce repetitions. As these subjects do not have high rates of speech error such as repetitions, the perceptual system does not appear to be implicated in speech control.

b. Does speech recovered over the external loop carry sufficient information to determine whether an overt error has occurred?
It is not clear that speakers can recover sufficient sound information from speech output to determine whether an error has been made. The sound of the voice is degraded through internal sources of noise generated during the articulatory processes. The main source of this internal noise is bone-conducted sound generated during articulation. The bone-conducted sound also has heavily attenuated formant structure that reduces its intelligibility (Howell & Powell, 1984). The degraded bone-conducted sound is loud enough to mask the unadulterated information regarding articulation that occurs in the air-conducted sound (von Bekesy, 1960, estimated that bone-conducted sound is at approximately the same level as sound transmitted through air). These influences lead to the external loop having little information about a speaker's speech output and would not supply reliable information for the monitor to determine whether an error had been made.

c. An analysis of perceptual representations that could be supplied to the monitor based on Levelt's view.
Levelt's account is attractive in that it uses an existing perceptual mechanism (Postma, 2000), so no extra processes are required for dealing with the speaker's own voice. Conversely, for perception to do "what it always does" (Postma, 2000), the perceptual system must process the speaker's own speech returned over internal or external loops like any other speech they hear. The presence of bone-conducted components in self-generated auditory feedback suggests that perception would have to remove the distortions to make this speech the same as that of others, so the perceptual system has to do different things for speech from different sources. The perceptual system also has to process speech recovered from the internal and external loops differently.

The internal loop is examined first. Information is obtained by the perception system about the features of covert repairs, discussed earlier, that were attributed to responses to errors at different levels in the language process. The speaker needs to pinpoint the level at which the error occurred, and there is an advantage in doing this as quickly as possible. In Levelt's model, production proceeds in a top-down manner, so the representations at each level can be supplied to perception over the internal loop immediately after they are generated. This seems to be in agreement with Levelt's view of the representation supplied to perception from production, which is "parsed speech, a representation of the input speech in terms of its phonological, morphological, syntactic, and semantic composition" (1989, p. 13). The lemma and phonological forms generated during production could, for instance, constitute the syntactic and phonological attributes (respectively) of this parsed representation. Two properties are highlighted and similar points apply at other levels in the hierarchy. (1) The lemma representation is abstract and has no phonological information (the latter is not available when lemmas are generated). (2) The lemma representation would be available before the phonological information because the latter is available at a lower level in the hierarchical processing proposed by Levelt.

The external loop is examined next. Whereas the production system works in top-down fashion, the perception system when working on auditory input builds the higher level representations in part from the lower forms (although there are also top-down influences). Processing information bottom-up over the external loop would allow lemma forms to have associated phonological information. However, the abstract form of the representation supplied over the internal loop does not allow associated lower level representations, so would not be allowed over the external loop if the representations are equivalent. One way of making the representations in the perception system equivalent would be for the perceptual representation based on auditory output (external loop) to have; for instance, the lower level phonological information stripped away when the lemma form is generated. Such abstract representations would seem to deny both bottom-up and top-down influences between representational levels in speech perception, which are influences that have been documented in speech perception (Klatt, 1976; Samuel, 1996).

As mentioned, the internal loop has representations from the higher levels in production available in perception before representations at lower levels have become available. With the external loop, in contrast, representations from lower levels would be available to the monitor before the higher level representations, assuming some degree of bottom-up processing again. Either the perceptual system has separate representations for the internal and external loops (leaving the representation from the internal loop having different timing to that generated when there is auditory input, and making it atypical of ordinary perception) or the information arriving over the two loops would need to be integrated at each representational level. The latter would involve buffering to align the representations and processing to combine the internal- and external-loop representations. Such additional processing would not be needed when the perceptual system is doing its ordinary job of dealing with other speakers' speech, so this seems unlikely to be a built-in feature of the perceptual system.

The ad hoc assumption has been made that the inner loop, rather than supplying information to perception in the order in which representations are computed, supplies (syllabified) phonological representations as they unfold in time (Levelt, Roelofs, & Meyer, 1999). Perception could then, for instance, recompute the lemmas that underlie those phonological representations to see whether they are in error. As representations would need to be generated down to the syllable level before they can be transmitted over the internal loop, timing differences between the internal and external loops would be reduced (but not removed). Also, generating representations down to the syllable level would lead to processing that is closer to that which takes place over the external loop. However, these advantages are not obtained without the generating cost. In addition the syllables generated in the production process would have to be analyzed to locate any errors and determine at what level they occurred.

It may not be necessary, in Levelt's view, to "integrate" information from the two loops, thus avoiding the necessity to deal with the offsets between internal and external loops—as they could be treated like two different voices (Hartsuiker, personal communication, 2003). For this proposal to work, it would have to be consistent with the way the perceptual system keeps external voices separate and would have to work for the voices on each loop. Acoustic information seems to be essential to keep external voices separate (Duifhuis, Willems, & Sluyter, 1982). Duifhuis and colleague's harmonic sieve could be applied to separate voices received over the external loop but the speech over the internal loop would not have harmonic information that could be used to keep it separate from other voices.

The Monitor

In this section it is assumed that the monitor receives accurate information about articulation although, as seen above, this is questionable.

a. Error detection by the monitor.

The monitor has to detect a discrepancy between intended forms (production) and forms supplied about speech output over the internal and external loops (perception). Given that, according to the preceding analysis, separate representations of each linguistic level are fed back over each of the loops, the monitor must have a representation of each of these forms to compare and detect any discrepancy (even assuming that it can deal with inputs at each level that are available asynchronously). To make this comparison, like must be compared with like, so it has to be assumed that the monitor has multiple intended representations for comparison equivalent to the actual forms produced at all stages during output of a message. Based on these assumed inputs, many questions arise: How does the conceptualizer know the right answer before the processes in production that compute these outputs yield their results? If the errorless versions exist in the conceptualizer, why are they not used by the production system? Until these questions are answered directly or by giving details of different architectures for the perception-monitoring systems, the task faced is at least as complicated as the problem that it was originally intended to explain (Howell, 1996; Howell & Harvey, 1983).

b. Output of the monitor into the production system.
The monitor takes corrective action when a difference is detected between intended and actual versions (only the actual version is assumed to be in error). On detection of an error, on-going production would have to be interrupted and the utterance restarted. If a retrace occurs, then that would have to be replanned if the representation of the original non-altered speech is lost after it is used (as seems likely given the length of time an overall correction takes; Hartsuiker & Kolk, 2001). Prosody is organized differently between the reparandum and alteration to empha-size the alteration (Howell & Young, 1991) so the same conceptual input does not appear to have been provided to the production system to make the repair. No specifications are given as to how reinitiating the origi-nal conception could result in different prosodic output forms (Levelt, 1989). The solution to this problem might be that the conceptual input is changed after an error, otherwise the feedback that eventually returns to the monitor will indicate an error when the original conceptual form is compared with the feedback of the revised form. The latter step is tantamount to saying that when an error is detected, a completely novel articulation is produced and the usefulness of the recursion (that could use the initial representation in the conceptualizer for monitoring for errors) is lost. Once again, the apparent explanatory power places mas-sive constraints on how a monitor can work to produce output to make a correction, and there is little information on how it could achieve the result required.

The perceptual processes that supply information for the monitor to work with and the monitor process do not appear to be specified in suf-ficient detail for the roles they need to fulfill. It might be retorted that many assumptions have been made in drawing this conclusion. While this is true, this in itself underlines the underspecification of the moni-tor. Placing a monitor that works on perceptual inputs at other points in the process does not seem to be a solution to the problems high-lighted above. If the monitor reinitiates production, it should be located in the conceptualizer (where the message starts). The monitor can then sort out errors at all lower levels. There is no advantage to proposing multiple monitors (Postma, 2000) as, in addition to the problems indi-cated here that would apply to each of the monitors, there are additional issues concerning how the information from the individual monitors is collated.

In summary (1) speakers can tolerate errors they produce and these are probably not detected and demonstrably not corrected, (2) it is not possible to recover information about production accurately by the perception mechanism, and (3) there are many unanswered questions about the monitor.

The Covert Repair Hypothesis (CRH)

In the discussion of Levelt's work, it was seen that pauses and repetitions, which are features commonly seen in stuttered speech, were attributed to covert repair behavior. Levelt himself did not investigate covert repairs because the presumed source of error is unknown. Kolk and Postma (1997) argued that speakers who stutter have high rates of covert repairs of errors relative to fluent speakers because they have slow phonological processing. The CRH model uses Dell's spreading activation account to illustrate how slow processing leads to word errors (see Chapter 9). When a speaker makes a lexical selection, several candidate words and other phonologically related words are activated (Figure 22.2). Activation for all words increases over time and the activation level for the intended word is greatest when there is sufficient time to reach full activation (at point S in Figure 22.2). When there is time pressure, because the experimenter stresses fast responding or because a speaker has a slow phonological system, decisions are made some time before the word is fully activated (at point S- in Figure 22.2). As shown, on some occasions an intruder word sometimes has higher activation than the intended word and the wrong word is selected. If produced, this word would be heard as an error. The CRH adds the Leveltian monitoring process that allows production of the word to be suppressed by feeding back an indication of which word was uttered to the monitor via the internal loop. Pauses and word repetitions

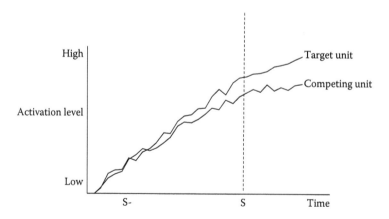

FIGURE 22.2 Activation versus time for target and competing word candidates. Two points where output commences are shown, normal (S) and early (S-).

(features of covert repairs, but not errors in themselves) are a result of the repair processes and signify that a selection error occurred.

According to our definition, covert repairs do not contain errors. Levelt (1989) partly acknowledges this for dysfluent event-types seen in covert repairs insofar as he disregards covert repairs in his extended discussion of putative errors in different types of repair. Other authors have noted that errors (consistent with our definition) are infrequent (Garnham, Shillcock, Brown, Mill, & Cutler, 1981) and often go unrepaired (Hartsuiker et al., 2005). The CRH suffers from some of the same problems as does Levelt's model because it invokes the internal monitoring process (which has been criticized above). Also, the model has not addressed the full range of questions about stuttering outlined in the introduction, so even if it did not have these problems, it would be incomplete as a theory. The main omissions concern developmental aspects of stuttering (why is there an association between stuttering and periods linked to rapid syntactic development, why is the rate of recovery high in childhood but low after teenage?).

THE VICIOUS CYCLE ACCOUNT

Bernstein Ratner (1997) also argued that stuttering is a linguistic-encoding problem, specifically associated with syntax, which leads to speech errors. Her evidence is that stuttering does not occur when children produce one-word utterances but does so when multi-word utterances occur (the stage at which children are usually regarded as starting to produce grammatical utterances). At the latter stage function words occur (prior to this, only content words were used). A logical flaw in her coincidence argument is that because things occur at the same time (here stuttering and use of function words), they are not necessarily causally related. Also, the supposition that stuttering starts when speakers first use function words is contradicted by empirical findings. The average age that children start to use function words is about 24 months (Labelle, 2005), whereas Yairi and Ambrose (2005) report that the average rage of stuttering onset is 33 months (p. 53).

Bernstein Ratner and Wijnen (2007) have developed Bernstein Ratner's original idea about stuttering as a language problem. The hypothesis is that "stuttering [is] connected to a maladaptive setting of the monitoring parameters," in particular, people who stutter invest too much time in monitoring their own speech. They use evidence from delayed auditory feedback (DAF) to support this idea. Under DAF, speakers hear their speech shortly after they produce it and this causes speech to suffer dramatically. A possible explanation is that the speaker hears his or her speech and this is sent as feedback to the linguistic system where a check is made that the correct sound was uttered. When a sound is delayed, the language system receives erroneous feedback and acts to correct this (producing an error). However, the view that DAF provides evidence for linguistic monitoring is flawed. Monitoring linguistic content before proceeding to the next speech sound is not consistent with speech rates that are achievable (Borden, 1979). As discussed above, auditory feedback is not accurate as the sound the speaker hears is not a veridical representation of the sound that is output (Howell & Powell,

1984). Young speakers could not use auditory feedback like this as the target and produced forms do not correspond due to lags in phonological development. Thus, the information supposed to be used to establish whether an error occurred would not be appropriate.

Like Levelt, Bernstein Ratner and Wijnen consider the motor processes passively translate linguistic input to speech output when they say about stuttering "what we believe to be a problem in language encoding can lead to apparent motor execution difficulties." In contrast, evidence presented later in this chapter shows that some problems experienced by people who stutter arise in the motor processes (e.g., coordination between articulators).

To summarize, the above accounts focus on language as the source of fluency problems. They all invoke monitoring and consider that the motor system responds passively to whatever input it receives. As has been seen, all these assumptions are questionable. For this reason, in our model, we leave out monitoring and give the motor system, as well as the language system, an active role in stuttering.

EXPLAN THEORY

Theories We Draw On

One theory that we draw on is Dell's (1986) spreading activation account. We use this as the activation module in EXPLAN. Dell's theory was developed to explain how speech errors (consistent with the definition used earlier) arise in the language system. CRH used the activation module to supply information to the monitor over the internal loop. We use the activation module but do not link it to a monitoring process. Multiple word candidates are activated and we use this to account for occasional errors that occur (Howell & Akande, 2005). However, we simplify consideration by focusing on the situation where the single correct word candidate is activated (the word that is usually selected). We also hypothesize that activation rate varies with the complexity of the material (so a word like "scramble" that starts with a consonant string, is activated slower than a word like "ramble," which does not).

We have also made extensive use of PW, as described by Selkirk (1984). A PW is a prosodic unit that she defines as a single content word nucleus with function words as satellites (see below for examples). She considers PW to be elements at the lower end of the prosodic hierarchy within the linguistic system, but as will be considered fully when our model is described, we interpret them differently and use them to reflect different processes. For us the alternation between easy and difficult materials in PW shows how the interface between linguistic and motor programming/execution works.

We also employ the notion that speech is represented as gesture in the linguistic system, which is inherent in Saussure's (1966) structuralism (although we do not embrace structuralism per se). Saussure characterized continuous speech as a sequence of states with different degrees of aperture of the vocal tract. Seven different apertures were proposed (from 0—minimum aperture as in /p/, through to 6—maximum as in /a/). Thus speech is reflected in terms of opening and clos-ing gestures (implosions and explosions) that lead to syllable impressions. Thus passing from an implosive gesture to an explosive one marks a syllable bound-ary. Saussure uses gesture at the linguistic level. Authors who only examine the motor system, also propose that gestures are used to generate speech output (Max & Caruso, 1997). Gestures could be output from the language system and input to the motor system. Gestures could then be a unit that communicates across the language–speech interface.

Outline of EXPLAN Theory

To account for fluency control, monitoring is only needed if errors occur fre-quently in speech and if covert repairs are the result of such errors (and even then a full linguistic analysis would not necessarily be required). However, event-types 1–6 (including those associated with covert repairs) do not contain errors. This is not to deny that occasional errors occur (Dell, 1986), some of which could be detected by a monitor like that described by Levelt (1989). However, the ideas that language is continuously monitored for errors in real time and that speech progresses fluently until one is detected (Levelt, 1989) presents many problems. If language monitoring is discarded as a proposal for online control, the perceptual mechanism need not necessarily be linked to production during speech control. The fundamental characteristic of our model is that it does not require feedback monitoring for on-going speech control.

Like Levelt and those that follow him, we assume that language planning (PLAN) and speech-motor programming and execution (EX) are independent processes. The name EXPLAN is used to signify that both processes are impli-cated in fluent speech control. PLAN generates a symbolic representation that takes different amounts of time, depending on the complexity of the units, and EX implements each representation motorically and realizes it as vocal output.

The independence assumption, allows planning for future words to continue while a speaker utters the current one. Fluency problems arise when the plan for material is not ready in time. This arises in two ways: (1) If the speaker utters the prior material fast and needs the problem material early; (2) If the problem material is particularly difficult to generate, its plan may not be ready irrespective of the rate on the lead-in sequence. Fluency problems are most likely when both influences occur in a stretch of speech.

The PW units, as originally defined by Selkirk, are a unit within which the interacting processes can be examined. From the current perspective, the impor-tant features of PW are: (1) that each of them has a single locus of difficulty (the content word is the problem), and (2) the difficult word can be preceded by func-tion words that are simple to execute so the content word is approached rapidly.

The speaker can deal with the situation where the linguistic plan is not ready in time either by stalling or advancing, each of which has characteristic forms of dysfluency associated with them. Stalling delays the move to output the difficult word by pausing prior to the content word or repeating the motor plans for the simple function word or words that have been output previously (leading to word or phrase repetitions). In stallings, the speaker deals with the situation where the content word plan is not ready by increasing the time taken up before its execution starts. Advancing involves starting the difficult word with the part of its plan already available. This results in part-word repetitions, prolongations, and word breaks when the plan runs out. According to EXPLAN, PW incorporate adjustments to motor rate (initial function words) and planning difficulty (on the content word). To put this another way, a PW is a unit that has elements that span between PLAN and EX processes. This interpretation of PW contrasts with the view that they are the last prosodic level within the linguistic system (Selkirk, 1984).

EXPLAN has been formulated in terms of time for activation to build up (representing planning) and decay over the time that the word was executed. The goal of this was to show how serially organized inputs representing the words in a PW could lead to elements being triggered out of order that corresponded with stalling and advancing dysfluency patterns. Assumptions were made about the rate of activation/decay of function and content words in PW. A criterion was specified about which word, or part of a word, would be executed next.

It was assumed activation built up linearly at different rates and to different extents for words that differed in difficulty (function words rapidly and content words gradually). Activation decayed from its maximum as the inverse of the build-up rate. The rise to full activation (representing planning) and decay over the time to execute this word is shown for the function word in the PW "he stood" as the inverted tick at the left of Figure 22.3a. When execution is complete, the element with the highest activation is selected next (this is the next one in sequence when speech is progressing fluently).

Planning of words in a PW takes place in parallel and the planning-onsets of the words is offset so they are in the order they appear in the intended utterance. Activation of the initial function word occurs at a rapid rate. As content words like "stood" are, generally speaking, linguistically more complex and longer than function words, their activation profiles build up more gradually and they reach higher levels of activation.

Execution involves all the processes concerned with generating output, starting with the gestural input supplied from the planning process. During time for execution, the activation of a word that has reached its maximum decays. The activation level after it has been uttered depends on how long the word takes to execute and the decay rate of activation. The word that has the highest activation is produced. Thus, in the example in Figure 22.3a, the function word has been produced, its activation has decayed, the content word is fully activated, and will be produced next in sequence.

Two key concepts that explain how dysfluency arises in EXPLAN are (1) the next word has highest, although not necessarily full, activation (this also means the next word produced may not be the next one in the intended sequence), and (2) the plans of previously produced words or parts of words can be reactivated and reexecuted if their activation is highest.

Stalling occurs after the initial function word in a PW has been produced, some of its activation has decayed but its activation level is higher than that of the

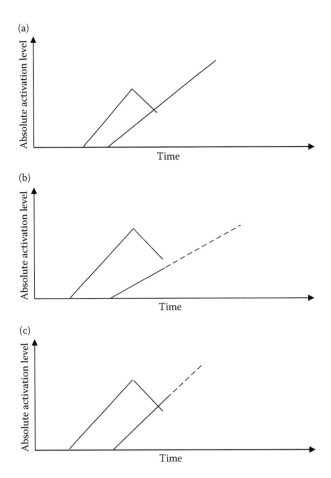

FIGURE 22.3 Part (a) shows activation build up and decay representing two function words and a content word. Part (b) shows activation and decay parameters for the situation leading to stalling for an utterance consisting of a function word preceding a content word. Part (c) shows activation and decay parameters for the situation leading to advancing for an utterance consisting of a function word preceding a content word.

subsequent content word being planned (whose activation is still building up but has not reached its maximum). Figure 22.3b shows the situation where the function word has been uttered once. Note that at this point, activation for the content word is lower than that of the function word.

Advancings occur when the content word in the planned sequence has highest, but not full activation (as shown in Figure 22.3c). Here the content word has the highest activation level, so it will be produced next in the sequence. As its activation is not full, only the first part of the plan will be available. This situation can lead to the different forms of advancings considered earlier (Howell, 2007b).

Supporting Evidence for EXPLAN

Difficulty

EXPLAN maintains that language and motor factors are both important in leading to stuttering. In this and the following section, work on the relationship between difficulty (language factor) and speech rate (motor factor) in stuttering in spontaneous utterances is reviewed. My group used phonological and phonetic measures to quantify different levels of difficulty within function and content word classes. Content words are the material that is difficult (phonetically and phonologically). One way of showing the difficulty of content words is by comparison of their phonetic properties with function words. Figure 22.4 shows the incidence of manner, word length, and contiguous consonants, and that these vary across the age range from 6 years to adulthood (shown separately for content and function words). Figure 22.4a shows significant increases over ages in use of each factor for content words while Figure 22.4b shows no such increase for function words. The change over word type and ages for content words shows that content words that are acquired later are more complex than those acquired earlier.

When words are phonetically difficult, stuttering rate increases for content words. This is shown in Figure 22.5 where phonetic difficulty is represented as the sum total over eight features marked as easy/difficult by Jakielski (1998). For example, words containing a contiguous string of consonants score a point, but words with just singletons score zero. There is a significant correlation for content but not function words.

Figure 22.5 also shows that function words have a more limited range of phonetic difficulty. The lack of correlation with the difficulty measure for the function words underlines the importance of examining word types separately. To summarize, planning difficulty, as indicated by this phonetic measure, correlates with stuttering rate.

Rate

Variation in speech rate has been examined to see whether it affects stuttering in the way EXPLAN predicts. Timing control can be represented in different ways in language and speech-motor processes. At the language level, timing information could be represented as being linked with or separate from the symbolic linguistic representation. At the speech-motor level, it has been proposed that there are external timing inputs that modulate speech rate (as in Guenther's, 2001, DIVA model). In this section, speech-motor rate control alone is examined.

Generally speaking, if speech is slowed, there is less likelihood of planning getting out of alignment with execution. When dysfluencies start to occur, rate adjustments are needed, but only around the points where difficulty is high (local). Global changes are necessary when speakers have to make a long-term adjustment to rate (as for instance, when a speaker continuously makes advancings).

Howell, Au-Yeung, and Pilgrim (1999a) provided evidence that rate control operates locally in utterances. Spontaneous speech of adults who stutter was segmented into tone units (TU) and these were separated into those that were

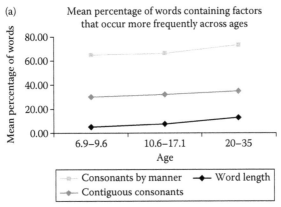

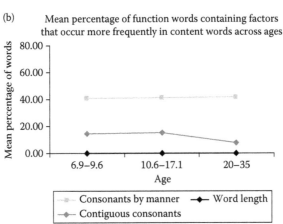

FIGURE 22.4   Mean percentage of (a) content, and (b) function words containing difficult manners, long words or contiguous consonants that occur more frequently in the speech of speakers who stutter aged 18 +.

stuttered and those that were fluent. Syllable rate was measured in the section prior to the stuttering (the whole segment in the case of fluent TU). The TU were classified into fast, medium, and slow rate categories based on the rate in the fluent section. The TU that were spoken slowly had a lower rate of stuttering than those spoken more rapidly. These findings support the idea that fluency problems arise when speech rate is high locally to the content word (possibly because approach rate taxes planning of difficult words).

Howell and Sackin (2000) examined whether local rate change can occur independently of global rate change for conditions known to affect the fluency of speakers who stutter. Fluent speakers repeated the sentence "Cathy took some cocoa to the teletubbies" several times under frequency shifted feedback (FSF), in normal listening conditions, and when speaking and singing. The plosives in the utterance were marked and the duration of the intervals between the first and each

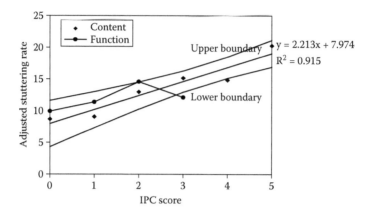

FIGURE 22.5   Adjusted stuttering rate (ordinate) versus number of times the four factors marked as difficult occurred (abscissa) for speakers aged over 18 years. The straight line is fitted to the content words and the upper and lower bounds around this line are indicated by the dashed line. The function word points are connected by a solid line.

of the subsequent plosives was measured. The interval-distributions were plotted for every interval and for all speaking conditions. Global slowing between speaking conditions occurs when the mean of the distribution shifts to longer durations. Local slowing between conditions occurs when there are fewer intervals at the short duration end of the distribution, but no shift in the overall mean. One statistic that reflects shifts at the lower end of the distribution is the 25th percentile.

The differences between the means of the distributions were significant for all pairs of speaking conditions (showing global slowing) except speaking versus singing in normal listening conditions. Howell and Sackin then calculated the time where the 25% fell, and repeated the earlier analyses, this time to see whether the fast intervals shifted between the different conditions. Of particular note was the finding that there was a significant shift of the 25% when speaking was compared with singing in normal listening conditions (singing produced local slowing). Thus local slowing occurred between these conditions, although there had been no global slowing. This suggests that these are two distinct modes of changing rate. EXPLAN specifically requires speakers to have the option of making local rate changes to deal with fluency problems. Singing is known to enhance the fluency of speakers who stutter and this would have to derive from the local rate changes that speakers make in this mode of vocal control.

Pauses

Pauses are a form of stalling. EXPLAN predicts that pauses should occur prior to the content word in a PW (the positions where they can delay onset of the following content word). To fill this role, pauses should tend to appear at the start of PW more often than they occur at the start of syntactic units (as some other authors have maintained). Pinker (1995) used the examples "[The baby]$_{np}$ [ate [the slug] $_{np}]_{vp}$" and "[He]$_{np}$ [ate [the slug]$_{np}]_{vp}$" to show that pauses do not occur at syntactic boundaries. He stated that pausing is allowed after the subject NP "the baby," but not after the subject NP, in the pronominal "he." Note that both these positions involve the same major syntactic boundary, a subject NP, so syntactic factors alone cannot account for this difference in pause occurrence.

It is possible that pauses occur at PW boundaries as they do not always coincide with syntactic boundaries. The PW boundaries in the examples are "[The baby]$_{PW}$ [ate]$_{PW}$ [the slug]$_{PW}$" and "[He ate]$_{PW}$ [the slug]$_{PW}$," respectively. If the PW boundaries in the two sentences are examined, pausing between "baby" and "ate" is allowed in the first sentence (as Pinker observed), as they are in two separate PW. Pausing should not occur in the second sentence (again as Pinker observed) because there is no PW boundary at the corresponding point. Thus it seems that PW are preferred units for specifying boundaries where pauses occur. Gee and Grosjean (1983) offer a related analysis to the current one using units related to PW. It has also been proposed that pause-location is determined by both syntactic and prosodic factors (Ferreira, 1993; Watson & Gibson, 2004). A full analysis comparing different models for predicting pause location is required.

To summarize, pauses and word repetition are things that speakers do in anticipation, or as a result of material that is time-consuming to prepare (consistent with EXPLAN). They do not signify error as required in CRH and Bernstein Ratner's work. Next we look at EXPLAN's prediction about the distribution of dysfluencies, and then consider some experimental tests and scanning evidence.

Dysfluency-Distribution

The proposal that whole word repetition serves the role of delaying the time at which the following word is produced, has been made by several authors working on fluent speech (for example, Blackmer & Mitton, 1991; Clark & Clark, 1977; Maclay & Osgood, 1959; MacWhinney & Osser, 1977; Rispoli, 2003). However, these accounts have not linked them to function words nor examined how word repetition depends on the position they occupy in PW contexts. For word repetition to work as stalling, only the function words before the content word should be involved, as reported in a number of studies on stuttering (Au-Yeung, Vallejo Gomez, & Howell, 2003, for Spanish; Dworzynski, Howell, Au-Yeung, & Rommel, 2004, for German; and Howell, Au-Yeung, & Sackin, 1999b, for English). The same has been reported for selected constructs for fluent English speakers (Strenstrom & Svartvik, 1994). The latter authors reported that subject pronouns (which appear before verbs in English, i.e., PW-initial) have a greater tendency to be produced dysfluently than object pronouns (which appear after verbs in English). Overall, word repetitions tend to appear in the position in PW that EXPLAN requires.

Stalling/Advancing Reciprocity

EXPLAN predicts a reciprocal relationship between stalling on function words and advancing on content words. If a speaker stalls, there should be no need to advance and vice versa. Early findings confirmed this relationship as stalling and advancing occurred rarely in the same PW (Howell et al., 1999b).

It has been found for a number of languages (Au-Yeung et al., 2003; Dworzynski et al., 2004; Howell et al., 1999b) that speakers who stutter show more dysfluency on function words (stalling) than on content words (advancing) in early development, but the opposite in later development (termed an exchange relation). This suggests that older speakers stop stalling and start advancing. Howell et al. (1999b) noted that the exchange to advancing at older ages corresponded with a reduced chance of recovering from stuttering and suggested that the advancing pattern may be a factor implicated in this change. This would suggest that a change in speech-planning occurs when speakers persist.

Howell et al. (1999b) examined the link of dysfluency rate with *word type* so they could use PW to investigate language–speech interactions. There are several other ways of characterizing the points where simple and complex material alternate. For example, Howell (2004) looked at stressed and unstressed words. He reported that stressed function words and unstressed content words produced an exchange relation. From this, it also appears that stressing a word (irrespective of lexical type) can result in the exchange first reported on content and function words. Some authors have argued that word frequency effects could account for the exchange pattern (exchanges would then be expected between low and high frequency items). This account seems problematic in connection with stuttering, as word frequency is particularly difficult to measure in childhood and varies markedly between speakers at these early stages of language development.

The EXPLAN account maintains that exchanges reflect a change from stalling to advancing with age. Consequently, Howell (2007a) examined these dysfluency categories directly in a longitudinal study on children who stuttered aged from about eight years up to teenage. They were independently assessed at teenage to see whether they were still stuttering (persistent) or not (recovered). For recovered speakers, the absolute level of dysfluencies decreased as they get older, but the ratio of stallings, to advancings remained constant. Speakers whose stuttering persisted, on the other hand, showed a reduced rate of stalling and an increased rate of advancing. This is consistent with the EXPLAN predictions, but not CRH, which would predict that the pattern of dysfluencies produced by children whose stuttering persists would always differ from children who recover or who have always been fluent because they plan speech more slowly.

Priming

Priming techniques are a way of manipulating planning time. An auditory sentence or syllable is presented (the prime). Participants then describe a picture (the probe) and speech initiation time (SIT) are measured. When the auditory prime matches some aspect of the probe, the planning time needed for the production of different elements in the phrase is reduced. Past work has shown that SIT is shorter for children who stutter than children who do not stutter for material that is primed phonologically and syntactically (Anderson & Conture, 2004; Melnick, Conture, & Ohde, 2003) but not lexically (Pellowski & Conture, 2005).

All previous priming investigations look for effects at the language level whereas EXPLAN stresses the importance of PW units that reflect operation at the language-motor interface. Savage and Howell used PW like "He is swim-ming" and "She is running" (both consist of two function words followed by a content word) in a priming study that tested EXPLAN. On a trial, a child was primed either with a function word (e.g., they heard and repeated "he is") or a content word (e.g., they heard and repeated "swimming"). A cartoon (the probe) was then displayed depicting an action that had to be described, and SIT and dys-fluency rate were measured. When the auditory prime matched an aspect of the probe (e.g., "he is" was primed and the picture was of a boy, or "swimming" was primed and this was the action), the planning time needed for the production of different elements in the phrase would be reduced.

EXPLAN predicts that priming either the function or the content word (the elements in PW) will have opposite effects (Savage & Howell, 2008). Priming a function word should reduce its planning time, allowing it to be produced more rapidly. When rate of production of a function word is increased, pressure is placed on having the content word plan ready earlier. If it is not ready, this increases the chance of stalling or advancing dysfluencies. Priming the content word reduces its planning time (as with function words). But this time priming should reduce the dysfluency rate on function and content words (priming the content word acceler-ates planning and decreases the chances of plan unavailability, which should be reflected in a reduction of stalling and/or advancing). In addition to the asym-metric effects of function and content word priming, EXPLAN predicts that there will be bigger effects in participants who stutter than in fluent controls though both speaker groups should show priming effects.

Savage and Howell confirmed these predictions in children who stuttered and controls (mean age 6 years). Priming function words increased dysfluencies on function and content words whereas priming content words reduced dysfluencies on function and content words. The additional prediction that these effects should be true of both groups of speakers was also confirmed though the effects for the children who stutter were bigger.

The findings suggest that the same process underpins the production of dys-fluencies for both children who stutter and controls, and that it takes the form of a timing misalignment between planning and execution. The primed production of a content word immediately before using it in a picture description reduced the time needed to plan the content word online by activating its plan (so that it was available in advance). This reduced the discrepancy between the time needed to plan the content word (relatively long) and the time needed to execute the func-tion words (relatively short), and in turn decreased the likelihood of speaking dysfluently.

Central Nervous System (CNS) Underpinning

Stalling and advancing are mediated by motor and language processes, respec-tively and consequently, when each occurs activity should be seen in different parts of the CNS. According to EXPLAN, stalling is a motor-timing adjust-ment and as such is likely to involve the cerebellum (Howell, 2002). Advancing reflects planning processes and would involve Broca's area. The fact that there is different activity in both cerebellar and Broca's area between fluent controls and people who stutter (Watkins, Smith, Davis, & Howell, 2008) is in general agreement with EXPLAN. A further test would be to classify scans obtained immediately after either stalling or advancing has occurred and see whether cerebellar and cerebral activity dominates the CNS patterns. Subsequent work should then look at children and older speakers who stutter to ascertain whether there is a change from activity in cerebellar (indicates stalling predominates at younger ages) to cerebral areas (indicates advancing predominates at older ages).

Reasons were given earlier that DAF does not support feedback to the linguistic level. However, DAF must affect some CNS structures, as there is little doubt about the influences of this on the fluency of speakers who stutter (fluency improves) and controls (fluency is reduced). The DAF could have these effects on both groups of speaker if it slows speech. Slowing would make fluent speakers' speech sound less fluent. Speakers who stutter would also be slowed, but as they have dysfluencies that are due to over-rapid speech, these would be reduced. DAF could slow speech if it affected a motor (not linguistic) level in the CNS and this would avoid the problems discussed earlier. One way DAF could do this is if it produced a second rhythmic signal that disrupts cerebellar timing mechanisms (Howell, Powell, & Khan, 1983).

Recently, there has been behavioral support for the proposal that DAF affects cerebellar timing processes. Howell and Sackin (2002) used a speech version of the Wing and Kristofferson (1973) metronome tapping, and analysis procedure and marked onset of the consonants. Howell and Sackin recorded speakers uttering a CV syllable at a metronome rate. They marked onset of the consonants. Wing and Kristofferson's analysis procedure takes such sequences and decomposes variance into components associated with motor (Mv) and timing or clock (Cv) variance. The analysis procedure assumes that if the motor system leads to an action being placed at the wrong point in time, it is compensated for in the next interval. This gives rise to Mv that can be estimated from the lag one autocovariance. The other source of variance identified in the model is Cv. This can be estimated by subtracting Mv from the overall variance that leaves an estimate of Cv. In work with patients, Ivry (1997) showed that Mv and Cv arose in the cerebellum, as lateral lesions of the cerebellum affected Cv, and medial lesions affected Mv. Howell and Sackin used fluent speakers speaking isochronously at several different DAF delays. The Mv remained constant across DAF delays but Cv increased with delay. From this it appears that DAF specifically affected Cv.

The interpretation that DAF affects cerebellar regions (Howell & Sackin, 2002) has received some support from fMRI work in which speakers who stutter speak under DAF. These speakers showed increased activity in the cerebellum (e.g., Watkins et al., 2008). Other data that are consistent with a functional cerebellar deficit in people who stutter are provided by behavioral work using the posture/balance and complex movement tasks that Dow and Moruzzi (1958) introduced for assessing cerebellar defects (Howell, Au-Yeung, & Rustin, 1997; Howell et al., 2008).

What Does the Speech Motor System Do
That Is Not Linguistic-Symbolic?

Most of the work reviewed in this chapter has been concerned with the language level. However, the assumption that the language system is independent from the motor system needs to be demonstrated, as does the distinctive processing that the motor system does. Our recent work has used Smith's spatiotemporal index (STI) to this end (see Smith & Goffman, 2004, for a review). The STI quantifies variability over a set of repetitions of the same phrase after each repetition has been time- and amplitude-normalized. Smith's original work used a lower-lip kinematic signal for this analysis. Howell, Anderson, Bartrip, and Bailey (2009) showed that the same procedure can be used on an acoustic signal (speech energy in their case). They also measured lower-lip movement so that they could verify their measurement techniques against reported results. The availability of two signals allowed them to show that intercoordination between lips and energy was worse in speakers who stutter than controls (Howell, Anderson, & Lucero, in press) using newly developed metrics related to STI. Articulatory intercoordination is likely to be done in the motor system.

FURTHER WORK

Some areas, where further work is required, are listed. First, further specification is needed about what is meant by a "part-plan." Is it incomplete in extent; that is, properly coarticulated to a particular point (Howell & Dworzynski, 2005) but stops abruptly. Alternatively, some features are absent at the point where speech halts (consistent with the view that coarticulated features of the same utterance are propagated at different rates). Howell and Huckvale (2004) presented some examples where speech was interrupted but coarticulation for the following vowel was appropriate (e.g., the prolonged /s/ in a word subsequently realized as "CD" was appropriate for /i/). This offers slight support for the first proposal about part-plans but more is needed. Other procedures that may be used to obtain evidence for part-plans is the tip-of-the-tongue phenomenon that Howell and Sackin (2001) proposed may be related to stuttering.

Second, more work is needed to determine whether the changes that occur in the speech of children who stutter over development are due to development of the language (Bernstein Ratner & Wijnen, 2007) or motor system (van Lieshout & Namasivayam, 2010) in both systems or is due to some different aspect of behavior entirely (e.g., anxiety changes with age). Finally, space has not permitted discussion of the relation of stuttering to other developmental speech disorders (Howell, 2007b). This issue also deserves further attention.

CONCLUSIONS

This chapter addressed a number of questions that an adequate theory about stuttering should address. The answers that EXPLAN offers are summarized next.

1. Fluent episodes of speech are interspersed with dysfluent events because local speech rate and difficulty of the content words interact to heighten the chance of fluency breakdown.
2. EXPLAN provides a theoretical reason why the two classes of dysfluency type (stalling and advancing) ought to be distinguished. The need to subgroup dysfluency types is often recognized as being necessary (Yairi & Ambrose, 2005). However, all other schemes subgroup dysfluencies based on empirical observation. EXPLAN suggests that the stalling and advancing dysfluency classes reflect different psychological processes that depend on motor (stalling) and linguistic (advancing) operations, respectively.
3. Errors are not assumed to disrupt ongoing control in the EXPLAN account. Consequently, the concept of a monitor (which is problematic) is discarded. It is recognized that errors can occur on occasions in all speakers but speakers do not monitor for them to control on-going production.
4. Any speaker can stall or advance when dealing with fluency problems similar to those seen in stuttering.
5. Diagnosis of stuttering is aided by looking at the relative incidence of stalling and advancing dysfluency event-types.
6. The incidence of stuttering is at its peak when language development is maximal because speakers start to produce speech that allows language–speech interaction to be observed. Stuttering onset has nothing to do with receptive syntactic development (Howell, Davis, & Au-Yeung, 2003) although conceivably expressive syntax could contribute to fluency failure because it increases language complexity.
7. There is a high rate of recovery in early development because these speakers predominantly stall. This type of dysfluent event permits development into fluent control.
8. There is a reduced chance of recovery in later development when speakers shift to advancing.

ACKNOWLEDGMENTS

This work was supported by grant 072639 from The Wellcome Trust awarded to Peter Howell. Thanks to Stavroula Thaleia Kousta for helpful comments on this manuscript.

REFERENCES

Anderson, J., & Conture, E. (2004). Sentence-structure priming in young children who do and do not stutter. *Journal of Speech, Language, and Hearing Research, 47,* 552–571.
Andrews, G., & Harris, M. (1964). *The syndrome of stuttering.* London, UK: Heinemann Medical Books.

Au-Yeung, J., Vallejo Gomez, I., & Howell, P. (2003). Exchange of disfluency from function words to content words with age in Spanish speakers who stutter. *Journal of Speech, Language, and Hearing Research, 46*, 754–765.

Bernstein Ratner, N. (1997). Stuttering: A psycholinguistic perspective. In R. Curlee & G. Siegel (Eds.), *Nature and treatment of stuttering: New directions* (2nd ed., pp. 99–127). Boston, MA: Allyn & Bacon.

Bernstein Ratner, N., & Wijnen, F. (2007). The vicious cycle: Linguistic encoding, self-monitoring and stuttering. In J. Au-Yeung & M. M. Leahy (Eds.), *Research, treatment and self help in fluency disorders: New horizons. Proceedings of the Fifth World Congress on Fluency Disorders* (pp. 84–90). Dublin, Ireland: The International Fluency Association.

Blackmer, E. R., & Mitton, J. L. (1991). Theories of monitoring and the timing of repairs in spontaneous speech. *Cognition, 39*, 173–194.

Bond, Z. S. (1999). *Slips of the ear: Errors in the perception of casual conversation*. San Diego, CA: Academic Press.

Borden, G. J. (1979). An interpretation of research on feedback interruption in speech. *Brain & Language, 7*, 307–319.

Clark, H. H., & Clark, E. (1977). *Psychology and language. An introduction to psycholinguistics*. New York, NY: Harcourt.

Cutler, A. (1982). The reliability of speech error data. *Linguistics, 19*, 561–582.

Dell, G. S. (1986). A spreading activation theory of retrieval in sentence production. *Psychological Review, 93*, 283–321.

Dow, R. S., & Moruzzi, G. (1958). *The physiology and pathology of the cerebellum*. Minneapolis, MN: University of Minnesota Press.

Duifhuis, H., Willems, L. F., & Sluyter, R. J. (1982). Measurement of pitch in speech: An implementation of Goldstein's theory of pitch perception. *Journal of the Acoustical Society of America, 71*, 1568–1580.

Dworzynski, K., Howell, P., Au-Yeung, J., & Rommel, D. (2004). Stuttering on function and content words across age groups of German speakers who stutter. *Journal of Multilingual Communication Disorders, 2*, 81–101.

Ferreira, F. (1993). Creation of prosody during sentence production. *Psychological Review, 100*, 233–253.

Garnham, A., Shillcock, R. C., Brown, G. D. A., Mill, A. I. D., & Cutler, A. (1981). Slips of the tongue in the London-Lund corpus of spontaneous conversation. *Linguistics, 19*, 805–817.

Gee, J. P., & Grosjean, F. (1983). Performance structures: A psycholinguistic and linguistic appraisal. *Cognitive Psychology, 15*, 411–458.

Guenther, F. (2001). Neural modeling of speech production. In B. Maassen, W. Hulstijn, R. Kent, H. F. M. Peters, & P. H. M. M. van Lieshout (Eds.), *Speech motor control in normal and disordered speech* (pp. 12–15). Nijmegen, The Netherlands: Uttgeverij Vantilt.

Hartmann, R. R. K., & Stork, F. C. (1972). *Dictionary of language and linguistics*. London, UK: Applied Science Publishers.

Hartsuiker, R. J., & Kolk, H. H. J. (2001). Error monitoring in speech production: A computational test of the perceptual loop theory. *Cognitive Psychology, 42*, 113–157.

Hartsuiker, R. J., Kolk, H. H. J., & Martensen, H. (2005). The division of labor between internal and external speech monitoring. In R. J. Hartsuiker, R. Bastiaanse, A. Postma, & F. Wijnen (Eds.), *Phonological encoding and monitoring in normal and pathological speech* (pp. 187–205). Hove, UK: Psychology Press.

Howell, P. (1996). Producing and perceiving speech. In D. Green et al. (Eds.), *Cognitive science* (pp. 120–147). Oxford, UK: Blackwell.

Howell, P. (2002). The EXPLAN theory of fluency control applied to the treatment of stuttering by altered feedback and operant procedures. In E. Fava (Ed.), *Pathology and therapy of speech disorders* (pp. 95–118). Amsterdam, The Netherlands: John Benjamins.

Howell, P. (2004). Comparison of two ways of defining phonological words for assessing stuttering pattern changes with age in Spanish speakers who stutter. *Journal of Multilingual Communication Disorders, 2,* 161–186.

Howell, P. (2007a). Signs of developmental stuttering up to age eight and at 12 plus. *Clinical Psychology Review, 27,* 287–306.

Howell, P. (2007b). A model of serial order problems in fluent, stuttered and agrammatic speech. *Human Movement Science, 26,* 728–741.

Howell, P., & Akande, O. (2005). Simulations of the types of disfluency produced in spontaneous utterances by fluent speakers, and the change in disfluency type seen as speakers who stutter get older. In J. Veronis & E. Campione (Eds.), *Disfluency in Spontaneous Speech* (pp. 93–98). Edinburgh, Scotland: ISCA Tutorial and Research Workshop.

Howell, P., Anderson, A. J., Bartrip, J., & Bailey, E. (2009). Comparison of acoustic and kinematic approaches to measuring utterance-level speech variability. *Journal of Speech, Language and Hearing Research, 52,* 1088–1096.

Howell, P., Anderson, A., & Lucero, J. (in press). Motor timing and fluency. In B. Maassen & P. H. H. M. van Lieshout (Eds.), *Speech motor control: New developments in basic and applied research.* Oxford, UK: Oxford University Press.

Howell, P., Au-Yeung, J., & Pilgrim, L. (1999a). Utterance rate and linguistic properties as determinants of speech dysfluency in children who stutter. *Journal of the Acoustical Society of America, 105,* 481–490.

Howell, P., Au-Yeung, J., & Rustin, L. (1997). Clock and motor variance in lip tracking: A comparison between children who stutter and those who do not. In W. Hulstijn, H. F. M. Peters, & P. H. H. M. van Lieshout (Eds.), *Speech production: Motor control, brain research and fluency disorders* (pp. 573–578). Amsterdam, The Netherlands: Elsevier.

Howell, P., Au-Yeung, J., & Sackin, S. (1999b). Exchange of stuttering from function words to content words with age. *Journal of Speech, Language and Hearing Research, 42,* 345–354.

Howell, P., Davis, S., & Au-Yeung, J. (2003). Syntactic development in fluent children, children who stutter, and children who have English as an additional language. *Child Language Teaching and Therapy, 19,* 311–337.

Howell, P., Davis, S., & Williams, R. (2008). Late childhood stuttering. *Journal of Speech, Language and Hearing Research, 51,* 1–19.

Howell, P., & Dworzynski, K. (2005). Planning and execution processes in speech control by fluent speakers and speakers who stutter. *Journal of Fluency Disorders, 30,* 343–354.

Howell, P., & Harvey, N. (1983). Perceptual equivalence and motor equivalence in speech. In B. Butterworth (Ed.), *Language production* (Vol. 2, pp. 203–224). New York, NY: Academic Press.

Howell, P., & Huckvale, M. (2004). Facilities to assist people to research into stammered speech. *Stammering Research, 1,* 130–242.

Howell, P., & Powell, D. J. (1984). Hearing your voice through bone and air: Implications for explanations of stuttering behaviour from studies of normal speakers. *Journal of Fluency Disorders, 9,* 247–264.

Howell, P., Powell, D. J., & Khan, I. (1983). Amplitude contour of the delayed signal and interference in delayed auditory feedback tasks. *Journal of Experimental Psychology: Human Perception and Performance, 9,* 772–784.

Howell, P., & Sackin, S. (2000). Speech rate manipulation and its effects on fluency reversal in children who stutter. *Journal of Developmental and Physical Disabilities, 12,* 291–315.

Howell, P., & Sackin, S. (2001). Function word repetitions emerge when speakers are operantly conditioned to reduce frequency of silent pauses. *Journal of Psycholinguistic Research, 30,* 457–474.

Howell, P., & Sackin, S. (2002). Timing interference to speech in altered listening conditions. *Journal of the Acoustical Society of America, 111,* 2842–2852.

Howell, P., & Young, K. (1991). The use of prosody in highlighting alteration in repairs from unrestricted speech. *Quarterly Journal of Experimental Psychology, 43*(A), 733–758.

Ivry, R. (1997). Cerebellar timing systems. *International Review of Neurobiology, 41,* 555–573.

Jakielski, K. J. (1998). *Motor organization in the acquisition of consonant clusters.* PhD thesis, University of Texas at Austin. Ann Arbor, Michigan, UMI Dissertation services.

Johnson, W. & Associates. (1959). *The onset of stuttering.* Minneapolis, MN: University of Minnesota Press.

Klatt, D. H. (1976). Speech perception: A model of acoustic phonetic analysis and lexical analysis. *Journal of Phonetics, 7,* 279–312.

Kolk, H., & Postma, A. (1997). Stuttering as a covert repair phenomenon. In R. F. Curlee & G. M. Siegel (Eds.), *Nature and treatments of stuttering: New directions* (pp. 182–203). Needham Heights, MA: Allyn & Bacon.

Labelle, M. (2005). The acquisition of grammatical categories: A state of the art. In H. Cohen & C. Lefebvre (Eds.) *Handbook of categorization in cognitive science* (pp 433–457). Amsterdam, The Netherlands: Elsevier.

Levelt, W. (1983). Monitoring and self-repair in speech. *Cognition, 14,* 41–104.

Levelt, W. (1989). *Speaking: From intention to articulation.* Cambridge, MA: Bradford Books.

Levelt, W., Roelofs, A., & Meyer, A. (1999). A theory of lexical access in speech production. *Behavioral and Brain Sciences, 22,* 1–75.

Maclay, H., & Osgood, C. E. (1959). Hesitation phenomena in spontaneous English speech. *Word, 15,* 169–182.

MacWhinney, B., & Osser, H. (1977). Verbal planning functions in children's speech. *Child Development, 48,* 978–85.

Max, L., & Caruso, A. J. (1997). Acoustic measures of temporal intervals across speaking rates: Variability of syllable- and phrase-level relative timing. *Journal of Speech, Language and Hearing Research, 40,* 1097–1110.

Melnick, K., Conture, E., & Ohde, R. (2003). Phonological priming in picture naming in young children who stutter. *Journal of Speech, Language, and Hearing Research, 46,* 1428–1443.

Menyuk, P., & Anderson, S. (1969). Children's identification and reproduction of /w/, /r/, and /l/. *Journal of Speech and Hearing Research, 12,* 39–52.

Nooteboom. S. (2005). Listening to oneself: Monitoring speech production. In R. Hartsuiker, G. Bastiaanse, A. Postma, & F. Wijnen (Eds.), *Phonological encoding and monitoring in normal and pathological speech* (pp. 167–186). Hove, UK: Psychology Press.

Pellowski, M. W., & Conture, E. G. (2005). Lexical priming in picture naming of young children who do and do not stutter. *Journal of Speech, Language and Hearing Research, 48,* 278–294.

Pinker, S. (1995). Language acquisition. In L. R. Gleitman, M. Liberman, & D. N. Osherson (Eds.), *An invitation to cognitive science* (2nd ed., Volume 1: Language). Cambridge, MA: MIT Press.

Postma, A. (2000). Detection of errors during speech production: A review of speech monitoring models. *Cognition, 77,* 97–131.

Quirk, R., Greenbaum, S., Leech, G., & Svartvik, J. (1985). *A comprehensive grammar of the English language.* London, UK: Longman.

Rispoli, M. (2003). Changes in the nature of sentence production during the period of grammatical development. *Journal of Speech, Language and Hearing Research, 46,* 818–830.

Roelofs, A. (2004). Error biases in spoken word planning and monitoring by aphasic and non-aphasic speakers: Comments on Rapp and Goldrick (2000). *Psychological Review, 111,* 561–572.

Samuel, A. (1996). Phoneme restoration. *Language and Cognitive Processes, 11,* 647–653.

Saussure, F. de. (1966). *Course in general linguistics.* New York, NY: McGraw-Hill. (Original work published 1916).

Savage, C., & Howell, P. (2008). Lexical priming of content and function words with children who do and do not stutter. *Journal of Communication Disorders, 41,* 459–484.

Selkirk, E. (1984). *Phonology and syntax: The relation between sound and structure.* Cambridge, MA: MIT Press.

Smith, A., & Goffman, L. (2004). Interaction of motor and language factors in the development of speech production. In B. Maassen, R. Kent, H. Peters, P. van Lieshout, & W. Hulstijn (Eds.), *Speech motor control in normal and disordered speech* (pp. 227–252). Oxford, UK: Oxford University Press.

Strenstrom, A.-B., & Svartvik, J. (1994). Imparsable speech: Repeats and other nonfluencies in spoken English. In N. Oostdijk & P. de Haan (Eds.), *Corpus-based research into language.* Amsterdam-Atlanta, GA: Rodopi.

Van Lieshout, P.H.H.M., & Namasivayam, A. K. (2010). Speech motor variability in people who stutter. In B. Maassen & P. H. H. M. Van Lieshout (Eds.), *Speech motor control: New developments in basic and applied research* (pp. 191–214). Oxford, UK: Oxford University Press.

von Bekesy, G. (1960). *Experiments in hearing.* New York, NY: McGraw Hill.

Watkins, K., Smith, S., Davis, S., & Howell, P. (2008). Structural and functional abnormalities of the motor system in developmental stuttering. *Brain, 131,* 50–59.

Watson, D., & Gibson, E. (2004). The relationship between intonational phrasing and syntactic structure in language production. *Language and Cognitive Processes, 19,* 713–755.

Wing, A. M., & Kristofferson, A. B. (1973). Response delays and the timing of discrete motor responses. *Perception & Psychophysics, 14,* 5–12.

World Health Organization. (1992). *International statistical classification of diseases and related health problems,* Tenth revision (ICD-10). Geneva, Switzerland: World Health Organization.

Yairi, E., & Ambrose, N. G. (2005). *Early childhood stuttering.* Austin, TX: PRO-ED.

23 An Approach to Differentiating Bilingualism and Language Impairment

Sharon Armon-Lotem and Joel Walters

INTRODUCTION

Bilingualism presents a weighty challenge to clinical assessment in general and to the analysis of language impairment (LI) and neurological disorders in particular. A wide range of linguistic and social phenomena converge in the bilingual person in ways that are often difficult to differentiate. Simply analyzing and comparing the two languages of a bilingual may be insufficient for determining impairment or identifying disorder (although this alone would be a major improvement of much current practice that generally addresses only a single language, often, the second language). From a research perspective, clinical disorders offer numerous challenges to the study of bilingualism, in particular: what it means theoretically to know a language, the notion of completeness in linguistic knowledge, and the relationship between a language user's two languages. From a practitioner's point of view, theory and method in bilingualism can help inform clinical decisions that may make a large difference in people's lives.

This chapter on bilingualism and neurolinguistic disorders centers on whether diagnosis is necessary in both languages or whether it is sufficient to look at a single language. The two populations we choose to look at here, children with LI and adults with schizophrenia, share the fact that impairment is manifested in both languages. A further question arises as to whether bilingualism exacerbates the linguistic manifestation of the impairment; that is, whether it makes linguistic performance worse or makes it harder to diagnose, and so forth. The two populations potentially differ in several ways: (1) age (children vs. adults); (2) the nature of the impairment (for LI children more grammatically indicated/diffuse across linguistic domains, for schizophrenia more focused on lexical/pragmatic phenomena); and (3) different manifestation due to typological differences versus similar manifestation (schizophrenia). It will be argued that it may be sufficient to diagnose and treat a single language in adult schizophrenics, but it is crucial to look at both languages in the case of developmental language impairment such as Specific Language Impairment (SLI).

Two Sets of Questions for the Study of Bilingualism and Language Impairment

At the outset, we contrast two perspectives: bilinguals with LIs or language impaired individuals who happen to be bilingual. The researcher in bilingualism is drawn to the former; the clinician–educator naturally gravitates to the latter. We are motivated here to integrate these two perspectives in an attempt toward dialogue between researchers and clinicians.

One set of questions relates to social aspects of bilingualism, in particular to social identity and attitudes. Again we ask: Are we talking about bilinguals with language disorders or language impaired individuals who happen to be bilingual? These alternative formulations of the question bring us to the heart of the difference/deviance debate. In the study of bilingualism, especially subtractive bilingualism in children (Lambert, 1990) but also the relative prestige of a bilingual's two languages, the relevant constructs include ethnolinguistic vitality, language status, and attitudes toward the second language and its speakers (e.g., Allard & Landry, 1994). In the area of language-related learning disabilities, intentions and goals are critical notions for proper assessment, along with affective factors, such as self-esteem and self-confidence.

In bilingual acquisition, Pearson (2007) reviews a variety of studies (e.g., De Houwer, 2003; Pearson, Fernandez, Lewedag, & Oller, 1997) in search of social factors to explain why approximately 25% of bilingual children from bilingual environments do NOT acquire the home/minority language. The factors examined include: input, language status, access to literacy, immigrant status, and community support. She concludes that "quantity of input has the greatest effect on whether a minority language will be learned," but that both status and attitudes also make a difference. In showing the importance of language status; that is, the difference between minority and majority languages, Pearson presents the intuitive observation: "if one does not speak a language well, one will not use it. If one reports using a language often, we can infer the person has some skill in that language." But then she goes on to show that this adage may not be true for the majority language, citing Hakuta and D'Andrea (1992) who showed language attitudes to be a better predictor of language use than proficiency in Mexican-American teenagers. Finally, in the context of community support for the minority language and the economic benefits of ethnolinguistic enclaves, Pearson states that "It is crucial to have contact with monolingual speakers of the minority language," but goes on to report that "the effect of language of instruction at school could more than counterbalance the effect of less Spanish in the home." She argues strongly for either simultaneous bilingualism or early second language acquisition both as a means to maintaining the minority language and for its presumed cognitive, social, and affective benefits (Bialystok, 2001; Bialystok & Senman, 2004; Cummins, 1976; Pearson, 2008).

Questions on social aspects of bilingualism and LI include:

a. How are both bilingualism and LI expressed in a speaker's social identity?
b. How do positive attitudes to a bilingual's native and/or second language and its speakers contribute to achievement in L2 (additive bilingualism)? How do negative attitudes to L1 and its speakers and positive attitudes to L2 and its speakers contribute to or impede achievement in L2 (subtractive bilingualism)?
c. What are some of the goals and beliefs of bilinguals with language disorders about their bilingualism and language disabilities, and how are those goals and beliefs expressed in their perceptions of self, in the way they conceive of language and communication, and in their language behavior. In particular, how do the intentions and speech acts of bilingual language disordered individuals reflect their social identities, attitudes, goals, and beliefs?

A second set of questions is an attempt to disentangle bilingualism and language impairment (LI) by identifying the relative contribution of each to language performance. In doing so, we hope to shed light on theoretical issues in bilingualism and neurolinguistics as well as on clinical practice, asking:

a. How can linguistic indicators of LI be identified in both languages in SLI/schizophrenia? More specifically, to what extent are the manifestations of LI similar/different across the two languages?
b. How can the manifestations of LI and typically developed (TD) bilingualism be differentiated given the fact that some of the same linguistic markers are characteristic of both bilingualism and LI?

The motivation for these questions is both practical and methodological. Practically, we are interested in knowing what to recommend to teachers, and clinicians regarding educational planning and programming for children or family members regarding supportive frameworks for adult schizophrenics. A second motivation comes from our research bias favoring individual analysis, personal design, and case studies and rejecting approaches that rely on large samples, group means, and comparisons of monolinguals and bilinguals. We do not expect that answers to these questions will be easy to attain, certainly not as easy as the "monolingual" solution, recommending that the child be spoken to in one language only at home or at school.

To address these questions, we ideally need demographic and ethnographic information about language use, language choice, language preferences, and language attitudes in the home, neighborhood, and school environments in *both* languages, sampling a range of topics, with a variety of listeners/interlocutors. We need to combine this information with a variety of language tasks, conducted in *both* languages, including spontaneous speech and focused probes of a range of morphosyntactic, lexical, and pragmatic stimuli, tasks, and response measures. Within this mass of data, we pay special attention to bilingual phenomena such as codeswitching, interference, and fluency and how they interact with pragmatic phenomena such as certainty and confidence, insecurity and defensiveness.

REPRESENTATION AND PROCESSING IN BILINGUALISM: A SELECTIVE REVIEW

Two theoretical constructs inform this work: representation and processing. Representations of syntactic and lexical structure may be incomplete or different for both bilingual and LI children, but are assumed to be unimpaired in schizophrenia. Processing of linguistic information, however, may differ for both groups. LI in children has been considered a result of impaired representations and/or impaired processing in terms of duration, rate, and salience, showing up as difficulties in temporal integration, word-finding, morphosyntactic substitution, syntactic permutation errors and in tasks with heavy memory demands. Schizophrenic language processing difficulties have been reported primarily in the lexical and pragmatic domains as wordsalad, an overabundance of lexical rather than anaphoric cohesion, and prevalence of exophoric reference. Developing bilinguals may show evidence of linguistic representations that differ from those of monolinguals, and may also experience difficulties in processing related to their lexical knowledge or reduced exposure to each language. Adult second language learners, however, are assumed to transfer linguistic representations from L1, especially with regard to morphology and syntax; lexical knowledge and declarative memory are said to be more involved in adult language learning than grammatical knowledge and procedural memory (Ullman & Pierpont, 2005).

Linguistic representations and processing of linguistic structures in the literature on bilingualism, especially from the laboratories of Green and Kroll, are the foundational constructs of Walters's (2005) sociopragmatic–psycholinguistic model of bilingualism. The review in this section begins with the work of Kroll and Green and then presents a brief outline of the structural and processing components of Walters's sociopragmatic psycholinguistic (SPPL) model, concluding with three issues deemed most relevant to the study of bilingualism: typological differences, codeswitching, and code interference.

FOCUS ON BILINGUAL LEXICAL REPRESENTATION

Lexical representation has been widely investigated in bilingualism, in particular to address the question of shared versus separate representational systems. Kroll's model of bilingual lexical production (Kroll & De Groot, 1997; Kroll & Tokowicz, 2005) contains different levels of representation for concepts, lemmas, and phonology. Language specific information is claimed to be available at the conceptual level in the form of language cues (cf. language tags) and at the lemma level, where language information is "distinct for words in each of the bilingual's languages" (p. 539). The phonological level consists of features shared between the two languages, activating representations from both languages. This model argues for an integrated set of lemmas to account for comprehension processes in word recognition.

Kroll and Tokowicz (2005) criticize some models of bilingualism for not distinguishing "among different levels of representation," maintaining that bilingualism does not need to be represented in the same way at each level. Their review analyzes studies of a wide range of linguistic domains (e.g., orthography, phonology, lexical semantics). Bilingual stimuli in these studies include cognates, translation equivalents, interlingual homographs, orthographic neighbors, semantically related words, concrete and abstract nouns and tasks such as word recognition, priming, lexical decision, Stroop-type picture–word production, translation, word association, and semantic ratings. In contrast to morphology and syntax, where typological differences may argue for more separate systems (Emmorey, Borinstein, Thompson, & Gollan, 2008; Meisel, 2004; Paradis & Genesee, 1997; Pyers & Emmorey, 2008), Kroll and Tokowicz (2005) amass a broad range of support on behalf of the notion that the "lexicon is integrated across languages, and that lexical access is parallel and nonselective" (p. 534).

BILINGUAL PROCESSING MODELS: KROLL AND GREEN

In terms of processing, the most prevalent constructs in bilingual research are storage and retrieval/access, activation/inhibition, and control. Of the two most influential models, Kroll's model focuses on lexical processing and Green's is more broadly scoped. The specifically bilingual aspects of these models are highlighted here.

In Kroll's Conceptual Features Model (Kroll & De Groot, 1997) *interference* is determined by similarity in features across languages and by similarity in within-language and cross-language mappings from meaning to form, with more similarity reflecting less interference. *Codeswitching* in recognition and lexical decision tasks (Grainger & Beauvillain, 1987; Li, 1996) is explained in terms of activation of both languages. *Cross-language priming* effects (e.g., Grainger & Dijkstra, 1992) are claimed to come from activation of both lemmas and lexical features, while studies that showed no evidence for cross-language priming were apparently due to activation of the lemma only. Data on codeswitching at all linguistic levels from phonotactics to discourse (e.g., Clyne, 2003; Walters, 2005) provide strong evidence for this account.

Green's Model of Inhibitory Control

Green (1998, 2000) poses the main question in bilingual processing as a problem of control under conditions of multitasking, comparing bilingual production to a Stroop task. Phrased differently: How do bilinguals avoid speaking in L1 when they want to speak in L2? Green's (1993) model proposes to account for a broad range of bilingual data, including involuntary speech errors, interference, and fluent codeswitching and for findings in picture naming tasks.

The core structural constructs in the model are lemmas and language tags. The model involves two processes, *activation* of the lemma and *retrieval* of the lexeme, with *control* specified as one of three states of activation. The processing notions in control include competition, selection, and inhibition as well as schemas and goals. The multilevel nature of control is explained as follows: "first, one level of control involves language task schemas that compete to control output; second, the locus of word selection is the lemma level ... and selection involves the use of language tags; third, control at the lemma level is inhibitory and reactive." Two conditions are involved in control: explicit intentions and language tags on both word meanings (lemmas) and word forms (lexemes). Green discusses how this works for steady-state production in a second language and for codeswitching, arguing: In L2 production, activation of both lemmas and lexemes in L2 is increased, while L1 lexemes are suppressed when phonological information is retrieved. In codeswitching, there is competition at the stage of phonological assembly, and the lexeme that "reach[es] threshold first" is the one produced.

In Green's model, an executive processor, the Supervisory Attentional System (SAS) activates language task schemas (e.g., for translation and word naming), which compete to control output. These schemas exercise control by activating and inhibiting language tags at the lemma level via functional control circuits. The "functional control circuits" regulate activation and inhibition to handle competition between language task schemas. Green illustrates this process with an example of a bilingual aphasic who was able to translate into a language he could not speak spontaneously. The functional control circuit for this phenomenon is called a translation schema (L1 = > L2), which increases activation of a word production schema (for L2) and suppresses L1. Codeswitching "costs" in studies of numeral naming (Meuter & Allport, 1999) are also explained in terms of inhibitory control. He cites experimental research on translation, codeswitching, Stroop effects, and cross-language competitive priming as further evidence for his model.

Our work differs in several ways. First, our interest in codeswitching and code interference is more restricted. We focus on morphosyntactic rules and typological differences across languages in LI in children and in lexical as well as pragmatic issues in schizophrenia. The SPPL model presented below takes a more dynamic view of bilingual representation in terms of where L1 and L2 information is specified in the model and offers a different perspective on processing.

REPRESENTATION OF SOCIOPRAGMATIC AND PSYCHOLINGUISTIC STRUCTURE

The SPPL model of bilingualism contains seven structural/information sources and a set of processing mechanisms to describe how information flows between these components during bilingual speech (Figure 23.1). Two modules (depicted vertically at the sides of the model) indicate that L1 and L2 *language choice* and *affective* information are available at every stage of language production. Interaction of the *language choice* module with the other information components provides an account for codeswitching, code interference, and fluency. The

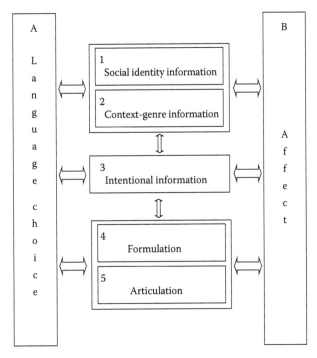

FIGURE 23.1.   A sociopragmatic–psycholinguistic (SPPL) model of bilingualism.

upper components of the model characterize sociopragmatic information, and the lower components represent psycholinguistic information. The sociopragmatic–psycholinguistic partition distinguishes impairment, which is more communicative, for example, in schizophrenia, from language disorders such as SLI.

The *language choice module* is responsible for making L1 and L2 information available to the bilingual speaker: (1) for expressing one's social identity; (2) in the choice of where to speak and in preferences for interlocutors and genres; (3) in conceiving intentions; (4) in retrieving and formulating concepts and words; and finally (5) in articulating an utterance. The language choice module selects, regulates, and retrieves information from these components and integrates them with the speaker's linguistic choices. This module has been used to account for a distinction between sociopragmatically and psycholinguistically motivated codeswitching in healthy bilingual adults (Altman, Schrauf, & Walters, under review) and in sequential bilingual children (Raichlin & Walters, 2005).

The *affective module* has an analogous framework for distinguishing sociopragmatically motivated discourse markers and those which are used to convey fluency and other discourse formulation functions. It characterizes differences between more affectively motivated slips of the tongue (of the Freudian type) and more phonetically and phonologically based tip-of-the-tongue phenomena. It is currently the source of research attempting to distinguish social from linguistic indicators of schizophrenia.

Five internal components represent information sources and stages in language production, moving from expression of social identity to articulatory output.

Social identity information, the lead component, shows that bilingualism is grounded in the social world of the speaker. Social identity is constructed when the bilingual makes new friends, switches jobs, and integrates language choices regarding accent, names, and greetings with these elements of social life. Social identity information is relevant to both LI in children and adult schizophrenia, in part due to social ostracizing and in part due to identities grounded in communication difficulties.

The *contextual/genre component* specifies setting, participants, topic and genre information in conversational interaction. It addresses the classical sociolinguistic question of "who speaks that language to whom, where, and about which topic" (Fishman, 1965). It accounts for bilingual code alternation between immigrant parents and their native-born children. The genre subcomponent distinguishes scripted language, for example, in doctor–patient exchanges, from spontaneous conversation. For both LI and schizophrenia, this component accounts for language choices, with preferences for "safe" listeners, topics, and perhaps more scripted language than spontaneous conversation.

The central component of the model is responsible for identifying *speaker intentions* and their bilingual features. It is informed by speech act theory and research on discourse markers (e.g., *well, like, ya' know*), greetings, and lexical choice, and bridges the upper sociopragmatic sources of information with lower psycholinguistic sources. A speaker's intention (to request, promise, deceive, or blame) is peppered with bilingual information, from subtle indicators of the speaker's identity latent in discourse markers or the prosodic shape of the utterance to lexical preferences influenced by psycholinguistic factors such as interference, lexical gaps, and word frequency.

The *formulator*, locus of most psycholinguistic research on bilingual processing, gets at the heart of lexical representation, or how words are stored in the mind. Monolingual models of lexical processing posit a universal, dictionary-like lemma containing syntactic and semantic information that maps into a morphophonological lexeme. In contrast, lexical formulation in the SPPL Model contains pragmatic information as well as structural features from *both* languages. Representations are highly variable, both within and across speakers. In addition to lexical information, the formulator specifies discourse patterns to handle relevance, cohesion, and sequencing of information. This discourse component is where schizophrenics have been shown to be impaired in their first language (Fine, 2006) and are assumed to be impaired in their second language as well.

The SPPL approach to formulation accounts for variability and incompleteness in a bilingual's knowledge. All bilinguals (and even monolinguals) experience lexical near-misses, which the listener perceives as malapropisms. The model attempts to characterize this variability by incorporating pragmatic and discourse information in the formulator and by making bilingual information available from the language choice module.

Finally, the bilingual *articulator,* accounts for the fact that bilinguals, even those without a trace of an accent, show evidence (sometimes only via precise acoustical measurements) of a merged system of sounds. The Spanish–English bilingual produces neither the sounds of Spanish nor the sounds of English (Caramazza, Yeni-Komshian, Zurif, & Carbone, 1973; Obler 1982). The SPPL Model and its bilingual articulator attempt to characterize this uniqueness as well as variability within and across speakers.

PROCESSING IN SPPL

Four general cognitive processing mechanisms are found in the SPPL framework: imitation, variation, integration, and control. Their generality enables an account of both sociopragmatic and psycholinguistic information. These mechanisms are supported by a set of basic processes, including: attention, discrimination, recognition, identification/recall, classification/sorting, and categorization. Imitation and variation, grounded conceptually in linguistics, are elaborated on here. Integration and control draw from Anderson's (1996) Functional Theory of Cognition and Powers's (1973, 1978) Perceptual Control Theory, respectively, and are beyond the scope of this chapter (but see Walters, 2005).

Imitation drives both sociopragmatic and psycholinguistic information. Language production begins with an innate representation that is defined by a set of structural features; that is, phonemes, morphemes, syntactic, and semantic structures. These features are selected, copied, and adapted, in order to express social, psychological, and linguistic preferences. Among the basic level processes that support this mechanism, *recognition* and *recall* are most prominent.

By way of example, the selection of names and use of greetings are among the most salient ways to project *social identity.* If schizophrenics are impaired in the social domain, their impairment could be manifested in the imitation mechanism. In contrast, language impaired children may show use of lexical imitation, for example, use of social routines or a fixed verb stem, as a strategy to compensate for limitations in morphosyntactic processing.

Imitation is also vital in generating *intentions.* A speech act selected to encode an intention is assumed to involve social identity, contextual, and genre information. It is conceived here as having been copied from a mental inventory of available intentions and integrated with an appropriate propositional content. In bilingual processing, copies of L1 speech act forms are sometimes combined with L2 propositional content (or vice versa) to yield utterances with code interference. When the Israeli speaker of English responds "Not right" in order to express mild disagreement, imitation is at work in replicating the speech act and the propositional content from each of the bilingual speaker's languages. Intentions are not expected to be impaired in either schizophrenia or SLI, but the expression of intentions in terms of speech act form and its link to propositional content should present different kinds of problems for each population.

In the *formulator,* imitation is the processing mechanism that takes the abstract information in a concept and lemma and copies or maps it onto morphophonological information to yield the lexeme. In bilingual lexical processing, information can be said to be copied from different linguistic levels and integrated to yield transfer errors; that is, forms with code interference as well as codeswitching. For example, Hebrew does not lexicalize the difference between process and result like English does in the distinction between "*study*" and "*learn*." Thus, native Hebrew speakers of English typically use the word "learn" in a context that requires use of the word "study" (e.g., "I am learning English at school.") In terms of the imitation mechanism, the speaker has selected the syntactic and semantic information from the Hebrew lemma "*lmd*" (to learn) and copied it onto the English lexeme, resulting in the word "learn." Studies of codeswitching might ignore this phenomenon, since on the surface only a single language appears in the example above. In the present context, codeswitching and code interference show evidence of the same underlying imitation process.

Variation. The approach to variation taken here builds on notions of diversity or richness of linguistic forms, strategies, and patterns from sociolinguistics, adding a psycholinguistic perspective on variation as a mechanism in language use. The claim is: richer variation will allow a speaker to generate more language, more varied language and in more contexts. When the bilingual speaker produces codeswitching or code interference, a variant is produced. The mechanism by which choices are made is variation—variation in presentation of self, in deciding who to interact with, in choosing a topic, in selecting a speech act, in accessing a lexical representation. The variation mechanism allows the speaker to select from a range of linguistic options and manipulate them to fit his/her social identity and specific intentions. The variation mechanism is grounded in the basic processes of *discrimination* and *classification*.

In both schizophrenia and SLI, processing demands in other domains (e.g., lexical selection in schizophrenics, temporal integration in SLI) may lead to impairment in the variation mechanism, which in turn may have similar or different manifestations in the two phenomena.

REPRESENTATION AND TYPOLOGICAL DIFFERENCES

Insight into abstract linguistic representations can be attained by taking advantage of contrasting typological differences between a bilingual's two languages, particularly in the areas of morphology and syntax. For example, English is morphologically "sparse" and requires an overt sentence subject, whereas Russian, Hebrew, and Spanish are relatively rich in their inflectional morphologies. Russian has a rich morphological case system; English, Hebrew, and Spanish do not. All four languages have prepositions, some which are governed by verbs (and obligatory) and others used to introduce adverbial prepositional phrases, such as locatives, temporals, and instrumentals. Syntactically, English, Russian, Hebrew, and Spanish are all SVO languages, but show different degrees of freedom in word order, with English and Spanish less flexible than Russian and Hebrew. Russian, Hebrew, and Spanish all allow null subjects, but English does not. The use of null subjects in Hebrew is more limited than its use in Spanish. On the borders of syntax, semantics, and pragmatics, English and Spanish have both definite and indefinite articles, Hebrew has only a definite article, and Russian has neither, but marks definiteness by demonstratives and changes in word order.

These typological differences lead to code interference in bilinguals. For example, Russian speakers' omission of definite articles in English and Hebrew suggests that a slot for this morpheme is missing in their underlying representation. Inappropriate insertion of definite articles in these languages may show that a speaker has acquired a representation for grammatical definiteness, but may not yet have acquired all of the semantic and pragmatic constraints on their use, as found in monolingual acquisition (Avram, 2007)

Typological differences have also been found in the clinical markers for SLI. In English, widespread use of root infinitives is a clinical marker for SLI (Rice & Wexler, 1996), whereas in Hebrew, SLI children show weakness in some aspects of the inflectional system, but this is not a diagnostic for SLI. A combination of inflectional and derivational factors seems to offer a better tool (Dromi, Leonard, Adam, & Zadunaisky-Ehrlich, 1999; Ravid, Levie, & Avivi-Ben-Zvi, 2001). In a Hebrew–English bilingual child, use of root infinitives in English and difficulties with Hebrew verb morphology could be the result of code interference between very different systems rather than indicators of LI, as is reported for learners of English with different first languages (Paradis, 2007).

The interface of bilingualism and LI requires that we distinguish processing from representation, and more specifically, differentiate cross-linguistic influence from clinical markers of SLI. Typological variation can lead to different manifestations of (impaired) linguistic representation and can be differentiated from bilingual representation by the quantity and type of errors the bilingual child produces. In general, impaired representation is expected to yield omissions, while bilingual representation is expected to yield substitutions due to shared storage. In contrast, bilingual schizophrenics should present a relatively intact morphosyntactic system in their native language and the same kind of code interference as nonimpaired bilinguals in their second language.

CODESWITCHING AND CODE INTERFERENCE

Codeswitching is motivated by sociopragmatic and psycholinguistic factors. These motivations can be distinguished in terms of intentionality and directionality. For example, a Russian immigrant to the United States might codeswitch into English to show how much she understood about her new job but would codeswitch back to Russian to describe a particular kind of existential frustration because English doesn't have a term with Soviet flavor. Similarly, an Argentinean-born ivy-league professor who feigns a nonnative accent in English in order to project her minority identity in faculty meetings, might converse in accentless, idiomatic English with her native English-speaking graduate students. Sociopragmatic codeswitching is goal-driven and motivated by identity as well as external, contextual factors. Structural-psycholinguistic codeswitching stems from individual linguistic and mental factors, in particular difficulties in finding words and lack of structural equivalence across languages, when the bilingual is confronted with word finding and fluency issues. In processing terms, codeswitching is characterized as involving the mechanisms of imitation and variation.

In early bilingual acquisition, codeswitching occurs across speakers and intrasententially. Despite 50 years of scientific research on codeswitching, folk wisdom says that it causes confusion and leads to problems in school. But, as Zentella (1997) states so strongly, the pediatrician, school official, or other "professional" makes this kind of assessment based on very limited data. The child is usually assessed in the majority language. The diversity of patterns of bilingualism and socialization in the home, in the neighborhood, and in the schoolyard are often ignored (but see Bedore & Peña, 2008).

Structural properties of codeswitching (e.g., where it occurs syntactically) alone cannot say unequivocally whether a bilingual's two languages are represented in like fashion or whether they are differentiated. Neither can structural and distributional features of codeswitching in the environment, for example, how much and where family members codeswitch, directionality from L1→L2 or L2→L1, tell the whole story about questions of representation. However, coupled with information about identity, context, genre, and intention, this structural information can offer a wider picture of the role of codeswitching in bilingualism, and as claimed here, as a diagnostic of LI. We have found directionality and psycholinguistic motivations for codeswitching to be excellent indicators of language dominance in both schizophrenics and SLI children.

Code interference is closely related to codeswitching. Three constructs are relevant here: completeness, fluency, and automaticity. Completeness is grounded in the structural or representational aspects of language. The products of one or both languages in bilinguals are incomplete because their linguistic representations are incomplete. In the lexical domain, bilingual lemmas, perhaps more so than their monolingual counterparts, are not full-scale *Oxford English Dictionary* (OED) entries. Rather, they are potentially "incomplete"—phonologically, syntactically, semantically, and pragmatically.

Fluency and automaticity are processes, reflections of incompleteness. Fluency is linguistically defined; automaticity cuts across perceptual and cognitive domains. Along these lines, dysfluency results when:

- information from the two languages has not been accurately or appropriately copied from memory (due to deficiencies in storage, search, or retrieval),
- there is underuse, overuse, inappropriate use of the imitation, and/or variation mechanisms,
- imitation and variation are out of balance; that is, when the control mechanism indicates disturbances (e.g., unstable relations between intentions and perceptions).

Dysfluency manifests itself as hesitations, pauses, false starts, repetitions, and use of discourse markers as space fillers and lexical inventions. Two additional bilingual phenomena related to code interference and fluency are *size of lexicon* and *rate of speech*. Bilinguals' vocabulary size, both children and adults, is marked by lexical gaps and size limitations, which lead to word-finding difficulties. Vocabulary size is a structural issue, and rate of speech is a processing phenomenon. Both contribute to fluency.

RESEARCH ON BILINGUAL SLI AND SCHIZOPHRENIA

Our research on bilingualism and LI in SLI and schizophrenia is marked by its wide range of linguistic indicators, including morphosyntactic features of verbs and prepositions, lexis, pragmatics, and social factors. Due to space limitations, we focus on verbal morphosyntax, prepositions, and narrative abilities in SLI and clinical as well as linguistic indicators in schizophrenia.

VERBAL MORPHOSYNTAX

For SLI, the bilingual children were all successive bilinguals, immigrant children with at least 2 years of exposure to the L2 in Hebrew-speaking preschool programs. All children were screened again, at time of study, for both languages using standardized instruments where available, for example, CELF 2 Preschool for English (Wiig, Secord, & Semel, 2004), and Goralnik Diagnostic Test for Hebrew (Goralnik, 1995). The cutoff point for atypical development (A-TD) was set at one SD below norm for the CELF and 1.5 SD below norm for the Goralnik. This screening distinguished between children who showed typical development (TD) in both languages (A-TD) in both languages, and TD in one language (English: E-TD; Hebrew: H-TD).

In one paper (Armon-Lotem, Adam, Saiege-Hadded, & Walters, 2008), we examined the use of verbal inflections by 15 English–Hebrew preschool bilinguals, ages 4–7: six typically developing (TD) bilinguals from regular preschools and nine language impaired bilinguals placed in "language preschools" following standardized speech and language pathologist (SLP) assessments. Using a case studies approach and multiple tasks (sentence completion, sentence imitation, and productions/enactment), we found similar errors for all bilinguals, with a significance difference in quantity across the different groups. In English, both TD bilinguals and E-TD bilinguals tended to use root infinitives in up to 20% of the relevant contexts. By contrast, A-TD bilinguals showed the same kind of errors in 50–60% of the relevant contexts, like monolingual children with SLI. In Hebrew, the TD bilinguals used the wrong person inflection in 16% of the contexts, which targeted verbs inflected for 1st and 2nd person. A-TD bilinguals substituted 1st and 2nd person forms like TD bilinguals, but did so in 50–60% of the relevant contexts. By contrast, E-TD children opted for the bare form, omitting person morphology altogether in 50–60% of the relevant contexts.

These findings raise the question as to whether quantitative differences are enough to diagnose LI in bilinguals. Is the high ratio of root infinitives indicative of SLI in the A-TD bilinguals? Does this mean that the E-TD group is not SLI? Is the high ratio of person substitution indicative of SLI in the A-TD group? Are the omissions of person morphology in Hebrew indicative of SLI in the E-TD group?

We propose that since the E-TD bilinguals perform like TD children in their L1, they are not SLI by definition, but rather slow second language learners, who have not mastered the inflectional system of their L2. More specifically, their errors reflect a strategy that is unlike Hebrew typical and impaired acquisition. The E-TD bilinguals had difficulties with the uninterpretable person features that are not available in their L1. These features are sensitive to critical period (White, 2003), and so the E-TD bilinguals show an error pattern that reflects the acquisition of L2 after the critical period. For the A-TD children, though tense-marking may not be a qualitative clinical indicator of SLI in bilingual populations, the quantity of errors, when manifested in both languages, is a potential indicator. That is, quantitative and qualitative differences when found in both languages can be indicative of SLI, while a qualitative difference only in the second language is not.

PREPOSITIONS

Twelve children with LI who attended special "language preschools" after being diagnosed as language impaired by an SLP and seven TD who attended regular preschools were tested. Children's ages ranged from 4.0 to 7.4, and they all came from the same bilingual neighborhood and same (middle-high) SES. Seven children were A-TD while four were E-TD, and the 12th child was H-TD. Our case study approach made it possible to start profiling the different groups.

Data were analyzed for quantity of errors, according to the following categories:

- Substitution with code interference: The baby laughed *on* the clown.
- Substitution with no code interference: The baby laughed *to* the clown.
- Omission with code interference: The elephant pulled *(down)* the zebra's pants.
- Omission with no code interference: The baby laughed *(at)* the clown

Findings showed better performance on spontaneous speech than imitation and that the children in the language preschools had more errors in English than in Hebrew, reflecting higher proficiency in Hebrew, and a tendency toward more code interference in English. Both TD and LI children had errors in prepositions due to code interference, but LI children also showed substitutions of prepositions that could not be explained by code interference. This was true for both languages, with verb governed prepositions being more problematic than locatives and temporals in English. There were very few omission errors, which were mostly restricted to the A-TD group.

Follow-up work on prepositions with 50 children shows about half of the children are dominant in one language, scoring within norms for only one of their languages. These children are not discussed here, since they are assumed either to have not yet acquired L2 or show evidence of L1 language loss. This left us with more homogeneous groups of 15 children with LI who were A-TD (six male, nine female) and 11 TD children (three male, eight female).

Findings showed evidence of code interference for both typically developing and language impaired bilingual children, as manifested by substitution errors. Different performance on restricted (verb-governed) and free prepositions (locatives and temporals) distinguished LI and TD bilinguals, with LI children performing better on free than restricted prepositions and TD children showing no difference on these two forms. Moreover, LI children's omissions were not traceable to code interference. In addition, language specific effects emerged in English, with restricted prepositions posing greater difficulty than the Hebrew prepositions in this category. Finally, sentence length influenced the proportion of bilingual errors but not LI errors. The findings contribute to the discussion of ways to generate bilingual language samples that are comparable across languages despite structural differences and further suggest a possible new indicator for SLI among bilingual children.

- Only LI children omitted prepositions where there was no code interference.
- Both TD and LI children show unsystematic substitutions that are not due to code interference, with a quantitative difference between the two groups.
- Utterance length had a different influence on the two types of prepositions and errors.

NARRATIVE AND DISCOURSE ABILITIES

Narrative and discourse abilities are elicited with multiple stimulus materials, including response to picture books, retelling of stories presented orally and via interactive role playing. In storytelling the child is first given a picture book to look through on his/her own and then asked to tell a narrative, following the pictures.

Mlodinov (2007) investigated the narratives of 11 Russian–Hebrew-speaking bilingual children, ages 6–6.9 with 1–3.5 years of exposure to L2, five of them diagnosed with language problems, and six TDs. Two narratives were elicited from each child, one in each language, using the same six black and white pictures depicting a story of "A fox and a crow" in both languages. She found that the LI children used more codeswitching and made more morphosyntactic errors than the TD children.

A cross-linguistic difference was found between the two languages, with better performance in L2/Hebrew, as indicated by the use of more connectors per proposition, and a smaller percentage of morphosyntactic errors than the Russian narratives. Moreover, TD children told longer narratives in Hebrew, and in both languages their narratives were more fluent and included more temporal markers and fewer "unclear" referents than the narratives of the LI children. Hebrew narratives also included less codeswitching and a lower percentage of unclear references than the Russian ones. On the other hand, the Russian narratives included more propositions and were more fluent than the Hebrew narratives.

Schizophrenia in Two Languages

Our approach to the relation between schizophrenia and bilingualism parallels the work in bilingual SLI. We want to identify linguistic indicators that may be unique to schizophrenia, which are not influenced by second language use. We examine clinical indicators (blocking, topic shift) and a range of linguistic markers (exophoric reference, lexical repetition, incomplete syntax, unclear reference) of schizophrenia and two bilingual discourse phenomena (codeswitching, discourse markers) in order to begin disentangling bilingualism and schizophrenia.

Recently, cognitive dysfunction has been found to correlate better with schizophrenic phenomena than traditional diagnostic criteria such as delusions, hallucinations, and flat affect (Park, Puschel, Sauter, Rentsch, & Hell, 2003; Perry et al., 2001). Cognitively schizophrenia includes executive functions and working memory. Linguistically, the illness is defined and diagnosed by disorganized speech and thought, for example, topic switching, alogia, derailment, incoherence, blocking, poverty of content of speech, thought-disorder, loose associations, incoherence, and word salad. Avolition and affective disturbance are also expressed to some extent in language, leading to social dysfunction. While current thinking in research and clinical practice labels schizophrenia a cognitive disorder, all aspects of the illness involve language behavior (Fine, 2006). Current research offers a number of explanatory proposals that shed light on the role of language in schizophrenia, among them diminished lateralization (Liddle, White, & Francis, 2007) attention and sequencing difficulties (Docherty, 2005), and impaired ability to build up context verbally and nonverbally.

In one study (Bersudsky, Fine, Gorjaltsan, Chen, & Walters, 2005) eight diagnosed Russian–Hebrew bilingual schizophrenics were matched with healthy Russian–Hebrew bilinguals for age, gender and educational level, and spontaneous speech data were collected in L2 Hebrew via sociolinguistic interviews and transcribed for analysis. One clinical measure and four linguistic measures that have shown differences between schizophrenics and different control groups (Caplan, Guthrie, Tang, Komo, & Asarnow, 2000; Goren, Fine, Manaim, & Apter, 1995; Rochester & Martin, 1979) were applied to the data.

The clinical measure, blocking (sudden inability to participate in the interview due to word or thought retrieval difficulties) successfully distinguished the two populations, only the schizophrenics showing evidence of blocking. Of the linguistic measures, incomplete syntax, lexical repetition, and unclear reference revealed virtually no differences between schizophrenics and healthy second language learners. One other measure, exophoric reference (to the physical context of the interaction), did appear more in the transcripts of the patient group, but this may have been an artifact of the interview procedure. Thus, based on clinical diagnosis (PANNS) and linguistic measures showing differences between clinical and typical populations, we concluded that our eight schizophrenics were very similar to other immigrant language learners. Next, approaching the data from a second language/bilingual perspective, we looked at three additional indicators from the areas of morphosyntax, lexis, and pragmatics/discourse.

Morphosyntax

Structures based on typological similarities and differences between Russian and Hebrew were examined. Gender agreement for nouns and adjectives, preposition use and verb tense morphology showed appropriate use in both schizophrenics and healthy immigrants. At the other end of the difficulty scale, the definite article does not exist in Russian and thus poses major difficulties due to its presence as a prefix on Hebrew nouns. It is also a highly frequent form in Hebrew. Appropriate use of definite articles in Hebrew, then, is a good indicator of the extent to which Russian native speakers have acquired Hebrew. In the present study, contexts in which the definite article was obligatory were counted and proportion of appropriate obligatory use was calculated. On the whole, schizophrenics afforded themselves fewer opportunities to use definite articles, and their error patterns (both omissions and substitutions) were very similar to those of the controls. For schizophrenics appropriate use of definite articles ranged from 13 to 82% of obligatory uses of the article (M = 58.9%); for healthy immigrants appropriate use ranged from 47 to 90% (M = 72.6%). Individual analyses revealed that four healthy immigrants performed better than the schizophrenics, but four other schizophrenics performed equal to or better than the controls.

Lexis

Type-token ratios, measures of lexical diversity were calculated for both an overall estimate of diversity and for diversity of content words. In Hebrew, a morphologically rich language, prepositions, pronouns, and determiners appear both as prefixes and suffixes attached to nouns and verbs as well as independent function words. The data for schizophrenics and healthy L2 learners differed very little, the data showing very similar mean lexical diversity (0.36 vs. 0.39, respectively) and range (0.12 vs. 0.19).

Pragmatics/Discourse

Four markers were selected to cover a range of discourse and pragmatic functions (*az* "so," *ze* "this," *em* "um," *eh* "uh"). Only one group difference emerged, schizophrenics producing almost twice as many fluency markers (*eh*) as healthy immigrants. Moreover, a very large proportion of these forms came during blocking, the clinical indicator of schizophrenia. The picture that emerges, then, from these discourse and pragmatic data continues to show that immigrant schizophrenics use language very much like their healthy counterparts.

For the bilingual measure examined (codeswitching), there were again no differences between schizophrenics and healthy language learners, and only six participants (three in each group) codeswitched at all. The very limited use of codeswitching during the interviews attests to the fact that even schizophrenics were well aware of the social norms of the interview situation (despite the fact that they knew the interviewer to be bilingual in Russian and Hebrew). Finally, both groups presented the same range of language learner phenomena, including interference/translation strategies, use of routine phrases, and self-monitoring.

A second study was aimed to avoid the inherent variability in comparing small numbers of patients with healthy subjects and take advantage of bilingualism as an opportunity to implement a within-subject design.

From a pool of 60 patients diagnosed clinically (PANNS evaluation), 12 (10 males and 2 females) ranging in age from 25 to 59 (M = 33.8), who met the following criteria were identified: (1) clear signs of thought disorder in their schizophrenic diagnosis; (2) homogeneity in terms of age, age at the time of immigration, length of residence in Israel; and (3) age at the onset/diagnosis of illness. These patients participated in two sessions, one in their preferred language (Russian) and the other in Hebrew/L2, with a bilingual interviewer.

A range of clinical and linguistic indicators of schizophrenia and two bilingual discourse phenomena were examined. These included: blocking, topic shifting, exophoric reference, lexical repetition, unclear reference, and incomplete syntax. Exophoric reference (percentage of phoric nominal groups) was the only indicator to show within-subject cross-linguistic differences, and even then only four of the patients accounted for the higher level of exophora in Hebrew. The bilingual discourse measures on the other hand, revealed three times as much codeswitching from Russian to Hebrew and six times as many discourse markers in Russian than in Hebrew. The codeswitching is indicative of greater salience of Hebrew in the hospital environment where the study was conducted as well as higher frequency of Hebrew lexis, especially for nouns, where most CS occurs. The finding for DMs belies the fact that patients preferred Russian and the experimenter who conducted both Russian and Hebrew interview sessions reported better Russian than Hebrew. It may, however, hint at an impairment in social skills grounded in language. More detailed analyses are needed to clarify this speculation.

To conclude, the disorder in schizophrenia cuts across the two languages. This finding is important for assessment. The characteristics of language that lead to the diagnosis of schizophrenia are roughly equal in both languages of these fairly adept bilingual speakers, even though they learned their second language as adults. However, there were patients (different for each of the indicators) who showed more markers of schizophrenia in L2. One possible explanation for this additive effect of bilingualism and schizophrenia is that short-term memory and monitoring of language output may be under particular stress with the double burden of schizophrenia and communicating in a second language. On the other hand, (1) the more low level task of processing syntax was similar in the two language, and (2) fluency markers and the social awareness of interacting in a conversation were even elevated in the second language; speakers used their second language to achieve fluency by code-switching, and they used discourse markers in their first language to create rapport with the interviewer in the first language that was in fact the minority language in the culture. Docherty et al. (2006) point out that schizophrenia language problems are not unitary but rather there are many ways that the speech may be unclear (see Fine, 2006, for extensive detail). Thus the discovery of a subgroup of speakers who show relatively greater difficulty in the second language is not surprising. These speakers have relatively greater difficulty in using a second language in the context of the cognitive and social difficulties underlying the schizophrenia.

RESEARCH AND ASSESSMENT STRATEGY

The methodological approach we use is based on large amounts of data, collected with a variety of tasks and procedures from relatively small numbers of subjects from bilingual backgrounds, matched with typically developing bilinguals for age and language for children and for education and occupation for adults. In order to deal with the heterogeneity of bilingualism and neurolinguistic disorders, we conduct within-subject, cross-language case studies of a range of linguistic phenomena. Data analyses proceed in stages, focusing first on the individual subject, with comparisons across languages, linguistic markers, and tasks; next on comparisons of bilingual impaired subjects matched linguistically and chronologically with unimpaired bilingual subjects, and finally on group comparisons, across languages, linguistic features, and tasks.

Three general principles guide this approach. One essential requirement is to assess and collect data in *both languages*. This practice follows the principle that LI in children and psychiatric disorders in adults should be manifested in both languages of a bilingual. Second, since a bilingual is more than a sum of her two languages, assessing one language can be highly misleading, especially if the assessment is done in the less dominant language. Thus, the individual is the primary unit of analysis, and group data are examined only after labor-intensive analyses of individual cases (see Guendouzi, 2003, on the importance of individual analysis). A third principle is that assessment measures should not be literal translations of words and structures; rather they need to be developed and constructed by taking into account the typological differences and similarities manifested in the two languages.

Beyond these general guidelines, methodological choices in studies of bilingual language acquisition and use involve several sampling decisions. These choices include:

1. the specific linguistic structures to investigate,
2. the tasks and response measures needed to elicit those structures,
3. which bilingual speakers to choose to examine.

The question of which linguistic structures to examine poses a problem of whether to aim for depth or breadth. Linguistic studies tend to aim for depth in their quest for answers to focused research questions (e.g., Genesee, 2001, for bilingualism; Rice & Wexler, 1996, for SLI), while clinical, psychoeducational studies, and standardized measures of language seek breadth (e.g., Stuart-Smith & Martin, 1999) and tend to use standardized measures. Tasks and response measures are crucial to creative research and offer the most potential for breakthroughs in treatment of communication disorders (cf. melodic intonation therapy in aphasia). Once relevant structures and functions in the two languages have been selected, tasks and response measures can be derived from the theoretical constructs. Nevertheless, the problem of comparing impaired bilinguals and "typically developing bilinguals" still remains the problem that introduces the largest source of variance to the study. The unpredictability in these sources of variance and the inherent confounding in designing studies that can keep track of all of them favor a "bilingual" approach based on large amounts of data, gathered in both languages, from relatively small numbers of bilinguals, each individual offering a relatively self-contained basis for analysis and interpretation. In the terminology of design and statistics, each subject in effect serves as his or her own control. Thus, bilingualism offers a unique opportunity to avoid the pitfalls of group comparisons and between-subject designs that are inevitably victims of the kind of heterogeneity discussed above with regard to defining bilingualism. The remainder of this section outlines the choices we make in terms of: identification of participants, selection of stimuli, tasks and procedures, and data analyses.

SUBJECT SELECTION

For the study of bilingual SLI, we focus on children ages 4–7 with bilingual backgrounds in English–Hebrew and Russian–Hebrew, conducting cross-linguistic, intrasubject comparisons on a case by case basis. Within-subject comparisons reduce the impact of the sociocultural differences. We choose children from similar SES and from L2 (Hebrew-speaking) preschools with a majority of native speakers of the target language. We select subjects from among LI children rather than from among bilinguals, since LI children represent a clinically referred population, whereas bilinguals are not, and there is less consensus about defining criteria for bilinguals. Given the heterogeneity in the bilingual population, we have limited our work to early successive bilinguals, where the child is exposed to one language at home and another in preschool prior to the age of three; that is, early L2 acquirers. We include only early bilinguals who are able to carry on a conversation in both languages and whose two languages are balanced for a range of linguistic measures (e.g., MLU), excluding late bilinguals who began acquiring L2 after the age of three. Finally, all participants are cognitively, emotionally, and neurologically unimpaired but show primary language disorder, being at least 1–1.5 SD (depending on the specifics of the standardized measure and conventional practice in using it) behind typically developing bilinguals for both languages. In addition to placement in special "language preschools," all subjects are tested on standardized measures in both languages where available. Where a standardized measure does not exist (e.g., Russian), we have developed two screening measures: an age appropriate sentence imitation task and a nonword repetition task, designed in both languages to reflect the contrastive structures of the two languages. These were supplemented by parental input on L1 proficiency and concerns.

For schizophrenia, we identify patients from a hospital environment, choosing subjects from a larger outpatient pool who have been evaluated with standardized instruments (PANNS) and clinical interviews, focusing on language-based indicators: disorganized speech, derailment, or alogia. Language proficiency in both languages is evaluated by bilingual research assistants in three domains: lexis, grammar, and fluency.

STIMULUS SELECTION BASED ON CONTRAST ACROSS LANGUAGES

Typological differences and similarities serve as the theoretical basis for development of stimuli. Target structures include those which are similar in both languages and those which are contrastive, allowing investigation of transfer as well as code interference. For example, in the area of verbal morphosyntax we targeted present and past tense morphemes in English, tense, number, gender, and conjugation (pattern) morphology in Hebrew, and tense and aspect in Russian. For prepositions, we distinguish "restricted" prepositions lexically or grammatically selected by the verb from "free" prepositions that introduce adverbial (locative/temporal) preposition phrases with parallel and contrastive stimuli across language pairs.

Due to the exploratory nature of research on schizophrenic language and findings of largely intact grammatical systems in the second language, our research has relied primarily on naturalistic data collection, including sociolinguistic interviews and narrative recall. Planned studies will investigate lexical and pragmatic deficits along the same lines described here for bilingual SLI children.

TASKS AND PROCEDURES

Each subject is tested with a wide range of tasks. In addition to the studies presented above, we have used:

1. Guided play with a uniform set of toys in two settings: kitchen and playground; the former represents the home environment and is expected to elicit more spontaneous speech in the home language and the latter represents the school environment and is expected to elicit more spontaneous speech in the school language.
2. Sentence imitation and sentence completion targeting cross-linguistic interference in verbal morphosyntax, prepositions, case marking, and definiteness as well as a wide range of higher syntactic structures that involve changes in word order (Porat, 2009).
3. Narrative elicitation based on familiar and unfamiliar stories, with and without picture stimuli; and bilingual retelling, where the subject retells narratives presented in different languages to three listeners, one who speaks only the native language, one who speaks only L2, and one who is bilingual (Raichlin & Walters, 2005; Walters, Iluz-Cohen, & Armon-Lotem, 2009).
4. A pragmatic-discourse task involving role playing, for example, a doctor–patient situation. In this task the context is constrained by the role relationship, allowing examination of pragmatic choices and sociolinguistic appropriateness (Andersen, 2000; Oz, Altman, Armon-Lotem, & Walters, 2009).

5. Social identity as elicited via person perception and ethnolinguistic identity procedures (Armon-Lotem, Adam, & Walters, 2008) (Armon-Lotem, Gagarina, Altman, Burstein-Feldman, Gordishevsky, Gupol, & Walters, 2008).

This range of tasks serves as the basis for bilingual profiles, allowing comparison across languages and examination of task effects both within and across languages.

DATA ANALYSES: FROM INDIVIDUAL PROFILES TO GROUP PATTERNS

Data analyses include some measures that cut across tasks (e.g., omission and substitution errors) and others that are unique to certain tasks (e.g., story grammar categories for narratives, discourse markers for spontaneous speech). With the individual subject as the primary unit of analysis, comparisons across languages, linguistic markers, and tasks are conducted only when we are sure we have homogeneous groups of subjects, be they typically developing or impaired.

Cross-Language Measures

In order to prepare linguistic data for analyses, we first identify all the obligatory contexts for a particular structure. For verbal morphology and prepositions, these are the contexts in which a particular verb form is expected to appear. For prepositions, the procedure is the same. For narrative structure, obligatory contexts are not as clear-cut, notwithstanding findings from story grammar research. Thus, we opt to transcribe the narratives, pair the subject's utterances with the picture or oral stimuli and then identify the narrative categories. Beyond each separate linguistic domain, we also examine performance across domains, for example, lexical abilities in spontaneous speech, role playing and narrative; verbal inflections and prepositions in these tasks as well as in story completion, sentence imitation and other tasks that specifically target these structures; social identity indicators such as names, pronouns, and discourse markers in actual language use as well as in reported language use.

Error analyses are particularly useful. We have looked at: (1) the quantity of errors; (2) comparisons of omissions and substitutions; (3) qualitative assessment of errors that can be traced to code interference; and (4) errors that are unique and cannot be traced to either of the child's languages.

Additional cross-language measures comparing individual performance for each individual include: (1) proficiency as indicated by standardized language tests, MLU/MPU, verb-based utterances (%V/U), subjective ratings of lexis, grammar, and fluency, pragmatic variation, nonword repetition designed to capture typological contrasts in morphophonology; (2) structure of the lexicon (e.g., content/function word distributions) and lexical diversity; and (3) fluency measures (e.g., discourse markers, pauses, repetitions).

Measures of Bilingualism

Measures include: (i) code-switching (analyses based on frequency, grammatical category, directionality, and motivations) in narrative, retelling, and role-playing tasks; and (ii) background information including age, gender, birth order, length, and amount of exposure to L1 and L2.

REFERENCES

Allard, R., & Landry, R. (1994). Subjective ethnolinguistic vitality: A comparison of two measures. *International Journal of the Sociology of Language, 108,* 117–144.

Altman, C., Schrauf, R.W., & Walters, J. (under review). *Bilingualism in autobiographical memory: Crossovers, codeswitching and functions of codeswitching.*

Andersen, E. (2000). Exploring register knowledge: The value of 'controlled improvisation.' In L. Menn & N. Ratner (eds.), *Methods for Studying Language Production.* London: Erlbaum, 225–249.

Anderson, N. H. (1996). *A functional theory of cognition.* Mahwah, NJ: Lawrence Erlbaum Associates.

Avram, I. (2007). *The Autonomous Contribution of Syntax, Semantics and Pragmatics to the Acquisition of the Hebrew Definite System and the Relation to Theory of Mind.* PhD dissertation, Bar-Ilan University.

Armon-Lotem, Sh., Gagarina, N., Altman, C., Burstein-Feldman, Zh., Gordishevsky, G., Gupol, O. & J. Walters. (2008). Language acquisition as a window to social integration among Russian language minority children in Israel. *Israel Studies in Language and Society, 1*(1), 155–177.

Bedore, L. M., & Peña, E. D. (2008). Assessment of bilingual children for identification of language impairment: Current findings and implications for practice. *International Journal of Bilingual Education & Bilingualism, 11*(1), 1–29.

Bersudsky, Y., Fine, J., Gorjaltsan, I., Chen, O., & Walters, J.(2005). Schizophrenia and second language acquisition. *Progress in Neuro-Psychopharmacology and Biological Psychiatry, 29,* 535–542.

Bialystok, E. (2001). *Bilingualism in development: Language, literacy, and cognition.* New York, NY: Cambridge University Press.

Bialystok, E., & Senman, L. (2004). Executive processes in appearance-reality tasks: The role of inhibition of attention and symbolic representation. *Child Development, 75,* 562–579.

Caplan, R., Guthrie, D., Tang, B., Komo, S., & Asarnow, R. F. (2000). Thought disorder in childhood schizophrenia: Replication and update of concept. *Journal of the American Academy of Child & Adolescent Psychiatry, 39*(6), 771–778.

Caramazza, A., Yeni-Komshian, G., Zurif, E., & Carbone, E. (1973). The acquisition of a new phonological contrast: The case of stop consonants in French-English bilinguals. *Journal of the Acoustical Society of America, 54,* 421–428.

Clyne, M. (2003). *Dynamics of immigrant language contact.* Cambridge, UK: Cambridge University Press.

Cummins, J. (1976). The influence of bilingualism on cognitive growth: A synthesis of research findings and explanatory hypotheses. *Working Papers on Bilingualism, 9,* 1–43.

De Houwer, A. (2003). Home languages spoken in officially monolingual Flanders: A survey. In K. Bochmann, P. Nelde, & W. Wolck (Eds.), *Methodology of conflict linguistics* (pp. 71–87). St. Augustin, Germany: Asgard.

Docherty, N. M. (2005). Cognitive impairments and disordered speech in schizophrenia: Thought disorder, disorganization, and communication failure perspectives. *Journal of Abnormal Psychology, 114*(2), 269–278.

Docherty, N. M., Strauss, M. E., Dinzeo, T. J., & St-Hilaire. A. (2006). The cognitive origins of specific types of schizophrenic speech disturbances. *The American Journal of Psychiatry, 163*(12), 2111–2118.

Dromi, E., Leonard, L., Adam, G., & Zadunaisky-Ehrlich, S. (1999). Verb agreement morphology in Hebrew-speaking children with specific language impairment. *Journal of Speech, Language and Hearing Research, 42,* 1414–1431.

Emmorey, K., Borinstein, H. B., Thompson, R., & Gollan, T. H. (2008). Bimodal bilingualism. *Bilingualism: Language and Cognition, 11,* 43–61.

Fine, J. (2006). *Language in psychiatry: A handbook of clinical practice.* London, UK: Equinox.

Fishman, J. A. (1965). Who speaks what language to whom and when? *La Linguistique, 2,* 67–88.

Genesee, F. (2001). Bilingual first language acquisition: Exploring the limits of the language faculty. *Annual Review of Applied Linguistics, 21,* 153–168.

Goralnik, E. (1995). *Goralnik Diagnostic Test for Hebrew. Matan,* Even Yehuda (In Hebrew).

Goren, A. R., Fine, J., Manaim, H., & Apter, A. (1995). Verbal and nonverbal expressions of central deficits in schizophrenia. *Journal of Nervous and Mental Disease, 183,* 715–719.

Grainger, J., & Dijkstra, A. (1992). On the representation and use of language information in bilinguals. In R. J. Harris (Ed.), *Cognitive processing in bilinguals* (pp. 207–220). Amsterdam, The Netherlands: Elsevier Science Publishers B.V.

Green, D. W. (1993). Towards a model of L2 comprehension and production. In R. Schreuder & B. Weltens (Eds.), *The bilingual lexicon* (pp. 249–277). Amsterdam, The Netherlands: John Benjamins.

Green, D. W. (1998). Mental control of the bilingual lexico-semantic system. *Bilingualism: Language and Cognition, 1*(2), 67–81.

Green, D. W. (2000). Concepts, experiments and mechanisms. *Bilingualism: Language and Cognition, 3*(1), 16–18.

Guendouzi, J. (2003). 'SLI', a generic category of language impairment that emerges from specific differences: A case study of two individual linguistic profiles. *Clinical Linguistics and Phonetics, 17*(2), 135–152.

Hakuta, K., & D'Andrea, D. (1992). Some properties of bilingual maintenance and loss in Mexican background high-school students. *Applied Linguistics, 13,* 72–99.

Kroll, J. F., & De Groot, A. M. B. (1997). Lexical and conceptual memory in the bilingual: Mapping form to meaning in two languages. In A. M. B. De Groot & J. F. Kroll (Eds.), *Tutorials in bilingualism: Psycholinguistic perspectives* (pp. 169–199). Mahwah, NJ: Lawrence Erlbaum Publishers.

Kroll, J. F., & Tokowicz, N. (2005). Models of bilingual processing and representation: Looking back and to the future. In J. F. Kroll & A. M. B. De Groot (Eds.), *Handbook of bilingualism: Psycholinguistic approaches* (pp. 531–554). Oxford, UK: Oxford University Press.

Lambert, W. E. (1990). Issues in foreign language and second language education. *Proceedings of the First Research Symposium on Limited English Proficient Student Issues.* Washington, DC: Office of Bilingual and Multicultural Education.

Liddle, P., White, T., & Francis, S. (2007). Diminished lateralization and focalization of cerebral function in schizophrenia. *Schizophrenia Research, 98,* 19–20.

Meisel, J. M. (2004). The bilingual child. In T. K. Bhatia & W. C. Ritchie (Eds.), *The handbook of bilingualism.* New York, NY: Blackwell.

Mlodinov, D. (2007). The production of narratives by bilingual Russian-Hebrew speaking children with and without language impairment. Ms. Bar Ilan University.

Meuter, R. F., & Allport, A. (1999). Bilingual language switching in naming: Asymmetrical costs of language selection. *Journal of Memory and Language, 40*, 25–40.

Obler, L. K. (1982). The parsimonious bilingual. In L. K. Obler & L. Menn (Eds.), *Exceptional language and linguistics*. New York, NY: Academic Press.

Oz, H., Altman, C., Armon-Lotem, Sh. & Walters, J. (2009). Social Identity, Language Proficiency, Ethnic Identity and Social Preferences of Russian-Hebrew Sequential Bilinguals. Paper presented at the International Society for Bilingualism (ISB7), Utrecht.

Paradis, J. (2007). Bilingual children with specific language impairment: Theoretical and applied issues. *Applied Psycholinguistics, 28*, 512–564.

Paradis, J., & Genesee, F. (1997). On continuity and the emergence of functional categories in bilingual first language acquisition. *Language Acquisition, 6*, 91–124.

Park, S., Puschel, J., Sauter, B. H., Rentsch, M., & Hell, D. (2003). Visual object working memory function and clinical symptoms in schizophrenia. *Schizophrenia Research, 59*(2–3), 261–268.

Pearson, B. Z. (2007). Social factors in childhood bilingualism in the United States. *Applied Psycholinguistics, 28*(3), 399–410.

Pearson, B. Z. (2008). *Raising bilingual children: A parents' guide*. New York, NY: Random House.

Pearson, B. Z., Fernandez, S., Lewedag, V., & Oller, D. K. (1997). Input factors in lexical learning of bilingual infants (ages 10 to 30 months). *Applied Psycholinguistics, 18*, 41–58.

Perry, W., Heaton, R. K., Potterat, E., Roebuck, T., Minassian, A., & Braff, D. L. (2001). Working memory in schizophrenia: Transient "online" storage versus executive functioning. *Schizophrenia Bulletin, 27*(1), 157–176.

Porat, S. (2009). The use of structures involving syntactic movement by English-Hebrew Bilingual children with Specific Language Impairment (SLI). Poster presented at the Research Conference on Bilingualism and SLI, Jerusalem, Israel, February.

Powers, W. T. (1973). *Behavior: The control of perception*. Chicago, IL: Aldine.

Powers, W. T. (1978). Quantitative analysis of purposive systems: Some spadework at the foundations of scientific psychology. *Psychology Review, 85*(5), 417–435.

Pyers, J. E., & Emmorey, K. (2008). The face of bimodal bilingualism: Grammatical markers in American Sign Language are produced when bilinguals speak to English monolinguals. *Psychological Science, 19*(6), 531–536.

Raichlin, R. & Walters, J. (2005). Codeswitching among Russian-Hebrew Bilingual Children: Psycholinguistic vs. sociopragmatic motivations. Paper presented at the International Society for Bilingualism (ISB5), Barcelona.

Ravid, D., Levie, R., & Avivi-Ben-Zvi, G. (2001). Hebrew adjectives in language-impaired and typically developing grade schoolers. In L. Verhoeven (Ed.), *Classification of developmental language disorder: Theoretical issues and clinical implications*. Mahwah, NJ: Erlbaum.

Rice, M., & Wexler, K. (1996). Toward tense as a clinical marker of specific language impairment in English-speaking children. *Journal of Speech and Hearing Research, 39*, 1239–1257.

Rochester, S., & Martin, J. (1979). *Crazy talk: A study of discourse of schizophrenic speakers*. New York, NY: Plenum.

Stuart Smith, J., & Martin, D. (1999). Developing assessment procedures for phonological awareness for use with Panjabi-English bilingual children. *International Journal of Bilingualism, 3*, 55–80.

Ullman, M. T., & Pierpont, E. I. (2005). Specific language impairment is not specific to language: The procedural deficit hypothesis. *Cortex, 41*, 399–433.

Walters, J. (2005). *Bilingualism: The sociopragmatic-psycholinguistic interface.* Mahwah, NJ: Erlbaum.

Walters, J., Iluz-Cohen, P. & Armon-Lotem, Sh. (2009). Telling Stories in Two Languages: Narratives of Bilingual Children with SLI. Paper presented at the 3rd International Symposium Communication Disorders in Multilingual Populations, Agros, Cyprus.

White, L. (2003). *Second language acquisition and universal grammar.* Cambridge, UK: Cambridge University Press.

Wiig, E. H., Secord, W. A., & Semel, E. M. (2004). *Clinical evaluation of language fundamentals: Preschool 2.* San Antonio, TX: Harcourt/Psych Corp.

Zentella, A. C. (1997). *Growing up bilingual: Puerto Rican children in New York.* Malden, MA: Blackwell.

24 Nonlinear Phonology: Clinical Applications for Kuwaiti Arabic, German, and Standard Mandarin

B. May Bernhardt, Joseph Stemberger,
Hadeel Ayyad, Angela Ullrich, and Jing Zhao

INTRODUCTION

The following chapter outlines major characteristics of nonlinear phonological theories and implications for clinical application across four languages: English, Kuwaiti Arabic, German, and Standard Mandarin. Because the first clinical applications were developed for English (e.g., Bernhardt, 1990; Bernhardt & Stemberger, 2000), the chapter first reviews nonlinear phonology and clinical applications for English. Key phonological aspects of each of the other languages are then described, with adaptations of the English analyses suggested for clinical application.

Phonological assessment and intervention have benefited from the application of phonological and psycholinguistic theories. The current approach to phonological description is constraints-based nonlinear phonology. Nonlinear phonological theories describe the hierarchical representation of phonological form from the phrase to the individual feature. Constraints-based theories focus on limitations in the output (e.g., fricatives are impossible or marginal) and what happens when a speaker attempts to produce a word that is beyond those limitations (e.g., contains a fricative). The perspective taken by the current authors (e.g., Bernhardt & Stemberger, 1998) emphasizes the grounding of constraints in the processing of words and the access of phonological elements during the learning process, where only a subset of a language's possible phonological output forms have yet been learned, and differential accuracy on different elements in the target word lead to the access of some target elements but not others.

The present chapter presents an overview of theories and clinical applications, beginning with English. Adaptations are presented for three other languages: (Kuwaiti) Arabic, German, and Mandarin. Because many readers of this volume will be more familiar with English, we draw attention to aspects of the other languages that differ substantively from English.

BACKGROUND: CONSTRAINTS-BASED NONLINEAR PHONOLOGICAL THEORIES

Nonlinear phonological theories evolved from "linear" theories in generative phonology. A basic premise of generative phonology is that phonological alternations
reflect context: for example, A → B/_C (A is pronounced as B when it precedes C
and is right next to [adjacent to] C). Linear theories can explain alternations of *surface*-adjacent elements with one-to-one relationships (i.e., at the level of articulatory
implementation). For example, in English nasal-stop sequences, the nasals take on
the place of articulation of the following surface-adjacent stop, for example, *want*
(Coronal) versus *donkey* (Dorsal). However, linear theories cannot easily account
for (a) patterns in which the relationship between the underlying representation and
surface forms is other than one-to-one, or (b) interactions of phonological elements
that are not immediately surface-adjacent. Goldsmith (1976) demonstrated that
the one-to-many association between phonological elements could be explained
by positing independent (*autosegmental*), hierarchically organized phonological
elements (his analysis focusing on tones and vowels). Clements and Keyser (1983)
further posited independent tiers (levels) for consonants and vowels. The latter
assumption clarified *surface-distant* consonant or vowel assimilations (harmonies)
such as /tʰeɪk/ → [kʰeɪk] or /beɪbi/ → [bibi]; if vowels and consonants are independent from each other, vowels are immediately adjacent on the vowel tier, and
consonants on the consonant tier, allowing vowel–vowel or consonant–consonant
interactions. The concept of nonlinear hierarchical representation was extended to
all aspects of phonological form. Figures 24.1 and 24.2 depict the various levels of
the phonological hierarchy from the phrase to the individual feature.

Figure 24.1 describes prosodic or word structure representations. At the highest level, words are grouped into rhythmic phrasal units with various levels of
prominence reflecting morphosyntax, pragmatics, and/or phonology. A phrase is
made up of prosodic words, each of which has one primary stress (level of prominence); relative prominence above the prosodic word is malleable, unpredictable,
and difficult to transcribe (for English at least). Making up the prosodic word are
the "feet," metrical groupings of syllables (the next level down in the hierarchy).
In English, feet can be composed of one syllable (a *degenerate* foot) or up to four
(wSww, as in the word *degenerate*) and are described in terms of direction of
acoustic prominence; that is, which part of the foot is stressed. The left-prominent
foot (Strong–weak, trochaic), as in *bucket*, is the most frequent foot type cross-
linguistically. This contrasts with a right-prominent (weak–Strong, iambic) foot as
in *bouquet* (borrowed with the right-prominent foot structure of French). The syllables that make up the foot also can be characterized as containing hierarchical
structure; that is, with onsets and rimes and/or timing units (Kenstowicz, 1994).
The *rime* includes the most sonorous element of the syllable (*nucleus* or *peak*) and
any postnuclear consonants (*coda*); the *onset* includes all prenuclear consonants.
For example, *black* is subdivided into the onset /bl/ and the rime /æ:k/, which is
subdivided into the nucleus /æ:/ and the coda /k/. Most nonlinear descriptions
also posit a timing tier (Hayes, 1990). The timing tier accounts for patterns in

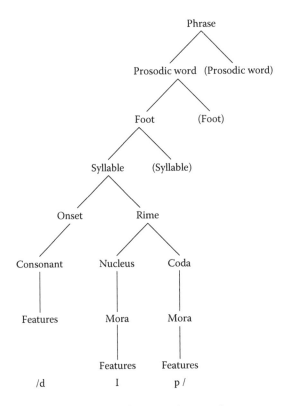

FIGURE 24.1   The prosodic hierarchy from the phrase to the mora.

which syllable duration is maintained by lengthening one element when another is deleted, usually in the rime; that is, vowel lengthening after coda deletion in *what* /wʌt/ → [wʌ:]. Special status has been accorded to timing units within the rime (*weight units* or *moras*). Weight units appear to relate to stress assignment in *quantity-sensitive* languages (Hayes, 1989, 1995). That is, short (often lax) vowels are posited to have one mora, and long vowels or diphthongs, two. In some languages (e.g., English, Arabic), coda consonants can also be moraic, especially if the vowel is short/lax; for example, the English word *what* has two moras, one for the vowel and one for the coda (/t/).

Below the timing tier are the segments (consonants and vowels), which are composed of hierarchically organized features (Figure 24.2 and Table 24.1; see also Bernhardt & Stemberger, 1998, 2000; McCarthy, 1988; Sagey, 1986).

The specific features and their assigned values vary somewhat in the literature. However, phonologists generally agree that there are three major organizing features (*nodes*); that is, *Place, Laryngeal,* and *Root (Manner)*, which dominate specific features. Manner features are directly linked through the Root node to the segmental tier. In Table 24.1 for English, the following set of manner features is assumed: [consonantal] (distinguishing true consonants and glides), [continuant]

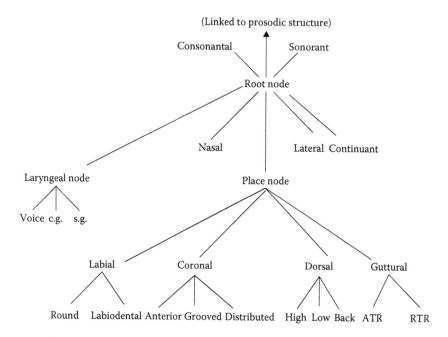

FIGURE 24.2 The feature hierarchy: Manner (Root), Laryngeal, and Place features. Note. s.g. = spread glottis, c.g. = constricted glottis; ATR = advanced tongue root, RTR = retracted tongue root. The Root node links upward to the prosodic tiers and downward to all features. The [Guttural] place node is particularly relevant for Arabic (also called [Radical] or [Pharyngeal]).

(distinguishing stops, fricatives, and affricates), [nasal] (accounting for /m/, /n/, /ŋ/), [lateral] (accounting for /l/). Laryngeal features distinguish between voiced and voiceless obstruents (stops, fricatives, and affricates) and the state of the glottis ([spread], [constricted]). In most approaches, features dominated by the Root and Laryngeal nodes are binary (+, −). The Place node dominates three single-valued features: [Labial] (pertaining to the lips), [Coronal] (pertaining to the tongue tip and blade) and [Dorsal] (pertaining to the back of the tongue). These are designated as privative ("on-off") rather than binary, because the absence of one of these features (e.g., [Labial]) does not create a similarity between different phonemes that underlies phonological patterns in human languages. Under [Labial], [labiodental] accounts for the distinction between bilabials and labiodentals, and [round] for the distinction between /w/ and the other labials. Subsidiary features of [Coronal] designate tongue position relative to the front portion of the oral cavity ([+anterior], as in /t/, or [−anterior], as in /ʃ/), tongue shape (as [+grooved], e.g., /s/, or [−grooved], e.g., /θ/, [grooved] being functionally equivalent to the acoustically based feature [strident]), and degree of contact between the tongue tip or blade and the passive articulators ([distributed]). [Dorsal] subsumes binary features of tongue body height ([high], [low]) and backness ([back]). The same place features are used for consonants (C-Place) and vowels (V-Place). Glides have more than one place feature.

TABLE 24.1
Manner, Laryngeal and Place Features of English and Corresponding Consonants

Manner Features	Consonants
[+consonantal]	p b t d k g m n ŋ f v θ ð s z ʃ ʒ tʃ dʒ l
[–consonantal]	w j ɹ h (ʔ)ᵃ
[+lateral]	l
[+nasal]	m n ŋ (ŋ syllable-final only)
[–continuant]	p b t d k g (ʔ)ᵃ m n ŋ
[+continuant] (& [–sonorant])	f v θ ð s z ʃ ʒ
[–continuant, +continuant]	tʃ dʒ

Laryngeal Features	
[+voiced] obstruents	b d g ð v z ʒ dʒ
[–voiced] obstruents	p t k f θ s ʃ tʃ
[+spread glottis]	pʰ tʰ kʰ f θ s ʃtʃ h
([+constricted glottis])ᵃ	(ʔ)

Place Features	
Labial	p b m f v (w ɹ)ᵇ
Labial [+labiodental]	f v
Coronal [+anterior]ᶜ	t d n θ ð s z l
Coronal [–anterior]ᵇ	ʃ ʒ tʃ dʒ (j ɹ)
Coronal [+grooved]	s z ʃ ʒ tʃ dʒ
Coronal [–grooved]	θ ð (t d n l)
Dorsalᵇ,ᶜ	k g ŋ (ɫ j ɹ w)
Labial & Dorsal	w
Coronal & Dorsalᶜ	j (ɫ)
Labial & Coronal & Dorsal	ɹ

Note: The table is based on the feature table in Bernhardt and Stemberger (2000, p. 168), with some changes.
Underlined features are considered adult defaults (unmarked).
ᵃ The glottal stop is included here for completeness but is not an underlying phoneme.
ᵇ The /w/, /j/ and /ɹ/ have more than one place feature.
ᶜ The /l/ is velarized in postvocalic positions.

Throughout the phonological hierarchy, a distinction is made between what is frequent/less-complex (*unmarked* or *default*) and infrequent/complex (*marked* or *nondefault*). Default word and syllable structures include simple onsets, nuclei, rimes, and feet. For consonants, the features of /t/ are generally considered defaults in most adult languages; however, children may have default features that differ from those of the ambient language (Bernhardt & Stemberger, 1998). Developmentally, the unmarked, default elements tend to appear before the marked, nondefault elements and to replace them in phonological patterns (Bernhardt & Stemberger, 1998). The general constraints for an early phonological system involve a tension between defaults and nondefaults. Early in acquisition, the inability to produce a given element (markedness constraint) often outranks the ability to produce it (survival or faithfulness constraints).

CLINICAL APPLICATION

Since 1990, there have been several studies investigating the application of nonlinear phonology to intervention for English (reported in, e.g., Bernhardt, 1990, 1992; Bernhardt, Brooke, & Major, 2003; Bernhardt & Gilbert, 1992; Bernhardt & Major, 2005; Bernhardt & Stemberger, 1998, 2008; Edwards, 1995; Major & Bernhardt, 1998; Von Bremen, 1990) Through these investigations, a clinical methodology was devised for data analysis and goal-setting, both quantitative (Masterson & Bernhardt, 2001) and qualitative (described in detail in Bernhardt & Stemberger, 2000). Elements of the phonological hierarchy are systematically evaluated in turn (in both inventory and relational analyses), beginning with syllable and word structures (word length, stress patterns, and word shapes in terms of CV sequences), and proceeding through segments (taking into account word position) and features. (Table 24.1 shows the feature-consonant correspondence for evaluation across word positions; Table 24.2 shows an example from Bernhardt & Stemberger, 2000, of key elements for word structure analysis.)

Features are examined as independent elements (e.g., all [Dorsal] consonants), in various combinations (e.g., [Dorsal]&[+voiced]) and in sequence

---

TABLE 24.2

Key Word Structures for Assessment of English Prosodic Structure in Phonological Development

Word Length	Stress Patterns			Word Shapes	
1. syllable	S			(?)V(V)	(C)V(V)CV(V)
2. syllables	Sw	Ss		(?)V(V)C	CV(V)CV(V)C
3. syllables	Sww	Sws	Ssw	CV(V)	CV(V)CCV(V)C
4. syllables	wS	wSw	swS	CV(V)C	Other
Other	Other			(C)V(V)CC	
				CCV(V)(C)	

Note: Table 2 is based on a table in Bernhardt and Stemberger (2000, p. 167) for word and syllable structure analysis.

S = strong or primary stress; s = secondary stress; w = weak or unstressed;
C = consonant, V = vowel; parentheses indicate optionality

(e.g., Labial-Dorsal). Both established elements (strengths) and unestablished elements (needs) are identified. Established elements (defaults and acquired non-defaults) are often incorporated into intervention as a foundation from which to address the needs (the negatively constrained, marked nondefaults), particularly for children with needs outside the phonological system (social, linguistic, familial, developmental). Thus, taking a constraint-based view of phonological intervention, the general objective is to promote the nondefaults and help the child overcome the overuse of defaults, at all levels of the phonological hierarchy.

Until recently, most clinical applications of nonlinear phonology have focused on English and readers are directed to, for example, Bernhardt and Stemberger (2000) for detailed descriptions. However, a project is underway that is investigating phonological acquisition and impairment from a constraint-based nonlinear perspective for other languages. For three of these, German (Ullrich & Bernhardt, 2005), Kuwaiti Arabic (Ayyad & Bernhardt, 2008; Ayyad, Bernhardt, & Stemberger, 2006), and Mandarin, elicitation word lists and analysis methods have been worked out. We present an introduction to nonlinear phonological analysis for these languages as a foundation for other languages.

(KUWAITI) ARABIC

Arabic is an Afro-Asiatic Semitic language spoken by over 150 million people. Modern Standard Arabic (MSA) is derived from (but not identical to) Classical Arabic of the Qur'an, and is used in educational contexts and the media. However, in descriptions of Arabic, the issue of diglossia is prominent (e.g., Amayreh & Dyson, 1998). Diglossia refers to the differences between colloquial spoken Arabic of the various regions (with over 30 dialects) and "standard" Arabic (either Classical or MSA). Pronunciation differences affect, for example, the uvular stop {q} of MSA, which has variable realizations, for example, /g/ or emphatic /gˤ/ (Kuwait, Jordan), /dʒ/ or even /j/ (Kuwait).* Further, in Cairene Arabic, /s/, /z/, and /zˤ/ are used in place of MSA /θ/, /ð/, and /ðˤ/ (Amayreh & Dyson, 2000). Vowels differ, too, across regions. The root of the word "salt" in MSA is /mlħ/, pronounced as /mɪlħ/ in Kuwaiti Arabic, and as /malħ/ in Egypt and parts of Jordan. Lexical differences are also noted. For example, "sock" is [əð̣ˈlaʁ] in Kuwaiti Arabic, but /ʃʌrab/ in Saudi Arabia and Egypt, and /dʒraːb/ in Jordan, Syria, and Palestine. (Syntactic differences are beyond the scope this chapter.)

SYLLABLE AND WORD STRUCTURES OF KUWAITI ARABIC

Kuwaiti Arabic has the following syllable shapes:

1. CV: a light syllable, as in the prefix /tə/ (feminine present singular)
2. CVC: a heavy syllable, as in /sˤədʒ/ ("true")

---

* The emphatics are represented with a pharyngeal superscript. However, they may be more uvularized than pharyngealized in some dialects. Note that we use {} for MSA, // for the adult colloquial dialect phonemes, and [] for narrow pronunciation.

3. CVV: a heavy syllable as in /li:/ ("mine"; Kuwaiti Arabic)
4. CVCC: a super-heavy syllable, as in /bərd/ ("cold outside"). There are a variety of word-final clusters, some of which come from morphologically derived forms, for example, /nt/ as in /bɪnt/ ("girl"), /ht/, as in /taht/ ("under"), [mʃ] as in [ʔɛmʃ] ("Walk" [imperative]) and [bt] as in [jɪb̥t] ("I brought").
5. CVVC: a super-heavy syllable, as in /leiʃ/ ("why"; Kuwaiti Arabic)

Omar (1991) also suggests that CVVCC can exist in some Arabic dialects but this is disputed by Anis (1961) and Hassan (1950). Hassan (1950) also includes VC (for the definite article /al/).

Kuwaiti Arabic has medial consonant sequences (primarily heterosyllabic), but in addition, there are a variety of syllable- and word-initial two-element clusters as a result of morphological alternation, for example, [hn] in [hnud] (plural of /hɪnd/ "man from India"); [χj] in [χjut̥] (plural of /χejt̥/ "thread"); or [b̥ʃ] in [b̥ʃut] (plural of /bɪʃt/ "man's robe").

Words in Kuwaiti Arabic are typically one to three syllables in length, but can be up to at least five syllables long (especially in words of foreign origin). A foot is typically composed of one or two syllables (with an extra unstressed syllable possible in word-final position or involving affixes and clitics). Stress in Kuwaiti Arabic is predictable and reflects the following general principles:

1. Generally, epenthetic schwa is not stressed.
2. Primary stress is on the final syllable of a word if that syllable is super-heavy; that is, either CVVC or CVCC; for example, /nas.tə.ˈʕe:n/ ("seek for help") and /jes.tə.ˈquir:/ ("to settle").
3. If the final syllable is not super-heavy, primary stress falls on the penultimate syllable if that syllable is heavy (CVC, CVV). For example, /ʔəs.ˈtəj.ham/ ("to enquire") and /ju.ˈna:di:/ ("calling") do not have a super-heavy final syllable, but do have a heavy penultimate syllable (CVC and CVV, respectively), which is therefore stressed.
4. Primary stress falls on the third syllable from the last (antepenultimate) if the penultimate is short, and the final syllable is not super-heavy, for example, /ˈʕəl.lə.mɛk/ ("teach you").

No data are currently available regarding word structure development for monolingual Kuwaiti Arabic-learning children. However, a Kuwaiti Arabic–English bilingual child (Ayyad et al., 2006), aged 2.4, produced words of up to four syllables, showing mastery of stress patterns such as (s)wSw and Swsw. Word shapes for the child included codas, vowel length distinctions, medial geminates and sequences, and word-initial clusters (no word-final cluster targets were in the target words elicited). Dyson and Amayreh (2000), although focusing primarily on segmental acquisition in Jordanian Arabic, observed low percentages of syllable deletion, coda deletion, and sequence simplification in their sample of

2- to 4-year-old children (less than 5–10% of such patterns by age 4). Thus, structurally complex words can occur fairly early in Arabic development, with simplification patterns resembling those for other languages. Much more information is needed on this topic, however.

SEGMENTS AND FEATURES OF KUWAITI ARABIC

The Kuwaiti Arabic segmental inventory is similar to that of other spoken dialects of Arabic and MSA, with differences noted earlier and described further below.

Vowels

Like MSA, the Kuwaiti Arabic vowel system has the three cardinal vowels (short and long variants): /i(:)/, /a(:)/, /u(:)/, and the diphthongs /aj/ and /aw/. However, other vowels are also used, for example, [oː], as a variant of /aw/,* the diphthong /ej/ and the epenthetic schwa (used to break up consonant sequences, and after a prepausal word-final geminate). Vowels may show contextual effects, for example, lowering in the context of uvulars, pharyngeals or glottals, and fronting in the context of front consonants, giving phonetic variants such as [ɛ], [ɨ], [æ], or [ʌ]. Detailed information is not available on vowel development in Arabic, but vowel length would appear to be an important parameter for development, as would the contextual influences on vowels (lowering, fronting).

Consonants

Consonants in Kuwaiti Arabic are produced across the vocal tract from the lips to the glottis, and include uvulars, pharyngeals, glottals, and "emphatics." Emphatics are consonants with a secondary uvular or pharyngeal articulation, which results from retraction of the tongue dorsum (and/or root) toward the back wall of the pharynx.† Table 24.3 shows the correspondences between features and consonants of Kuwaiti Arabic (using the format of Table 24.1 for English.)

Manner features for Kuwaiti Arabic are as follows:

1. [+consonantal]: all but the [−consonantal] glides /w/, /j/, glottals /h/, and phonemic /ʔ/
2. [+nasal]: /m/, /n/, and the allophone [ŋ] (produced before velar stops only)
3. [−continuant]: stops /b/, /t/, /d/, /k/, /g/, /ʔ/ (and for some speakers using MSA, [q]), the nasals and the "emphatics" /tˤ/, /dˤ/, /gˤ/. (The lack

---

* In Cairene Arabic, according to Watson (2002), /o/ has replaced /aw/ more pervasively than in Kuwaiti Arabic.
† Bin-Muqbil (2006) claims that the secondary articulation of emphatics is [Dorsal] rather than pharyngeal, thereby distinguishing emphatics from the uvulars, pharyngeals, and glottals. He suggests that uvulars have a [Dorsal] secondary articulation, and a primary pharyngeal articulation (like the other gutturals). The /q/, however, acts similarly to the emphatics and is thus designated as primarily [Dorsal]. Bin-Muqbil's data were from MSA-speaking male adults from Saudi Arabia (Riyadh dialect), and it is not known whether the same is true for Kuwaiti Arabic.

TABLE 24.3

Manner, Laryngeal and Place Features of Kuwaiti Arabic and Corresponding Consonants

Manner Features	Consonants
[+consonantal]	b t(ˤ) d(ˤ) k g(ˤ) m n [ŋ] {q}ᵃ f θ ð(ˤ) s(ˤ) z ʃ tʃ dʒ χ ʁ ħ ʕ l(ˤ) r
[−consonantal]	w j ʔ h
[+lateral]	l
[+nasal]	m n [ŋ] (ŋ syllable-final before /k/)
[−continuant]	b t d k g {q}ᵃ ʔ m n [ŋ]
[+continuant] (& [−sonorant])ᵇ	f θ ð(ˤ) s(ˤ) z ʃ χ ʁ ħ ʕ
[−continuant, +continuant]	tʃ dʒ

Laryngeal Features	
[+voiced] obstruents	b d(ˤ) g(ˤ) ð(ˤ) z dʒ ʁ ʕ
[−voiced] obstruents	t(ˤ) k f θ s(ˤ) ʃ tʃ χ ħ
[+spread glottis]	t(ˤ)ʰ kʰ f θ s(ˤ) ʃ tʃ χ ħ h
[+constricted glottis]	ʔ

Place Features	
Labial	b m f w
Labial [+labiodental]	f
Coronal [+anterior]	t(ˤ) d(ˤ) n θ ð(ˤ) s(ˤ) z l(ˤ) r
Coronal [−anterior]	ʃ tʃ dʒ f
Coronal [+grooved]	s(ˤ) z ʃ tʃ dʒ
Coronal [−grooved]	θ ð(ˤ) (t(ˤ) d(ˤ) n l(ˤ) r)
Dorsalᶜ	k g {q}ᵃ [ŋ] (j w)
Guttural (Radical, Pharyngeal)ᶜ	χ ʁ ħ ʕ ʔ h (tˤ dˤ g ðˤ sˤ lˤ)ᶜ
Labial & Dorsal	w
Coronal & Dorsal	j

Note: Underlined features are considered adult defaults (unmarked).

ᵃ The {q} is from Modern Standard Arabic and is sometimes used in colloquial Kuwaiti Arabic. It may or may not pattern with the other [Guttural] consonants.

ᵇ The pharyngeal fricatives have minimal turbulence and may be alternatively designated as approximants ([+continuant]&[+sonorant]).

ᶜ The features of the emphatic consonants are as yet unstudied for Kuwaiti Arabic. They may have a secondary [Dorsal], [−low] (uvular) articulation or a secondary [Guttural] articulation.

of */p/ plus use of emphatics and phonemic/contrastive /ʔ/ distinguish Arabic from English.)

4. [+continuant](&[−sonorant]) fricatives and [−continuant]–[+continuant] affricates: Fricatives are produced across the vocal tract. The pharyngeal pair (/ʕ/ and /ħ/) are sometimes considered approximants

([+continuant]&[+sonorant]) in MSA rather than fricatives because of lack of turbulence (Bin-Muqbil, 2006). Affricates include palatoalveolars /tʃ/ and /dʒ/, as in English.

Laryngeal features comprise both values [voiced] for obstruents (including contrasts among emphatics, but not */p/ or */v/). As in English, voiceless fricatives, affricates and /h/ are [+spread glottis], but the voiceless stops appear to vary in use of aspiration (i.e., [+spread glottis] or [–spread glottis]). Glottal stop is phonemic (contrastive) in Arabic ([+constricted glottis]).

Kuwaiti Arabic [Labial], [Coronal], and [Dorsal] place features resemble English in their correspondences, with some exceptions: (1) [Labial] does not include */p/ or */v/; (2) [Coronal] includes emphatic /tˤ/, /dˤ/, /ðˤ/, /sˤ/, and /lˤ/; and (3) [Dorsal] includes emphatic /gˤ/ and uvulars ([–high], [–low]) /χ ʁ/ and ([q]). In some words and contexts, /l/ can also have a [Dorsal] or [Guttural] secondary articulation. Here we follow McCarthy (1994) and Watson (2002) by including [Guttural] (also called [Radical] or [Pharyngeal]); this feature includes the uvulars /χ ʁ/, the pharyngeals /ħ ʕ/, and the glottals /h ʔ/. The emphatics are considered to have a secondary uvularized ([Dorsal]) or pharyngealized ([Guttural]) feature (footnote c). Bin-Muqbil (2006) also suggests that [q] is not designated as [Guttural] because it acts more like an emphatic. Whether the glottals actually have a pharyngeal constriction (thus being [Guttural] as opposed to placeless) is unknown for Kuwaiti Arabic.

Although no data exist for Kuwaiti Arabic monolingual development, preliminary data are available for two Arabic–English bilingual brothers (between ages 2.4 and 2.10 and 4.9 and 5.2, respectively). Both showed production of all manner, laryngeal and place features across the consonantal inventory of Arabic. The latest developing consonants were the uvular stop [q] and the interdentals, acquired by 5.2 for the older brother and by 2.10 for the younger brother (who had more exposure to MSA through a babysitter). Gutturals and [q] were produced by the younger brother by age 2.4, although emphatics were inconsistent by 2.10; at that age, he also showed inconsistent production of /r/ and sibilants (with place inconsistency between alveolars and postalveolars for sibilants). For other dialects of Arabic, reports indicate later acquisition of gutturals, emphatics, interdentals, and /dʒ/ (up to age 8), for example, Amayreh (2003) and Ammar and Morsi (2006). The later acquisition of interdentals, exact sibilant place, secondary articulation, and /r/ matches development for other languages. It appears that gutturals can be learned before age 3, however.

NONLINEAR PHONOLOGY AND ASSESSMENT OF (KUWAITI) ARABIC-SPEAKING CHILDREN

No matter what Arabic dialect a client speaks, evaluation needs to take into account the extent to which the client has been exposed to MSA, diglossia being a prevalent aspect of Arabic usage. A tool for nonlinear phonological assessment of Kuwaiti Arabic is under development, which includes a word list for elicitation (Ayyad et al., 2006). Word structure analysis necessarily will include a focus on: (a) syllable types (as in English, i.e., light, heavy, super-heavy) and their relation to stress; (b) medial consonants (geminates, and more extensive sequences than for English); (c) vowel length distinctions (more extensive than for English); and (d) morphological alternations that create syllable-initial clusters or geminates (unlike English). The feature inventory in Table 24.3 can serve as a basis for both independent and relational analysis (with the addition of word position and sequence evaluations). Particular attention is needed for place of articulation, especially gutturals, emphatics, and later-developing fricatives. For vowels, the dialect variants beyond the three cardinal vowels of Standard Arabic are a necessary part of elicitation and evaluation, as are potential contextual effects of consonants on vowel production. Although the current development of a nonlinear phonological assessment tool is for the Kuwaiti dialect, findings and methodologies will have implications for other dialects of Arabic because of commonalities across dialects. The rich consonant inventory (including gemination) and morphonological alternations create specific challenges for phonological development and will make an interesting basis for comparison with other languages with and without such features as more data are collected, from children with typical or protracted phonological development.

GERMAN

German is a West Germanic Indo-European language spoken by approximately 123 million people in 15 countries. In Germany, Austria, parts of Switzerland, Liechtenstein, and Luxembourg, German is the official state language (Fox, 2007). Standard German (Hochdeutsch or "High German") derives from a north German variant. This section of the chapter provides an overview of Standard German phonology and highlights key parameters for nonlinear phonological assessment, referring to the assessment tool Nichtlineare Phonologische Diagnostik (NILPOD, Ullrich 2008 = Nonlinear phonological assessment).

PROSODIC STRUCTURE

German is similar to English in terms of prosodic structure (see Table 24.4). German words can be composed of one to eight (or more) syllables, with longer words including many compounds. The trochaic (stressed–unstressed) stress pattern is most frequent as in /ˈʔan.ʁuj/ (Anruf, "phone call") or /ˈlam.pə/ (Lampe, "lamp"), but words can also begin with an unstressed syllable (especially in words of foreign origin or containing a prefix), for example, /piˈʁaːt/ (Pirat, "pirate") or /baˈnaː.nə/ (Banane, "banana").

Frequent word shapes in terms of C and V sequences include CVV (/ʃuː/, Schuh, "shoe") and CVC (/ɡɪb/, gib, "give!"). Unstressed syllables can be monomoraic (a short vowel and no coda). Stressed syllables (at least in monosyllabic words) are considered to be minimally bimoraic; that is, containing a short lax vowel plus

TABLE 24.4
Basic Word Shapes in German

Word Length	Parameter	Word Shapes	Examples
1 syllable	Simple onset, no coda	CVV	/diː/ *die* 'the'
	Simple onset and coda	CV(V)C	/ˈfɪʃ/ *Fisch* 'fish'
			/ˈbaɪn/ *Bein* 'leg'
	Cluster word-initial, optional coda(s)	$C_{2\text{-}3}V(V)C_{0\text{-}4}$	/ˈglaːs/ *Glas* 'glass'
			/ˈʃtaʊp/ *Staub* 'dust'
	Cluster word-final, optional onset #	$C_{1\text{-}3}V(V)C_{2\text{-}4}$	/ˈzaft/ *Saft* 'juice'
			/ˈdɛŋkst/
			denkst 'think' (2sg)
2 syllables	Simple onsets, no coda	CV(V).CV(V)	/ˈkʰyçə/
			Küche 'kitchen'
	Simple onsets, simple word-final coda	CV(V).CV(V)C	/pʰiˈʁaːt/
			Pirat 'pirate'
			/ˈbɪliç/
			billig 'cheap'
	Cluster word-initial, optional coda #	$C_{2\text{-}3}V(V)C_{0\text{-}3}.CV(V)$ $C_{0\text{-}3}$	/ˈʃtaiɡn̩/ *steigen* 'climb'
	Cluster medial,[a] optional coda, onset #	$C_{1\text{-}3}V(V). \, C_{2\text{-}3}V(V)C_{0\text{-}3}$	/ɡəˈʃpɛnst/ *Gespenst* 'ghost'
	Cluster word-final, optional onset #	$C_{1\text{-}3}V(V).C_{1\text{-}3}V(V)C_{2\text{-}4}$	/ɡəˈʃpɛnst/ *Gespenst* 'ghost'
3 or more syllables	Simple onsets, no codas	CV(V).CV(V). CV(V)....	/ˌmɐ.məˈlaː.də/ *Marmelade* 'jam'
	Simple onsets, coda	CV(V).CV(V)..... CV(V)C	/ˈtsaʊ.bɛh.kʰaɪt/ *Zauberkeit* 'magic'
	Cluster word-initial, optional coda #	$C_{2\text{-}3}.V(V)C_{0\text{-}3}.CV(V).$ $C_{0\text{-}3}...$	/ˈʃtʁʊmpf.ˌhoːzə/ *Strumpfhose* 'tights'
	Cluster medial, optional coda, onset #	$C_{1\text{-}3}V(V)C_{2\text{-}4}V(V)$ $C_{2\text{-}4}V(V) ...$	/ˈtʰa.ʃn̩.ˌlam.pə/ *Taschenlampe* 'flashlight'
	Cluster word-final, optional onset #	$C_{1\text{-}3}V(V).C_{1\text{-}3}V.$ $C_{1\text{-}3}V...C_{2\text{-}4}$	/(ʔ)e.le.ˈfant/ *Elefant* 'elephant'

Note: Parentheses indicate optionality. Subscripts indicate potential numbers of consonants.

coda (/bɛt/ Bett "bed"), or a long tense vowel or diphthong (/ʃɔɪ/ scheu "shy"; Féry, 1995). Furthermore, stressed syllables are considered by some linguists (e.g., Wiese, 1996) to be maximally trimoraic; that is, containing a long vowel or diphthong plus a coda (e.g., /maɪn/, *mein*, "my"), or a short vowel plus a syllable-final cluster (e.g., /hʊnt/, *Hund*, "dog"). Wiese (1996) designates any additional syllable-final consonants as an appendix. (If the extra cluster consonants are coronal obstruents, up to four consonants can appear in the rime, e.g., /dɛŋkst/, *denkst*, "think [2sg].") Some accounts (e.g., Wiese, 1996) controversially treat intervocalic consonants after lax vowels as ambisyllabic, for example, the medial /n/ in /ʃpɪnə/ (*Spinne*, "spider"). The majority of syllables contain an onset, and apparently vowel-initial stressed syllables begin with a glottal stop, even word medially, unlike in English (e.g., Lleó & Vogel, 2004; e.g., /tsaːn.ʔaːtst/, *Zahnarzt*, "dentist"). Word initial consonant sequences are also frequent; there are 22 two-element clusters and two common three-element consonant clusters (/ʃpʁ/, /ʃtʁ/) with additional uncommon three-element clusters that mainly appear in words of foreign origin, for example, /skl/, /spl/, /ʃpl/, /skʁ/). Word medially and finally, many consonant sequences occur because of compounding (which results in many heterosyllabic word-medial sequences) and affixation.

In terms of acquisition, codas can appear relatively early in typically developing German-speaking children (Kehoe & Lleó, 2003b, 2003c); consonant clusters and iambic stress patterns tend to occur later, as in English. Children with phonological impairment tend to show difficulty with complex structures such as clusters, iambic stress patterns, and codas, similar to English-learning children (Fox & Dodd, 2001). The extent of the similarities between the two Germanic languages developmentally is not yet known, however.

SEGMENTS AND FEATURES OF GERMAN

Vowels

The German vowel system is larger than that of English, consisting of 15 monophthongs and three basic diphthongs /aɪ, aʊ, ɔɪ/, with additional diphthongs created by sequences of a vowel and the vocalic realization of the postvocalic "rhotic" [ɐ] (e.g., [bɛɐk], *Berg*, "mountain"). As in English: (a) monophthongs include front unrounded vowels (/iː/ vs. /ɪ/, /eː/ vs. /ɛ/) and back rounded vowels (/uː/ vs. /ʊ/, /oː/ vs. /ɔ/) that contrast in length and tenseness; (b) the mid central vowel /ə/ is restricted to unstressed syllables; and (c) other lax vowels do not appear in unstressed open syllables. Unlike English, the only German low vowel is /a/ and there is a series of front rounded vowels contrasting in length and tenseness (/yː/ vs. /ʏ/, /øː/ vs. /œ/). Kehoe and Lleó (2003a, 2003b) conducted evaluations of four German-learning children on vowel development. Tense and lax (long and short) vowels and diphthongs were observed before age 2, with lax vowels produced accurately in advance of the other vowel types, and diphthongs produced accurately earlier than tense vowels (where length and tenseness were both required for accuracy, however). The unstressed vowel schwa was later-developing, approximately by age 2.6 (Kehoe & Lleó, 2003a). Although vowel mismatches have been reported for children with protracted phonological development (Fox & Dodd, 2001), insufficient information is available on vowel development. We expect that children with protracted phonological development may have difficulty learning schwa, diphthongs, and tense-lax contrasts as noted above for typically developing children, plus the marked front rounded vowels.

Consonants

Standard German contains 23 consonant phonemes plus glottal stop (preceding apparently vowel-initial, word-initial, and/or stressed syllables). The correspondence between nonlinear features and German consonants is displayed in Table 24.5.

TABLE 24.5
**Manner, Laryngeal and Place Features of German
and Corresponding Consonants**

Manner Features	Consonants
[+consonantal]	p b t d k g m n ŋ f pf v s z ts ʃ (ʒ tʃ dʒ) ç x ʁ[a] l
[–consonantal][b]	j h (ʔ)
[+ lateral]	l
([+trilled])	(ʀ r)[a]
[+nasal]	m n ŋ
[–continuant]–[–nasal]	p b t d k g (ʔ)
[+continuant] (& [–sonorant])	f v s z ʃ (ʒ)[c] ç x ʁ
[–continuant, + continuant]	pf ts (tʃ dʒ)[c]
Laryngeal Features	
[+voiced] stops and fricatives	b d g v z̩ (ʒ dʒ) ʁ[a]
[–voiced] stops and fricatives	p t k f pf s ts ʃ (tʃ) ç x
[+spread glottis]	pʰ tʰ kʰ f pf s ts ʃ (tʃ) ç x h
([+constricted glottis])[b]	(ʔ)
Place Features	
Labial	p b m f pf v
Labial [+labiodental]	f v pf
Coronal [+anterior][d]	n t d s z ts l
Coronal [–anterior][c,e]	ʃ (ʒ tʃ dʒ) (ç j)
Coronal [+grooved]	s z ts ʃ (ʒ tʃ dʒ)
Dorsal[f]	k g ŋ ç x ʁ (j)
Dorsal [–low] [–high][f]	ʁ
Dorsal [+back][f]	k g ŋ x ʁ
Dorsal [–back]	ç j
Coronal & Dorsal	ç j

Note: Underlined features are considered adult defaults (unmarked).
a Dialectal variants are trilled uvular /ʀ/ and trilled alveolar /r/.
b The glottal stop is included here for completeness but is not an underlying phoneme.
c The palatoalveolars /tʃ dʒ ʒ/ appear in words of foreign origin.
d The /ç/ and /j/ are both [Coronal] and [Dorsal].
e Plus dialectal variant /r/.
f Plus dialectal variant /ʀ/.

In terms of manner categories, German, like English, includes stops, nasals, fricatives, affricates, a lateral, and a rhotic. Among the stops, /g/ can appear as a fricative [ç] word finally. Sonorants can be syllabic in unstressed syllables, as in English. There are three main dialectal variations of the rhotic consonant: the uvular fricative [ʁ] (Standard German), the coronal trilled [r], and the uvular trilled [R] (Wiese, 1996). Postvocalic "rhotics" (in the spelling) are produced as the vowel [ɐ]. Among the fricatives and affricates, there are no interdentals, but there are the additional affricates /pf/, /ts/ (sometimes realized as [f] or [s]; Durell, 1992), and the dorsal fricatives /x/ and /ç/ and the rhotic uvular fricative. The palatoalveolars /ʒ/, /tʃ/, and /dʒ/ occur primarily in words of foreign origin.

Laryngeal features include both values of [voiced] syllable initially (though there is rarely voicing during the closure or constriction of obstruents), but only [-voiced] obstruents syllable-finally (unlike English, which has a voicing contrast across word positions). The feature [+spread glottis] applies to voiceless fricatives and affricates, /h/ and voiceless stops word initially, as onsets to medial stressed syllables, and before pause (as in English). The glottal stop ([+constricted glottis]) obligatorily appears before word-initial and/or stressed vowel-initial syllables (even in connected speech and after prefixes, unlike English).

Place features include [Labial], [Coronal], and [Dorsal]. The [Labial] category includes stops /p/ and /b/, fricatives /f/ and /v/, and the affricate /pf/. In comparison with English, there is no [w], and the rhotic is not labial; however, /v/ is far more frequent. Coronals include both values of [anterior], with stops, nasals, fricatives, and /l/ being [+anterior] as in English, but also including /ts/. The /l/ is alveolar in all contexts with minimal or no velarization. The coronal fricatives differ from English in that: (a) word-initial /s/ is very rare as a singleton and in clusters; (b) word-initial /z/ is very high frequency; (c) there are no interdentals; and (d) /ʃ/ is the common sibilant in word-initial clusters (e.g., /ʃp/). Rhotics are [Dorsal] except for the dialectal variant, alveolar trilled [r]. The [Dorsal] category includes the stops /k/ and /g/ and syllable-final nasal /ŋ/ but in comparison with English, also the fricatives /x/ (in the context of back vowels) and /ç/ (usually in the context of front vowels), and the rhotic fricative /ʁ/.

Developmental challenges for consonants include the fricatives and affricates, as in English (Fox & Dodd, 2001) and syllable-initial voicing contrasts. For children with protracted phonological development, Fox and Dodd (2001) note frequent occurrence of velar fronting, stopping, and intrusive consonants. However, the additional [Dorsal] phonemes may also promote earlier learning of [Dorsal] (Ullrich, 2004), and of "backing"; that is, default use of [Dorsal] (Fox & Dodd, 2001; Ullrich, 2004). The more frequent use of /v/ may promote earlier acquisition of [v] in German than in English; similarly, the unvelarized alveolar /l/ may result in earlier acquisition of [l] in German and different patterns of substitution (stops rather than the glide [w]; Romonath, 1991). In addition, sequences of consonants across vowels or sequences of vowels across consonants may present developmental challenges, resulting in consonant or vowel harmony, assimilation or metatheses (Fox & Dodd, 2001; Ullrich, 2004).

Nonlinear Phonology and Assessment of German-Speaking Children

The discussion above highlighted major aspects of German phonology that need to be considered in a nonlinear phonological assessment. An assessment tool, NILPOD (Ullrich, 2008), has been developed for German, utilizing a nonlinear phonological framework as a basis for analysis and providing both inventory (independent) analyses and comparisons with adult targets (relational analyses). The analysis is primarily qualitative (to facilitate efficiency in the clinic), but the assessor can quantify various aspects of the analysis if needed. In addition, NILPOD includes a wordlist for elicitation of speech samples that covers all aspects of the phonological hierarchy. Depending on severity level, either 75 or 105 items are presented to the client in a picture-naming task.

Because German and English are similar structurally, prosodic analyses for German can follow those for English (as they do in NILPOD). However, the greater frequency of compounds and word-initial clusters necessitates elicitation of more multisyllabic words and words with word-initial clusters. Table 24.4 shows word shape examples for German, focusing on the most relevant clinical (developmental) considerations (clusters, codas, word length).

For segments, similarities to and differences from English were discussed above, with developmental challenges noted. A nonlinear assessment requires an evaluation of consonants, vowels, their features, and sequences (as is done in NILPOD). Table 24.5 is a basis for consonant feature analysis (word position not included here but an essential component of evaluation). If a client shows frequent assimilation, coalescence or metathesis, evaluation of consonant sequences will be a vital aspect of the analysis (both for immediately surface-adjacent elements and more distant elements). Consonants and vowels share place features according to nonlinear feature theories; thus, any assimilations or dissimilation of place features across consonants and vowels can be evaluated in terms of place features across the two categories.

A major purpose of nonlinear phonological assessment is to determine goals for treatment that will address the phonological hierarchy and the child's positive and negative constraints on production (markedness and faithfulness constraints). The NILPOD analysis leads to selection of three types of goals (compared with four in the Bernhardt & Stemberger approach, 2000). Goals address prosodic structure, segments (and features), and interactions between segments and prosodic structure (positional constraints, sequences). A recent evaluation study of NILPOD was conducted with 60 clinicians in Germany (Ullrich, Romonath, & Bernhardt, 2008). Results confirm the clinical relevance of these analyses for goal selection, especially for children with moderately to severely protracted phonological development.

STANDARD MANDARIN

Standard Mandarin (also known as Pŭtōnghuà, Guóyǔ, and Huáyǔ) is a Sino-Tibetan language spoken by over 800 million people. It is the language of government in China and Taiwan, and is widely used in educational institutions and national media, and as a means of communication between speakers of different dialects or languages. In addition to their local dialect or language, almost every citizen of China learns Standard Mandarin. Mandarin is a tone language, with a segmental inventory of average size, but relatively simple word and syllable structure.

PHONOLOGY OF STANDARD MANDARIN

PROSODIC STRUCTURE

Tones and Tone Sandhi

Tone is an obligatory characteristic of words in Standard Mandarin. There are five tones and several tone alternations (tone sandhi). Tones include:

1. Tone 1 (T1): high (H) level, for example, /ma^{H}/ "mother"
2. Tone 2 (T2): mid-rising (MH), for example, /ma^{MH}/ "hemp"
3. Tone 3 (T3): mid-low-mid "dipping," for example, /ma^{MLM}/ "horse" (with the variant ML in nonphrase-final position, at least in some dialects)
4. Tone 4 (T4): high-low falling (HL), for example, /ma^{HL}/ "scold"
5. Neutral tone (T0), for example, /wo^{MLM}tə^{0}/ "mine" (*restricted to unstressed syllables*)

(The "neutral" tone generally appears in noninitial syllables, and has a different but predictable variant similar to tones 1–4 after each preceding tone, but it is difficult to describe the variation as assimilation. We denote neutral tone with a superscript "0.")

   T3 sandhi is perhaps the best-known alternation: a dipping tone changes to a rising tone when it occurs before another dipping tone (i.e., T3→T2/_T3), for example, for the word "ant" /ma^{MLM}ji^{MLM}/→ [ma^{MH}ji^{MLM}]; the two component characters of the word "ant" are both pronounced with a dipping tone in isolation, but when they are put together for the word "ant," the first dipping tone is changed to a rising tone. Regarding acquisition, Jeng (1979), Li (1977), Li and Thompson (1977), and Zhu and Dodd (2000a, b, c) note that children appear to master tone and tone sandhi earlier than the full segmental inventory.

SYLLABLE STRUCTURE, WORD LENGTH AND STRESS

In terms of syllable types, Standard Mandarin includes open syllables V, VV, CV, CVV, CVVV, and closed syllables VC, CVC, and CVVC (where VV = diphthong and VVV = triphthong). Consonant clusters do not occur word initially or finally, although sequences of consonants can occur word medially (e.g., [nʂ] in /tia^{HL}nʂi^{HL}ti^{H}/ "television"). (However, note that Duanmu, 2000, suggests that, for some variants of Mandarin, the first vowel of the diphthong or triphthong may be a prenuclear glide and part of the onset, i.e., CG).

There are many monosyllabic and disyllabic words in children's early vocabularies, some trisyllabic words (e.g., /tia^{HL}nsi^{HL}ti^{H}/ "television"), and few tetrasyllabic words (the maximum; e.g., /ko^{H}ŋko^{HL}ŋtɕ^{h}i^{HL}tş^{h}ɤ^{H}/ "public bus"). Most common words are either monosyllabic or disyllabic, for example, /ɕie^{MH}/ and /ɕie^{MH}tsə^{0}/ (which both mean "shoes" in adult Mandarin). Mandarin is cross-linguistically unusual in that, in addition to using tones to differentiate lexical meanings, words of two or more syllables can show different levels of prominence or stress. Duanmu (2000) argues that stress is trochaic. Unstressed syllables often occur in suffixes such as /tsə/ in [pi^{MH}tsə^{0}] "nose," particles such as the possessive /tə/ in /wo^{MLM}tə^{0}/ "mine" and the second syllable of some disyllabic words such as /pa^{MLM}şou^{0}/ "handle" (cf. /şou^{MLM}/ "hand"). Unstressed syllables show vowel reduction (to schwa) and/ or tone neutralization.

In terms of phonological development, the Mandarin inventory of word shapes may be earlier acquired in Mandarin than in English because of the restricted number of codas (/n/, /ŋ/) and absence of word-initial or word-final consonant clusters. However, the greater set of complex nuclei may take longer to learn than English diphthongs. Development of word stress, appears to be delayed relative to development of tone (Zhu, 2002). Furthermore, whereas English-speaking children often use weak syllable deletion to resolve markedness constraints on word length, this may not be the case for Mandarin-learning children, because unstressed syllables may not be as reduced as in English. However, much research remains to be done about the development of word structure in Mandarin.

SEGMENTS AND FEATURES

Vowels

Vowels are the obligatory tone-bearing units in Mandarin. There are eight monophthongs: /i, u, y, a, o, ə, ɤ, ɻ /. The /ɻ/ is a retroflexed central vowel that can occur in isolation such as / ɻ ^{HL}/ "two" or in rhotacization. Schwa only occurs in unstressed syllables. Mandarin has nine diphthongs, with either rising sonority as in /ai, ei, ou, ao/ or falling sonority as in /ia, ua, uo, ie, ye/, and four triphthongs /iao, iou, uai, uei/. (However, see the note above about Duanmu's, 2000, treatment of the first vowel of the diphthong or triphthong for some variants of Mandarin.)

Consonants

Standard Mandarin has an inventory of 24 consonants. (See Table 24.6.) All consonants except the velar nasal /ŋ/ can occur syllable initially, whereas only /n/ and /ŋ/ can occur syllable finally. There are few disagreements in the literature about the consonant inventory, except for classification of /w/ and /j/ (included as consonants by Lee & Zee, 2003, but not by Zhu & Dodd, (2000c), who treat /j/ as an allophone of /i/ and /w/ as an allophone of /u/).

TABLE 24.6

Manner, Laryngeal and Place Features and Corresponding Consonants for Mandarin

Manner Features	Consonants
[+consonantal]	p pʰ t tʰ k kʰ m n ŋ f s ʂ ɕ x ts tsʰ tʂ tʂʰ tɕ tɕʰ l R
[−consonantal]	w j
[+sonorant][+cons][−nasal]	l ɻ
[+nasal]	m n ŋ
[−continuant][−nasal]	p pʰ t tʰ k kʰ
[+continuant]−[−sonorant]	f s ʂ ɕ x
[−continuant]−[+continuant]	ts tsʰ tʂ tʂʰ tɕ tɕʰ

Laryngeal Features	
[−voiced] [−spread glottis]:	p t k ts tʂ tɕ
[−voiced] [+spread glottis]:	pʰ tʰ kʰ tsʰ tʂʰ tɕʰ f s ʂ ɕ x

Place Features	
Labial	p pʰ m f w
Coronal [+anterior]	t tʰ n s ts tsʰ l
Coronal [−anterior]	ʂ ɕ tʂ tʂʰ tɕ tɕʰ ɻ j
Coronal [+grooved]	s ʂ ts tsʰ tʂ tʂʰ ɻ
Coronal [−grooved]	t tʰ n ɕ tɕ tɕʰ l j
Dorsal	k kʰ ŋ x w j

Table 24.6 (following the feature system in Bernhardt & Stemberger 1998, 2000) shows the features and associated Mandarin consonants. Manner categories include:

1. [+consonantal]: all but the [−consonantal] glides /w/, /j/;
2. [+nasal]: across all places of articulation (with word position restrictions as noted earlier);
3. [−continuant]: oral stops and nasals across all places of articulation;
4. [+continuant]&[−sonorant]: fricatives across all places of articulation; and
5. [−continuant]−[+continuant]: a number of coronal affricates (see below).

Although there are no comparative reports concerning this topic, the higher type-frequency of affricates in Mandarin than in English (six versus two) may result in earlier acquisition of Mandarin affricates (as high token frequency does in Quiche Mayan: Pye, Ingram, & List, 1987). Resolution of the constraint prohibiting affricates (i.e., prohibiting two values of [continuant] in one segment) may also differ statistically in these two languages. In preliminary data for 4-year-old Mandarin-learning children, we have observed frequent replacement of affricates with fricatives, for example, /tɕiao^MLM/ "foot" → [ɕiao^MLM] and /tsʰai^HL/ "vegeta-ble" → [sai^HL] (whereas English-learning children more often replace affricates with stops, Bernhardt & Stemberger, 1998).

For laryngeal features, [-voiced] obstruents include the same set as in English, but the laryngeal *contrast* for stops and affricates is voiceless aspirated versus voiceless unaspirated (rather than voiced versus voiceless). Whether the laryngeal contrast would for this reason develop earlier or later than in English is unknown. Unlike English, there are no voiced fricatives. The [+spread glottis] feature applies to voiceless fricatives and aspirated stops and affricates as in English, but there is no */h/ in Mandarin.

Mandarin [Labial], [Coronal], and [Dorsal] place features are similar to those of English, with some notable exceptions. [Labial] includes /p pʰ m f w/ but not */b v/; [Coronal] includes the alveolars ([+anterior]) [-grooved] /t tʰ n l/ and [+grooved] /s/ but also the [+grooved] affricates /ts tsʰ/. The [-anterior] seg-ments include /j/ (as in English), but no palatoalveolars; rather, the inventory has [+grooved] retroflexes /ʂ tʂ tʂʰ ɻ/ and [-grooved] alveopalatals /ɕ, tɕ tɕʰ/. [Dorsal] includes the stops /k kʰ/ (but not */g/), the nasal /ŋ/, and the glides /w/ and /j/ (i.e., similar to English), but also the velar fricative /x/.

Some disagreements exist regarding details of place of articulation. Lee and Zee (2003) state that /t tʰ n/ are *dento-alveolar*; that is, [+distributed] in Standard Mandarin, unlike in English, where they are [-distributed] (Bernhardt & Stemberger, 1998). Furthermore, because /s/ is apico-*laminal* in Mandarin, it may not be produced with the same degree of grooving as the English apical /s/. Mandarin postalveolar segments may or may not be actually retroflexed, but chil-dren are traditionally taught to curl their tongue when pronouncing these sounds to make obvious the distinctions among the alveolar affricates and fricatives. (In addi-tion, lips are protruded for these segments, i.e., they have a noncontrastive [+round] feature, similar to palatoalveolars in many languages, including English.)

In terms of development, children generally acquire the coronal retroflexes, /ʂ tʂ tʂʰ ɻ/ later than other segment types. In our recent study of 4-year-old typically developing children, a common pronunciation of /ʂɤ^MH/ "snake" was /sɤ^MH/ and of /tʂʰi^H/ "eat" was '[tsʰi^H] (substitution of dento-alveolars, similar to English-learning children's "fronting" of palatoalveolars to alveolars). Although there are no comparative data available, the presence of the velar fricative /x/ may affect the timing of acquisition of [Dorsal] for consonants (i.e., earlier than in English, as noted for German: Ullrich, 2004).

NONLINEAR PHONOLOGY AND ASSESSMENT OF MANDARIN-SPEAKING CHILDREN

The discussion of Mandarin above highlighted some of the similarities and dif-ferences with English. A tool for nonlinear phonological assessment of Mandarin (including a word list for elicitation) has been piloted with 4-year-old children (both typically developing and those with protracted phonological development).

TABLE 24.7

Tones and Tone Sequences in Mandarin

Individual Tones	H, MH, ML(M), HL, 0 (Neutral)
Tone sequences	H-0, MH-0, ML(M)-0, HL-0
	H-H, H-MH, H-ML(M), H-HL
	MH-MH, MH-H, MH-ML(M), MH-HL
	ML(M)-ML(M)
	ML(M)-ML(M) → MH- ML(M) (expected tone sandhi or change)
	ML(M)-H, ML(M)-MH, ML(M)-HL
	HL-HL, HL-H, HL-MH, HL- ML(M)
	Other

Note: Tone patterns: H = high, Tone 1; MH = mid-high rising, Tone 2; MLM = mid-low-mid dipping, Tone 3 (may be ML in some dialects if not phrase-final before a pause); HL = high-low falling, Tone 4; 0 = neutral tone (in unstressed second syllables, predictable from previous tone).

For Mandarin, prosodic structure evaluation necessarily requires elicitation and analysis of all tones and major tone sandhi, in addition to evaluation of word length, shape, and stress as in English. (A table listing tones and tone sequences is presented in Table 24.7 as a basis for tone assessment.) It is predicted that children with protracted phonological development may show difficulty with complex nuclei, complex tone patterns (e.g., T3), and stress-tone interactions (i.e., features associated with the vowel system). Thus, these require special attention in assessment.

In terms of consonants, the affricates, the unaspirated-aspirated contrast for stops and affricates, and the retroflexes stand out as the key elements that may present particular challenges for development other than those expected cross-linguistically (later development of fricatives, liquids, velars). For vowels, diphthongs and triphthongs will presumably be challenging and require special focus in assessment.

CONCLUSION

As phonological theories develop, greater insights can be gained concerning phonological acquisition, whether typical or protracted. Much remains to be done cross-linguistically concerning the application of (nonlinear) phonological theory to assessment and intervention with children with protracted phonological development. The current chapter focuses on English, German, Arabic, and Mandarin, the first four languages from a larger cross-linguistic study of protracted phonological development from a nonlinear perspective. It is expected that the emerging database will be a strong source of evidence about patterns in protracted phonological development and that the constraints-based nonlinear theories will provide a comprehensive framework from which to view the patterns.

ACKNOWLEDGMENTS

The authors would like to acknowledge the children in Canada, Germany, Kuwait, and Shanghai whose pronunciations contributed to this article and their families.

REFERENCES

Amayreh, M. M. (2003). Completion of the consonant inventory of Arabic. *Journal of Speech, Language, and Hearing Research, 46*(3), 517–529.

Amayreh, M. M., & Dyson, A. T. (1998). The acquisition of Arabic consonants. *Journal of Speech, Language, and Hearing Research, 41*(3), 642–653.

Amayreh, M. M., & Dyson, A. T. (2000). Phonetic inventories of young Arabic-speaking children. *Clinical Linguistics and Phonetics, 14*(3), 193–215.

Ammar, W., & Morsi, R. (2006). Phonological development and disorders: Colloquial Egyptian Arabic. In H. Zhu & B. Dodd (Eds.), *Phonological development and disorders in children: A multilingual perspective* (pp. 204–232). Clevedon, UK: Multilingual Matters.

Anis, I. (1961). *Al-Aswat-l-lughawiyya* [The sounds of language] (3rd ed). Cairo, Egypt: Dar-l-Nahda-l-arabiyya Press.

Ayyad, H., & Bernhardt, B. M. (2008, June). The phonological development of a Kuwaiti Arabic child with hearing impairment compared with a typically developing age peer and younger child. *International Conference of the Clinical Phonetics and Linguistics Association,* Istanbul, Turkey.

Ayyad, H., Bernhardt, B. M., & Stemberger, J. P. (2006, November). *Bilingual phonological acquisition of Kuwaiti Arabic and English in siblings.* Poster presented at the annual ASHA conference, Miami, FL.

Bernhardt, B. (1990). *Application of nonlinear phonological theory to intervention with six phonologically disordered children.* Unpublished doctoral dissertation, University of British Columbia.

Bernhardt, B. (1992). The application of nonlinear phonological theory to intervention. *Clinical Linguistics and Phonetics, 6,* 283–316.

Bernhardt, B., Brooke, M., & Major, E. (2003, July). *Acquisition of structure versus features in nonlinear phonological intervention.* Poster presented at the Child Phonology Conference, UBC, Vancouver, BC.

Bernhardt, B., & Gilbert, J. (1992). Applying linguistic theory to speech-language pathology: The case for nonlinear phonology. *Clinical Linguistics and Phonetics, 6,* 123–145.

Bernhardt, B., & Major, E. (2005). Speech, language and literacy skills three years later: Long-term outcomes of nonlinear phonological intervention. *International Journal of Language and Communication Disorders, 40,* 1–27.

Bernhardt, B., & Stemberger, J. P. (1998). *Handbook of phonological development: From a nonlinear constraints-based perspective.* San Diego, CA: Academic Press.

Bernhardt, B., & Stemberger, J. P. (2000). *Workbook in nonlinear phonology for clinical application.* Austin, TX: Pro-Ed.

Bernhardt, B. M. & Stemberger, J. P. (2008, June). *Changes in vowels after intervention focusing on consonants and word structure*. International Conference of Clinical Linguistics and Phonetics Association, Istanbul.

Bin-Muqbil, M. S. (2006). *Phonetic and phonological aspects of Arabic emphatics and gutturals*. Unpublished doctoral dissertation, University of Wisconsin-Madison.

Clements, G. N., & Keyser, S. J. (1983). *CV phonology*. Cambridge, MA: MIT Press.

Duanmu, S. (2000). *The phonology of standard Chinese*. New York, NY: Oxford University Press.

Durell, M. (1992). *Using German*. Cambridge, UK: Cambridge University Press.

Dyson, A. T., & Amayreh, M. M. (2000). Phonological errors and sound changes in Arabic-speaking children. *Clinical Linguistics & Phonetics, 2000, 14*(2), 79–109.

Edwards, S. M. (1995). *Optimal outcomes of nonlinear phonological intervention*. Unpublished MA thesis, University of British Columbia.

Féry, C. (1995). Alignment, syllable, and metrical structure in German. Seminar für Sprachwissenschaft (SFS-Report-02-95, Habilitationsschrift), University of Tübingen.

Fox, A. (2007). German speech acquisition. In S. McLeod (Ed.), *The international guide for speech acquisition* (pp. 386–397). Clifton Park, NY: Thomson Delmar Learning.

Fox, A., & Dodd, B. (2001). Phonologically disordered German-speaking children. *American Journal of Speech-Language Pathology, 10*(3), 291–303.

Goldsmith, J. (1976). *Autosegmental phonology*. Doctoral dissertation: MIT. [Published by Garland Press, New York, 1979].

Hassan, T. (1950). *Manahij-l-bahth fi-l-lugha* [Research methods in language]. Cairo, Egypt: Ar-Risala Press.

Hayes, B. (1989). Compensatory lengthening in moraic phonology. *Linguistic Inquiry, 20*, 253–306.

Hayes, B. (1990). Diphthongization and coindexing. *Phonology, 7*, 31–71.

Hayes, B. (1995). *Metrical stress theory: Principles and case studies*. Chicago, IL: The University of Chicago Press.

Jeng, H. (1979). The acquisition of Chinese phonology in relation to Jackobson's laws of irreversible solidarity. *Proceedings of the 9th International Congress of Phonetic Sciences* (pp. 155–161). Copenhagen, The Netherlands: University of Copenhagen.

Kehoe, M., & Lleó, C. (2003a). A phonological analysis of schwa in German first language acquisition. *The Canadian Journal of Linguistics/La Revue Canadienne de Linguistique, 48*(3–4), 289–327.

Kehoe, M., & Lleó, C. (2003b). The acquisition of nuclei: A longitudinal analysis of phonological vowel length in three German-speaking children. *Journal of Child Language, 30*, 527–556.

Kehoe, M., & Lleó, C. (2003c). The acquisition of syllable types in monolingual and bilingual German and Spanish children. In B. Beachley, A. Brown, & F. Conlin (Eds.), *BUCLD 27 Proceedings* (pp. 402–413). Somerville, MA: Cascadilla Press.

Kenstowicz, M. (1994). *Phonology in generative grammar*. Cambridge, MA: Blackwell.

Lee, W.-S., & Zee, E. (2003). Standard Chinese (Beijing). *Journal of the International Phonetic Association, 33*, 109–112.

Li, C. N., & Thompson, S. A. (1977). The acquisition of tone in Mandarin-speaking children. *Journal of Child Language, 41*, 185–199.

Li, P. J.-K. (1977). Child language acquisition of Mandarin phonology. In R. Cheng, Y. C. Li, & T. Tang (Eds.), *Proceedings of the symposium on Chinese linguistics: 1977 Linguistic Institute of the Linguistic Society of America* (pp. 295–316). Taipei, Taiwan: Student Books.

Lleó, C., & Vogel, I. (2004). Learning new segments and reducing domains in German L2 phonology: The role of the Prosodic Hierarchy. *International Journal of Bilingualism, 8*(1), 79–104.

Major, E., & Bernhardt, B. (1998). Metaphonological skills of children with phonological disorders before and after phonological and metaphonological intervention. *International Journal of Language and Communication Disorders, 33*, 413–444.

McCarthy, J. J. (1988). Feature geometry and dependency: A review. *Phonetica, 43*, 84–108.

McCarthy, J. J. (1994) The phonetics and phonology of Semitic pharyngeals. In P. Keating, (Ed.), *Papers in laboratory phonology III: Phonological structure and phonetic form* (pp. 191–233). Cambridge, UK: Cambridge University Press.

Masterson, J., & Bernhardt, B. (2001). *Computerized articulation and phonology evaluation system (CAPES)*. San Antonio, TX: The Psychological Corporation.

Omar, A. M. (1991). *A study on linguistic phonology*. Cairo, Egypt: Alam-l-kutub.

Pye, C., Ingram, D., & List, H. (1987). A comparison of initial consonant acquisition in English and Quiché. In K. Nelson & A. van Kleeck (Eds.), *Children's Language* (Vol. 6, pp. 175–190). Hillsdale, NJ: Erlbaum.

Romonath, R. (1991). *Phonologische Prozesse an sprachauffälligen Kindern, eine vergleichende Untersuchung an sprachauffälligen und nichtsprachauffälligen Vorschulkindern* [Phonological processes of children with phonological disorders: A comparative investigation of preschool children with and without speech disorders]. Berlin, Germany: Edition Marhold.

Sagey, E. (1986). *The representation of features and relations in non-linear phonology*. Doctoral dissertation, MIT [Published by New York, NY: Garland Press, 1991.]

Ullrich, A. (2004). *Nichtlineare Analyse des phonologischen Systems deutschsprachiger Kinder* [Nonlinear analyses of the phonological systems of German-speaking children]. Unpublished Master's thesis, Julius-Maximilans-Universität Würzburg.

Ullrich, A. (2008). *Nichtlineare phonologische Diagnostik (NILPOD)* [Nonlinear phonological assessment]. Unpublished manuscript, University of Cologne, Germany.

Ullrich, A., & Bernhardt, B. (2005). Neue Perspektiven der phonologischen Analyse - Implikationen für die Untersuchung phonologischer Entwicklungsstörungen [New perspectives in phonological analysis – Implications for the investigation of developmental phonological impairments]. *Die Sprachheilarbeit, 5,* 221–233.

Ullrich, A., Romonath, R., & Bernhardt, B. M. (2008). Nonlinear scan analysis in German: An evaluation by practicing German speech-language pathologists and logopedists. *International Association of Child Language Congress*, July, 2008, Edinburgh.

Von Bremen, V. (1990). *A nonlinear phonological approach to intervention with severely phonologically disordered twins*. Unpublished MA thesis, University of British Columbia.

Watson, J. (2002). *The phonology and morphology of Arabic*. Oxford, UK: Oxford University Press.

Wiese, R. (1996). *The phonology of German*. Oxford, UK: Clarendon Press.

Zhu, H. (2002). *Phonological development in specific contexts: Studies of Chinese-speaking children*. Clevedon, UK: Multilingual Matters Ltd.

Zhu, H., & Dodd, B. (2000a). Development and change in the phonology of Putonghua-speaking children with speech difficulties. *Clinical Linguistics and Phonetics, 14*, 351–368.

Zhu, H., & Dodd, B. (2000b). Putonghua (Modern Standard Chinese)-speaking children with speech disorders. *Clinical Linguistics and Phonetics, 14,* 165–191.

Zhu, H., & Dodd, B. (2000c). The phonological acquisition of Putonghua (Modern Standard Chinese). *Journal of Child Language, 27,* 3–42.

25 Bilingual Children With SLI: Theories, Research and Future Directions

Maria Adelaida Restrepo, Gareth Morgan, and Ekaterina Smyk

INTRODUCTION

Bilingualism and specific language impairment (SLI) are at the crossroads of linguistic and psycholinguistic accounts of language. This chapter merges theoretical and research accounts of both areas to explain the limited information available on bilingual children with SLI. The SLI is a developmental language disorder characterized by primary deficits in language, not explained by sensory, gross neurological damage, emotional, or cognitive deficits (Leonard, 1998, 2009). Language difficulties of children with SLI tend to occur on grammatical aspects, although several language aspects can be compromised, such as difficulties in word learning and retrieval, semantic development, and phonological working memory (e.g., Dollaghan & Campbell, 1998; Edwards & Lahey, 1998; Gray, 2003, 2004, 2005). This chapter will discuss how bilingualism interfaces with SLI from the theoretical point of Dynamic Systems Theory (DST; Herdina & Jessner, 2002). We then address theories of SLI from linguistic and processing accounts, and review research evidence of SLI crosslinguistically and from bilingual populations. We conclude with some future directions.

In our work, we use a DST of language, bilingualism, and SLI (Herdina & Jessner, 2002; Kohnert, 2008) because it allows for the interaction of multiple languages, linguistic aspects, and contexts with the different cognitive processes involved in language. Language is a dynamic system; that is, it is a complex system, which is fluid and always changing (Kohnert, 2008). In the context of bilingualism, DST helps us to understand the role of variable linguistic input in different social and cultural contexts, while at the same time acknowledging the interactions across languages and linguistic abilities in terms of language proficiency, and typical or atypical development (Evans & McWhinney, 1999; Herdina & Jessner, 2002; Kohnert, 2008). In DST, language abilities in multilingual children change depending upon the quantity and quality of input needed to induce a change. When the input is strong, language changes can be positive on all the languages that the child speaks, but they can also be negative for one language and positive for the other (Herdina & Jessner, 2002; Kohnert, 2008). The fluid nature of language can respond to change any time there is sufficient input to induce a change. A visit of a family member, schooling in a new language, or new social relationships, for example, can induce change in a child's developing languages. Therefore, DST can account for great variability even in children with similar backgrounds but different language experiences. In addition, using DST we can still examine the processing and linguistic accounts of SLI to help us understand and describe this complex and dynamic system. DST has been used to account for both SLI and bilingualism, and researchers are beginning to use it to explain the two and their interactions (e.g., Kohnert, 2008; Kohnert & Derr, 2004).

Kohnert (2008) uses DST as one aspect of her theoretical framework, which acknowledges the convergences of several theories: connectionism, social constructivism, DST, general interactive processing, and functionalism. For purposes of this chapter, we focus on DST and cognitive interactive processes of language to explain some of the phenomena observed in bilingual children with SLI. Nevertheless, we must acknowledge current linguistic theories that attempt to explain the nature of SLI and second language acquisition.

Language knowledge in bilinguals is distributed across the languages they speak in terms of semantic, pragmatic, and grammatical skills (Kohnert, Windsor, & Ebert, 2008; Peña & Kester, 2004). Sequential and simultaneous bilingual children can demonstrate language influences across the different grammars in the languages they acquire. Theories explaining these influences are beyond the scope of this chapter, but we acknowledge that errors, for example, in bilingual discourse can reflect dynamic changes in a language due to transfer from a first language to a second language, from a second language to a first language, or the interlanguage that children develop while acquiring a second language (Gass & Selinker, 2008). Therefore, in addition to SLI characteristics, bilingual children with SLI can have characteristics typical for sequential and simultaneous language learners.

Theoretical accounts of SLI can be categorized in two general domains: linguistic and processing theories (Leonard, 1998; Schwartz, 2009; Ullman & Pierpont, 2005). Linguistic theories hypothesize that SLI deficits are due to limitations in linguistic knowledge, but differ on the locus of the impairment. Processing theories hypothesize that SLI deficits are due to limitations in processing linguistic information, but differ on what specific processes are impaired and whether they are in general domains or specific domains (Schwartz, 2009). To our knowledge, there is limited information on how these theories account for bilingual SLI characteristics and language performance, and thus, research on this population is largely descriptive.

PROCESSING ACCOUNTS OF SLI

Processing accounts can be categorized in two strands, general cognitive processing limitations that affect linguistic and nonlinguistic processes and specific cognitive possessing limitations that affect specific linguistic processes (Leonard, 1998;

Schwartz, 2009). In terms of general processing accounts, the primary account of SLI is the Limited Processing Capacity (LPC) Hypothesis; for a review see Leonard (1998, 2009). The LPC hypothesis considers limitations in three different areas: limited space, such as limits in memory capacity; limited attention/ energy, such as an inability to complete a task because the energy has already been spent; and limited processing speed, such as an inefficiency to process information fast enough, and thus the information is vulnerable to decay or interference from new incoming information (Leonard, 1998; Schwartz, 2009). More specifically, LPC theory hypothesizes that children with SLI have limitations in working memory capacity (Gutierrez-Clellen, Calderon, & Weismer, 2004; Weismer, 1996; Weismer, Evans, & Hesketh, 1999; Weismer & Hesketh, 1998), which in turn leads to limitations in processing input and output. In this theory, children with SLI present with difficulties processing complex material (Gillam, Cowan, & Marler, 1998). As stimuli become more complex (linguistically, cognitively, or an increase in attention demands) performance deteriorates, especially in comparison to controls. For example, Gillam et al. (1998) found that typical and SLI groups performed similarly on a recall task when audiovisual stimuli were paired with a spoken response. This was an expected effect as visual input is rapidly converted into phonological forms ready for rehearsal, which would be facilitated by the spoken response; however, children with SLI had significantly poorer recall when audiovisual stimuli were paired with a pointing response. The authors do not attribute this difference in performance by children with SLI to any deficits in language, but instead to the cross modal aspect of the task. In other words, children with SLI were not able to retain the word in memory or use phonological codes, or both when the task demanded cross modal operations like audiovisual stimuli paired with a motor task like pointing.

One criticism of the different LPC hypotheses is that they do not directly address the limitations in the linguistic profile of children with SLI (Schwartz, 2009). This is especially true when discussing those who are bilingual, although correlations have been observed between processing skills and language performance in monolingual populations, such as between processing complex sentences, and phonological memory and vocabulary development (Archibald & Gathercole, 2006; Montgomery, 2003). Further, interpreting research that addresses processing limitations across languages (monolingual vs. bilingual) and across classification (typical vs. atypical) can be complicated because of differential demands in processing across the different groups on similar tasks (Kohnert, Windsor, & Yim, 2006). Using a DST may help researcher to better understand these complex processes in multilingual contexts.

The General Slowing Hypothesis (GSH; Kail, 1994), posits that children with SLI demonstrate slower reaction times, lexical access, and learning skills in general. It is particularly applicable to investigate SLI as it uses speed of processing as a method to measure processing capacity and assumes that speed is equal to the amount of work that can be completed in a particular amount of time. Evidence in support of this hypothesis has been reported in slower reaction times or additional time required to complete a task by children with SLI when compared to matched peers, which is consistent with a DST as well (e.g., Hill, 2001; Leonard et al., 2007; Schul, Stiles, Wulfeck, & Townsend, 2004; Windsor & Hwang, 1999). Although children with SLI as a group perform slower than age and language matches, not all children with SLI demonstrate this pattern and both speed and processing skills have been shown to each account for unique variance in language performance (Leonard et al., 2007). The GSH hypothesizes that slower processing skills interfere with processing of complex sentences for example (e.g., Montgomery, 1995), but also with the access of lexical information in tasks such as rapid automatic naming (e.g., Catts et al., 2005), word learning (e.g., Gray, 2004, 2005) and fast mapping (e.g., Gray, 2003). Studies on bilingual SLI in these areas are sparse; however, differences in reaction times in identifying words between typical bilingual Spanish–English children and monolingual English children with language impairments (LI; Windsor & Kohnert, 2004) and in rapid naming (Morgan, Srivastiva, Restrepo, & Auza, 2009) have been found. Such differences can be mistaken as SLI and therefore, research in this area indicates that there is a great need to understand the role of a bilingual's two languages or the acquisition of a second language on the processing skills of typical bilingual children. Competition between languages can account for slower processing times in bilinguals; however, the question remains whether it applies to all fluent bilinguals, to only sequential bilinguals in additive or subtractive language contexts, or to only late sequential bilinguals. In addition, research explaining the relationship of how processing speed affects bilingual children with SLI remains undetermined.

Specific cognitive processing accounts of SLI have hypothesized that a reduction in skills such as phonological working memory (Campbell, Dollaghan, Needleman, & Janosky, 1997; Dollaghan & Campbell, 1998; Gathercole & Baddeley, 1990) or temporal processing (Tallal & Newcombe, 1978) can account for the linguistic difficulties of children with SLI. In the phonological working memory domain, Girabau and Schwartz (2008) tested Spanish–English bilinguals with and without LI on a nonword repetition task; typical bilinguals outperformed bilinguals with LI. An effect of syllable length was observed where performance decreased across both groups as nonwords became longer; however, only six of the 11 typical bilinguals scored below 100% (no less than 95%) syllables correct on all nonwords regardless of length. Bilinguals with LI went from 95% syllables correct for single syllable words to 9% syllables correct for five syllable words. This dramatic decrease in syllable accuracy provides evidence that children with LI have limitations in the amount of information that they can attend to, which in this case supports a deficit in phonological working memory.

Kohnert et al. (2006) measured children who were typically developing monolingual English speakers (EO), typical bilingual Spanish–English speaking children (BI), and monolingual English speaking children with LI (ELI) on the Competing Language Processing Task (CLPT; Gaulin & Campbell, 1994), a measure of verbal working memory capacity, and the nonword repetition task (NWR), which was developed by Dollaghan and Campbell (1998). They found similar differences to Girabau and Schwartz (2008) on the NWR, where all children showed decreasing accuracy in syllables correct as the nonword length increased; similarly, ELI children showed the most dramatic decrease in accuracy. Kohnert et al. also found that the EO children outperformed ELI children on both tasks, but that BI children did not differ significantly from ELI children on the CLPT. The nonword repetition task, which used nonwords that followed the phonotactics of English (Dollaghan & Campbell, 1998), revealed significant group separation amongst all three groups at the four-syllable nonword level (EO outperformed all groups and BI outperformed the ELI group); however, there was significant group overlap for nonwords with fewer than four syllables. These results provide evidence that children with LI have a reduction in specific skills like verbal working memory and phonological working memory, but that language experience is a mitigating factor when comparing monolinguals and bilinguals.

Gutierrez-Clellen et al. (2004) examined verbal working memory (VWM) in typical bilingual Spanish–English speaking children, typical English-proficient with limited Spanish speaking children and, typical Spanish-proficient with limited English speaking children. English and Spanish versions of the CLPT and Dual Processing Competing Language Test (DPCT) were used to measure VWM in the three groups. Results indicated no differences on measures of VWM between the three groups nor between languages. Conversely, in two experiments Thorn and Gathercole (1999) observed the effect of vocabulary knowledge on phonological short-term memory in French–English bilinguals as compared to their monolingual English and English speaking children learning French as a second language peers. Results indicated a strong relationship between vocabulary knowledge and short-term memory. Multiple regression analyses revealed English vocabulary significantly accounting for 9% of the variance in English nonword repetition performance and French vocabulary significantly accounting for 38% of French NWR; these results support the existence of a language effect in processing measures such as nonword repetition. In terms of processing capacity as a measure by phonological working memory, English speaking children learning French as a second language performed equally on the French nonword repetition task to younger, yet proficient bilingual French–English children matched for performance in French vocabulary. It would be expected that older children (mean age difference of 2 years 6 months) would exhibit a larger phonological working memory advantage; however, this finding suggests that despite the age difference, the contribution of language-specific knowledge provides a possible advantage in phonological working memory for the younger proficient bilinguals.

The use of processing measures has been advocated as a tool that is free of language and cultural experience to identify language impairment in language minority populations. Nevertheless, research evidence suggests caution when choosing processing measures for nonmainstream children because these measures contain components that are sensitive to language and cultural experiences. Moreover, norms for such tasks must be validated with bilingual populations.

LINGUISTIC ACCOUNTS OF SLI

Linguistic accounts of SLI share the underlying hypothesis of linguistic knowledge deficits that result in problems with morphosyntax. Although these accounts differ in the assumed locus of deficits, they are centered on domain-specific linguistic knowledge, in contrast with domain-general processing accounts (e.g., Leonard, 1998; Paradis, 2007; van der Lely, 2005).

The Functional Category Deficit Account is based on the concept of acquisition of functional categories, such as determiners, complementizers, and inflections, in typically developing (TD) children. Radford (1988, 1990) has argued that children begin to acquire functional categories around 2 years of age, thus, the early grammar can be described only in terms of lexical categories. According to this account, children with SLI have greater difficulties with grammatical morphology due to slower development of functional categories. In particular, the grammatical morphemes that appear to be problematic for English-speaking children with SLI are associated with the use of functional categories (e.g., Leonard, Eyer, Bedore, & Grela, 1997). However, the reported differences between children with SLI and MLU-matched children in the use of functional categories relate to the differences in the degree of use (Leonard, 1998).

The functional category deficit account has been extended to studies in other languages. Italian-speaking children with SLI are more likely to omit direct object clitics than MLU-matched children (e.g., Leonard, Bortolini, Caselli, McGregor, & Sabbadini, 1992; Leonard, Sabbadini, Volterra, & Leonard, 1988). In contrast with Italian, French-speaking children with SLI were reported to use articles to the same extent as MLU-matched children (Le Normand, Leonard, & McGregor, 1993). Omissions and incorrect use of grammatical morphemes were found in Spanish-speaking children with SLI (Restrepo, 1998), specifically, articles have been documented as a primary area of difficulty (Anderson & Souto, 2005; Restrepo & Gutierrez-Clellen, 2001). However, studies on Spanish-speaking children suggest that grammatical morphemes associated with lexical categories such as the noun plural inflection could also be problematic for children with SLI (Bedore & Leonard, 2001; 2005; Merino, 1983), although the differences are not clinically significant.

The Extended Optional Infinitive Account considers problems with tense-bearing morphology as the source of deficits in children with SLI (Rice & Wexler, 1996; Rice, Wexler, & Cleave, 1995). Wexler (1994) described the Optional Infinitive (OI) stage in early grammar of TD children as a period when the infinitival form of a verb is optionally used instead of the finite form, although children possess the grammatical properties of finiteness. The OI stage was accounted by the Agreement/Tense Omission Model (ATOM; Wexler, Schütze, & Rice, 1998), according to which either agreement and/or tense could be optionally omitted in child grammar. Although, this proposal accounted for instances of missing subject–verb agreement in English, it did not apply to null-subject languages such as Italian or Spanish. To address this issue, Wexler (1998, 2003) proposed the Extended Unique Checking Constrain (EUCC), according to which the OI stage existed in early child grammar only in the non-null subject languages. In particular, in non-null subject languages both the category tense (TNS) and subject agreement (AGRS) have a noninterpretable determiner (D) feature. Grammatical subjects represented as determiner phrases (DP) contain the interpretable D feature, and therefore, the D feature needs to be checked against AGRS and TNS. In null subject languages only TNS has the noninterpretable D feature and, thus, checking is only limited to the TNS, which is not affected in these languages (Leonard, 2009). Wexler's account explains difficulties with function words such as auxiliaries, clitics, and article omissions, but not for their substitutions.

Children with SLI are assumed to have the extended period of the optional infinitive stage (Rice, Wexler, & Cleave, 1995). However, it is not clear how long children with SLI remain in the extended OI stage and what proportion of finite forms indicates the emergence from the OI stage. Because the OI stage is manifested by the omissions of finiteness markings, it is not always evident in English whether the underlying problem refers to the selection of infinitival forms in finite contexts or other factors resulting in omissions of grammatical morphemes. Although cross-linguistic data supported the OI stage in a variety of Romance and Germanic languages (e.g., in French: Paradis & Crago, 2001; in German: Rice, Noll, & Grimm, 1997; in Swedish: Hansson & Nettelbladt, 1995), not all studies are consistent with this account. In particular, Italian- and Hebrew-speaking children with SLI use the finite forms to the comparable extent as MLU-matched children (e.g., Bortolini & Leonard, 1996; Dromi, Leonard, & Shteiman, 1993). Research with bilingual children with SLI is still needed to account for their variability in the representation of the deficit across languages. For example, how the account handles the use of a place holder article in bilingual children undergoing language loss, or how language influence impacts the types of errors observed in some children (Restrepo, 2003).

Implicit Grammatical Rule Deficit Account describes the core problem of SLI as a deficit in learning, representation, and/or processing of implicit morphological rules (e.g., Gopnik, 1990; Ullman & Gopnik, 1999). Originally this account was based on the feature-deficit hypothesis, according to which tense, number, person, case, and gender features are absent in the underlying grammar of children with SLI (Gopnik, 1990). Ullman and Gopnik (1999) suggested the three-level explanation of morphological deficits in SLI: The procedural memory deficit that affects nonlinguistic functions could possibly cause an inability to learn implicit rules; the selection of the appropriate word form relies on conceptual system, which depend on declarative memory; individuals with SLI may employ a compensatory strategy by adding suffix-like endings to forms retrieved by conceptual system.

Two options are available to compensate for the deficit in acquiring morphological rules. The relatively intact lexical memory provides a compensatory way of memorizing the inflected verb forms as unanalyzed lexical items. Taking into account the appropriate age, individuals with SLI could be taught morphological rules. Lexical learning should eventually result in acquiring the inflected forms, especially in English with relatively few inflections; however, this assumption was not supported by data from adults with SLI (Gopnik & Crago, 1991). As pointed out by Leonard (1998), individuals with SLI are characterized by rather inconsistent use of inflections with the same lexical item, which cannot be predicted by this account. Moreover, Swisher, Restrepo, Plante, and Lowell (1995) found that children with SLI made greater gains in generalizing trained bound morpheme to untrained vocabulary item under an implicit-rule learning condition rather than an explicit-rule learning condition. This finding is also inconsistent with the implicit rule deficit account.

Morehead and Ingram (1973) found that children with SLI are limited in the scope of syntactic categories and syntactic rules that can be applied, which is in contrast with the implicit rule deficit account. This finding is supported by studies in other languages and in bilingual SLI children undergoing language loss. In particular, Leonard, Bortolini, Caselli, McGregor, and Sabbadini (1992) found that Italian-speaking children with SLI used articles and clitics to a lesser degree than TD MLU-matched children. Restrepo and Gutierrez-Clellen (2001) reported article omissions and gender agreement substitution as the most common types of article errors in Spanish-speaking children with SLI.

Other linguistic accounts assumed that grammatical difficulties in SLI are the result of problems in establishing structural relationships (e.g., Clahsen, Bartke, & Göllner, 1997; Rice & Oetting, 1993; Rothweiler & Clahsen, 1993; van der Lely, 1998). The Missing Agreement Account proposed that children with SLI have difficulties in establishing agreement relations between the two phrase-structure categories (Clahsen 1989, 1993; Clahsen & Hansen, 1997; Rothweiler & Clahsen, 1993). Although this claim was originally applied to German-speaking children, studies on other languages were derivable from this account (Clahsen & Hansen, 1997; Leonard, 1998). According to this approach, the following grammatical areas are problematic for children with SLI: the use of subject–verb agreement (e.g., third person singular in English; number markings on finite verbs in German and Italian), auxiliaries, gender markings on determiners and adjectives, and case markings (in German). In contrast, crosslinguistic data on Italian articles do not seem to support this proposal: Clitics and articles are reported to be used with lower percentages by children with SLI, however, when these forms are produced, they show the correct agreement marking in most cases (e.g., Leonard et al., 1992).

Van der Lely and colleagues (e.g., Bishop, Bright, James, Bishop, & van der Lely, 2000; van der Lely, 1994, 1996) proposed that there is a homogeneous subtype of SLI, which is characterized by a representational deficit for dependent relationships. In particular, children with SLI have difficulties forming or understanding structures that mark syntactic dependencies (e.g., subject–verb agreement or a pronoun case marking in English). Marshall and van der Lely (2007) extended this approach as the Computational Grammatical Complexity Hypothesis, according to which the core deficit in the representation of structural linguistic complexity is at the syntactic, morphological, and phonological levels. They argued that because problems in the three levels apply to the realization of tense, it could be a reliable marker of SLI.

In summary, despite differences among linguistic accounts, their proponents argue that individuals with SLI have language difficulties due to limitations in the grammatical knowledge. Although linguistic accounts seem to capture language characteristics of SLI crosslinguistically, not all studies are consistent with their predictions and no single approach seems to account for the wide range of cross-linguistic differences in individuals with SLI (Leonard, 2009). Further, Morgan, Restrepo, and Auza (2009) found that Spanish-speaking monolingual children with SLI demonstrated a variable linguistic profile where no single deficit in clitics, subjunctives, articles, or derivational morphemes could be identified as a clinical marker. These results therefore suggest that linguistic accounts often reflect the performance errors that are better explained through processing accounts of SLI. Further, given the variability in the SLI profile in a language such as Spanish, finding a linguistic marker as in English for bilingual SLI may not be a productive endeavor given the variability observe in bilingual and Spanish SLI. This variability may be better understood within DST and cognitive interactive processes (Kohnert, 2008).

RESEARCH IN BILINGUAL POPULATIONS WITH SLI

Despite a growing number of crosslinguistic studies, research on SLI in bilingual populations remains rather limited. Several theoretical issues can be raised with regard to bilingual individuals: the characteristics of dual-language acquisition in individuals with SLI, the linguistic and processing differences between monolingual and bilingual children with SLI, and the specific characteristics of SLI that would be used in assessment and treatment of bilingual populations. One particular phenomenon in bilingual SLI children is the role of the sociolinguistic context in the continued development of the languages the children speak. Bilingual children with SLI who attend programs in which both of the languages are stimulated, also called additive bilingual programs, demonstrate similar characteristics to those of monolingual children and no greater severity in their language (Bruck, 1982). On the other hand, children who are in subtractive language environments, where their native language is not stimulated, are at a great risk of demonstrating native language attrition (Anderson, 2004; Restrepo, 2003). However, it is possible that for some, the second language acquisition process is slowed down. To date, there are very few longitudinal studies that help us understand language acquisition in these children.

Restrepo and Kruth (2000) investigated a grammatical profile of a Spanish–English bilingual child with SLI in comparison with a TD bilingual age-matched child. Using spontaneous language samples in both languages, they found differences in the use of verb forms, tenses, pronouns, and prepositions in English and in the use of definite articles, pronouns, and prepositions in Spanish. Additionally, the language productions of the bilingual child with SLI were characterized by decreased MLU and limited syntactic complexity. The authors argued that although there is no universal marker of SLI in bilingual populations and no single theory could account for a variety of crosslinguistic characteristics, there are qualitative differences in the use of grammatical morphology that are not due to dual-language development. Further, Restrepo (2003) examined the language profiles of two bilingual children with SLI undergoing language loss. The children attended first grade in an English-only educational system and came from homes where they only spoke Spanish. One child demonstrated a decrease in syntactic length and complexity in Spanish, whereas the other child demonstrated an increase in syntactic length, but also an increase in the number of grammatical errors per sentence in Spanish. Both children demonstrated a limited variety of syntactic, morphological, and lexical forms in Spanish. Their English skills on the other hand, while they were highly ungrammatical, they had greater sentence length and complexity than Spanish, their first language. Restrepo's case studies suggest that bilingual children with SLI who live in subtractive language environments are at a great risk of losing grammatical skills in their native language indicating an interaction between linguistic and processing deficits, best explained within a DST.

Research examining sequential bilingual children's second language performance indicates that this language can have some of the same characteristics as monolingual children with LI. In addition, there can be qualitative differences from those of monolingual populations. For example, Jacobson and Schwartz (2005) investigated the English performance in bilingual children with SLI and found that they exhibited past tense difficulties, like monolingual English-speaking children do. However, they also found that the pattern of errors differed between typically developing and those with SLI. Children with SLI scored relatively better on irregular verbs and worse on novel verbs; they also exhibited more nonproductive errors such as bare stem verbs. Similarly, some of the characteristics in Restrepo's case studies indicate some errors occur only in bilingual populations like the replacement of the Spanish articles with the English "the" as in "the casa" (the house) or the form "le," which is a clitic, but the form was used as an article in one of the case studies. Both examples indicate that the children were simplifying the article system in Spanish.

These studies suggest that bilingual SLI children presents unique challenges that linguistic and processing accounts of SLI have not considered. Consistent with processing accounts and with the DST, these results are not surprising and indicate that bilingual children with language impairment in subtractive environments demonstrate different language patterns in their native language, while they continue to acquire their second language. These patterns are not predictable yet, until we conduct further longitudinal group studies.

An important issue with language impairment in bilinguals is how we differentiate language impairment from the language performance of second language learners. Paradis and colleagues (Paradis, 2007; Paradis, Crago, & Genesee, 2006; Paradis, Crago, Genesee, & Rice, 2003) investigated whether bilingual French–English-speaking children with SLI differed from monolingual age-matched children in each language in acquisition of grammatical morphology. According to the linguistic account, the core deficit of SLI is internal to the linguistic system, and therefore, it was predicted that bilingual children with SLI would not be delayed in comparison with monolingual age-matched children with SLI. Using spontaneous language samples, bilingual children with SLI were compared with monolingual speakers of French and English with and without SLI in the productions of grammatical morphemes that mark tense and nontense features. Results revealed that bilingual and monolingual children with SLI had greater difficulties with tense and nontense morphemes than TD age peers. However, there were no significant differences between bilingual and monolingual SLI groups in the use of grammatical morphemes in either language. Results were consistent with the linguistic account confirming that bilingual children with SLI performed poorly in comparison with TD monolingual children in each language, but to the same extent as monolingual age peers with SLI.

In a subsequent study, Paradis et al. (2006) investigated the use of direct object clitics in French–English bilingual and monolingual children with and without SLI. Additionally, a language-matched TD bilingual group was included to account for any possible acquisition differences between monolingual and bilingual conditions. Results revealed that bilingual children with SLI used object clitics in French to the same extent as the language-matched TD bilingual children, but significantly more often than monolingual French-speaking children with SLI. The authors concluded that because bilingual participants were not lagging behind monolingual children with SLI, the difficulties with direct object pronouns were not due to the acquisition of the two languages.

In a more recent study, we examined performance comparing Spanish language skills between monolingual children from Mexico and bilingual children in the United States attending schools in subtractive language environments. Results indicated that the bilingual children shared deficits in the same areas as monolinguals with SLI; however, the bilinguals still outperformed the monolinguals with SLI. In this case, areas that we predicted to be problematic for monolingual Spanish-speaking children with SLI also seemed to be difficult for bilinguals living in a subtractive language environment: articles, clitics, subjunctives, derivational morphemes, and rapid naming. These results indicate that norms in bilingual populations are necessary for differential diagnosis of SLI and typical language. To this end, examination of qualitative differences in the native and second language will be helpful.

Linguistic and processing accounts of SLI do not account for the language characteristics of bilingual children with SLI. Nevertheless, these accounts fit within the DST framework of language and bilingualism, which accounts for variability, the competition, and the changes within one child depending on the input and context at any given time. Bilingual children with SLI present with the same linguistic and processing difficulties that monolinguals do. However, bilingual populations in general do not perform like monolingual in some processing skills, such us working memory (Kohnert et al., 2006). Further, bilingual children educated in subtractive language environments are at risk of losing native language skills, which in turn can complicate differential diagnosis. To date, there is no evidence that this is the case for bilingual children with SLI living and educated in additive bilingual environments. In fact, research indicates that bilingual children with SLI perform as well as monolingual children with SLI (Bruck, 1982; Thordardottir, Weismer, & Smith, 1997), which seems to be the case with other populations with language impairment, such as in children with Down Syndrome (Kay-Raining Bird et al., 2005).

Future research needs to describe characteristics in bilingual children with SLI better, and theories must account for these characteristics. Moreover, information on what characteristics of bilingual SLI are universal and those that are language-specific would help in defining the population in general and in understanding the nature of the disorder. This in turn, would lead to better intervention and diagnostic protocols for these children. In addition, intervention research would benefit from examining what skills transfer crosslinguistically and what skills do not. To date, very little research is available to make informed decisions on how to best serve bilingual children with SLI.

REFERENCES

Anderson, R. T. (2004). First language loss in spanish-speaking children: Patterns of loss and implications for clinical practice. In B. Goldstein (Ed.), *Bilingual language development & disorders in Spanish-English speakers* (pp. 187–212). Baltimore, MD: Brooks Publishing.

Anderson, R., & Souto, S. M. (2005). The use of articles by monolingual Puerto Rican Spanish-speaking children with specific language impairment. *Applied Psycholinguistics, 26,* 621–647.

Archibald, L. M. D., & Gathercole, S. E. (2006). Short-term and working memory in specific language impairment. *International Journal of Language & Communication Disorders, 41,* 675–693.

Bedore, L., & Leonard, L. (2001). Grammatical morphology deficits in Spanish-speaking children with specific language impairment. *Journal of Speech, Language, and Hearing Research, 44,* 905–924.

Bedore, L., & Leonard, L. (2005). Verb inflections and noun phrase morphology in the spontaneous speech of Spanish-speaking children with specific language impairment. *Applied Psycholinguistics, 26,* 195–225.

Bortolini, U., & Leonard, L. (1996). Phonology and grammatical morphology in specific language impairment: accounting for individual variation in English and Italian. *Applied Psycholinguistics, 17(1),* 85–104.

Bishop, B., Bright, P., James, C., Bishop, S., & van der Lely, H. (2000). Grammatical SLI: a distinct subtype of developmental language impairment? *Applied Psycholinguistics, 21,* 159–181.

Bruck, M. (1982). Language impaired children's performance in an additive bilingual education program. *Applied Psycholinguistics, 3,* 45–60.

Campbell, T., Dollaghan, C., Needleman, H., & Janosky, J. (1997). Reducing bias in language assessment: Processing-dependent measures. *Journal of Speech, Language, and Hearing Research, 40,* 519–525.

Catts, H., Adlof, S., Hogan, T., & Ellis Weismer, S. (2005). Are specific language impairment and dyslexia distinct disorders? *Journal of Speech, Language, and Hearing Research, 48,* 1378–1396.

Clahsen, H. (1989). The grammatical characterization of developmental dysphasia. *Linguistics, 27,* 897–920.

Clahsen, H. (1993). Linguistic perspectives on specific language impairment. *Working Papers Series "Theorie des Lexikons"*, 37.

Clahsen, H., & Hansen, D. (1997). The grammatical agreement deficit in Specific Language Impairment: Evidence from therapy experiments In M. Gopnik (Ed.), *The inheritance and innateness of grammars* (pp. 141–160). Oxford University Press.

Clahsen, H., Bartke, S., & Göllner, S. (1997). Formal features in impaired grammars: A comparison of English and German SLI children. *Journal of Neurolinguistics, 10*(2–3), 151–171.

Dollaghan, C., & Campbell, T. F. (1998). Nonword repetition and child language impairment. *Journal of Speech, Language, and Hearing Research, 41,* 1136–1146.

Dromi, E., Leonard, L. B., & Shteiman, M. (1993). The grammatical morphology of Hebrew speaking children with specific language impairment: some competing hypotheses. *Journal of Speech and Hearing Research, 36,* 760–771.

Edwards, J., & Lahey, M. (1998). Nonword repetitions of children with specific language impairment: Exploration of some explanations for their inaccuracies. *Applied Psycholinguistics, 19(2),* 279–309.

Evans, J., & McWhinney, B. (1999). Sentence processing strategies in children with expressive and expressive-receptive specific language impairments. *International Journal of Language & Communication Disorders, 34,* 117–134.

Gass, S. & Selinker, L. (2008). *Second language acquisition. An introductory course.* NY: Routledge.

Gathercole, S. E., & Baddeley, A. D. (1990). Phonological memory deficits in language disordered children: Is there a causal connection? *Journal of Memory and Language, 29(3),* 336–360.

Gaulin, C., & Campbell, T. (1994). Procedure for assessing verbal working memory in normal school-age children: Some preliminary data. *Perceptual and Motor Skills, 79,* 55–64.

Gillam, R., Cowan, N., & Marler, J. (1998). Information processing by school-age children with specific language impairment: Evidence from a modality effect paradigm. *Journal of Speech, Language, and Hearing Research, 41,* 913–926.

Girbau, D., & Schwartz, R. G. (2008). Phonological working memory in Spanish–English bilingual children with and without specific language impairment. *Journal of Communication Disorders, 41,* 124–145.

Gopnik, M. (1990). Feature blindness: a case study. *Language Acquisition,* 1, 139–164.

Gopnik, M., & Crago, M. (1991). Familial aggregation of a developmental language disorder. *Cognition, 39,* 1–50.

Gray, S. (2003). Diagnostic accuracy and test-retest reliability of nonword repetition and digit span tasks administered to preschool children with specific language impairment. *Journal of Communication Disorders, 36,* 129–151.

Gray, S. (2004). Word learning by preschoolers with specific language impairment predictors and poor learners. *Journal of Speech, Language and Hearing Research, 47*(5), 1117–1132.

Gray, S. (2005). Word learning by preschoolers with specific language impairment effect of phonological or semantic cues. *Journal of Speech, Language and Hearing Research, 48*(6), 1452–1467.

Gutierrez-Clellen, V., Calderon, J., & Weismer, S. E. (2004). Verbal working memory in bilingual children. *Journal of Speech and Hearing Research, 47,* 863–876.

Hansson K., & Nettelbladt, U. (1995). Grammatical characteristics of Swedish children with SLI. *Journal of Speech, Language and Hearing Research, 38,* 589–598.

Herdina, P., & Jessner, U. (2002). *A dynamic model of multilingualism.* Clevedon, UK: Multilingual Matters LTD.

Hill E.L. (2001). Non-specific nature of specific language impairment: A review of the literature with regard to concomitant motor impairments. *International Journal of Language and Communication Disorders, 36,* 149–171.

Jacobson, P. F., & Schwartz, R. G. (2005). English past tense use in bilingual children with language impairment. *American Journal of Speech-Language Pathology, 14,* 313–323.

Kail, R. (1994). A method for studying the generalized slowing hypothesis in children with specific language impairment. *Journal of Speech, Language and Hearing Research, 37*(2), 418.

Kay-Raining Bird, E., Cleave, P., Trureau, N., Thordardottir, E., Sutton, A., & Thorpe, A. (2005). The language abilities of bilingual children with down syndrome. *American Journal of Speech-Language Pathology, 14,* 187–199.

Kohnert, K. (2008). *Language disorders in bilingual children and adults.* San Diego, CA: Plural Publishing.

Kohnert, K., & Derr, A. (2004). Language intervention with bilingual children. In B. Goldstein (Ed.), *Bilingual language development and disorders in Spanish-English speakers* (pp. 315–343). Baltimore: Brookes.

Kohnert, K., Windsor, J., & Ebert, K. D. (2008). Primary of "specific" language impairment and children learning a second language. *Brain and Language,* 1–11.

Kohnert, K., Windsor, J., & Yim, D. (2006). Do language-based processing tasks separate children with language impairment from typical bilinguals? *Learning Disabilities Research & Practice, 21,* 19–29.

Leonard, L. B. (1998). *Children with specific language impairment.* Cambridge, MA: The MIT Press.

Leonard, L. B. (2009). Crosslinguistic studies of child langauge disorders. In R. G. Schwartz (Ed.), *Handbook of child langauge disorders* (pp. 308–324). New York, NY: Taylor & Francis.

Leonard, L., Bortolini, U., Caselli, M. C., McGregor, K., & Sabbadini, L. (1992). Morphological deficits in children with specific language impairments: The status of features in underlying grammar. *Language Acquisition, 2,* 151–179.

Leonard, L., Bortolini, U., Caselli, M. C., McGregor, K., & Sabbadini, L. (1992). Some influences of the grammar of English- and Italian-speaking children with specific language impairment. *Applied Psycholinguistics, 9,* 39–57.

Leonard, L. B., Ellis Weismer, S., Miller, C. A., Francis, D. J., Tomblin, J. B., & Kail, R. V. (2007). Speed of processing, working memory, and language impairment in children. *Journal of Speech, Language, and Hearing Research, 50,* 408–428.

Leonard, L., Eyer, J., Bedore, L., & Grela, B. (1997). Three accounts of the grammatical morpheme difficulties of English-speaking children with specific language impairments. *Journal of Speech, Language and Hearing Research, 40,* 741–753.

Leonard, L. B., Sabbadini, L.,Volterra, V., & Leonard, J. S. (1988). Some influences on the grammar of English- and Italian-speaking children with specific language impairment. *Applied Psycholinguistics, 9,* 39–57.

Le Normand, M. T., Leonard, L., & McGregor, K. (1993). A cross-linguistic study of article use by children with specific language impairment. *European Journal of Disorders of Communication, 28,* 153–163.

Marshall, C. R., & van der Lely, H. (2007). Derivational morphology in children with grammatical-specific language impairment. *Clinical Linguistics and Phonetics, 21*(2), 71–91.

Merino, B. (1983). Language development in normal and language handicapped Spanish-speaking children. *Hispanic Journal of Behavioral Sciences, 5,* 379–400.

Morehead, D., & Ingram, D. (1973). The development of base syntax in normal and linguistically deviant children. *Journal of Speech, Language and Hearing Research, 16*, 330–352.

Morgan, G., & Morgan, S. (2009). Software for randomly generating Spanish nonwords and calculation of their phonotactic probability and neighborhood density.

Morgan, G., Restrepo, M. A., Auza, A. (2009) Variability in the grammatical profiles of Spanish-speaking children with specific language impairment. In *Hispanic Child Languages: Typical and Impaired Development.* (ed.) Grinstead, J.

Montgomery, J. W. (1995). Sentence comprehension in children with specific language impairment: The role of phonological working memory. *Journal of Speech, Language and Hearing Research, 38*(1), 187.

Montgomery, J. W. (2003). Working memory and comprehension in children with specific language impairment: What we know so far. *Journal of Communication Disorders, 36*, 221–231.

Paradis, J., & Crago, M. (2001). The morphosyntax of specific language impairment in French: Evidence for an Extended Optional Default account. *Language Acquisition, 9*, 269–300.

Paradis, J. (2007). Bilingual children with specific language impairment: Theoretical and applied issues. *Applied Psycholinguistics 28*, 551–564.

Paradis, J., Crago, M., & Genesee, F. (2006). Domain-specific versus domain-general theories of the deficit in SLI: Object pronoun acquisition by French–English bilingual children. *Language Acquisition, 13/14*, 33–62.

Paradis, J., Crago, M., Genesee, F., & Rice, M. (2003). Bilingual children with specific language impairment: How do they compare with their monolingual peers? *Journal of Speech, Language and Hearing Research, 46*, 1–15.

Peña, E., & Kester, E. S. (2004). Semantic development in Spanish-English bilinguals: Theory, assessment, and intervention. In B. Goldstein (Ed.), *Bilingual language development & disorders in Spanish-English speakers* (pp. 105–128). Baltimore, MD: Paul H. Brookes.

Radford, A. (1988). Small children's small clauses. *Transaction of the Philological Society, 86*, 1–46.

Radford, A. (1990). *Syntactic theory and the acquisition of English syntax.* Oxford:Blackwell.

Restrepo, M.A. (1998). Identifiers of predominantly Spanish-speaking children with language impairment. *Journal of Speech, Language, and Hearing Research, 41*, 1398–1411.

Restrepo, M. A. (2003). Spanish language skills in bilingual children with specific language impairment. In S. Montrul & F. Ordoñez (Eds.), *Linguistic theory and language development in Hispanic languages. Papers from the 5th Hispanic Linguistics Symposium and the 4th Conference on the Acquisition of Spanish and Portuguese* (pp. 365–374). Summerville, MA: Cascadilla Press.

Restrepo, M. A., & Gutierrez-Clellen, V. F. (2001). Article production in bilingual children with specific language impairment. *Journal of Child Language, 28*, 433–452.

Restrepo, M. A., & Kruth, K. (2000). Grammatical characteristics of a bilingual student with specific language impairment. *Journal of Children's Communication Development, 21*, 66–76.

Rice, M., Noll, R. K., & Grimm, H. (1997). An extended optional infinitive stage in German-speaking children with SLI. *Language Acquisition, 6(4)*, 255–296.

Rice, M., & Oetting, J. (1993). Morphological deficits in children with SLI: Evaluation of number marking and agreement. *Journal of Speech and Hearing Research, 36*, 1249–1257.

Rice, M., Wexler, K., & Cleave, P. (1995). Specific language impairment as a period of extended optional infinitive. *Journal of Speech, Language and Hearing Research, 38*, 850–863.

Rice, M., & Wexler, K. (1996). Toward tense as a clinical marker of specific language impairment in English-speaking children. *Journal of Speech, Language and Hearing Research, 39*, 1239–1257.

Rothweiler, M., & Clahsen, H. (1993). Dissociations in SLI children's inflectional systems: A study of participle inflection and subject-verb-agreement. *Logopedics Phoniatrics Vocology, 18(4)*, 169–179.

Schwartz, R. G. (2009). Specific language impairment. In R. G. Schwartz (Ed.), *Handbook of child language disorders* (pp. 3–43). New York, NY: Taylor & Francis.

Schul, R., Stiles, J., Wulfeck, B., & Townsend, J. (2004). How 'generalized' is the 'slowed processing' in SLI? The case of visuospatial attentional orienting. *Neuropsychologia, 42*, 661–671.

Swisher, L., Restrepo, M. A., Plante, E., & Lowell, S. (1995). Effects of implicit and explicit "rule" presentation on bound-morpheme generalization in specific language impairment. *Journal of Speech, Language and Hearing Research 38*, 168–173.

Tallal, P., & Newcombe, F. (1978). Impairment of auditory perception and language comprehension in dysphasia. *Brain and Language, 5*, 13–24.

Thordardottir, E. T., Weismer, S. E., & Smith, M. E. (1997). Vocabulary learning in bilingual and monolingual clinical intervention. *Child Language Teaching and Therapy, 13*, 215–227.

Thorn, A. S. & Gathercole, S. E. (1999). Language-specific knowledge and short-term memory in bilingual and non-bilingual children. *Quarterly Journal of Experimental Psychology, 52A*, 303–324.

Ullman, M.T, & Gopnik, M. (1999). Inflectional morphology in a family with inherited specific language impairment. *Applied Psycholinguistics, 20*, 51–117.

Ullman, M. T., & Pierpont, E. (2005). Specific language impairment is not specific to language: The procedural deficit hypothesis. *Cortex, 41*, 399–433.

van der Lely, H. (1994). Canonical linking rules: forward versus reverse linking in normally developing and specifically-language impaired children. *Cognition, 51*, 29–72.

van der Lely, H. (1996). Specifically language impaired and normally developing children: verbal passive vs. adjectival passive interpretation. *Lingua, 98*, 243–272.

van der Lely, H. (1998). SLI in children: movement, economy, and deficits in the computational-syntactic system. *Language Acquisition, 7(2–4)*, 161–192.

van der Lely, H. (2005). Domain-specific cognitive systems: insight from grammatical-SLI. *Trends in Cognitive Sciences, 9(2)*, 53–59.

Weismer, S. E. (1996). Capacity limitations in working memory: The impact on lexical and morphological learning by children with language impairment. *Topics in Language Disorders, 17*, 33–44.

Weismer, S., Evans, J., & Hesketh, L. (1999). An examination of verbal working memory capacity in children with specific language impairment. *Journal of Speech Language Hearing Research, 42*, 1249–1260.

Weismer, S. E., & Hesketh, L. (1998). The impact of emphatic stress on novel word learning by children with specific language impairment. *Journal of Speech and Hearing Research, 41*, 1444–1458.

Wexler, K., (1994). Optional infinitives, head movement and the economy of derivations. In D. Lightfoot and N. Hornstein (Eds.), *Verb movement* (pp. 305–350). Cambridge: Cambridge University Press.

Wexler, K. (1998). Very early parameter setting and the unique checking constraint: A new explanation of the optional infinitive stage. *Lingua, 106(1–4)*, 23–79.

Wexler, K. (2003). Lennenberg's dream: Learning, normal language development, and specific language impairment. In Y. Levy & J. Schaeffer (Eds.), *Language competence across populations. Towards a definition of specific language impairment* (pp. 11–62). Mahwah, NJ: Erlbaum.

Wexler, K., Schütze, C. T., & Rice, M. (1998). Subject case in children with SLI and unaffected controls: evidence for the Agr/Tns Omission Model. *Language Acquisition, 7*(2–4), 317–344.

Windsor, J., & Hwang, M. (1999). Testing the generalized slowing hypothesis in specific language impairment. *Journal of Speech, Language, and Hearing Research, 42*(5), 1205–1218.

Windsor, J., & Kohnert, K. (2004). The search for common ground: Part 1. Lexical performance by linguistically diverse learners. *Journal of Speech, Language, and Hearing Research, 47,* 877–890.

Section III

Acquired Disorders

26 Apraxia of Speech: From Psycholinguistic Theory to the Conceptualization and Management of an Impairment

Rosemary Varley

INTRODUCTION

The processes involved in word production are usually classified into a tripartite division of linguistic encoding, speech programming, and motor execution. The parallel division of acquired speech production disorders into those of aphasic, apraxic, or dysarthric origin mirror these processing phase distinctions. This chapter will explore conceptualizations of the processes involved in speech programming and their implications for the understanding and management of acquired apraxia of speech. This phase of encoding is usually viewed as postlinguistic, where the conceptual-semantic and phonological processing have been completed. The speaker has achieved an *abstract* phonological representation for an output. However abstract representations cannot drive the hardware of the speech production system. What is needed now is a process that converts the abstract representation into a neural code that can initiate the multiple movements of the articulatory system, all of which must be integrated with each other and precisely timed and targeted.

Within the community of scholars who study the process of speech programming it is possible to identify two broad families. One family can be characterized by an emphasis upon computation and assembly of speech tokens from more basic subcomponents each time a particular word is used. This type of approach is influenced by generative linguistic traditions. By this view, each time I say a word such as my name, the unconscious speech processing mechanisms in my mind activate the various subcomponents of the word and combine them together in the correct order to produce the output "Rosemary." These types of models are often described as elegant and parsimonious as they require storage of only a small number of subelements (such as the various vowel and consonants of a particular language) and from these a potentially infinite number of outputs can be generated. Hence words such as "roam," "rare," "mare" can be built out of the very same subcomponents that were the source of "Rosemary." One of the earliest elaborations of such assembly models was the slots and fillers model of Shattuck-Hufnagel (1979), where the process of speech control was seen as the generation of a set of slots for the word and a parallel but independent activation of the segments (or fillers) of the candidate lexical item. In a separate processing stage, the segments are assigned to the appropriate slot in the developing syllable structure.

The second family of scholars adopt a view of speech control that is influenced by diverse traditions such as cognitive linguistics, movement science, and neurobiological approaches. A key differentiator from assembly approaches is the weight that is given to factors such as the frequency with which a behavior occurs. Consistent with other forms of movement learning, if an action is performed frequently (e.g., a backhand shot in tennis), then a movement memory is formed that chains together the complex series of subcomponent movements. With regard to speech, if a word is said with some frequency, then a complete movement pattern (sometimes called a gestalt or schema) for that word is established, consolidated, and stored. Hence saying my name does not require me to assemble it from its subcomponent segments each time I say it. Because it is a word I have used with some frequency over the years, I simply have to activate the gestalt. Such models may not appear elegant and economical as they place greater demands upon memory capacity. However, the human brain has a very large storage capacity and costs of storage are offset by a massive reduction in demands for online computation.

This introductory sketch has outlined two broad approaches to the issue of speech control. However, the task of the novice in reading and understanding the literature on models of speech control is more complex than evaluating two opposing approaches. Like any healthy community, there is intermarriage between the two families with each tradition borrowing insights from the other. For example, in a series of articles Levelt described a dual-route model of speech control (Cholin, Levelt, & Schiller, 2006; Levelt, Roelofs, & Meyer, 1999; Levelt & Wheeldon, 1994), recognizing that different mechanisms of speech control might be involved in producing high frequency, over-learned syllables as compared to novel or low frequency ones. However, the theoretical debates have not always permeated through to discussions of the underlying psycholinguistic impairment in apraxia of speech (AOS). In the clinical arena, segmental assembly models have dominated the conceptualization and the management of AOS. In this chapter, I will explore the value of dual-route models of speech control for AOS. I will also argue that while other domains of psycholinguistic enquiry, such as models of lexical processing, have been illuminated by evidence from speech and language pathology, the area of speech control would also benefit from greater address to the evidence from AOS.

APRAXIA OF SPEECH

AOS is an impairment of speech production that can occur following damage to the movement control areas of the language dominant hemisphere. Typical sites of damage include premotor or motor association cortex and the areas to which this region is interconnected (e.g., basal ganglia and parietal somatosensory cortex, Dronkers, 1996; Luria, 1966). AOS often co-occurs with aphasia, but can also be present as an isolated disorder. It is differentiated from dysarthria through inconsistencies between the voluntary movements of speech and in the involuntary movements of the oral–laryngeal systems associated with actions such as chewing and facial expression. While the dysarthrias lead to impairment of all movements whether they are volitional or automatic, apraxia is an impairment of skilled volitional movements. The differentiation of AOS from aphasia often rests on the striking loss of speech fluency that is evident in apraxia. The speaker with AOS appears to have activated the correct word form, but then struggles and gropes toward a realization of that word. In the process of effortful construction of speech, there are multiple errors that reduce intelligibility. The temporal basis of speech is altered, with prolongation of steady-state components of speech segments and increased intersyllabic pauses. There is an overall disruption in the prosodic contour of the utterance (Kent & Rosenbek, 1983; Varley & Whiteside, 2001). In severe cases, speakers may be virtually nonverbal with only a small inventory of previously high frequency utterances available to them (e.g., "yes," "no," "bye"; Varley, Whiteside, Windsor, & Fisher, 2005).

The traditional conceptualization of the underlying psycholinguistic impairment in AOS is of a difficulty in activating segmental movement plans and combining them in order to create cohesive syllables (e.g., Darley, Aronson, & Brown, 1975). Such characterizations are entirely consistent with the observed surface behavior of speakers with AOS. The struggle and groping for articulatory positions suggests a loss of the spatial coordinates and temporal parameters of a particular segment. In the terms of segmental assembly models, the speaker with AOS appears to have an impairment of the processes involved in activating particular fillers and assigning them to their correct slot in the syllable frame. The view of AOS as a segmental access and assembly deficit has led to the development of highly principled therapies for the condition, which Square-Storer (1989) neatly characterized as *microstructural* therapies. These interventions involve redeveloping a set of segment-sized movement plans. The speaker with AOS is presented with multisensory information on the starting points of an articulatory gesture. This might involve diagrams, use of mirrors, pictures, and signs to cue the starting position for a segment. Alternatively, technology such as electropalatography might provide insight into both the starting point and the dynamics of an articulatory movement. Once the patient has acquired a basic repertoire of gestures, the patterns are combined in order to improve the capacity to form cohesive syllables. The evidence for the effectiveness of such interventions is sparse and the available evidence suggests that while microstructural therapies might result in improved performance on trained items, there is disappointing evidence for the generalization of improvements to untrained items or to more spontaneous speech (Wambaugh, Duffy, McNeil, Robin, & Rogers, 2005, 2006).

There are many reasons why an intervention may be of limited effectiveness. For example, some impairments might be intractable because they result from damage to a mechanism that is very narrowly localized within the brain. If the system is not distributed across neural sites then, in the event of damage to the processing hub, there is less potential for the rerouting of information through undamaged components. However, another reason for ineffective interventions might be that the underlying theory of a disorder is not fully correct, and if we modify the theory and motivate new therapies, then the treatment outcomes might improve.

An exploration of AOS from the perspective of gestalt or schema models might therefore be fruitful. One intriguing component of AOS symptoms is that most speakers display islands of preserved speech accuracy and fluency. The number of retained utterances might be small in speakers with severe AOS, but in cases with moderate impairment there can be a substantial inventory of fluent utterances (Varley et al., 2005). These utterances represent a conundrum for segmental assembly models of AOS. By this approach, segmental access and concatenation is necessary in converting abstract phonological representation to phonetic output. In this way, the speech control mechanism is a "final common pathway"—a term used in neurobiology to refer to the route from central control mechanisms via motor neurons to peripheral muscles. If the final common pathway is damaged, there is no pathway for the central system to communicate with the effector systems. In the case of speech, how is it that some output (e.g., "yes" but not "yacht") can jump from the central, abstract level to the effector level if the conversion mechanism is damaged? One solution to the problem is to explore the syllable or word frequency values of the preserved output. In counts of spoken word frequency "yes" has a value of 3840 per million and "yacht" is so infrequent it is not listed in the database of spoken word frequencies given by Leech, Rayson, and Wilson (2001). It would appear that higher frequency bestows protective properties to a word form, making it less susceptible to apraxic disruption. This is an indication within the overt behaviors demonstrated by people with AOS that the notion of dual mechanisms of speech control deserves exploration.

ASSEMBLY MODELS OF SPEECH CONTROL

It seems very obvious that words are made up of individual segments and that "cat" is produced from the concatenation of "c," "a," and "t." But this apparently very obvious insight is not shared by all speakers. People who have never learned to read (not because of dyslexia but because of limited access to formal education) do not share the notion that a spoken word consists of a string of segments (de Santos et al., 2004; Morias, Cary, Alegria, & Berterlson, 1979). Similarly individuals who have learned only a logographic writing system such as Chinese have difficulty making correct decisions when asked "What word do you get if you add [tʃ] to the end of the word 'purr'?" (Read, Zhang, Nie, & Ding, 1986). In addition, the segmental judgments of speakers (or more importantly, readers and writers) of languages with alphabetic spelling systems do not always reflect phonetic realities. For example, many will judge that "apple" contains five sounds and that there are five vowel sounds in spoken English. It is clear that such decisions regarding segmental composition are based upon knowledge of the orthographic coding of the word form, and these conscious judgments may provide little insight into the unconscious or implicit mechanisms of speech control.

Knowledge of an orthographic writing system might introduce bias into perceptions of the compositionality of words. However, there is a substantial body of evidence from the errors of healthy speakers that segments are important at some level of speech control and at least for some word forms. In particular, transposition, (or exchange or switch) errors such as "tog and froad" for "frog and toad," where the onsets of the two syllables have switched, indicate that at some phase in the speech control process segments are individually represented (Shattuck-Hufnagel, 1979). An assumption made in models such as the slots and fillers is that this phase is a central processing level at which conversion from the abstract phonological representation to a motoric phonetic representation takes place. In Shattuck-Hufnagel's seminal model, the activation of a representation in the phonological output lexicon results in a parallel creation of a matching syllable structure (the slots) and activation of segments that ultimately will fill the syllable slots (the fillers). In subsequent processing, segments are mapped to their appropriate slot. However, segments can be misassigned to a slot resulting in errors such as "tog and froad." Notice that the exchange error has occurred between the two syllable onsets and across word boundaries. This is typical of errors of this type, and exchanges within a syllable (e.g., changing "cat" to "tac") are rare. This would suggest that the process of phonological-to-phonetic conversion occurs only when the components of the emerging phrase or clause are simultaneously active in an output buffer. Dell (1988) proposes that the between-syllable constraint on exchange errors occurs because the nodes for individual phonemes are segregated by syllable position. Hence for English, /t/ would have two independent nodes as it can occur in syllable initial and final positions. By contrast, /h/would only occur once as it can only occur in a syllable initial position. The error of "cat" to "tac" would not occur as, following the selection of the phonological representation, the subsequent segmental activation would involve only /k/-initial, but not /k/-final. In an exchange error, /k/-initial might be assigned to another initial slot, but it is barred from entering a syllable final slot. This is a neat theoretical solution, but notice it begins to proliferate demands on storage resources and compromises the computational elegance of segmental assembly models. In addition, it blurs the distinction between slots and their fillers from the initial elaboration of this segmental model (e.g., Shattuck-Hufnagel, 1979). While the model proposed autonomy between these components, tagging fillers with slot information inevitably compromises the independence of the two elements of processing. Essentially, slots now come "for free" once the segment inventory is constrained and segregated by syllable position.

The evidence in support of segmental assembly models is drawn very largely from the errors made by healthy speakers either in naturalistic situations or in experimental manipulations where errors are induced through tongue-twister tasks (Motley & Baars, 1976). Meyer (1992) is cautious about the use of evidence that is dependent upon listeners' perceptual judgments. She points out that some of the characteristic features of exchange errors, such as their occurrence in stressed syllables or in word onsets might be due to listeners noticing errors in these perceptually prominent locations and failing to notice them in less prominent locations such as word final or unstressed positions. There are other reasons to be cautious about exchange error data. There is a remarkable absence of such errors in early child speech production and in the speech of people with various neurogenic speech and language disorders (Stemberger, 1989; Varley & Whiteside, 2001). One would predict that a young child learning to use a segmental assembly mechanism would make many errors of segmental assignment. However transposition errors appear in child speech at around the ages of six to seven, and at the same time that literacy develops. Similarly, we might expect "transpositional aphasia" to have been described. However, in impaired speech it is possible to observe many substitution errors, deletions, and contextually motivated errors such as assimilation and dissimilation, but exchange errors are uncommon. It may well be that a key factor in exchange errors is the simultaneous activation of large amounts of phonetic-phonological information; that is, all elements of the developing clause are highly activated and therefore potentially in competition with each other. In the case of pathology, less linguistic information is active as a consequence of disturbed lexical and syntactic processing, as well as postlexical impairments such as AOS. As result, there is less competing activation and therefore few exchange errors.

The predilection for exchange errors to occur across word boundaries rather than within words is important. One account for the distributional characteristics of exchange errors might be that they occur after the process of phonological-to-phonetic programming has been completed. If this were the case, then exchange errors might tell us little about the transfer of information from the phonological to the phonetic level and the processes specifically involved in word formation. Instead they might reflect the interference and interaction of simultaneously active information as a clause is fully encoded with its necessary lexical, morphophonemic, and prosodic specifications. This phase of processing is often described as an output buffer in stage models of language processing. If the source of exchange errors is from interaction of fully specified word forms in the output buffer, it remains possible that complete word forms or gestalts are inserted into the developing clause structure. Instead of transposition errors providing a window on the processes of word construction, the insight that they provide is into a postspecification process.

In summary, exchange errors provide important insights into the processes of speech control. However, the distributional characteristics of such errors—that they occur across word boundaries—indicates that there should be some caution in how we interpret them and use them to build models of the processes involved in speech control. In particular, we cannot infer that all words necessarily undergo assembly from more basic subword units. Transposition errors might occur after the process of phonological-to-phonetic conversion has occurred.

DUAL-ROUTE MODELS OF SPEECH CONTROL

Dual-route models can be found in many areas of psycholinguistics, and also in more general models of human cognition. For example, Norman and Shallice (1980) suggest that for behaviors we do repeatedly, we form scripts and schemas. These learned assemblies of behavior allow us to operate in a complex environment without having to compute everything afresh each time we do it. For example, expert clinicians have various scripts that they can activate when talking with patients—scripts for taking case histories, for breaking bad news, for describing the results of tests. However, we require a duality of behavioral control. As well as being placed in situations that are familiar, we also need resources to deal with novelty. We have to be able to generate new behaviors and to adapt to situations we have not encountered before. The expert clinician was once a novice and had to go through a demanding phase of developing a repertoire of scripts and schemas. During that phase, the novice made mistakes, was slow and nonfluent, and needed the feedback and guidance of mentors in order to learn.

In the case of language, this general notion of duality of behavioral control has not always been at the forefront of scientific enquiry. Since the 1960s, linguistics has been dominated by a generative tradition, with focus of computation of infinite outputs from a finite set of stored units (Chomsky, 1964). Within this tradition, the role of storage was minimized and the computational component maximized. This influence can be seen in assembly models of speech control. From an inventory of subunits, words can be generated afresh each time they are used. Storage could be reduced down to the inventory of phonemes/segments that a language used, or even further reduced down to atomic elements of phonemes such as distinctive features (Chomsky & Halle, 1968).

However, this generative tradition ignores two major biologically real cognition. First, the human brain has a large storage capacity—so why is there a need to minimize demands on storage? It is difficult to determine the size of the productive vocabulary of adult speakers. For example, Oldfield (1963) estimated 75,000 words for university undergraduates, while Levelt (1989) suggested 30,000 words for most adults. These are estimates of active vocabulary (i.e., words that the speaker uses), but there are also words the speaker understands but does not use (passive vocabulary). Presumably these estimates can be doubled, or trebled, for bilingual and trilingual speakers. Clearly there is a very large capacity for storing lexical information in the human mind. Second, the generative tradition ignores the fact that a successful information processor is capable of learning. If a complex action is required repeatedly, an efficient information processor will wire together its subcomponents into a complex assembly. Contrast the performance of a child learning to tie his or her shoelaces to that of an adult. A tutor might break down the complex action into subcomponent stages or segments in order to assist the child's learning. The novice's actions are slow and errorful. But once learning has occurred, the expert initiates a gestalt or cohesive action plan that is fast and fluent. The action plan has a beginning and an end point, but the skilled actor will be unable to describe the subcomponent segments of the plan. Indeed, such subcomponents no longer exist as the boundaries have been subsumed into the cohesive action plan.

Can these same notions of duality of behavioral control be applied to speech? By some accounts, speech and language is the unique achievement of the human species. From this view, "speech is special" and not subject to the same constraints and parameters that govern other domains of movement control such as shoelace-tying. But given the growing evidence of continuities between the capacities of humans and nonhuman species even in domains that were previously seen as the exclusive property of humans such as word learning (Kaminski, Call, & Fischer, 2004), the knowledge states of others (Santos, Nissen, & Ferrugia, 2006), or learning recursive patterns in auditory signals (Gentner, Fenn, Margoliash, & Nusbaum, 2006), it becomes more difficult to sustain claims that speech is special.

A dual-route speech control model proposes that linguistic units are encoded differently depending on the frequency with which they are used. High frequency units would be stored as wholes, with no requirement for assembly from subcomponent units. Linguistic items that are novel or used infrequently have to undergo some constructional work. If they begin to be used frequently, then a movement gestalt will form. In this way, a dual-route model distinguishes expert from novice performance, and the fluent speaker from the learner. Activation of a stored plan brings a number of advantages. It guarantees error-free production. Assembling a word each time it is used creates the possibility for introduction of errors, while retrieving a gestalt means that phonetic errors can be eliminated at least until the buffer phase of processing. Once encoding is error-free, there is a reduced need for feedback and checking the accuracy of outputs. Because encoding proceeds from activation rather than online computation, it is likely to be faster. Encoding via activation of macroschemata also simplifies the process of speech control. The online control of speech production is a massive (if not impossible) computational problem. Speech is fast, with fluent speech being produced at around a rate of four to six syllables per second. The speech effector system involves multiple subcomponents, the actions of which have to be constrained. Keller (1987) suggests that control of 60 individual muscle groups is required for speech. This is a computational problem with massive "degrees of freedom"—the potential to make an error is very large. If production proceeds from activation of stored gestalts, this control problem is simplified, particularly if the linguistic units that make up much of an utterance can be encoded in this way.

An influential dual-route model was proposed by Levelt and collaborators (Levelt et al., 1999; Levelt & Wheeldon, 1994). Levelt proposed the existence of a "syllabary"—a store of phonetic plans for frequently used syllables. Levelt (1992, p. 10) identifies a "paradox" that lies at the heart of assembly models of speech production, such as the slots-and-fillers model:

In fact, the frame-filling notion seems quite paradoxical. Why would a speaker go to the trouble of first generating an empty skeleton for the word, and then filling it with segments? In some way or another both must proceed from a stored phonological representation, the word's phonological code in the lexicon. Isn't it wasteful of processing resources to pull these apart first, and then to combine them again (on the risk of creating a slip).

In a complex experimental manipulation with healthy speakers, Levelt and Wheeldon provided evidence for the notion of the syllabary. They showed that the durations of high frequency syllables were shorter than phonetically similar low frequency syllables. The duration of the syllable is thought to shorten as a result of the overlap and cohesion in articulatory gestures that occurs during gestalt formation and consolidation.

Other studies have not always replicated syllable frequency influences on speech performance (Crompton, 1981). For example, Wilshire and Nespoulous (2003) found no influence of syllable frequency on the repetition and reading aloud performance of two participants with fluent aphasia. However, there were differences between studies in the analysis of speech tokens. While Levelt and Wheeldon used sensitive temporal measures, Wilshire and Nespoulous utilized perceptual judgments of error. But the nonreplication of syllable frequency effects highlights a paradox within Levelt's formulation of a dual-route model. Once frequency becomes a critical variable in determining the mechanism by which a linguistic unit is encoded, then it is not clear why the influence of frequency should be limited to a linguistic unit of predetermined size such as a syllable. Some frequently co-occurring speech gestures may correspond to syllable-sized chunks (e.g., "the"), some are multisyllable words (e.g., "goodbye"), others are phrases ("cup of tea"), and others are simple or complex clauses ("have a nice day"; "you know what I mean"). Shattuck-Hugnagel (1992) provided some early evidence that word rather than syllable structure was central in the phonological encoding process. In an experiment in which transposition errors were induced via tongue twisters, errors were significantly more frequent when the error pair shared word position ("*parade fad*"), as opposed to syllable and stress position ("re*peat fad*").

A dual-route model of speech control allows for large amounts of a speaker's outcome to be produced by the activation of stored gestalts, particularly when frequency is the determinant of encoding and there is no limit as to the size of the encoded chunk. This results in a significant simplification of the computational task confronting the speaker. Levelt and Wheeldon label production from storage as an "indirect" route of speech processing. However, in other areas of psycholinguistics where dual-route models have been explored such as reading and morphology (Coltheart, Curtis, Atkins, & Haller, 1993; Stemberger & MacWhinney, 1986) activation of information stored in lexicons is termed "direct," while processing involving computation from subunits is labeled "indirect." For purposes of consistency and clarity, the term "direct-route" is preferred here to describe activation of stored gestalts. But not all output is overlearned and the speaker must have mechanisms for dealing with novelty. Even the most frequent units in speech output were novel at some point in the genesis of a word production system. The demand for a mechanism to deal with novel outputs is at its highest at the period in the life span of peak vocabulary acquisition, typically in childhood and adolescence (Bloom, 2000). However, word learning continues throughout the life span, although the efficiency of these mechanisms and the plasticity of the phonetic learning system may reduce with age (Crompton, 1981). These are "indirect-route" resources, involving assembly from subword elements. It is not clear how indirect route processing is achieved. Levelt and Wheeldon propose that it uses assembly routines consistent with slots-and-fillers formulations of the process of speech control. It is possible that the system uses any resources it has to hand. For example, if there is a stored syllable plan that can be incorporated into a new form then the mechanism will scavenge that and insert it into the novel item. Hence low frequency multisyllabic words that contain high frequency subcomponent syllables will inherit some of the processing advantages of their higher frequency cognate (Jescheniak & Levelt, 1994). It is also likely that the capacity to recode (or transcode) auditory representations into phonetic-motoric representations is important in creating novel outputs. The establishment of an auditory representation will precede the output representation. Once input representation has been established, this can then drive the creation of new phonetic forms.

A dual-route model of speech control provides an account of how learning influences the process of speech control. Under a segmental assembly view, even the healthy adult speaker is perpetually a novice and having to construct each word form from its base components each time it is used. By contrast, a dual-route approach allows for learning and differentiates between expert and novice performance. It makes the prediction that the products of the two encoding routes might be differentiated across a range of variables. For example, response latencies might be shorter to high frequency forms due to a reduction in planning time. However, faster response times to high frequency forms in repetition or naming tasks are difficult to interpret and attribute unambiguously to a phonetic processing level. The facilitation of response might stem from nonphonetic factors such as faster word recognition and access at a phonological-lexical level (Varley, Whiteside, & Luff, 1999). The clearer discriminators of the products of the two encoding routes might be specific phonetic metrics such as syllable or word duration and measures of the extent of coarticulation (Whiteside & Varley, 1998). The duration of high frequency forms may be shorter as their production proceeds from a consolidated gestalt (Levelt & Wheeldon, 1994). Similarly, greater overlap of articulatory gestures may result from gestalt-driven production and will be reflected in measures of coarticulation. As yet, the empirical evidence for dual-mechanism approaches to speech control is limited, but the experimental agenda is clear. Investigations with healthy speakers will undoubtedly contribute to the debate, but supplementing this evidence with investigations of pathology, AOS in particular, is important. There have been great advances in psycholinguistic theory in the fields of reading and lexical processing as a result of detailed studies of individuals with acquired dyslexia and anomia. Theory development in the field of speech encoding has proceeded largely without input from pathologies and incorporating two lines of evidence from healthy and impaired speakers can only assist the development of a robust evidence base for dual-route approaches, or indeed other approaches to speech control.

AOS WITHIN A DUAL-ROUTE MODEL

What are the implications for AOS of a dual-route model of speech control? The standard theoretical approach to AOS is currently couched within the conceptualizations of segmental assembly models. The speech errors, nonfluency and groping that is evident in apraxic behavior is seen as a consequence of struggle to access correct segmental plans and to combine individual plans into cohesive syllables. Microstructural interventions aim to assist the apraxic patient to rebuild segment plans and to practice assembly routines. The approach has some difficulty in accounting for why a [s] segment might be accurately produced in "yes," but that the person with apraxia has to struggle and strive in order to achieve this articulatory gesture in isolation or tasks requiring combination of this consonant with a range of vowels.

A dual mechanism model can account for the islands of preserved production within apraxic behavior, particularly when the residual forms are of high frequency. In addition, because the model makes a fundamental discrimination between learned or expert behavior, and novel or novice performance, it can begin to provide an account of the surface signs of AOS. Beyond the preserved gestalts, the speaker with AOS has difficulty activating previously established schemata. Assuming that there is clear conceptual-semantic activation underlying the target form, the speaker will attempt to compensate for the retrieval failure and to fill the utterance gap. One option might be to attempt to build an output representation "on the fly," perhaps under guidance from the auditory input representation of the word form. The speaker with AOS is now relying on indirect encoding mechanisms in order to construct speech output. Many of the characteristics that are observed in the surface behavior of speakers with AOS such as segmental omissions, distortions and errors, prosodic abnormalities and reduced gestural overlap (Ziegler & von Cramon, 1986) might be predictable from the massive computational task of online control of speech production.

The speaker with AOS is not in the same position as a child during the period of maximal vocabulary acquisition. First, the speaker with AOS is generally an older adult. Many of the mechanisms that are necessary for "fast-mapping" of new heard inputs to output forms (Bloom, 2000) are likely to have undergone some age-related decline. This is the case for healthy older speakers; for example, it becomes increasingly difficult to learn the speech forms of a new language without the influence of earlier learned language forms. Hence the degree of "accent" in the later acquired language increases with age (Piske, MacKay, & Flege, 2001). The speech system demonstrates less plasticity and is more "frozen" and locked into existing articulatory patterns. Second, the lesions that cause AOS rarely disrupt one processing mechanism alone. In the tightly interconnected speech processing network, a lesion at one point disrupts the dynamics of processing at remote but interconnected locations (Metter, Wasterlain, Kuhl,

Hanson, & Phelps, 1981). For example, the recent description of "mirror neuron" systems in the human brain demonstrates the interconnectedness of perceptual mechanisms with action control systems (Rizzolatti & Arbib, 1998). The fundamental interconnectedness of input and output mechanisms and the likelihood of disturbed dynamics of activation across a distributed networks means that there is no guarantee that the auditory and transcoding systems necessary for indirect speech encoding are available to the speaker with AOS. This results in inadequate compensation via indirect speech assembly systems in all but a small number of speakers with AOS (Varley, Whiteside, Hammill, & Cooper, 2006).

To a student or novice reader, theoretical debates and controversies can appear dry and remote. But in the case of clinical management of a speech or language impairment, theoretical debates are the starting point for the management of an impairment. Segmental assembly models motivate one approach to therapy, while dual mechanism models allow a choice of strategies. Alongside microstructural therapy approaches, Square-Storer (1989) described the use of whole word approaches or macrostructural strategies. In particular, she outlines a key word technique. This involves taking a word that remains within the individual's repertoire (in the terms of dual-route models perhaps a residual higher frequency schema that can still be activated) and then attempting to build further word forms on the back of that schema. For example, if "yes" can still be used, can the multisyllable form "yesterday" be reestablished? This approach involves looking for the islands of retained competence and using them to build foundations for increasing speech output. Theories motivate coherent therapies, while a-theoretical therapies, based on scraps of received wisdom, do not stand up to the current demand for evidence-based clinical interventions. There are situations in which microstructural interventions are the right therapeutic strategy; for example, in an instance where the patient has good auditory ability, and a capacity to transcode from auditory to phonetic coding. But clinicians have to be able to evaluate different theoretical and therapeutic options and provide a principled case for the strategies they adopt.

SUMMARY AND CONCLUSIONS

In this chapter, I have described two broad approaches to the processes that are involved in speech encoding. One model focuses on assembly of forms from subcomponent units each time they are used. The second, a dual mechanism model, account for novel outputs by assembly, but allows for learning within the speech movement control system and production via stored gestalts. Therefore different mechanisms mediate the production of novel as opposed to overlearned, high frequency outputs. The implications of these two approaches on understanding the underlying mechanisms of AOS were explored. In particular, the presence of islands of fluent and error-free production within apraxic speech was viewed as a problem for the assembly approach, while the dual mechanism model could account for this within-individual dissociation of word production. The dual mechanism model is in need of theoretical elaboration and development of its empirical base. However, it appears a productive model and one that can inform specific clinical issues such as choice of therapeutic strategies for an individual patient.

FURTHER READING

Forum on apraxia of speech. (2001). *Aphasiology*, *15*, 39–84.

REFERENCES

Bloom, P. (2000). *How children learn the meaning of words*, Cambridge, MA: Bradford Books.

Cholin, J., Levelt, W. J. M., & Schiller, N. O. (2006). Effects of syllable frequency in speech production. *Cognition*, *99*, 205–235.

Chomsky, N. (1964). *Current issues in linguistic theory*, The Hague, The Netherlands: Mouton.

Chomsky, N., & Halle, M. (1968). *The sound pattern of English*. New York, NY: Harper and Row.

Coltheart, M., Curtis, B., Atkins, P., & Haller, M. (1993). Models of reading aloud: Dual-route and parallel distributed processing approaches. *Psychological Review*, *100*, 589–608.

Crompton, A. (1981). Syllables and segments in speech production. In A. Cutler (Ed.), *Slips of the tongue and language production* (pp. 109–162). Berlin, Germany: Mouton.

Darley, F., Aronson, A., & Brown, J. (1975). *Motor speech disorders*. Philadelphia, PA: W.B. Saunders.

Dell, G. (1988). The retrieval of phonological forms in production: Test of predictions from a connectionist model. *Journal of Memory and Language, 27*, 124–142.

de Santos Loureiro, C., Braga, L. C., do Nascimento Souza, L., Filho, G. N., Queiroz, E., & Dellatolas, G. (2004). Degree of illiteracy and phonological and metaphonological skills in unschooled adults. *Brain and Language, 89*, 499–502.

Dronkers, N. (1996). A new brain region for coordinating speech articulation. *Nature, 384*, 159–161.

Gentner, T. Q., Fenn, K. M., Margoliash, D., & Nusbaum, H. C. (2006). Recursive syntactic pattern learning by songbirds. *Nature, 440*, 1204–1207.

Jescheniak, J. D., & Levelt, W. J. M. (1994). Word frequency effects in speech production: Retrieval of syntactic information and of phonological form. *Journal of Experimental Psychology: Learning, Memory and Cognition, 20*, 824–843.

Kaminski, J., Call. J., & Fischer, J. (2004). Word learning in a domestic dog: Evidence for 'fast mapping'. *Science, 304*, 1682–1683.

Keller, E. (1987). The cortical representations of motor processes of speech. In E. Keller & M. Gopnik (Eds.), *Motor and sensory processes of language*. Hillsdale, NJ: Lawrence Erlbaum Associates Inc.

Kent, R., & Rosenbek, J. (1983). Acoustic patterns in apraxia of speech. *Journal of Speech and Hearing Research, 25*, 231–249.

Leech, G., Rayson, P., & Wilson, A. (2001). *Word frequencies in written and spoken English*. Harlow, UK: Longman.

Levelt, W. J. M. (1989). *Speaking: From intention to articulation*. Cambridge, MA: MIT Press.

Levelt, W. J. M. (1992). Accessing words in speech production: Stages, processes and representations. *Cognition, 42,* 1–22.

Levelt, W. J. M., Roelofs, A., & Meyer, A. S. (1999). A theory of lexical access in speech production. *Behavioral and Brain Sciences, 22,* 1–75.

Levelt, W. J. M., & Wheeldon, L. (1994). Do speakers have access to a mental syllabary? *Cognition, 50,* 239–269.

Luria, A. R. (1966). *The higher cortical functions in man.* New York, NY: Basic Books.

Metter, E. J., Wasterlain, C. G., Kuhl, D. E., Hanson, W. R., & Phelps, M. E. (1981). [18]FDG positron emission computed tomography in a study of aphasia. *Annals of Neurology, 10,* 173–183.

Meyer, A. S. (1992). Investigation of phonological encoding through speech error analyses: Achievements, limitations, and alternatives. *Cognition, 42,* 181–211.

Morias, J., Cary, L., Alegria J., & Berterlson, P. (1979). Does awareness of speech as a sequence of phones arise spontaneously? *Cognition, 7,* 323–331.

Motley, M. T., & Baars, B. J. (1976). Laboratory indication of verbal slips: A new method for psycholinguistic research. *Communication Quarterly, 24,* 28–34.

Norman, D., & Shallice, T. (1980). Attention to action: Willed and automatic control of behaviour. In R. Davidson, G. Schwartz, & D. Shapiro (Eds.), *Consciousness and self-regulation: Advances in research and theory.* New York, NY: Plenum Press.

Oldfield, R. C. (1963). Individual vocabulary and semantic currency: A preliminary study. *British Journal of Social and Clinical Psychology, 2,* 122–130.

Piske, T., MacKay, I. R. A., & Flege, J. E. (2001). Factors affecting degree of foreign accent in an L2: A review. *Journal of Phonetics, 29,* 191–215.

Read, C., Zhang, Y., Nie, H., & Ding, B. (1986). The ability to manipulate speech sounds depends on knowing alphabetic writing. *Cognition, 24,* 31–44.

Rizzolatti, G., & Arbib, M. A. (1998). Language within our grasp. *Trends in Neuroscience, 21,* 118–194.

Santos, L. R., Nissen, A. G., & Ferrugia, J. A. (2006). Rhesus monkeys, *Macaca mulatta,* know what others can and cannot hear. *Animal Behaviour, 71,* 1175–1181.

Shattuck-Hufnagel, S. (1979). Speech errors as evidence for a serial-ordering mechanism in sentence production. In W. E Cooper & E. C. T. Walker (Eds.), *Sentence processing: Psycholinguistic studies presented to Merrill Garrett* (pp. 295–342). Hillsdale, NJ: Lawrence Erlbaum.

Shattuck-Hufnagel, S. (1992). The role of word structure in segmental serial ordering. *Cognition, 42,* 213–259.

Square-Storer, P. (1989). Traditional therapies for apraxia of speech reviewed and rationalized. In P. Square-Storer (Ed.), *Acquired apraxia of speech in adults.* Hove, UK: Lawrence Erlbaum Associates Ltd.

Stemberger, J. P. (1989). Speech errors in early child language production. *Journal of Memory and Language, 28,* 164–188.

Stemberger, J. P., & MacWhinney, B. (1986). Form-orientated inflectional errors in language processing. *Cognitive Psychology, 18,* 329–354.

Varley, R. A., & Whiteside, S. P. (2001). What is the underlying impairment in acquired apraxia of speech? *Aphasiology, 15,* 39–49.

Varley, R., Whiteside, S., Hammill, C., & Cooper, K. (2006). Phases in speech encoding and foreign accent syndrome. *Journal of Neurolinguistics, 19,* 356–369.

Varley, R. A., Whiteside, S. P., & Luff, H. (1999). Dual-route speech encoding in normal and apraxic speakers: Some durational evidence. *Journal of Medical Speech and Language Pathology, 7,* 127–132.

Varley, R., Whiteside, S. P., Windsor, F., & Fisher, H. (2005). Moving up from the segment: A comment on Aichert and Ziegler's syllable frequency and syllable structure in apraxia of speech. *Brain and Language, 96*, 235–239.

Wambaugh, J. L., Duffy, J. R., McNeil, M. R., Robin, D. A., & Rogers, M. A. (2005). Evidence-based guidelines for the management of acquired apraxia of speech: Technical report. American Academy of Neurologic Communication Disorders and Sciences.

Wambaugh, J. L., Duffy, J. R., McNeil, M. R., Robin, D. A., & Rogers, M. A. (2006). Treatment guidelines for acquired apraxia of speech: A synthesis and evaluation of the evidence. *Journal of Medical Speech Language Pathology, 14*, xv–xxxxiii.

Whiteside, S. P., & Varley, R. A. (1998). A reconceptualisation of apraxia of speech: A synthesis of evidence. *Cortex, 34*, 221–231.

Wilshire, C. E., & Nespoulous, J.-L. (2003). Syllables as units in speech production: Data from aphasia. *Brain and Language, 84*, 424–447.

Ziegler, W., & von Cramon, D. (1986). Disturbed coarticulation in apraxia of speech: Acoustic evidence. *Brain and Language, 29*, 34–47.

27 The Role of Memory and Attention in Aphasic Language Performance

Malcolm McNeil, William Hula,
and Jee Eun Sung

INTRODUCTION

There is a scientific paradigm (Kuhn, 1962) within which research in aphasia is conducted. This paradigm encompasses the tacit assumptions about the underlying nature of the disorder (aphasia in this case) and in general dictates the kind of the research questions and methods used for answering them that is acceptably conducted by its practitioners. The paradigm is determined by the majority of the scientists working in the discipline. Although there is the possibility of coexisting paradigms for the clinical practice in aphasia on the one hand and theory-driven investigation of aphasia on the other, the practice of science in most Western cultures dictates coherence between them and the theoretical perspective typically holds more capital than the clinical one. That is, because it is generally believed that theory is the guiding principle for practice, the theoretical paradigm typically has a strong and perhaps dominating influence on the clinical paradigm. Such is the case with clinical aphasiology. This theoretical paradigm may be best characterized as the *centers and pathways* paradigm and is a direct descendent of the Wernicke/Lichtheim model of aphasia (Eggert, 1977). It is based on the notion that there are language centers in the brain that house specific linguistic rules and representations and that these centers are connected to one another by direct pathways. To illustrate, within this centers and pathways conceptualization of aphasia, the arcuate fasciculus pathway connects the posterior temporal lobe (putative) language comprehension center (Wernicke's area) to the inferior and posterior two-thirds of the third frontal convolution (putative) speech production center (Broca's Area). These centers and this specific pathway allow the association of representations and the performance of specific linguistic computations and language tasks (e.g., speech repetition in this instance). The aphasia classification system adhered to by the majority of aphasiologists best represents this scientific paradigm and is firmly grounded in this "anatomical connectionist" (not to be confused with "computational connectionist") models of aphasia. Within this model of aphasia, damage to a specific center (e.g., Wernicke's area) or a specific pathway (e.g., the arcuate fasciculus) will yield a specific pattern of language (Wernicke's Aphasia) or modality (repetition deficit in "Conduction Aphasia") deficit respectively, which corresponds to a "classical" type or category of aphasia (Geschwind, 1965a, 1965b; Goodglass, Kaplan, & Barresi, 2001; Kertesz, 1979). In general, this model of aphasic deficits, and the adherents of its derived classification system have tended to view aphasia as a loss of representations subserving specific language functions due to the damaged language center or the damaged or disconnected pathway. In its strongest formulations, it is assumed that the rules and the representations have either been deleted from the patient's repertoire or become permanently inaccessible because of a structural lesion in the relevant neural substrates responsible for the language computation or association. This assumption is reflected in definitions of aphasia as a "loss" of language (Benson, 1979), and in some formal theories and hypotheses proposed to account for specific signs and symptoms of aphasia such as the "trace deletion hypothesis" of Grodzinsky (2000), which was proposed to account for the failure of specific syntactic operations. Proponents of the centers and pathways model have tended to emphasize the differences among persons with aphasia by dividing them into the model-derived behavioral categories arranged along modality and psycholinguistic dimensions.

There is another view of the underlying mechanisms of aphasia held by a relatively small minority of aphasiologists. This view holds that some other part of the cognitive apparatus (e.g., attention or memory) may serve as an explanatory mechanism. This view of aphasia has been described to be in opposition to the classical anatomical connectionist view. For example, a view of aphasia that incorporates attention as an important construct tends to have more in common with accounts that emphasize the commonality of impairments among persons with aphasia. This view regards aphasia as a disorder of performance in which representations are not lost, but access to representations or moment-to-moment failures to map obligatory components of the language system (the assembly of representations) is impaired. This view of language and aphasia suggests that components of language (e.g., phonology, morphology, syntax) are always the product of online computations involving much smaller units of information and complex mapping processes among them. From this perspective it follows that a failure of the processes used to build the relevant products can account for the observed linguistic disorders. Processing models of language such as that proposed by Saffran, Schwartz, and Marin (1980) and computational models such as that of Martin, Dell, Saffran, and Schwartz (1994) have provided converging evidence for some of the hypothesized mechanisms underlying the observed pathologies of language and have highlighted some of the processes for the online construction of representations. Process and computational models of language pathologies are generally favored by the research community and the rather simplistic "loss" view of language is infrequently adhered to by aphasia researchers. Nevertheless, the "loss" view of aphasia permeates the nonaphasiologists' views of aphasia and is with very rare exception, held among health care professionals outside of the aphasia research community (Craven & Hirnle, 2009). It also is the norm among rehabilitation specialists, including those charged with the treatment of aphasia. As summarized by Hula and McNeil (2008), it is recognized that one consequence of assuming that linguistic units are deleted or made permanently unavailable is that treatment is then directed toward the restoration of those units with the intent of replacing the lost components. Additionally, this position has promoted diagnostic tools that have focused on quantifying *how much* or *what specific representations* are left intact. This has lead clinicians to attempt to assay vocabulary (e.g., the number of words within specific word classes), or determine those specific phonemes, derivational morphemes, syntactic structures, or semantic categories that remain in the patient's repertoire. These assumptions have given rise to aphasia treatment as "teaching"; as one might structure linguistic experience for first language acquisition or as one would systematically expose a person to a second language by providing them the specific representations (e.g., the phonology or the lexical forms) and rules (e.g., the morphologic and syntactic structures; pragmatic or situational contextual rules) for assembly and usage. This type of treatment is frequently administered in a didactic format. However, the alternative view that language representations are preserved in aphasia and that aphasic language performance is due to an impaired processing mechanism suggests that specific representations, rules, or language content may not be the most appropriate targets for rehabilitation. Instead, the underlying processing deficits might be used to organize the content of treatment, and measurements of the impaired process(es) might become primary or intermediate outcome targets.

Consistent with the view of aphasia that holds that the language representations and the rules used for their assembly are fundamentally intact in persons with aphasia is the claim that the cognitive support system necessary for "doing" language or building the representations and forming the necessary mappings among components of the linguistic system is responsible for the impaired products. Variants of this view have been discussed as "processing" or "access" impairments, and have been explored within a number of psychological constructs, but most frequently and productively as "memory" and "attention."

While strong assumptions about the localization of the brain lesion underlying aphasia types are frequently made from the centers and pathways model (Weems & Reggia, 2007), the alternative *"processing"* approaches have tended* to minimize the connections between specific aphasic symptoms and circumscribed lesion sites and have emphasized both the similarities between persons with aphasia and the variability within them according to both internal and external factors.

---

* While considerably less effort has been expended investigating lesion correlates of impaired attention or memory deficits in persons with aphasia than has been devoted to the correlation of lesion localization with aphasia syndrome, there has been considerable investigation of the neural substrates of attention and memory, independent of pathologies ascribed to these cognitive processes (Botvinick, Nystrom, Fissell, Carter, & Cohen, 1999; Larson, Kaufman, & Perlstein, 2009; West, 2003; West & Alain, 2000).

The writings of Freud (1953), Marie (1906), and Head (1926; reviewed by: Caplan, 1987; Darley, 1982; Schuell, Jenkins, & Jimenez-Pabon, 1964) emphasized the unidimensionality of the disorder. These early aphasiologists have provided an important historical background for theories that are consistent with the view of aphasia as a disorder that affects language-specific cognitive operations but is itself not a primary disorder of language; a perspective that underlies a memorial, attentional, or impaired processing view of aphasia. In the processing view, the elemental language representations and the algorithms used for their construction are proposed to be essentially intact. Again, this is differentiated from primary language differences or impairments such as that seen in second language learners or individuals who have not yet acquired the rules and representations due to maturation, social/cultural deprivation, or with severe cognitive impairments as may occur in some persons with autism or mental retardation.

MOTIVATING ARGUMENTS FOR A *PROCESSING* VIEW OF APHASIA

An alternative to the *centers and pathways* view and definition of aphasia has been proposed because there are a number of observations about aphasia that suggest fundamentally preserved linguistics (both linguistic rules and representations) as well as preserved processing capacities that are adequate for successful language functioning in the presence of the observed language impairments. Several indirect sources of evidence have been proposed to support the notion and that a source for the "breakdown" in language performance must be explained by the cognitive mechanisms involved in building the representations and not the loss of any of the building blocks themselves. Additionally, these mechanisms cannot involve a permanent or static impairment in the ability to enlist the cognitive mechanisms necessary for accomplishing the construction of the linguistic representations. A search for the source of these impaired cognitive mechanisms has taken a variety of forms including the description and experimental manipulation of behavioral patterns of performance (Hageman & Folkstad, 1986; Hageman, McNeil, Rucci-Zimmer, & Cariski, 1982; McNeil, Hageman, & Matthews, 2005) as well as anatomical (Nelson, Reuter-Lorenz, Persson, Sylvester, & Jonides, 2009; Thompson-Schill, Bedny, & Goldberg, 2005; Thompson-Schill et al., 2002) and physiological indices (King & Kutas, 1998; Peach, Rubin, & Newhoff, 1994). In support of their proposal that aphasia is the result of impairments in the underlying cognitive apparatus that supports language (the ability to allocate attentional or processing resources supporting language in this specific instance), McNeil and colleagues (McNeil, 1982, 1988; McNeil & Kimelman, 1986; McNeil, Odell, & Tseng, 1991) appealed to several phenomena that are inconsistent with the centers and pathways paradigm. They observed that aphasia affects all domains (phonology, morphology, syntax, semantics) and modalities of language (see Darley, 1982 for review). McNeil et al. (1991), in particular, took issue with the idea that damage to specific linguistic operations (e.g., coindexing of pronouns) could account for aphasic performance, and furthermore challenged the empirical bases of single- and double-dissociations (Odell, Hashi, Miller, & McNeil, 1995), which constitute much of the evidence for such arguments. They proposed that the broad impairments typically observed in aphasia can only be accounted for by a "superordinate mechanism [that] is shared by linguistic processing units" (McNeil et al., 1991, p. 28). Results showing that the centers and pathways derived aphasia categories are not reliable predictors of the syntactic comprehension of different sen tence types (e.g., Caplan, Waters, & Hildebrandt, 1997) are consistent with this view.

Second, a variety of linguistic and nonlinguistic factors, such as word stress (Kimelman & McNeil, 1987; Pashek & Brookshire, 1982), phonemic, semantic, and phrase cueing (Podraza & Darley, 1977), perceptual redundancy of visual naming stimuli (Benton, Smith, & Lang, 1972; Bisiach, 1966), and rate of presentation of auditory stimuli (Gardner, Albert, & Weintraub, 1975; Weidner & Lasky, 1976) can stimulate correct or improved language performance in persons with aphasia (for review, see Darley, 1976, 1982; Duffy & Coelho, 2001). More recently, repetitive transcranial magnetic stimulation to the right-hemisphere homologue of Broca's area was claimed to improve naming in some persons with aphasia in the absence of other treatment (Naeser et al., 2005). This stimulability of aphasic persons for correct or improved performance in the absence of specific linguistic information can only be explained by a disorder of processing language in which the fundamental rules and representations are preserved.

McNeil (1982, 1983, 1988) and McNeil et al. (1991) also noted that persons with aphasia are highly variable in their performance and that this variability cannot be accounted for by a loss of representations or functions. The specific kind of variability to which they refer is the tendency of persons with aphasia to respond differently to the same stimulus under the same contextual conditions on repeated presentations over very short periods of time such as days, minutes, or even seconds. The recognition of this sort of variability is not new and evidence for it can be found prominently in the work of Kreindler and Fradis (1968), who concluded that variability was fundamental to the disorder. More recent work has documented substantial variability of performance over brief periods of time on the same or similar items on a variety of task such as auditory comprehension and naming performance. With regard to auditory comprehension, it has been demonstrated that persons with aphasia can vary widely in their performance across homogeneous items (McNeil & Hageman, 1979; McNeil, Odell, & Campbell, 1982) but with sufficient numbers of homogeneous stimuli, reliable patterns of variability can be captured (Hageman et al., 1982). Furthermore, this variability is not limited to the moment-to-moment fluctuations of performance. In one naming study (Freed, Marshall, & Chulantseff, 1996), five individuals with mild to moderate aphasia were presented with 100 pictures five times over five consecutive days. Across individuals, 10–38% of the pictures elicited correct responses on some administrations with incorrect responses on one or more others. On average, across subjects, approximately 23% of the pictures were named with inconsistent correctness/incorrectness over the five sessions. Other studies have produced similar results supporting the conclusion that, despite relatively consistent overall or averaged error rates on repeated trials of the same stimuli, success or failure at naming a particular item in one instance is not an especially reliable predictor of performance on that item on a subsequent occasion (Crisman, 1971; Howard, Patterson, Franklin, Morton, & Orchard-Lisle, 1984). More recently, Caplan, Waters, DeDe, Michaud, and Reddy (2007) appealed to the notion of processing resources to account for the prominent variability they observed in sentence comprehension in a large group of unselected individuals with aphasia.

One explanation for the large moment-to-moment or repeated trial variability across all tasks in persons with aphasia could be that individuals have a number of ways to solve linguistic computational requirements and that there is a great deal of flexibility in compensation or strategy selections*. However, this does not explain why individuals would routinely select suboptimal solutions, either consciously or unconsciously. Ultimately, the underlying mechanisms that account for this within-task variability are *not* consistent with a "loss" of linguistic representations, rules, or to the cognitive apparatus used for processing language. That persons with aphasia are variable has received increasing support (Caplan et al., 2007; Crisman, 1971; Freed et al., 1996; Howard et al., 1984; Kreindler & Fradis, 1968) since early suggestions that variability should play an important role in the understanding of the underlying mechanisms in aphasia (McNeil, 1982). Linguistic variability was viewed by Kolk (2007) as a "hallmark of aphasic behavior." Indeed, Kolk proposed, as others had before him (McNeil, 1982, 1988) that an interaction between the language and an executive system would be required to account for this variability. Additionally, he proposed that a processing cost account was necessary to explain aphasic variability in syntactic processing. We extend this necessity to all linguistic domains and processing modalities.

A fourth argument marshaled by McNeil (1982, 1988) in favor of aphasia as a performance deficit concerns the fact that aphasia can be transient. Ictal and post-ictal aphasia has been reported in patients with epilepsy (Hamilton & Matthews, 1979; Lebrun, 1994; Lecours & Joanette, 1980; Linebaugh, Coakley, Arrigan, & Racy, 1979) with return to normal linguistic and cognitive status surrounding the episode. Aphasia is not an uncommon sign, with rapidly resolving or intermittent appearance with transient ischemic attacks (Mlcoch & Metter, 2001) and other neurological conditions (Kaminski, Hlavin, Likavec, & Schmidley, 1992; Rahimi & Poorkay, 2000).

Finally, McNeil (1982, 1988) suggested that the qualitative similarity of language performance in normal and aphasic individuals provides evidence that aphasia is best considered a disorder in the efficiency with which language is constructed or representations are built rather than one in which linguistic rules

---

* A great deal of variability has also been demonstrated to occur across language modalities (gesturing, writing, talking, reading, and listening) and across components of language, however, psycholinguistic operations unique to each processing modality could account for a substantial proportion of this variability. This source of within-subject variability will not be discussed here.

or representations are lost or permanently inaccessible. The idea that aphasic language performance represents a low end on a continuum shared with normal performance is not a new realization and was embraced by earlier aphasiologists (e.g., Freud, 1953). A number of empirical studies have demonstrated that persons with aphasia and normal individuals produce similar patterns of responses on a variety of language comprehension (Bates, Friederici, & Wulfeck, 1987; Brookshire & Nicholas, 1980, 1984; Dick et al., 2001; Hageman, 1980; Kilborn, 1991; McNeil et al., 1982; Miyake, Carpenter, & Just, 1994; Nicholas & Brookshire, 1986; Shewan, 1976; Shewan & Canter, 1971), language production (Ernest-Baron, Brookshire, & Nicholas, 1987; Schwartz, Saffran, Bloch, & Dell, 1994; Silkes, McNeil, & Drton, 2004), and grammaticality judgment (Bates et al., 1994; Blackwell & Bates, 1995; Wilson, Saygin, Schleicher, Dick, & Bates, 2003) tasks. These patterns have been realized when the normal individuals are stressed by time pressure, task complexity, or competing tasks. The relevance of these observations and the normal-to-aphasic continuum (also called the "continuity hypothesis") for understanding the nature of aphasic language impairment is that a structural lesion or an impaired linguistic system is not necessary to produce linguistic behaviors indistinguishable from those that characterize and define aphasia. Further, the cognitive conditions under which these patterns can be elicited may provide models for testing mechanisms underlying specific aphasic behaviors as well as for assessing diagnostic and treatment methods.

IF NOT A DISORDER OF THE LINGUISTIC UNITS, WHAT THEN?

THE ROLE OF MEMORY IN APHASIC LANGUAGE DEFICITS

Aphasia is typically defined as a "language disorder" or more rarely as a disorder that affects language (McNeil & Pratt, 2001). Linguistic constructs are used for its description and linguistic theory is applied as explanation for the behaviors observed. Indeed, aphasia is a disorder that affects language-specific behavior and is separated from its clinical neighbors by the presence of these disorders in the context of other intact cognitive functions such as procedural memory, affective and personality characteristics, perception, visual–spatial abilities, movement or motor abilities, or general world knowledge. Aphasia can coexist with disorders in these other domains of knowledge or processing; however, its diagnosis requires strong evidence that it cannot be accounted for by impairments of affect, movement, musical or artistic ability or by primary impairments of memory. However, memory (in addition to attention and other conceptualizations of executive functions, discussed below) is always utilized for the activation of language representations, the application of linguistic rules and for the necessary integration of the many products derived from the multiple linguistic components of language construction. Therefore, deficits in the storage of linguistic information for comprehension and the retrieval of information for production define aphasia and are, by their very nature, impairments of memory for linguistic information. The *centers and pathways* paradigm requires acceptance of the proposition that the deficits are not within the operations of the memory system per se, but rather within the linguistic computations. This is required because it is assumed that memorial systems are general purpose processing devices that serve all cognitive systems and would, if impaired, obligatorily affect nonlinguistic cognitive operations as well as linguistic ones. The argument is that aphasia is not a disorder of memory (or attention), because these other domains of cognition (e.g., perception, motor, visual–spatial, nonlinguistic reasoning, etc.), are by definition excluded in aphasia. However, impairments of these cognitive functions could subtend the impairments within the language-specific domain in persons with aphasia if linguistic-specific memory and attention systems existed and if they could be differentially or selectively impaired. This proposition is certainly consistent with many models of linguistic processing that are integrated within the constructs of memory and attention (e.g., Baddeley's working memory model, discussed later in this chapter).

Several theories of memory have been proposed that account for many aspects of language performance (e.g., Gibson, 1998; Gibson & Pearlmutter, 2000) and for those behaviors that characterize aphasia (e.g., Martin & Saffran, 1997).[*] There is in fact a relatively long history of research into impaired memory systems in aphasia. One review of this research (McNeil, 1988) concluded that long-term memory (LTM; either episodic or semantic) was unrelated to the language impairments in aphasia; at least in the sense that persons with aphasia do not "forget" how to do things that they knew pre-morbidly (fix a motor, make a bed, drive a car, or bake a cake) and they do not forget world events, people that they know or how to get from point A to point B, or what they comprehended minutes or hours before. One source of evidence supporting this later claim comes from the work on immediate and delayed story retelling. Bayles, Boone, Tomoeda, Slauson, and Kaszniak (1989) for example, demonstrated that persons with aphasia performed similarly to normal elderly individuals, and significantly better than individuals with mild Alzheimer's disease (AD) on a story retelling following a 60-minute filled delay. While the amount of information retold in the immediate condition by persons with both aphasia and AD can be expected to vary considerably across individuals (and to correlate highly with the overall severity of their comprehension deficits in the persons with aphasia), the story information that was comprehended and stored by the persons with aphasia, unlike that also initially comprehended by the persons with AD, was clearly held in LTM by whatever mechanisms that were available (e.g., rehearsal, chunking strategies, association with LTM, etc.). Additionally, they were accessible for recall without substantive decrement (not greater than normal-nonimpaired individuals).

Such preservation of performance is not the case with short-term memory (STM) as measured by span tasks (Adamovich, 1978; Albert, 1976; Cermak & Moreines, 1976; Cermak & Tarlow, 1978; Flowers, 1975; Swinney & Taylor, 1971).

[*] It must be remembered that observed diminished performance, relative to normal or pathological control groups on most tasks used to assess memory for language can as easily be attributed to impairments of linguistic computation as to impaired mechanisms of storage and retrieval.

Indeed, a review of the STM literature suggests that span is always impaired in large unselected groups of persons with aphasia compared to nonbrain damaged control groups and in most studies yields language spans of approximately 50% ($\pm 30\%$; or approximately $3.5, \pm 1$) of the normal control population ($7, \pm 2$; or approximately 30% of the normal span) regardless of language task. Furthermore, span tasks do not appear to separate populations by aphasia type, even when the recall tasks are optimized to detect the suspected underlying grammatical (Broca) versus semantic (Wernicke) deficit (Caramazza, Zurif, & Gardner, 1978). They also do not separate normal from aphasic performance by the serial exhaustive versus self-terminating type of search (Warren, Hubbard, & Knox, 1977) or by the presence or absence of top-down strategies used for aiding STM (Lubinski & Chapey, 1978).

However, STM has been recognized as being only one integrally linked component of the memory system when engaged for language processing. An important development in the identification of independent components within the memory system was provided by Baddeley and Hitch (1974) as a working memory (WM) system. This model was later elaborated by Baddeley (1986, 1993), and Baddeley and Logie (1999) among many others and it has had a large and enduring impact on models of linguistic processing. It was originally proposed to contain two independent and cognitively autonomous systems: a "phonological loop," concerned with maintenance and processing of acoustic and verbal information, and the "visuospatial sketchpad," which supports the same functions for nonlinguistic visual and spatial information (Baddeley, 1986). The activities of these two components were proposed to be regulated and coordinated by a "central executive." This phonological loop was proposed as a STM or "storage" system within which linguistic processing or a computation (work) is performed. The STM buffer is limited in the quantity of information that it can hold and the timecourse over which the work of the computation can occur. The central executive system is responsible for supplying the necessary attention or effort for both the computations and maintenance of information within the STM buffer as well as the other necessary information processing operations (e.g., goal maintenance, response selection, etc.) required for linguistic comprehension and production. Critically, the STM, as well as the computational part of the model, require access to, and continuous support from the attentional component of the central executive. Failure or degraded performance on tasks considered to be valid measures of WM can occur because of a failure of any of the three components of the model. Importantly, the computations as well as the STM system are considered by the current authors to be relatively fixed properties of the architecture and have person-specific defined capacity limitations. However, the central executive component of the WM system is viewed as a resource that can be variably and proportionally allocated in service of the processing/computations and the storage components of the WM system. As such, in our view, it is only this component of the WM system that has the potential to account for the phenomena described above that the *centers and pathways* account cannot. Nonetheless, the study of, and identified impairment of WM has become synonymous with impairments of any component of the model. Within this frame of reference, an impairment of WM does not separate which component(s) of the model are impaired. This lack of specificity has not only confused the assignment of impairment within the functional architecture, but it has diminished the search for the underlying impairment in persons performing pathologically on tests of WM. Importantly, this conflation has been well recognized by Baddeley and colleagues and has received substantial experimental and theoretical attention by many cognitive scientists (e.g., Cowan, 1995, 1999; Engle, Kane, & Tuholski, 1999; Shah & Miyake, 1999).

It is important to discuss WM in the context of a chapter focused primarily on attention and aphasia. The popularity of WM models, the important role that the central executive is believed to play in the overall success of the models, and the conflation of the three elements of the WM models requires consideration. Considerable work on attention and resource allocation has been conducted within the WM framework as well outside of it. The remainder of this discussion will focus on the role of the attentional system (controlled and automatic) in language processing and its potential as a viable account for the phenomenology of aphasia.

WORKING MEMORY, ATTENTION, AND RESOURCE ALLOCATION

Several WM models subsequent to Baddeley and colleagues have developed the notion of the central executive by employing "capacity" or "resource" concepts from the attentional literature. Just and Carpenter (1992, p. 124), for example, described this component of the model as "an energy source," which was analogous to Kahneman's (1973) attention resource capacity and they placed their theory in the tradition of Kahneman's work. They defined WM capacity as the activation available for supporting either of the two functions (storage and processing). They suggested that a unitary pool of resources is engaged in both language computations and in the maintenance of information used for the computation and for the storage of their products.

Such a line of research arguing that there is a single pool of resources utilized for all verbally mediated tasks predicts that there should be a trading relationship (though not necessarily an equivalent cost between components) between storage and computation when the overall task demands are high enough to exceed the individuals' available resources (Just & Carpenter, 1992; King & Just, 1991; MacDonald, Just, & Carpenter, 1992; Miyake et al., 1994). One way in which this trading relationship has been demonstrated in the context of sentence comprehension is by means of reading span tasks (Daneman & Carpenter, 1980). This specific task requires participants to read sentences and at the same time remember the final word from each sentence presented within a given set. Listening span versions of the task also have been developed (e.g., Gaulin & Campbell, 1994; Tompkins, Bloise, Timko, & Baumgaertner, 1994) and unlike their reading counterparts, have received at least basic psychometric development. According to Just and Carpenter (1992), some individuals may have greater total capacity and/or use their available resources more efficiently. These persons are expected to score high on WM span tasks and demonstrate better performance on a variety of sentence processing measures. Conversely, individuals who have lower total capacity or who use WM resources less efficiently should score lower in WM span tasks and have slower and/or less accurate performance in sentence processing.

If WM impairment is a strong determinant of language performance in aphasia, then WM span measures should correlate with performance on standardized aphasia tests. Caspari, Parkinson, LaPointe, and Katz (1998) found a high correlation ($r = .79$) between listening span and performance on the *Western Aphasia Battery* (WAB; Kertesz, 1982) among 22 individuals with aphasia. Sung and colleagues (2009) recently found similar correlations in a group of 20 persons with aphasia between listening span and performance on the *Porch Index of Communicative Ability* (PICA; Porch, 2001; $r = .70$) and a computerized version (CRTT) of the *Revised Token Test* (McNeil & Prescott, 1978; $r = .60$). However, Caspari et al. (1998) and Sung et al. (2009) both noted that the strong correlations between the WM measures used and language performance in aphasia could be interpreted as evidence that both are general measures of the severity of language impairment. Nonetheless, the fact that the requirements among the correlated language tasks (overall scores on the CRTT, PICA, and WAB) and the WM tasks (a visual recognition version by Caspari et al., and the auditory version of the Daneman and Carpenter task by Sung et al.) vary considerably in both linguistic computational requirements and STM span requirements, leaves open the strong possibility that there may be a common underlying source for the shared variance in the third component of the WM model; the attentional or resource requirements. While this hypothesis has received experimental attention with normal nonaphasic populations (e.g., Engle, Tuholski, Laughlin, & Conway, 1999) it has not been investigated within the same pool of persons with aphasia, using the same measures of language computation, STM and attention; a test that appears necessary to evaluate the interrelationships and unique contributions of the three components of the WM model to the underlying abilities/impairments.

Another prediction relative to aphasia that is consistent with the WM model and with the normal → aphasia continuum (the continuity hypothesis) is that if comprehension deficits in persons with aphasia are the result of reduced resource availability, normal individuals should also perform similarly when operating with reduced available resources. Miyake et al. (1994) presented sentences of varying complexity to normal individuals under time pressure using a rapid serial visual processing procedure. They found that the ordering of sentence types by difficulty was similar to that previously observed in individuals with aphasia. The ordinal ranking of the sentences was derived empirically from previous studies of sentence comprehension in persons with aphasia (Caplan, Baker, & Dehaut, 1985; Naeser et al., 1987), and the ranking agreed with a complexity metric based on the dichotomous sentence characteristics of three versus two thematic roles for a single verb, two versus one verbs present in a sentence, and noncanonical versus canonical order of thematic roles. Furthermore, as predicted by the WM capacity model, linguistic complexity interacted with both speed and subjects grouped by

WM span (although there was no three-way interaction that would also be predicted by the model). In both cases, greater WM limitations were associated with larger decrements on complex than on simpler sentences. This study also reported performance in the normal lower WM group operating under capacity limitation that was similar to the persons with aphasia. The low WM group showed over-additive impairments on the more complex sentences as was shown by the group with aphasia. Based on this finding, Miyake et al. argued that the over-additive effect on the more complex sentences for the group with aphasia was not due to specific linguistic impairments for selected syntactic structures because the same pattern was also elicited by the normal individuals with lower WM performance. The authors also speculated that these differences could be due to randomness inherent in the comprehension system, individual differences in the efficiency of certain processes, or differences in preferred strategies for adapting to a heavy resource load.

Berndt, Mitchum, and Wayland (1997) examined the capacity hypothesis in relation to two linguistically based hypotheses of aphasic comprehension; the trace deletion hypothesis and the hypothesis that agrammatic aphasia causes selective difficulty processing grammatical morphemes. They administered a sentence-picture matching task to 10 persons with aphasia, five of whom were classified by the *Western Aphasia Battery* as having Broca's aphasia and five who were classified as anomic. The results failed to provide support for the trace deletion hypothesis, which predicts above chance performance on active and subject relative sentences and chance performance on passives and object relatives. Four of the five participants with Broca's aphasia performed above chance on both active and passive sentences, while the one subject who showed the predicted pattern on actives and passives performed at chance on both subject relative and object relative sentences. The results also failed to support the grammatical morpheme hypothesis, which predicts that active and subject relative sentences should be similarly well understood, with passive and object relative sentences showing a similar degree of increased difficulty. When the performance of the five persons labeled as Broca's was examined together, active and passive sentences were equally easy to understand, with subject relative sentences being harder and object relative sentences being the most difficult to understand. These results were interpreted as support for the capacity theory. In analyzing the performance of all 10 participants together, the ordinal pattern of sentence difficulty across types was the pattern predicted by capacity theory. In other words, performance degradation was most evident in all individuals with aphasia regardless of the type of aphasia; especially when the two complexity factors of sentence length and syntactic structure were combined.

As mentioned above, the most common model of WM assumes a single, shared pool of processing resources for the phonological loop. However, debate about single versus multiple pools of attentional resources has a long history (Friedman & Polson, 1981; Gopher, Brickner, & Navon, 1982; Kahneman, 1973; Wickens, 1980, 1984) but a more limited one in terms of verbal WM. Caplan and Waters proposed that WM resources are fractionated into at least two parts

(Caplan & Waters, 1995, 1996; Waters & Caplan, 1996a, 1996b, 2004). They differentiated the *interpretive* language processing characterized by initial, first-pass, unconscious, obligatory processing from the *post-interpretive* processing that is conscious, controlled, and verbally mediated (Caplan & Waters, 1999; Waters & Caplan, 2004). They argued that traditional verbal WM span tasks, which rely on post-interpretive processing, only predict performance on tasks that also require post-interpretive processing; but not on tasks that rely heavily on interpretive processing such as automatic syntactic parsing. Additionally, they argued that the single capacity theory necessarily predicts interactions between effects of WM capacity and syntactic complexity, and many studies have failed to find such interactions. They further argued that where interactions have been found, they were due to the number of propositions contained in a sentence, a factor they relegate to post-interpretive processing.

In order to further assess the single versus multiple WM resource hypothesis, Caplan and Waters (1996) administered a sentence comprehension task to a group of 10 persons with aphasia carefully chosen to have performance above chance but below ceiling on semantically reversible, syntactically complex sentences. Sentence types were systematically varied in terms of syntactic complexity (canonicity) and number of propositions, and were presented in single and dual-task conditions. In the dual-task conditions, subjects had to continuously repeat a random digit string with a length equal to their digit span and their digit span minus one while comprehending the sentence. They were instructed to give primary emphasis to the digit task when it was present. Analyses of sentence comprehension showed reliable effects of both canonicity and number of propositions, but no effect of digit load or an interaction. In analyzing digit recall, main effects of both sentence type and number of digits were found, but without a significant interaction. A finer-grained analysis separating out the effects of canonicity and propositional load revealed a null effect of canonicity and a positive effect of propositional load on digit recall. Caplan and Waters interpreted these results as evidence for the separation of resources dedicated to syntactic processing from those available to other kinds of language processing. However, without demonstrating a bidirectional trading effect, it is very difficult to invoke a "resource" explanation for the findings rather than a simple interference effect, or a number of other explanations.

Some proponents of the single capacity hypothesis have responded to the criticism outlined above by noting the problems inherent in using null findings as support for a theoretical position, especially when the effect in question involves interactions that may be difficult to detect (Miyake, Emerson, & Friedman, 1999). Others have suggested that a single language resource capacity could account for null effects of digit load on processing of complex syntax by highlighting the distinction between encoding and storage processes (Bates, Dick, & Wulfeck, 1999; Dick et al., 2001). They propose that some task manipulations may primarily affect encoding (e.g., time pressure or noise masking) while others may primarily affect maintenance (e.g., digit load), and that processing of low frequency word orders, for example, may be vulnerable only to the former while inflectional morphology may be affected by both.

Also relevant to this discussion of resource capacity limitations as an explanatory construct in aphasia are theories and models that directly relate resources and processing speed. Haarmann and Kolk (1991) hypothesized that sentence comprehension deficits in aphasia could be due to a reduction in the resources deployed per unit time to drive the computations responsible for parsing syntax. They further proposed that this reduction in resources was compatible with either slow activation or rapid decay of critical sentence elements. Haarmann and Kolk conducted a syntactic priming experiment to test these two hypotheses against each other and also a third alternative; that the size of aphasic individuals' processing buffer is reduced. The results supported the slow-activation hypothesis: participants with aphasia demonstrated significant priming only in the longest prime-target stimulus onset asynchrony (SOA) condition, whereas an age-matched control group showed priming effects across the entire range of SOAs tested (300–1100 ms). The authors argued that the participants with aphasia had not lost their syntactic knowledge, but rather that their comprehension deficits were due to processing inefficiency rendering them unable to perform linguistic computations within a necessary time frame. While the methods of their study were novel, their interpretation of the results as a slowed processing mechanism underlying the comprehension impairments in individuals with aphasia is not unique (Blanchard & Prescott, 1980; Blumstein, Katz, Goodglass, Shrier, & Dworetsky 1985; Campbell & McNeil, 1985; Salvatore, 1974; Weidner & Lasky, 1976) and is consistent with a reduced availability of resources account as demonstrated using the psychological refractory period experimental method (Hula & McNeil, 2008; Hula, McNeil, & Sung, 2007).

A number of other studies have been carried out to address the issue of whether the phenomenology of aphasia can be accounted for by a failure of an attentional/resource allocation system (Arvedson & McNeil, 1987; Erickson, Goldinger, & LaPointe, 1996; LaPointe & Erickson, 1991; Murray, 2000; Murray, Holland, & Beeson, 1997b; Murray, Holland, & Beeson, 1998; Slansky & McNeil, 1997; Tseng, McNeil, & Milenkovic, 1993). These studies have generally adopted the strategy of manipulating the presence, priority, or difficulty of competing language or nonlanguage tasks. One consistent finding from these studies is that the language performance in persons with aphasia is more vulnerable to the introduction of a competing task than language performance in normal individuals (Arvedson, 1986; Murray, 2000; Murray, Holland, & Beeson, 1997a; Murray, Holland, & Beeson, 1997c; Murray et al., 1998). Unfortunately, such single-to-dual task comparisons are difficult to interpret within the context of resource theory, and although this finding is consistent with the notion that individuals with aphasia have impairments of attentional resource allocation, it is amenable to other interpretations as well, including (but not limited to) a fundamental capacity reduction. Other studies that have held the dual-task requirements constant have found that individuals with aphasia are less responsive than normal individuals to task manipulations that putatively affect task priority or allocation ratio. For example, Tseng et al. (1993) asked normal and persons with aphasia to monitor word strings for semantic and phonological targets, and found that, while normal individuals showed expected increases in reaction time (RT) associated with decreases in target frequency, participants with aphasia showed no effects of target frequency on RT or accuracy. Slansky and McNeil (1997) obtained similar findings when manipulating the linguistic stress of category decision and lexical decision stimuli presented in a sentence context. These findings suggest that individuals with aphasia may be impaired in their ability to accurately evaluate task demands, and/or to appropriately mobilize resources to maximize performance in meeting those demands. The former possibility is consistent with other studies demonstrating that ratings of task difficulty by individuals with aphasia do not correlate well with their reaction times, in contrast to nonbrain-injured persons' ratings (Clark & Robin, 1995; Murray et al., 1997a).

One problem that has plagued much (though not all) of the literature on attentional explanations for aphasia is a tendency toward vague usage of resource terminology. While Kahneman (1973) and Navon and Gopher (1979, 1980) were quite specific in describing theoretical distinctions critical to resource theory (e.g., processing resources vs. processing structures, concurrence costs vs. interference costs, task difficulty vs. task demand, data limits vs. resource limits), many aphasiologists who have employed both resource theory and linguistic (primarily syntax) theory as motivating constructs have often conflated them or ignored them altogether. Part of this tendency toward vague usage of the term *resource* may be due to their use of Baddeley's working memory model as a motivating construct. While this model has been elaborated by Baddeley (1993, 1996, 1998) and many others since its original formulation, it remains rather nonspecific in its employment of the concept of the "central executive" and related concepts such as "controlled attention," "resources," and "capacity" as employed by many users. Fortunately, many researchers have recognized the construct's over-simplification and evidence has been assembled supporting the validity for its fractionation (cf. Fournier, Larigauderie, & Gaonac'h, 2004; Fournier-Vicente, Larigauderie, & Gaonac'h, 2008; Kane & Engle, 2003; Miyake et al., 2000). For example, Kane and Engle (2003) demonstrated the differential demands of "goal maintenance" relative to those of "task switching" in the Stroop task. Fournier et al. (2004) identified such general functions as "coordination" among constituents, "inhibition" and "long-term memory retrieval" (similar to Miyake et al., 2000) as relevant components of the attentional/central executive. Fournier and colleagues argued for six separable functions of the central executive component of the WM model (verbal storage-and-processing coordination, visuospatial storage-and-processing coordination, dual-task coordination, strategic retrieval, selective attention, and shifting). Using a group of 180 young college students, these researchers demonstrated that, through confirmatory factor analysis, five of the six functions were related but distinguishable from one another. Importantly for this discussion, these investigators measured selective attention for linguistic information with the naming Stroop task; a task closely tied by these and other authors to the construct of inhibition.

It is reasonable to suggest that since persons with aphasia have a language problem, any appropriate test of attention in this population might require its assessment using nonlinguistic stimuli. However, if one source of executive resources is specialized for linguistic processing, as proposed by the WM model and supported by a sizable experimental literature as discussed above, then the use of nonlinguistic tasks would not provide the appropriate test of or insight into a resource account as a mechanism subtending the observed language impairment. Alternatively, if one used an attentional task that requires language processing, any observed impairments could not be unambiguously attributed to the attentional demands of the task and would lead to the inevitable equivocal interpretation that the impairment was as likely derived from impairments in linguistic computations as from the attentional component of the task. The Stroop task offers one potential method for resolving this situation.

STROOP AND STROOP-LIKE TASKS

Without doubt, the Stroop task is the most frequently studied attention paradigm in existence and it is clear why it is considered the "gold standard" of attentional measures (MacLeod, 1992). Review articles (e.g., Jensen & Rohwer, 1966; MacLeod, 1991) have catalogued hundreds of Stroop-like tasks and perhaps thousands of studies investigating an incredible array of variables involved in their performance. The original Stroop task (Stroop, 1935) involved rapidly naming the color of the ink for a printed color word with colored ink under two conditions; where the ink is either congruent with color word (e.g., the word "red" printed in red ink) or incongruent (e.g., the word "red" printed in blue ink) with it compared to a neutral condition (e.g., naming a color patch or reading the color word in traditional black ink). The ubiquitous and robust effect reveal that naming the ink color in the incongruent condition is more difficult (produces long reaction times and creates more errors) than the neutral condition. Conversely, naming the ink color in the congruent condition is often facilitative (produces shorter reaction times and less errors) compared to the relevant neutral condition. The incongruent result is considered to be an "interference" effect and is generally considered to be due to the required inhibition of the "automatic" activation of the word compared to the "controlled" processing required to name the color. Stroop task variants have been used to investigate attentional functions/impairments in persons with aphasia, though perhaps surprisingly infrequently given their acceptance and popularity in general psychology.

The first "Stroop" task used to investigate aphasia appears to have been conducted by Cohen, Meier, and Schulze (1983).[*] They examined a version of the Stroop task (three-color, three-choice button response instead of the traditional

---

[*] Other investigators (e.g., Golden, 1976; Perret, 1974; Stuss, Floden, Alexander, Levine, & Katz, 2001) had investigated the Stroop effect in both left and right hemisphere damaged individuals but do not appear to have examined the effects of aphasia. Chmiel (1984) also used a Stroop task to investigate the locus of the presumed phonological deficit within the linguistic system for a single person with conduction aphasia under conditions of silent or concurrent articulation. Because the relevant results for this discussion were not reported in this study, it will not be discussed in this review.

oral naming task) and a nonlinguistic (three-position parallel line identification, three-choice button response) task in two groups with aphasia (21 persons with Broca aphasia, 10 with Wernicke aphasia) and two groups of brain damaged persons without aphasia (15 with right hemisphere damage and 15 with diffuse brain damage) that when combined, formed the control group. The results revealed that the nonlinguistic task was responded to significantly faster than the linguistic task for all groups with no difference between groups for the nonlinguistic task or the congruent condition of linguistic task. The persons with aphasia showed significantly less interference than the control group on the linguistic incongruent condition. Further, the severity of aphasia, as indexed by the number of errors on an unspecified version of a "token test," correlated negatively ($r = -.42$) with the size of the interference effect, whereas age, time post onset and score on the Trail Making test correlated poorly ($r = .10–.18$) with the interference effect. The conclusion was that persons with aphasia showed less Stroop interference than the other brain damaged control participants. Whether this means that they did not have automatic access to the word meaning, which is believed to create the interference, or whether they had superior inhibitory processes for the automatic color word was not discussed. No distinctions in performance were discussed relative to the two groups with aphasia; a finding that could inform the debate about preserved automatic processing in persons with Wernicke's aphasia and its impairment in Broca's aphasia (Blumstein, Milberg, & Shrier, 1982).

Revonsuo (1995) appears to have been the first to observe the expected Stroop interference and facilitative effects (reduced reaction times for the congruent condition—e.g., word "red" in red ink relative to the control condition) in a person with aphasia. These effects paralleled the control participant's patterns and exceeded them in the magnitude of the total Stroop effect (the difference between the RTs in the congruent and incongruent word conditions).

Ansaldo, Arguin, and Lecours (2002) used a nonlinguistic "orientation" Stroop task to investigate the hemispheric lateralization of language recovery in a single participant described as having "severe Broca's aphasia" (p. 287). While the results for the congruent and incongruent conditions were not reported relative to a control condition (the traditional comparison for determining the interference and facilitation effects), reaction times were longer and error rates higher in the incongruent condition relative to the congruent condition on four separate occasions over a 12-month recovery period. While no test–retest reliability was established for this task, there was considerable variability in reaction times across the four measurements.

Finally, Wiener, Connor, and Obler (2004) administered a computerized manual-response numerical version of the Stroop task to five individuals with Wernicke's aphasia and 12 nonbrain-injured controls. The results indicated a significantly larger interference effect for the group with aphasia relative to the control group. The facilitation effect and error rates were not significantly different between the groups. They also reported a significant and large negative correlation ($r = -.91$) between the interference effect and Token Test (from the *Neurosensory Center Comprehensive Examination for Aphasia*; Spreen and

Benton, 1969) score; indicating that the larger the Stroop interference effect, the lower the auditory comprehension test score. A nonsignificant correlation between the interference effect size and the Complex Ideational Material subtest from the *Boston Diagnostic Examination for Aphasia* (Goodglass & Kaplan, 1983) also was reported. The authors interpreted these results as support for their hypothesis that persons with Wernicke's aphasia have a deficit of inhibition at the lexical/ semantic level of language processing.

Although the total number of individuals with aphasia that has been assessed with a Stroop-like task is small, several tentative conclusions seem warranted from the data presented thus far. First, persons with aphasia can perform the Stroop and Stroop-like tasks, even persons with very severe aphasia as evidenced by very low error rates. Second, while brain damaged participants can be expected to have slowed reaction times relative to normal controls, a generalized cognitive slowing does seem to account for the differential pattern of findings across the studies. Third, the presence and degree of interference revealed by the incongruent task relative to a legitimate control condition has varied across studies. The largest study (Cohen et al., 1983) showed no interference effects, suggesting either impaired access to word meanings or a hyper-normal inhibition mechanism. The Wiener et al. (2004) study reported an abnormally large interference effect, suggesting an impaired inhibitory mechanism. Differences in participants and tasks are likely sources for these differences across the two studies. Fourth, interference effects have been demonstrated in both linguistic and nonlinguistic tasks and failures to find differences have also been reported. Fifth, the size of the interference effects shown in the persons with aphasia, regardless of the comparisons with control populations, correlates significantly and negatively with Token Test-like tasks and this is present in the absence of such correlations on other linguistic and nonlinguistic tasks.

SUMMARY

The dominant view of aphasia held by the overwhelming majority of researchers, aphasia clinicians and related healthcare professionals is that it is a language disorder that conforms to a neurological centers and pathways model. The model makes specific predictions about lesioned neural centers and pathways that yield to "classical" types of aphasia. Nearly blind adherence to this view of aphasia has perpetuated the notion that refined linguistic description, tied to increasing specificity of lesion localization has the power to explain the phenomenology of aphasia and make relevant predictions about the underlying mechanisms, potential for recovery and its most appropriate treatment. We have attempted to review some of the observed phenomena that are incompatible with such a view and have also argued that this view of aphasia has diminished the search for the cognitive mechanisms that subtend the observed language impairments that define the condition.

There are a relatively small, but perhaps growing number of aphasia researchers that have recognized that the cognitive apparatus required for "doing" language may be the source for the observed linguistic behavior in persons with aphasia and that an exploration of these mechanisms may offer explanation and prediction that the traditional view cannot. A focus on WM as a construct has been helpful to the challenge of the traditional and accepted paradigm. That is, the WM model focused on the separation and individual contributions of STM and executive attention as critical components of language processing, in addition to the specific linguistic computational task requirements that is the exclusive domain of the traditional paradigm. We have attempted to argue that the most parsimonious account for the disparate phenomena of aphasia is an impairment of a language dedicated (executive) attentional system, with secondary, rather than primary impairments of the linguistic computational or STM component of the WM system.

A brief review of the dual task aphasia literature has revealed consistent findings of impairments in language processing (though not always restricted to the linguistic domain) that are not easily reconciled with simple linguistic explanations but that are compatible with attentional/resource impairments. Further, while dual-task methods have shed light on the nature of the attentional mechanisms, the methods are difficult to implement and they have not found their way into the armamentaria of clinical aphasiologists.

A review of the known studies that have used a Stroop task to investigate attentional mechanisms and impairments in persons with aphasia yielded only two group investigations and the results were contradictory. Although Stroop and Stroop-like task(s) are technically also dual tasks, there is an extensive knowledge-base about them, and they appear to be relatively easy to implement into language assessment procedures that extend beyond the traditional word naming task. This method may provide a platform for evaluating attention-related facilitative, inhibitory and goal maintenance abilities, and impairments in persons with aphasia on a person-by-person basis; all cognitive mechanisms that have been implicated as sources for their linguistic impairments.

REFERENCES

Adamovich, B. L. (1978). A comparison of the process of memory and perception between aphasic and non-brain-injured adults. *Clinical Aphasiology, 8,* 327.

Albert, M. L. (1976). Short-term memory and aphasia. *Brain & Language, 3,* 28–33.

Ansaldo, A. I., Arguin, M., & Lecours, A. R. (2002). Initial right hemisphere take-over and subsequent bilateral participation during recovery from aphasia. *Aphasiology, 16,* 287–304.

Arvedson, J. C. (1986). *Effect of lexical decisions on auditory semantic judgments using divided attention in adults with left and right hemisphere damage.* Unpublished doctoral dissertation, University of Wisconsin-Madison.

Arvedson, J. C., & McNeil, M. R. (1987). Accuracy and response times for semantic judgments and lexical decisions with left and right hemisphere lesions. *Clinical Aphasiology, 17,* 188–200.

Baddeley, A. D. (1986). *Working memory.* Oxford, UK: Clarendon.

Baddeley, A. D. (1993). Working memory or working attention. In A. D. Baddeley & L. eiskrantz (Eds.), *Attention: Selection, awareness and control: A tribute to Donald Broadbent* (pp. 152–170). Oxford, UK: Oxford University Press.

Baddeley, A. D. (1996). Exploring the central executive. *Quarterly Journal of Experimental Psychology, 49A*, 5–28.

Baddeley, A. D. (1998). The central executive: A concept and some misconceptions. *Journal of the International Neuropsychological Society, 4*, 523–528.

Baddeley, A. D., & Hitch, G. J. (1974). Working memory. In G. H. Bower (Ed.), *The psychology of learning and motivation: Advances in research and theory* (pp. 47–89). New York, NY: Academic Press.

Baddeley, A. D., & Logie, R. H. (1999). Working memory: The multiple-component model. In A. Miyake & P. Shah (Eds.), *Models of working memory: Mechanisms of active maintenance and executive control* (pp. 28–61). Cambridge, UK: Cambridge University Press.

Bates, E., Devescovi, A., Dronkers, N., Pizzamiglio, L., Wulfeck, B., Hernandez, A. . . . Marangolo, P. (1994). Grammatical deficits in patients without agrammatism: Sentence interpretation under stress in English and Italian. Abstracts from the Academy of Aphasia 1994 annual meeting [Special issue]. *Brain and Language, 47*, 400–402.

Bates, E., Dick, F., & Wulfeck, B. (1999). Not so fast: Domain-general factors can account for selective deficits in grammatical processing. *Behavioral and Brain Sciences, 22*, 96–97.

Bates, E., Friederici, A., & Wulfeck, B. (1987). Comprehension in aphasia: A cross-linguistic study. *Brain and Language, 32*, 19–67.

Bayles, K. A., Boone, D. R., Tomoeda, C. K., Slauson, T. J., & Kaszniak, A. W. (1989). Differentiating Alzheimer's patients from normal elderly and stroke patients with aphasia. *Journal of Speech and Hearing Disorders, 54*, 74–87.

Benson, D. F. (1979). *Aphasia, alexia, and agraphia.* New York, NY: Churchill Livingstone.

Benton, A. L., Smith, K. C., & Lang, M. (1972). Stimulus characteristics and object naming in aphasic patients. *Journal of Communication Disorders, 5*, 19–24.

Berndt, R. S., Mitchum, C. C., & Wayland, S. (1997). Patterns of sentence comprehension in aphasia: A consideration of three hypotheses. *Brain and Language, 60*, 197–221.

Bisiach, E. (1966). Perceptual factors in the pathogenesis of anomia. *Cortex, 2*, 90–95.

Blackwell, A., & Bates, E. (1995). Inducing agrammatic profiles in normals: Evidence for the selective vulnerability of morphology under cognitive resource limitation. *Journal of Cognitive Neuroscience, 7*, 228–257.

Blanchard, S. L., & Prescott, T. E. (1980). The effects of temporal expansion upon auditory comprehension in aphasic adults. *British Journal of Disorders of Communication, 15*, 115–127.

Blumstein, S. E., Katz, B., Goodglass, H., Shrier, R., & Dworetsky, B. (1985). The effects of slowed speech on auditory comprehension in aphasia. *Brain and Language, 24*, 246–265.

Blumstein, S. E., Milberg, W., & Shrier, R. (1982). Semantic processing in aphasia: Evidence from an auditory lexical decision task. *Brain and Language, 17*, 301–315.

Botvinick, M., Nystrom, L. E., Fissell, K., Carter, C. S., & Cohen, J. D. (1999). Conflict monitoring versus selection-for-action in anterior cingulate cortex. *Nature, 402*, 179–181.

Brookshire, R. H., & Nicholas, L. E. (1980). Verification of active and passive sentences by aphasic and nonaphasic subjects. *Journal of Speech and Hearing Research, 23*, 878–893.

Brookshire, R. H., & Nicholas, L. E. (1984). Comprehension of directly and nondirectly stated main ideas and details in discourse by brain-damaged and non-brain-damaged listeners. *Brain and Language, 21*, 21–36.

Campbell, T. F., & McNeil, M. R. (1985). Effects of presentation rate and divided attention on auditory comprehension in children with acquired language disorder. *Journal of Speech and Hearing Research, 28,* 513–520.

Caplan, D. (1987). *Neurolinguistics and linguistic aphasiology.* Cambridge, MA: Cambridge University Press.

Caplan, D., Baker, C., & Dehaut, F. (1985). Syntactic determinants of sentence comprehension in aphasia. *Cognition, 21,* 117–175.

Caplan, D., & Waters, G. S. (1995). Aphasic disorders of syntactic comprehension and working memory capacity. *Cognitive Neuropsychology, 12,* 637–649.

Caplan, D., & Waters, G. S. (1996). Syntactic processing in sentence comprehension under dual-task conditions in aphasic patients. *Language and Cognitive Processes, 11,* 525–551.

Caplan, D., & Waters, G. S. (1999). Verbal working memory and sentence comprehension. *Behavioral and Brain Sciences, 22,* 77–126.

Caplan, D., Waters, G., DeDe, G., Michaud, J., & Reddy, A. (2007). A study of syntactic processing in aphasia I: Behavioral (psycholinguistic) aspects. *Brain and Language, 101,* 103–150.

Caplan, D., Waters, G. S., & Hildebrandt, N. (1997). Determinants of sentence comprehension in aphasic sentence-picture matching tasks. *Journal of Speech, Language, and Hearing Research, 40,* 542–555.

Caramazza, A., Zurif, E. B., & Gardner, H. (1978). Sentence memory in aphasia. *Neuropschologia, 16,* 661–669.

Caspari, I., Parkinson, S. R., LaPointe, L. L., & Katz, R. C. (1998). Working memory and aphasia. *Brain and Cognition, 37,* 205–223.

Cermak, L. S., & Moreines, J. (1976). Verbal retention deficits in aphasic and amnestic patients. *Brain & Language, 3,* 16–27.

Cermak, L. S., & Tarlow, S. (1978). Aphasic and amnesic patients' verbal vs. nonverbal retentive abilities. *Cortex, 16,* 32–40.

Chmiel, N. (1984). Phonological recoding for reading: The effect of concurrent articulation in a Stroop task. *British Journal of Psychology, 75,* 213–220.

Clark, H. M., & Robin, D. A. (1995). Sense of effort during a lexical decision task: Resource allocation deficits following brain damage. *American Journal of Speech-Language Pathology, 4,* 143–147.

Cohen, R., Meier, E., & Schulze, U. (1983). Spontanes Lesen aphasischer Patienten entgegen der Instruktion? (Stroop-Test). *Nervenarzt, 54,* 299–303.

Cowan, N. (1995). *Attention and memory: An integrated framework.* New York, NY: Oxford University Press.

Cowan, N. (1999). An embedded-processes model of working memory. In A. Miyake & P. Shah (Eds.), *Models of working memory and executive control* (pp. 62–101). Cambridge, UK: Cambridge University Press.

Craven, R. R., & Hirnle, C. J. (Eds.). (2009). *Fundamentals of nursing: Human health and function.* Philadelphia, PA: Lippincott, Williams, & Wilkins.

Crisman, L. G. (1971). *Response variability in naming behavior of aphasic patients.* Unpublished master's thesis, University of Pittsburgh.

Daneman, M. A., & Carpenter, P. A. (1980). Individual differences in working memory and reading. *Journal of Verbal Learning and Verbal Behavior, 19,* 450–466.

Darley, F. L. (1976). Maximizing input to the aphasic patient: A review of research. *Clinical Aphasiology, 6,* 1–21.

Darley, F. L. (1982). *Aphasia.* Philadelphia, PA: W.B. Saunders.

Dick, F., Bates, E., Wulfeck, B., Utman, J. A., Dronkers, N., & Gernsbacher, M. A. (2001). Language deficits, localization, and grammar: Evidence for a distributive model of language breakdown in aphasic patients and neurologically intact individuals. *Psychological Review, 108,* 759–788.

Duffy, J. R., & Coelho, C. A. (2001). Schuell's stimulation approach to rehabilitation. In R. Chapey (Ed.), *Language intervention strategies in aphasia and related neurogenic communication disorders* (4th ed., pp. 341–382). Baltimore, MD: Lippincott Williams & Wilkins.

Eggert, G. H. (1977). *Wernicke's works on aphasia: A sourcebook and review.* The Hague, The Netherlands: Mouton.

Engle, R. W., Kane, M. J., & Tuholski, S. W. (1999). Individual differences in working memory capacity and what they tell us about controlled attention, general fluid intelligence, and functions of the prefrontal cortex. In A. Miyake & P. Shah (Eds.), *Models of working memory and executive control* (pp. 102–134). Cambridge, MA: Cambridge University Press.

Engle, R. W., Tuholski, S. W., Laughlin, J. E., & Conway, A. R. A. (1999). Working memory, short-term memory, and general fluid intelligence: A latent variable approach. *Journal of Experimental Psychology: General, 128*(3), 309–331.

Erickson, R. J., Goldinger, S. D., & LaPointe, L. L. (1996). Auditory vigilance in aphasic individuals: Detecting nonlinguistic stimuli with full or divided attention. *Brain and Cognition, 30,* 244–253.

Ernest-Baron, C. R., Brookshire, R. H., & Nicholas, L. E. (1987). Story structure and retelling of narratives by aphasic and non-brain-damaged adults. *Journal of Speech and Hearing Research, 30,* 44–49.

Flowers, C. R. (1975). Proactive interference in short-term recall by aphasic, brain-damaged nonaphasic and normal subjects. *Neuropsychologia, 13,* 59–68.

Fournier, S., Larigauderie, P., & Gaonac'h, D. (2004). Exploring how the central executive works: A search for independent components. *Psychologica Belgica, 44,* 159–188.

Fournier-Vicente, S., Larigauderie, P., & Gaonac'h, D. (2008). More dissociations and interactions within central executive functioning: A comprehensive latent-variable analysis. *Acta Psychologica, 129,* 32–48.

Freed, D. B., Marshall, R. C., & Chulantseff, E. A. (1996). Picture naming variability: A methodological consideration of inconsistent naming responses in fluent and nonfluent aphasia. *Clinical Aphasiology, 26,* 193–205.

Freud, S. (1953). *On aphasia.* New York, NY: International Universities Press, Inc. (originally published in German, 1891).

Friedman, A., & Polson, M. C. (1981). Hemispheres as independent resource systems: Limited-capacity processing and cerebral specialization. *Journal of Experimental Psychology: Human Perception and Performance, 7,* 1031–1058.

Gardner, H., Albert, M. L., & Weintraub, S. (1975). Comprehending a word: The influence of speed and redundancy on auditory comprehension in aphasia. *Cortex, 11,* 155–162.

Gaulin, C. A., & Campbell, T. F. (1994). Procedure for assessing verbal working memory in normal school-age children: Some preliminary data. *Perceptual and Motor Skills, 79,* 55–64.

Geschwind, N. (1965a). Disconnexion syndromes in animals and man. Part I. *Brain, 88,* 237–294.

Geschwind, N. (1965b). Disconnexion syndromes in animals and man. Part II. *Brain, 88,* 585–644.

Gibson, E. (1998). Linguistic complexity: Locality of syntactic dependencies. *Cognition, 68,* 1–76.

Gibson, E., & Pearlmutter, N. J. (2000). Distinguishing serial and parallel parsing. *Journal of Psycholinguistic Research, 29,* 231–240.

Golden, C. J. (1976). Identification of brain disorders by the Stroop color and word test. *Journal of Clinical Psychology, 32,* 654–658.

Goodglass, H., & Kaplan, E. (1983). *The assessment of aphasia and related disorders* (2nd ed.). Philadelphia, PA: Lea & Febiger.

Goodglass, H., Kaplan, E., & Barresi, B. (2001). *The assessment of aphasia and related disorders* (3rd ed.). Baltimore, MD: Lippincott, Williams, & Wilkins.

Gopher, D., Brickner, M., & Navon, D. (1982). Different difficulty manipulations interact differently with task emphasis: Evidence for multiple resources. *Journal of Experimental Psychology: Human Perception and Performance, 8,* 146–157.

Grodzinsky, Y. (2000). The neurology of syntax. *Behavioral & Brain Sciences, 23,* 1–71.

Haarmann, H. J., & Kolk, H. H. J. (1991). Syntactic priming in Broca's aphasics: Evidence for slow activation. *Aphasiology, 5,* 247–263.

Hageman, C. F. (1980). *Attentional mechanisms underlying patterns of auditory comprehension brain-damaged aphasic, non-aphasic, and normal listeners.* Unpublished doctoral dissertation, University of Colorado.

Hageman, C. F., & Folkstad, A. (1986). Performance of aphasic listeners on an expanded revised token test subtest presented verbally and nonverbally. *Clinical Aphasiology, 16,* 226–233.

Hageman, C. F., McNeil, M. R., Rucci-Zimmer, S., & Cariski, D. M. (1982). The reliability of patterns of auditory processing deficits: Evidence from the Revised Token Test. *Clinical Aphasiology, 12,* 230–234.

Hamilton, N. G., & Matthews, T. (1979). Aphasia: The sole manifestation of focal status epilepticus. *Neurology, 29,* 745–748.

Head, H. (1926). *Aphasia and kindred disorders.* Vol. I, II. London, UK: Cambridge University Press.

Howard, D., Patterson, K., Franklin, S., Morton, J., & Orchard-Lisle, V. (1984). Variability and consistency in naming by aphasic patients. *Advances in Neurology, 42,* 263–276.

Hula, W. D., & McNeil, M. R. (2008). Models of attention and dual-task performance as explanatory constructs in aphasia. *Seminars in Speech and Language, 29,* 169–187.

Hula, W. D., McNeil, M. R., & Sung, J. E. (2007). Is there an impairment of language-specific processing in aphasia? *Brain and Language, 103,* 240–241.

Jensen, A. R., & Rohwer, W. D. (1966). The Stroop color-word test: A review. *Acta Psychologica, 25,* 36–93.

Just, M. A, & Carpenter, P. A. (1992). A capacity theory of comprehension: Individual differences in working memory. *Psychological Review, 99,* 122–149.

Kahneman, D. (1973). *Attention and effort.* Englewood Cliffs, NJ: Prentice-Hall.

Kaminski, H. J., Hlavin, M. L., Likavec, M., & Schmidley, J. W. (1992). Transient neurologic deficit caused by chronic subdural hematoma. *American Journal of Medicine, 92,* 698–700.

Kane, M. J., & Engle, R. W. (2003). Working-memory capacity and the control of attention: The contributions of goal neglect, response competition, and task set to Stroop interference. *Journal of Experimental Psychology: General, 132,* 47–70.

Kertesz, A. (1979). *Aphasia and associated disorders.* New York, NY: Grune & Stratton.

Kertesz, A. (1982). *Western aphasia battery.* New York, NY: Grune & Stratton.

Kilborn, K. (1991). Selective impairment of grammatical morphology due to induced stress in normal listeners: Implications for aphasia. *Brain and Language, 41,* 275–288.

Kimelman, M. D. Z., & McNeil, M. R. (1987). An investigation of emphatic stress comprehension in adult aphasia. *Journal of Speech, Language, and Hearing Research, 30,* 295–300.

King, J., & Just, M. A. (1991). Individual differences in syntactic processing: The role of working memory. *Journal of Memory and Language, 30,* 580–602.

King, J. W., & Kutas, M. (1998). Neural plasticity in the dynamics of human visual word recognition. *Neuroscience Letters, 244,* 61–64.

Kolk, H. (2007). Variability is the hallmark of aphasic behaviour: Grammatical behaviour is no exception. *Brain and Language, 101,* 99–102.

Kreindler, A., & Fradis, A. (1968). *Performances in aphasia: A neurodynamical diagnostic and psychological study.* Paris, France: Gauthier-Villars.

Kuhn, T. S. (1962). *The structure of scientific revolutions.* Chicago, IL: University of Chicago Press.

LaPointe, L. L., & Erickson, R. J. (1991). Auditory vigilance during divided task attention in aphasic individuals. *Aphasiology, 5,* 511–520.

Larson, M. J., Kaufman, D. A. S., & Perlstein, W. M. (2009). *Neuropsychologia, 47,* 663–670.

Lebrun, Y. (1994). Ictal verbal behaviour: A review. *Seizur, 3,* 45–54.

Lecours, A. R., & Joanette, Y. (1980). Linguistic and other psychological aspects of paroxysmal aphasia. *Brain & Language, 10,* 1–23.

Linebaugh, C. W., Coakley, A. S., Arrigan, A. F., & Racy, A. (1979). Epileptogenic aphasia. *Clinical Aphasiology, 9,* 70–78.

Lubinski, R., & Chapey, R. (1978). Constructive recall strategies in adult aphasia. *Clinical Aphasiology, 18,* 338–350.

MacDonald, M. C., Just, M. A., & Carpenter, P. A. (1992). Working memory constraints on the processing of syntactic ambiguity. *Cognitive Psychology, 24,* 56–98.

MacLeod, C. M. (1991). Half a century of research on the Stroop effect: An integrative review. *Psychological Bulletin, 109,* 163–203.

MacLeod, C. M. (1992). The Stroop task: The "gold standard" of attentional measures. *Journal of Experimental Psychology: General, 121,* 12–14.

Marie, P. (1906). Revision de la question de l'aphasie: la troisieme circonvolution forntale gauche ne joue aucun role speciale dans la function du langage. *Seminars in Medicine, 26,* 241–247.

Martin, N., Dell, G. S., Saffran, E. M., & Schwartz, M. F. (1994). Origins of paraphasias in deep dysphasia: Testing the consequences of a decay impairment to an interactive spreading activation model of lexical retrieval. *Brain and Language, 47,* 609–660.

Martin, N. & Saffran E. M. (1997). Language and auditory-verbal short-term memory impairments: Evidence for common underlying processes. *Cognitive Neuropsychology, 14,* 641–682.

McNeil, M. R. (1982). The nature of aphasia in adults. In N. J. Lass, L. V. McReynolds, J. L. Northern, & D. E. Yoder (Eds.), *Speech, language, and hearing (Vol. II): Pathologies of speech and language* (pp. 692–740). Philadelphia, PA: Saunders.

McNeil, M. R. (1983). Aphasia: Neurological considerations. *Topics in Language Disorders, 3,* 1–19.

McNeil, M. R. (1988). Aphasia in the adult. In N. J. Lass, L. V. McReynolds, J. Northern, & D. E. Yoder (Eds.), *Handbook of speech-language pathology and audiology* (pp. 738–786). Toronto, Canada: D.C. Becker, Inc.

McNeil, M. R., & Hageman, C. F. (1979). Auditory processing deficits in aphasia evidenced on the Revised Token Test: Incidence and prediction of across subtest and across item within subtest patterns. *Clinical Aphasiology, 9,* 47–69.

McNeil, M. R., Hageman, C. F., & Matthews, C. T. (2005). Auditory processing deficits in aphasia evidenced on the Revised Token Test: Incidence and prediction of across subtest and across item within subtest patterns. *Aphasiology, 19,* 179–198.

McNeil, M. R., & Kimelman, M. D. Z. (1986). Toward an integrative information-processing structure of auditory comprehension and processing in adult aphasia. *Seminars in Speech and Language, 7*, 123–146.

McNeil, M. R., Odell, K. H., & Campbell, T. F. (1982). The frequency and amplitude of fluctuating auditory processing in aphasic and nonaphasic brain-damaged persons. *Clinical Aphasiology, 12*, 220–229.

McNeil, M. R., Odell, K. H., & Tseng, C. H. (1991). Toward the integration of resource allocation into a general theory of aphasia. *Clinical Aphasiology, 21*, 21–39.

McNeil, M. R., & Pratt, S. R. (2001). Defining aphasia: Some theoretical and clinical implications of operating from a formal definition. *Aphasiology, 15*, 901–911.

McNeil, M. R., & Prescott, T. E. (1978). *Revised token test.* Austin, TX: Pro-Ed.

Miyake, A., Carpenter, P. A., & Just, M. A. (1994). A capacity approach to syntactic comprehension disorders: Making normal adults perform like aphasic patients. *Cognitive Neuropsychology, 11*, 671–717.

Miyake, A., Emerson, M. J., & Friedman, N. P. (1999). Good interactions are hard to find. *Behavioral and Brain Sciences, 22*, 108–109.

Miyake, A., Friedman, N. P., Emerson, M. J., Witzki, A. H., Howerter, A., & Wager, T. D. (2000). The unity and diversity of executive functions and their contributions to complex "frontal lobe" tasks: A latent variable analysis. *Cognitive Psychology, 41*, 49–100.

Mlcoch, A. G., & Metter, E. J. (2001). Medical aspects of stroke rehabilitation. In R. Chapey (Ed.), *Language intervention strategies in aphasia and related neurogenic communication disorders* (pp. 37–54). Baltimore, MD: Lippincott Williams & Wilkins.

Murray, L. L. (2000). The effects of varying attentional demands on the word retrieval skills of adults with aphasia, right hemisphere brain damage, or no brain damage. *Brain and Language, 72*, 40–72.

Murray, L. L., Holland, A. L., & Beeson, P. M. (1997a). Accuracy monitoring and task demand evaluation in aphasia. *Aphasiology, 11*, 401–414.

Murray, L. L., Holland, A. L., & Beeson, P. M. (1997b). Auditory processing in individuals with mild aphasia: A study of resource allocation. *Journal of Speech, Language, and Hearing Research, 40*, 792–808.

Murray, L. L., Holland, A. L., & Beeson, P. M. (1997c). Grammaticality judgments of mildly aphasic individuals under dual-task conditions. *Aphasiology, 11*, 993–1016.

Murray, L. L., Holland, A. L., & Beeson, P. M. (1998). Spoken language of individuals with mild fluent aphasia under focused and divided-attention conditions. *Journal of Speech, Language, and Hearing Research, 41*, 213–227.

Naeser, M. A., Martin, P. I., Nicholas, M., Baker, E. H., Seekins, H., Kobayashi, M., . . . Pascual-Leone, A. (2005). Improved picture naming in chronic aphasia after TMS to part of right Broca's area: An open-protocol study. *Brain and Language, 93*, 95–105.

Naeser, M. A., Mazurski, P., Goodglass, H., Peraino, M., Laughlin, S., & Leaper, W. C. (1987). Auditory syntactic comprehension in nine aphasia groups (with CT scans) and children: Differences in degree but not order of difficulty observed. *Cortex, 23*, 359–380.

Navon, D., & Gopher, D. (1979). On the economy of the human-processing system. *Psychological Review, 86*, 214–255.

Navon, D., & Gopher, D. (1980). Task difficulty, resources, and dual-task performance. In R. S. Nickerson (Ed.), *Attention and performance* (pp. 297–315). Hillsdale, NJ: Erlbaum.

Nelson, J. K., Reuter-Lorenz, P. A., Persson, J., Sylvester, C. Y., & Jonides, J. (2009). Mapping interference resolution across task domains: A shared control process in left inferior frontal gyrus. *Brain Research, 1256*, 92–100.

Nicholas, L. E., & Brookshire, R. H. (1986). Consistency of the effects of rate of speech on brain-damaged adults' comprehension of narrative discourse. *Journal of Speech and Hearing Research, 29,* 462–470.

Odell, K. H., Hashi, M., Miller, S. B., & McNeil, M. R. (1995). A critical look at the notion of selective impairment. *Clinical Aphasiology, 23,* 1–8.

Pashek, G. V., & Brookshire, R. H. (1982). Effects of rate of speech and linguistic stress on auditory paragraph comprehension of aphasic individuals. *Journal of Speech and Hearing Research, 25,* 377–383.

Peach, R. K., Rubin, S. S., & Newhoff, M. (1994). A topographic event-related potential analysis of the attention deficit for auditory processing in aphasia. *Clinical Aphasiology, 24,* 81–96.

Perret, E. (1974). The left frontal lobe of man and the suppression of habitual responses in verbal categorical behavior. *Neuropsychologia, 12,* 323–330.

Podraza, B. L., & Darley, F. L. (1977). Effect of auditory prestimulation on naming in aphasia. *Journal of Speech and Hearing Research, 20,* 669–683.

Porch, B. (2001). *Porch index of communicative ability.* Albuquerque, NM: PICA Programs.

Rahimi, A. R., & Poorkay, M. (2000). Subdural hematomas and isolated transient aphasia. *Journal of the American Medical Directors Association, 1,* 129–131.

Revonsou, A. (1995). Words interact with colors in a globally aphasic patient: Evidence from a Stroop-like task. *Cortex, 31,* 377–386.

Saffran, E. M., Schwartz, M. F., & Marin, O. S. M. (1980). Evidence from aphasia: Isolating the components of a word production model. In B. Butterworth (Ed.), *Language production* (pp. 221–240). London, UK: Academic Press

Salvatore, A. (1974). *An investigation of the effects of pause duration on sentence comprehension by aphasic subjects.* Unpublished doctoral dissertation, University of Pittsburgh.

Schuell, H., Jenkins, J. J., & Jimenez-Pabon, E. (1964). *Aphasia in adults: Diagnosis, prognosis, and treatment.* New York, NY: Harper and Row.

Schwartz, M. F., Saffran, E. M., Bloch, D. E., & Dell, G. S. (1994). Disordered speech production in aphasic and normal speakers. *Brain and Language, 47,* 52–88.

Shah, P., & Miyake, A. (1999). Models of working memory: An introduction. In A. Miyake & P. Shah (Eds.), *Models of working memory: Mechanisms of active maintenance and executive control* (pp. 1–28). Cambridge, UK: Cambridge University Press.

Shewan, C. M. (1976). Error patterns in auditory comprehension of adult aphasics. *Cortex, 12,* 325–336.

Shewan, C. M., & Canter, G. J. (1971). Effects of vocabulary, syntax, and sentence length on auditory comprehension in aphasic patients. *Cortex, 7,* 209–226.

Silkes, J., McNeil, M. R., & Drton, M. (2004). Simulation of aphasic naming performance in non-brain-damaged adults. *Journal of Speech, Language, and Hearing Research, 47,* 610–623.

Slansky, B. L., & McNeil, M. R. (1997). Resource allocation in auditory processing of emphatically stressed stimuli in aphasia. *Aphasiology, 11,* 461–472.

Spreen, O., & Benton, A. L. (1969). *Neurosensory center comprehensive examination for aphasia.* Victoria, Canada: University of Victoria, Department of Psychology, Neuropsychology Laboratory.

Stroop, J. R. (1935). Studies of interference in serial verbal reactions. *Journal and Experimental Psychology, 6,* 643–662.

Stuss, D. T., Floden, D., Alexander, M. P., Levine, B., & Katz, D. (2001). Stroop performance in focal lesion patients: Dissociation of processes and frontal lobe lesion location. *Neuropsychologia, 39,* 771–786.

Sung, J. E., McNeil, M. R., Pratt, S. R., Dickey, M. W., Hula, W. D., Szuminsky, N. J., & Doyle, P. J. (2009). Verbal working memory and its relationship to sentence-level reading and listening comprehension in persons with aphasia. *Aphasiology, 23,* 1040–1052.

Swinney, D. A., & Taylor, O. L. (1971). Short-term memory recognition search in aphasics. *Journal and Speech and Hearing Research, 14,* 578–588.

Thompson-Schill, S. L., Bedny, M., & Goldberg, R. F. (2005). The frontal lobes and the regulation of mental activity. *Current Opinion in Neurobiology, 15,* 219–224.

Thompson-Schill, S. L., Jonides, J., Marshuetz, C., Smith, E. E., D'Esposito, M., Kan, I. P., . . . Swick, D. (2002). Effects of frontal lobe damage on interference effects in working memory. *Cognitive, Affective, and Behavioral Neuroscience, 2,* 109–120.

Tompkins, C. A., Bloise, C. G. R., Timko, M. L., & Baumgaertner, A. (1994). Working memory and inference revision in brain-damaged and normally aging adults. *Journal of Speech and Hearing Research, 37,* 896–912.

Tseng, C.-H., McNeil, M. R., & Milenkovic, P. (1993). An investigation of attention allocation deficits in aphasia. *Brain and Language, 45,* 276–296.

Warren, R. L., Hubbard, D. J., & Knox, A. W. (1977). Short-term memory scan in normal individuals and individuals with aphasia. *Journal of Speech and Hearing Research, 20,* 497–509.

Waters, G. S., & Caplan, D. (1996a). Processing resource capacity and the comprehension of garden path sentences. *Memory and Cognition, 24,* 342355.

Waters, G. S., & Caplan, D. (1996b). The capacity theory of sentence comprehension: Critique of Just and Carpenter (1992). *Psychologica, 103,* 761–772.

Waters, G. S., & Caplan, D. (2004). Verbal working memory and on-line syntactic processing: Evidence from self-paced listening. *The Quarterly Journal of Experimental Psychology, 57A,* 129–163.

Weems, S. A., & Reggia, J. A. (2007). Simulating single word processing in the classic aphasia syndromes based on the Wernicke–Lichtheim–Geschwind theory. *Brain and Language, 98,* 291–309.

Weidner, W. E., & Lasky, E. Z. (1976). The interaction of rate and complexity of stimulus on the performance of adult aphasic subjects. *Brain and Language, 3,* 34–40.

West, R. (2003). Neural correlates of cognitive control and conflict detection in the Stroop and digit-location tasks. *Neuropsychologia, 41,* 1122–1135.

West, R., & Alain, C. (2000). Effect of task context and fluctuations of attention on neural activity supporting performance of the Stroop task. *Brain Research, 873,* 102–111.

Wickens, C. D. (1980). The structure of attentional resources. In R. S. Nickerson (Ed.), *Attention and performance VIII* (pp. 239–258). Hillsdale, NJ: Erlbaum.

Wickens, C. D. (1984). Processing resources in attention. In R. Parasuraman & D. R. Davies (Eds.), *Varieties of attention* (pp. 63–102). New York, NY: Academic Press.

Wiener, D. A., Connor, L. T., & Obler, L. K. (2004). Inhibition and auditory comprehension in Wernicke's aphasia. *Aphasiology, 18,* 599–609.

Wilson, S. M., Saygin, A. P., Schleicher, E., Dick, F., & Bates, E. (2003). Grammaticality judgment under non-optimal processing conditions: Deficits observed in normal participants resemble those observed in aphasic patients. Abstracts from the Academy of Aphasia [Special Issue]. *Brain and Language 87,* 67–68.

28 Remediation of Theory of Mind Impairments in Brain-Injured Adults

Kristine Lundgren and Hiram Brownell

INTRODUCTION

Successful communication requires much more than knowledge of word meaning, phonology, and syntax. Consider the following scenario. Sam calls in sick to work in order to attend opening day of the baseball season. The next day, while talking with his colleagues at lunch, Sam says, "I wish I could have gone to the game yesterday, but I was sick in bed all day." Some of his close friends who know the truth appreciate the humor of Sam's ironic remark. The colleagues who do not know the truth are deceived by the remark and console the "sick" speaker. The difference between coworkers' interpretations reflecting irony or deception rests on what they know and do not know about Sam's true state of health. Making sense of alternative interpretations requires appreciation that different people may hold different beliefs about the world, some of which may be false. Theory of Mind (ToM) is the term used to summarize the ability to use other people's thoughts, beliefs, and emotions to understand and predict their behavior (Dennett, 1978; Leslie, 1987; Premack & Woodruff, 1978).

One important distinction in ToM research is between the capacity for first-order belief; that is, what a person believes about the world, which appears relatively early on in normal development, and the capacity for the more complex second-order beliefs, what one person believes about the mental state of another person, which appears later. Second-order beliefs are particularly relevant to apprehending the difference between lies, mistakes, and irony (Wimmer & Perner, 1983; Winner, Brownell, Happé, Blum, & Pincus, 1998; see also Saxe, Carey, & Kanwisher, 2004, for a related distinction).

ToM is a skill that is essential to successful communication as well as for pretense and social cognition (e.g., Baron-Cohen, Tager-Flusberg, & Cohen, 2000). The following example of how ToM provides a foundation for communication also rests on assessing whether one person can distinguish between what he or she knows to be true and what someone else mistakenly believes to be true; that is, a false belief. For example, a woman places her new vase on a table. While the woman is out of the room, a man enters and accidentally knocks the vase off the table, breaking it. The man is unaware that the woman sneaks a look into the room and sees the broken vase. Later, in a different setting, the woman asks, "What do you think of my new vase?" The man could respond with what is true ("The vase is broken") or not true ("The vase looks great"). The critical question for understanding what the man is trying to accomplish—irony versus deception—is whether the man knows that the woman knows the truth about the vase. Brain-injured patients in research studies at times confuse the elements of the scenario and misinterpret the man's utterance (Winner et al., 1998). Patients with deficient ToM may also misuse or underuse mental state terms in their explanations.

ToM can be extended to include related notions from pragmatics and discourse, such as the importance of shared knowledge between participants in a conversation (e.g., "common ground," Clark & Marshall, 1981) or Grice's conversational postulates (e.g., supplying an appropriate but not excessive amount of information, Grice, 1975). The recent surge of interest in ToM can be in part attributed to the broad applicability of ToM across topics and across populations including adults and normally developing children, children with autism spectrum disorders, and adults with brain injury (Baron-Cohen, Leslie, & Frith, 1985; Griffin et al., 2006; Happé, Brownell, & Winner, 1999; Stone, Baron-Cohen, & Knight, 1998; Stuss, Gallup, & Alexander, 2001; Wellman, 1990).

In light of the centrality of speaker and listener beliefs to communication, ToM provides a useful framework for addressing many deficits exhibited by patients with right hemisphere brain damage (RHD) or with traumatic brain injury (TBI). Many patients with RHD or TBI (without aphasia) exhibit significant impairments with nonliteral language, humor comprehension, and conversational discourse that appear related to ToM (Bibby & McDonald, 2004; Brownell, Griffin, Winner, Friedman, & Happé, 2000; Channon, Pellijeff, & Rule, 2005; Coelho, DeRuyter, & Stein, 1996; Griffin et al., 2006; Happé et al., 1999; Levin, Goldstein, Williams, & Eisenberg, 1991; Lundgren, Moya, & Benowitz, 1984; Martin & McDonald, 2005; McDonald, 1993; McDonald, 1999; Murdoch & Theodoros, 2001; Myers, 1999).

REMEDIATION OF DEFICITS ASSOCIATED WITH RHD AND TBI

Therapies have been developed for impairments associated with RHD, such as inattention and neglect (Rizzo & Robin, 1996; Sohlberg & Mateer, 1987). In addition, Myers (1999) and Tompkins (1995) outline approaches to treatment that could be adapted for treatment of discourse comprehension deficits. Remediation for the cognitive-communication deficits associated with TBI, such as attention (Sohlberg & Mateer, 1987; Sohlberg et al., 2003), memory (Ownsworth & McFarland, 1999), problem solving (Levine et al., 2000; Rath, Simon, Langenbahn, Sherr, & Diller, 2003; Von Cramon, Matthes-von Cramon, & Mai, 1991) and socialization (Ylvisaker, Turkstra, & Coelho, 2005) also exist. However, the literature to date lacks an array of treatment options comparable to those available for individuals with aphasia. This gap in the clinical literature limits a clinician's ability to address the needs of individual patients with communication deficits secondary to acquired brain damage. In this chapter we will consider how ToM relates to the constellation of communication and cognitive impairments related to RHD and to TBI. We will also describe an approach to training ToM in patients with acquired brain injury that we have recently developed and provide some preliminary evidence illustrating the usefulness of the approach.

Although variations on false belief tasks have been used extensively to examine ToM, many authors have pointed out that a child or adult may fail a false belief task either due to a selective ToM problem (attributable to lack of development or to neurological disorder) or due to limitations that apply across domains such as immature or impaired executive function (Roth & Leslie, 1998; Saxe et al., 2004; Zelazo, Jacques, Burack, & Frye, 2002). The false belief tasks used to assess ToM are often complex and involve more than one character, movement of characters and objects, and many other details including who has perceptual access to the truth (e.g., Winner et al., 1998). Also, logically comparable tasks using contrasting photographic representations rather than false mental states reveal similar performance patterns in very young children (Zaitchik, 1990). There is, however, substantial support for the existence of a special ToM capacity that can be dissociated from performance on comparable false photograph tasks (Leslie & Thaiss, 1992) and for the separability of executive function from ToM.

Saxe and her colleagues have performed several studies using functional imaging (fMRI) with nonbrain-damaged adults to support the neurological separability of ToM. One approach was based on the use of a range of stories of equivalent length involving, for example, mechanical inferences such as what happens when a pot of water is left on a hot burner for a long period, as well as mental states (Saxe et al., 2004). Participants listened to several types of stories while in the scanner and then answered questions about each story. The primary result showed selective right parietal activation (and to a lesser extent, left parietal activation) associated with ToM stories, and this effect was distinct from components of executive function. In another study, Saxe and Kanwisher (2003) presented participants with one set of stimulus items under two different sets of task instructions, one of which encouraged participants to interpret the task in terms of ToM. The parietal activation was observed only when participants treated the items as requiring mentalist processing.

In contrast to the evidence supporting the dissociability of ToM from other components of cognition in adults with no history of brain injury, ToM impairments in patients with RHD or TBI have not been unambiguously isolated from, for example, working memory span, the inhibitory ability needed to focus attention on only one of conflicting "truths," and representational ability. One promising suggestion has been reported by Griffin et al. (2006). These authors asked patients with RHD to interpret cartoons, some of which required appreciation of ToM while others rested on physical humor. One relevant finding was that the scores of patients with RHD on a measure associated with executive function (Trails B minus Trials A test, Spreen & Strauss, 1998) correlated highly with the quality of their interpretations of the non ToM cartoon items, but did not correlate with the quality of their interpretations of the ToM items. Thus, at least one measure of general cognitive ability appears to be related to apprehending one form of humor, but not to successful use of ToM.

While Griffin et al.'s finding is intriguing, patients with large lesions or diffuse lesions often present with a variable constellation of deficits that will affect many domains within cognition, including some degree of executive system involvement, as well as attentional, visuospatial, and emotional deficits, and changes in affect, personality, and empathy (see Brownell et al., 2000; Heilman & Valenstein, 2003; Joanette, Goulet, & Hannequin, 1990; Kempler, 2005; Myers, 1999; Tompkins, 1995, for reviews).

The relevance of executive function for the TBI population is also based on the prevalence of frontal and prefrontal system involvement. Diffuse axonal shearing is typically widespread subsequent to moderate or severe TBI; however, the frontal regions including subcortical connections are particularly vulnerable. In addition, focal contusions occur at characteristic locations due to the shape of the skull and typical direction of brain movement within the skull. These areas of damage usually include frontal regions among others, and their impact is often amplified by disconnection due to widespread diffuse axonal shearing (see Chen, Abrams, & D'Esposito, 2006; Cicerone, Levin, Malec, Stuss, & Whyte, 2006; and Katz, 1997, for reviews).

The primary goal of the work summarized in this chapter is to evaluate whether a structured, intensive training program directed at ToM can result in improvement even while performance in other, possibly related domains remains static. Selective improvement would support the separateness of ToM in patients with acquired brain injury, as well as in adults with no history of brain injury. Evidence to support the usefulness of this training program would provide one option for the remediation of impaired communication in individuals with acquired brain injury.

EMPIRICAL FOUNDATION FOR TOM TRAINING

The first task in building a ToM training program was developing a practical means of assessing ToM performance. This required a large number of test items that people would find interesting and enjoyable, even after repeated exposure. Humor comprehension, specifically, cartoon interpretation, has been used previously to examine ToM and in patient-based studies (e.g., Griffin et al., 2006; Happé et al., 1999). We found the work of Gary Larson (e.g., *The Far Side*, Larson, 2003) to be most suitable. Many, though certainly not all, of Larson's cartoons rely on ignorance (first-order beliefs) or deception (second-order beliefs), and the availability of large numbers of these items all drawn by the same artist provided some control over style, graphic conventions, and visuospatial complexity. We selected sets of cartoons whose humor rested on first- or second-order beliefs. The primary dependent measure of performance obtained during pre- and postbaseline and training reflects the quality of patient's interpretation of these cartoons. When shown a cartoon from the stimulus set, a patient was asked to identify salient features in the picture, read the caption, and finally describe what most people would find amusing about the cartoon. It was not important that the patient thought the cartoon was funny, but that the patient understood what most people would identify as being humorous, which in all cases rested on mental states of the characters.

In order to score the responses with consistency and to provide an opportunity for demonstrating subtle changes in performance over time, we developed the ToM Cartoon Interpretation Scale (the ToMCIS) using explicit criteria (listed below) for scoring the patients' interpretations (Lundgren, Brownell, Cayer-Meade, & Spitzer, 2007). The scale extends from 0 to 5 for first-order belief cartoons and 0 to 6 for second-order belief cartoons, and can be used with high reliability (90% for independent raters) to reflect a patient's facility with the mental states of other people.

ToMCIS levels:

6. Complete and appropriate, identifies the second-order belief/mental state of the character(s).
5. Complete and appropriate, identifies the first-order belief/mental state of the character(s).
4. Complete and appropriate, identifies the mental state of the character(s) but (a) delayed (> 5 seconds before response initiation); (b) may contain self-corrections, or false starts but eventually gets to the correct response; or (c) may include some tangential comments and/or personalization.
3. Provides a mental state term relevant to the cartoon but inaccurate (i.e., wrong mental state, mental state of self rather than the character/wrong character) identification of the mental state.
2. Mentions oddness or incongruity of elements.
1. Indicates elements of understanding the incongruous nature of the critical elements of the cartoon and may describe the physical details in the picture, but does not identify the mental state of the character(s)
0. No response, "I don't know," or completely off-topic comments such as unrelated, personalized associations tangential to the cartoon.

Our second challenge was devising an empirical context to support interpretation of ToM ability by documenting connections to performance in other domains. Chief among the potential counter explanations for patients' difficulty on ToM tasks is weak central executive ability, often associated with frontal system dysfunction (see Chen et al., 2006; Cicerone et al., 2006; and Katz, 1997, for reviews). The executive function construct is very broad and may include inhibition, working memory, planning, set shifting, and more, and can be decomposed into subparts that do not always intercorrelate (Lehto, 1996).

The tactic we have adopted at this stage in our research is fairly general: using widely available assessment tools with normative data such as *The Delis-Kaplan Executive Function System* (Delis, Kaplan, & Kramer, 2001) to gain a broad perspective on the central executive. In addition, work by Tompkins and her colleagues with RHD patients (e.g., Tompkins, 1990; Tompkins, Bloise,

Timko, & Baumgaertner, 1994; Tompkins, Boada, & McGarry, 1992) has high-lighted the importance of one particular component of the executive system, working memory (Baddeley, 1986; Baddeley & Hitch, 1994; Caplan & Waters, 1999; Just, Carpenter, & Keller, 1996). Tompkins's work suggests that patients with RHD show apparently normal appreciation of, for example, metaphoric alternative meanings when the experimental context is designed to minimize any requirement for strategic planning or conscious effort by participants, but show deficits when the task requirements are altered to maximize strategic requirements. Additionally, Tompkins et al. (1994) have reported that capac-ity of working memory, often tied to prefrontal regions (Crosson et al., 1999; Smith & Jonides, 1999), correlates with discourse comprehension performance for patients with RHD.

The Tompkins Working Memory Span procedure is not as widely known as the others. Tompkins et al. (1994) adapted the classic reading (listening) span test of Daneman and Carpenter (1980) for use with patients with acquired brain-injury. This variant is a complex memory test that requires active processing of information in addition to simple retention: participants judge the truth value of sentences while retaining the final word in each of a set of sentences for later recall. One advantage of the span construct over other measures of executive function is that it has been related directly to the disrupted comprehension often observed in patients with acquired brain damage.

Test stimuli in the Tompkins et al. procedure are tape-recorded, simple active declarative sentences (e.g., "You sit on a chair") that end in a common, one-to-two syllable noun, verb, or adjective. After each sentence, a participant responds true or false and must retain the final word of a sentence for a spoken recall test. The sentences are presented in sets of varying size: Level 2 sets have just two sentences; Level 3 sets contain three sentences each; Level 4 sets contain four sentences each; and Level 5 sets contain five sentences each. A participant listens to the sentences in a set and, at the end of the set, recalls the final words of the sentences. There are three sets of sentences for each level. The items are blocked by level, and the three levels are presented in order of increasing difficulty. The test contains a total of 42 words to recall, and the primary dependent measure is the number of errors out of 42.

In addition to establishing the (lack of) connection between ToM performance and executive function, it is similarly useful to distinguish ToM from performance in a very different functional domain. Brain injury, particularly in posterior (pari-etal) regions of the right hemisphere and, to a lesser extent, in the left hemisphere, is often associated with visuospatial impairments that appear unrelated to ToM. (It is interesting to note that the work of Saxe and colleagues suggests that the parietal regions may be highly relevant to ToM ability.) We have used a short version of The Benton Line Orientation Task developed by Qualls, Bliwise, and Stringer (2000), which, with 15 items, correlates highly ($r = + .9$) with the long form. This test measures how well a person perceives a diagram of a line angle and then matches that angle with one of a set of alternatives presented with the model in view.

Another array of assessments reflect extensions beyond the ToM construct. Because the boundaries between the role of ToM in communication and the roles of related skills are not as yet clearly drawn, we have tried to chart how change in ToM performance relates to change in other domains in an exploratory spirit. Affect, for example, is another domain that can cause disruption to the adjustment of brain-injured patients as they recover. To provide a summary measure, we have adopted the Florida Affect Battery (Bowers, Blonder, & Heilman, 1999) designed for use with neurological populations to assess interpretation of emotion carried by facial expression and tone of voice. We also use Baron-Cohen and Wheelwright's *Empathy Quotient* (Baron-Cohen & Wheelwright, 2004; Lawrence, Shaw, Baker, Baron-Cohen, & David, 2004), which is a self-report measure. Patients read a sentence and then respond to how strongly they feel about the statement based on a four point scale ("strongly agree" to "strongly disagree").

A final extension of ToM changes is conversational language use. This different type of assessment is based on a 30 minute videotaped "first encounter" conversation in which a patient meets another person for the first time and talks to the person in order to get to know her (Kennedy, Strand, Edythe, Burton, & Peterson, 1994). The middle 20 minutes of this conversation is assessed in two ways, one, based on Kennedy and colleagues' (1994) work and, two, using the Prutting and Kirchner (1987) Pragmatic Protocol. Each pre- and posttraining conversation is transcribed and then analyzed by trained judges to provide a fine-grained assessment of discourse and a global assessment of pragmatic functioning, that is, the success of communication observed in a relatively natural context. In addition to the coding of discourse and pragmatic behaviors, the number of appropriate and inappropriate mental state terms spoken by the patient can be tabulated in order to determine whether the use of mental state terms transfers to other verbal tasks. In the child language literature, the use of mental state terms such as "think" and "believe" has been used as evidence of a child's understanding of mind (Zaitchik, 1990).

We use one other assessment that is not directly related to ToM, but that is relevant to the variable performance by patients with brain injury who often fatigue quickly and who may perform uncharacteristically on a given day due to extraneous factors. Particularly when a patient performs over many sessions, there will be day to day fluctuations in energy level and mood that might affect performance. To gain some traction on this fact of patient performance, we use a slightly modified version of the *Stroke and Aphasia Quality of Life* scale (SAQOL-39; Hilari, Byng, Lamping, & Smith, 2003). The battery contains four domain scales: a Physical score, Communication score, Psychosocial score, and Energy score. Two of these scales (Physical, Communication) are not expected to change for a patient from session to session. For example, the Physical scale includes questions such as "…how much trouble did you have walking?" The Communication scale, which is designed for people with aphasia, includes items such as "… how much trouble did you have speaking clearly enough to use the phone?" Other scales are more likely to show change from session to session if a patient is affected by some acute issue, such as a new health problem. The Psychosocial scale asks about symptoms associated with depression (e.g., "… did you have no interest in other people or activities?".) The Energy scale includes questions such as "… did you have to stop and rest often during the day?"

We have modified the time frame used for items in the original version of the battery slightly by substituting "yesterday and today" for "during the past week" for all items because we administer the battery to patients more than once per week. Each item is followed by a rating scale with five levels defined both verbally and numerically: Couldn't do it at all (1); A lot of trouble (2); Some trouble (3); A little trouble (4); and No trouble at all (5).

Our practice is to exclude data from a session if a patient scores more than two standard deviations below his or her baseline average for either the Psychosocial or Energy scale based on his or her other session scores. (Low scores also alert the clinician to consider whether further action is needed to protect the patient). Additional sessions can often be scheduled.

OVERVIEW OF TRAINING PROTOCOL

The foundation of the proposed training is to make explicit and concrete the ingredients for understanding ToM so that a patient can see exactly what he or she may not be consciously aware of, or able to remember and use without aid. Explicit provision of missing or weak links in a task has worked in other domains. For example, Wellman et al. (2002) have used thought bubbles (balloons used to convey thoughts of cartoon characters) in order to help some children with autism to perform ToM tasks with greater success. When mental states are represented in thought balloons, they become far more accessible: the once abstract and difficult concept of a mental state is now just another kind of sentence describing something about the world. This simple therapeutic device does not work for all individuals with autism, but it works for many. A similar approach used with patients with RHD has proven effective in a metaphor training protocol that uses circles with line segments to represent explicitly the semantic features that are or are not shared across word concepts (Lundgren, Brownell, Roy, & Cayer-Meade, 2006).

Thought bubbles provide a completely explicit, visual means to support strategies for thinking about mental states. Thought bubbles provide the opportunity to observe the similarities and differences between two people's thoughts, that is, false beliefs, which provide a basis for predicting and understanding behavior. In addition, in our visual materials (see Figure 28.2), the supporting graphic displays make explicit whether a character has or does not have direct perceptual access (line of sight) to the topic being discussed. In addition, this mode of graphic display, which is well within the visuospatial abilities of the vast majority of brain-damaged patients more than a few weeks post onset of their illness, allows easy tabulation of beliefs and thoughts such that the thoughts of individuals are available in concrete form for practice and review.

We have developed a structured ToM training protocol that provides a progression of tasks involving ToM abilities. Our program begins with first-order beliefs and progresses to second-order beliefs, including intentional deception. The protocol is designed to support mental state operations for (1) generating thoughts about a pictured object from another person's perspective; (2) evaluating the thoughts of one or two characters as an object changes form and the characters change location within a house; (3) evaluating differences between characters' thoughts and their eventual actions; and (4) inhibiting personalized thoughts unrelated to the beliefs of the characters. Different patients may have difficulty with one or more than one component, reflecting the complexity of the domain.

The training items are presented using one or two characters with bubbles placed above their heads to depict their thoughts about a variety of objects. The patient notes the thoughts of the character as they relate to the object and, in some situations, to the beliefs of another character. The patient is then asked to predict behavior based on the relevant mental state(s) of one or both characters. A detailed description of the protocol is included as an appendix.

EVALUATION OF TRAINING PROTOCOL

We take a two-fold approach to evaluation, the foundation of evidence-based practice. We want to assess whether individual patients make gains in ToM performance that can reasonably be atttributed to the training protocol, and we also want to understand, on a more theoretical level, how any gains do or do not relate to change in the other domains mentioned above. In light of the heterogeneity across patients with RHD and TBI in terms of symptom profiles and lesions, we have incorporated assessments of the domains outlined above into a variant of a single-subject experimental design (Barlow, Nock, & Hersen, 2009; Kearns, 1986, 2000; Olswang, Thompson, Warren, & Minghetti, 1990) for this phase II project (Golper et al., 2001; Robey & Schultz, 1998). The single subject approach, although it has limitations in terms of the statistical generality of results, provides a practical starting point for understanding how a range of patients with idiosyncratic cognitive-linguistic profiles will respond to the protocol. After a description of our approach, we present some illustrative results from one patient who has gone through a preliminary version of the protocol.

OVERVIEW OF THE PROCEDURES

1. *Informed Consent*: Consent is obtained by a speech-language pathologist with experience in communicating with individuals with cognitive-linguistic deficits.
2. *Pretraining Assessment and Posttraining Assessment Battery*: These tests provide beginning and end points for a patient's experience in the protocol and provide one way to evaluate whether there has been useful change. This battery includes the target of the training (i.e., cartoon interpretation of first- and second-order belief items), and, for comparison, line orientation that is not trained and is not expected to change. In addition, ancillary measures obtained include examination of executive function, empathy, pragmatic language, affect, and quality of life.

3. *Pretraining Baseline Probes*: The purpose of these pretraining probes is to supply a baseline of performance on the most critical measures, cartoon interpretation and line orientation. The baseline performances will indicate whether a patient's performances are stable over time or, in contrast, whether there is steady improvement that cannot logically be attributed to the intervention that lies in the future and that might be a result of practice or even spontaneous recovery. If a patient's performance from session to session is very stable, it will be easier to identify a change that coincides with the beginning of training. On the other hand, if there is a great deal of fluctuation from session to session in the Baseline phase, identifying important improvements in performance linked to training will be more difficult.

   For most patients, there are approximately 10 sessions, 3 per week for approximately 3.5 weeks, which include Cartoon Interpretation and Line Orientation tests, and also the SAQOL-39 to identify days on which a patient is behaving or feeling "Out of Sorts," in which case data from that session will be excluded from analysis. Some patients may receive an extended series of baseline assessments in order to make extra sure that even extended amounts (20 sessions) of practice interpreting cartoons does not by itself lead to improvement.

4. *Training and Probes*: Training starts immediately after completion of baseline sessions. Each training session includes assessment of Cartoon Interpretation and Line Orientation, as well as the SAQOL-39. The protocol supports extensive practice with mental state operations that tap (1) generating thoughts about pictured objects from another person's perspective; (2) evaluating the thoughts of one or two characters as objects change form and the characters change location within a house; (3) evaluating differences between characters' thoughts and their eventual actions; and (4) inhibiting personalized thoughts unrelated to the characters. Training items are presented using one or two characters with bubbles placed above their heads to depict their thoughts about a variety of objects. Sometimes the characters are depicted in the same room of a house and therefore as sharing beliefs, and sometimes they are in different rooms and not obviously sharing beliefs. The patient determines the beliefs of each character as they relate to a pictured object and, in some situations, to the beliefs of the other character in the house. The patient then predicts and/or interprets behavior based on the relevant mental state(s) of one or both characters. Our program begins with first-order beliefs and progresses to second-order beliefs, including intentional deception.

   Patients are seen three times weekly by a speech-language pathologist and receive homework assignments on two additional days to include a total of five training hours per week. The homework component is motivated by results showing that aphasia treatment outcomes are improved with increased intensity of treatment (Bhogal, Teasell, &

Speechley, 2003). A homework notebook is given to each patient for recording practice responses. The homework tasks are directly related to the training phase introduced in the previous training session. For example, if a patient is working on Phase II, the patient will be given multiple choice tasks in a homework notebook to reinforce the skills successfully achieved. Immediate feedback as to the accuracy of the response is presented to the patient on the next page of the homework notebook. Homework completion is recorded by the patient in the training log and reviewed with the speech-language pathologist on a weekly basis.

5. *Posttraining Baseline Probes*: The posttraining sessions provide extensive data on how well patients fare on cartoon interpretation after completing the training. The posttraining sessions also provide data on whether training gains fade shortly after the formal training ends. There are approximately10 sessions, 3 per week for approximately 3.5 weeks, which include Cartoon Interpretation and Line Orientation tests, and also the SAQOL-39 scale to identify days on which a patient is behaving or feeling "Out of Sorts," in which case data from that session will be excluded from analysis.

6. *Long-Term Follow Up*: Three to four months after the end of training, patients are seen once more for a brief session of cartoon interpretation and line orientation judgments and augmented quality of life to provide an indication of permanence of gains.

Booster Sessions. Following the final training session, a set of cartoons that have been correctly interpreted are given to the patient, and the patient is encouraged to share these cartoons and their meanings with family members, friends, and neighbors in order to continue to reinforce these skills. One of the advantages of using *Far Side* cartoons (Larson, 2003) is that they are interesting enough to support repeated examination.

Data Analysis. The major question is whether patients will show better (more mentalist) cartoon interpretations after the training, and whether performance on the line orientation task will not change. More to the point, the question is whether any improvement in ToM can be attributed to the training as opposed to other factors such as extensive practice with items.

Although a variety of procedures can be used to assess the efficacy of the intervention, a recurring issue in single subject designs is how to interpret inferential statistical tests carried out on repeated observations from a single individual. The inferential tests assume that the error term is based on independent observations; however, repeated observations from a single subject are typically not independent. We mention below just two of many different approaches, none of which is perfect. The goal is to assess whether initiation of training coincides with a real and important change in patients' cartoon interpretation and, as a comparison, with any change in their visuospatial performance as measured by Benton scores. Our prediction is that initiation of training is associated with change in cartoon interpretation but not with any change in Benton performance.

One approach is based on multiple regression techniques. A patient's score (cartoon interpretation, Benton) for each session provides the dependent variable. Predictor variables include X_1 session number (1 to approximately 30), which provides an index of time and any progressive change starting during the baseline phase and continuing into and beyond the training phase. The second predictor variable X_2 is "dummy coded": 0 is used for all pretraining baseline sessions and 1 for all training and posttraining sessions. The second, dummy coded predictor variable, which distinguishes pretraining baseline sessions from all later sessions, reflects overall change in level of performance before versus after initiation of training. Support for the effectiveness of treatment could take the following form. With X_1, session number, and X_2, pre- versus postinitiation of training, as the two predictor variables in a multiple regression analysis, a significant effect of X_2 (that is, a beta weight reliably greater than 0.0) indicates a reliable improvement in overall mean level of performance that coincides with initiation of training and that is completely separate from any steady improvement over sessions due to, for example, practice.

Interpreting the significance level associated with the training effect can be complicated by the statistical assumption of nonindependence across observations (see discussion by Crosbie, 1993). We assessed the independence in the residuals of the analysis; that is, the left over "error" that remains after effects of session number and training are removed. It is the residuals that make up the error term used in the analysis for evaluating the statistical significance of the training effect. In brief, we obtain the residuals from the multiple regression analyses described above and examine whether the residuals represent independent pieces of information by examining the autocorrelations among the residuals. (An autocorrelation of lag 1 is calculated by pairing the first of a patient's residual scores with the second, the second with the third, the third with the fourth, and so on. SPSS, version 16, includes an autocorrelation choice found under the Time Series menu option.) In this way, it is possible to assess whether or not the statistical assumption of independence is seriously violated. In practical terms, including session number as a predictor variable accounts for virtually all of the lack of independence present in the raw scores, resulting in very small autocorrelations among the residuals. Still, it is important to note that even a small (nonsignificant) autocorrelation may have an effect on actual significant levels: A small positive autocorrelation may inflate the actual alpha level slightly such that an apparent .05 alpha level may in fact be .07. Crosbie (1993) has provided some simulation data that provide a rough guide to how serious the problem is. [Crosbie has also written an analysis program ITSACORR that uses an estimation procedure to handle the problem of correlated error, but this program has been severely criticized (Huitema, 2004).] The bottom line is that we take into account the potential inaccuracy of alpha levels produced in the regression analysis and adjust our interpretation accordingly. The autocorrelations among the residuals in our analyses are typically quite small and not statistically significant. Most often, the important result concerning the impact of training is sufficiently clear that the interpretation is not greatly affected by a small amount of autocorrelation. For data sets that yield ambiguous results, other analytic procedures can shore up interpretation.

One alternative, for example, is based on a recent application of "bootstrapping" developed by Borckardt et al. (2008; see also McKnight, McKean, & Huitema, 2000) specifically to facilitate analysis of treatment effects from single subject designs with relatively small numbers of observations. These authors have made available a free, user-friendly, downloadable computer program (http://clinicalre-searcher.org) to carry out the analysis. In brief, one starts with a null hypothesis of no change in performance from pre- to postinitiation of training. The software computes the autocorrelation (lag 1) for the sample data collected from a patient. (The dependent measure is the same as used in the regression analysis.) Then, working with the assumption of no effect, the software draws a very large number (e.g., 10,000) of random samples of pre- and postinitiation of training data with that level of autocorrelation. By tabulating what happens in the 10,000 samples, one gets a very good idea of how large a difference in performance would happen by chance. The software can provide probabilities for observing a mean difference in performance from pre- to posttraining that is as large or larger than what was actually found. It is then simple to evaluate whether an improvement seen in a patient is greater than what one might expect on the basis of chance.

Other relevant information is whether there is change in working memory span or other executive function measures for individual patients who show improvement on the cartoon assessment. For patients who show improvement on cartoon assessment but not on executive function or working memory, the training would appear to affect a distinct domain (ToM) within cognition. After many patients are tested, it should be possible to generate hypotheses about why ToM gains are selective for some patients but not others, whose ToM impairments seem intertwined with other deficits. To gauge generalization of training gains, we examine changes in a patient's empathy test, perception of emotion, and conversational skill.

SAMPLE RESULTS

While we are still refining the design, we have begun to test patients on many of the ancillary measures outlined above and on the basic protocol. One illustrative patient, S1, was a high-school educated man in his early 60s who had sustained unilateral RHD due to a middle cerebral artery stroke several years prior to testing. He exhibited slight residual neglect and impaired understanding of nonliteral language. He completed the protocol without any trouble, which suggests that patients are willing to stay with the program for the needed length of time. The patient showed consistent performance levels pre- and posttraining on line orientation, as can be seen in Figure 28.1. Regression analysis confirmed that there was no reliable effect of pre- versus postinitiation of training on line orientation performance ($p = .732$). In contrast, patient S1 showed a very strong effect in his cartoon interpretations ($p = .005$). This patient, thus, shows a clear effect of the training protocol that does not appear due to other nonspecific change in overall cognitive function. In addition, for this man, ToM appears to be distinct from executive function (cf. Griffin et al., 2006): both pre- and posttraining the patient tested as severely impaired on one measure of executive function (Helm-Estabrooks, 2001), and his Working Memory

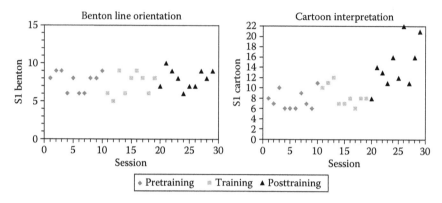

FIGURE 28.1   Results from Patient S1 for Benton Line Orientation (on the left) and Theory of Mind Cartoon Interpretation Scale scores (on the right).

Span score remained nearly identical. The patient's pre- versus postinitiation of training scores on other, more exploratory measures are more difficult to interpret. The patient's score on the Florida Affect Battery improved slightly but his Empathy score remained constant. Finally, something that needs to be explored is the best way to assess the introspective gains in quality of life that patients experience: the SAQOL self-report scale did not show improvement for this patient; it is not known whether the patient's significant others perceived any improvement.

CONCLUSION

This ToM training protocol represents the start of a long-term effort to augment the evidence-based treatment options available for patients with acquired brain-injury who present with cognitive-linguistic communication deficits. Preliminary results suggests that patients with RHD may benefit from this structured ToM training program, that the single subject approach for initial evaluation can work well, and that ToM performance can be usefully distinguished from performance in other cognitive domains. In time, accumulated evidence from this initial training study will provide a foundation for the design of larger studies focused on determining (1) whether patients with TBI, a growing population, respond in ways similar to patients with RHD; (2) whether specific lesion variables (e.g., etiology, size, and location) or functional considerations (e.g., initial severity of impairment) predict response to training; and (3) whether improvement on a specific ToM task can generalize to other aspects of communication or interpersonal competence.

ACKNOWLEDGMENT

The preparation of this chapter was supported by NIH grants R01DC009045 and P30DC0520702. This chapter reflects equal contributions by the authors, whose order was determined by a coin toss.

REFERENCES

Baddeley, A. D. (1986). *Working memory*. Oxford, UK: Oxford University Press.

Baddeley, A. D., & Hitch, G. J. (1994). Developments in the concept of working memory. *Neuropsychology, 8,* 485–493.

Barlow, D., Nock, M., & Hersen, M. (2009). *Single case experimental designs. Strategies for studying behavior for change* (3rd ed.). Boston, MA: Pearson.

Baron-Cohen, S., Leslie, A. M., & Frith, U. (1985). Does the autistic child have a "theory of mind?" *Cognition, 21,* 37–46.

Baron-Cohen, S., Tager-Flusberg, H., & Cohen, D. J. (Eds.). (2000). *Understanding other minds* (2nd ed.). Oxford, UK: Oxford University Press.

Baron-Cohen, S., & Wheelwright, S. (2004). The empathy quotient (EQ). An investigation of adults with asperger syndrome or high functioning autism, and normal sex differences. *Journal of Autism and Developmental Disorders, 34,* 163–175.

Bhogal, S. K., Teasell, R., & Speechley, M. (2003). Intensity of aphasia therapy: Impact on recovery. *Stroke, 34,* 987–993.

Bibby, H., & McDonald, S. (2004). Theory of mind after traumatic brain injury. *Neuropsychologia, 43*(1), 99–114.

Borckardt, J. J., Nash, M. R., Murphy, M. D., Moore, M., Shaw, D., & O'Neil, P. L. (2008). Clinical practice as natural laboratory for psychotherapy research. A guide to case-based time-series analysis. *American Psychologist, 63*(2), 77–93.

Bowers, D., Blonder, L. X., & Heilman, K. M. (1999). *Florida Affect Battery*, Center for Neuropsychological Studies Cognitive Neuroscience Laboratory, University of Florida Gainesville.

Brownell, H., Griffin, R., Winner, E., Friedman, O., & Happé, F. (2000). Cerebral lateralization and theory of mind. In S. Baron-Cohen, H. Tager-Flusberg, & D. J. Cohen (Eds.), *Understanding other minds* (2nd ed., pp. 306–333). Oxford, UK: Oxford University Press.

Caplan, D., & Waters, G. S. (1999). Working memory and sentence comprehension. *Behavioral and Brain Sciences, 22,* 77–126.

Channon, S., Pellijeff, A., & Rule, A. (2005). Social cognition after head injury: Sarcasm and theory of mind. *Brain and Language, 93,* 123–134.

Chen, A. J.-W., Abrams, G. M., & D'Esposito, M. (2006). Functional reintegration of prefrontal networks for enhancing recovery after brain injury. *Journal of Head Trauma Rehabilitation, 21,* 107–118.

Cicerone, K., Levin, H., Malec, J., Stuss, D., & Whyte, J. (2006). Cognitive rehabilitation interventions for executive function: Moving from bench to bedside in patients with traumatic brain injury. *Journal of Cognitive Neuroscience, 18,* 1212–1222

Clark, H. H., & Marshall, C. (1981). Definite reference and mutual knowledge. In A. K. Joshi, B. L Webber, & I. A. Sag (Eds.), *Elements of discourse understanding* (pp. 10–63). Cambridge, UK: Cambridge University Press.

Coelho, C. A., DeRuyter, F., & Stein, M. (1996). Treatment efficacy: Cognitive-communicative disorders resulting from traumatic brain injury. *Journal of Speech and Hearing Research, 39,* S5–S17.

Crosbie, J. (1993). Interrupted time-series analysis with brief single-subject data. *Journal of Consulting and Clinical Psychology, 61,* 966–974.

Crosson, B. R. , Rao, S. M. , Woodley, S. J., Rosen, A. C., Bobholz, J. A., Mayer A., . . . Stein, E. A. (1999). Mapping of semantic, phonological, and orthographic verbal working memory in normal adults with functional magnetic resonance imaging. *Neuropsychology, 13,* 171–187.

Daneman, M., & Carpenter, P. A. (1980). Individual differences in working memory and reading. *Journal of Verbal Learning and Verbal Behavior, 19,* 450–466.

Delis, D. C., Kaplan, E., & Kramer, J. H. (2001). *Delis-Kaplan executive function system (D-KEFS).* San Antonio, TX: The Psychological Corporation.

Dennett, D. (1978). Beliefs about beliefs. *Behavioral and Brain Sciences, 1,* 568–570.

Golper, L. A. C., Wertz, R. T., Frattali, C. M., Yorkston, K., Myers, P., Katz, R., . . . Wambaugh, J. (2001). Evidence-based practice guidelines for the management of communication disorders in neurologically impaired individuals: Project introduction. Academy of Neurologic Communication Disorders and Sciences, *Practice Guidelines Project: Introduction.*

Grice, H. P. (1975). The logic of conversation. In *Syntax and semantics, Vol. 3: Speech acts* (pp. 41–58). New York, NY: Seminar Press.

Griffin, R., Friedman, O., Ween, J., Winner, E., Happé, F., & Brownell, H. (2006). Theory of mind and the right cerebral hemisphere: Refining the scope of impairment. *Laterality, 11,* 195–225.

Happé, F., Brownell, H., & Winner, E. (1999). Acquired "theory of mind" impairments following stroke. *Cognition, 70,* 211–240.

Heilman, K. M., & Valenstein, E. (Eds.). (2003). *Clinical neuropsychology* (4th ed.). Oxford, UK: Oxford University Press.

Helm-Estabrooks, N. (2001). *CLQT Cognitive Linguistic Quick Test.* New York, NY: The Psychological Corporation.

Hilari, K., Byng, S., Lamping, D. L., & Smith, S. C. (2003). Stroke and Aphasia Quality of Life Scale-39 (SAQOL-39): Evaluation of acceptability, reliability, and validity. *Stroke, 34,* 1944–1950.

Huitema, B. E. (2004). Analysis of interrupted time-series experiments using ITSE: A critique. *Understanding Statistics, 3,* 27–46.

Joanette, Y., Goulet, P., & Hannequin, D. (1990). *Right hemisphere and verbal communication.* New York, NY: Springer-Verlag.

Just, M. A., Carpenter, P. A., & Keller, T. A. (1996). The capacity theory of comprehension: New frontiers of evidence and arguments. *Psychological Review, 103,* 773–780.

Katz, D. I. (1997). Traumatic brain injury. In M. V. Mills, J. W. Cassidy, & D. I. Katz (Eds.), *Neurologic rehabilitation: A guide to diagnosis, prognosis, and treatment planning* (pp. 105–143). Malden, MA: Blackwell Science.

Kearns, K. P. (1986). Flexibility of single-subject experimental designs. Part II: Design selection and arrangement of experimental phases. *Journal of Speech and Hearing Disorders, 51,* 204–214.

Kearns, K. P. (2000). Single-subject experimental designs in aphasia. In S. E. Nadeau, L. J. Gonzalez Rothi, & B. Crosson (Eds.), *Aphasia and language* (pp. 421–441). New York, NY: Guilford Press.

Kempler, D. (2005). *Neurocognitive disorders in aging.* Thousand Oaks, CA: Sage Publications, Inc.

Kennedy, M., Strand, W. B., Edythe, A., Burton, W., & Peterson, C. (1994). Analysis of first-encounter conversations of right-hemisphere-damaged adults. *Clinical Aphasiology, 22,* 67–80.

Larson, G. (2003). *The complete far side 1980–1994.* Kansas City, MO: Andrews McMeel Publishing, Inc.

Lawrence, E. J., Shaw, P., Baker, D., Baron-Cohen, S., & David, A. S. (2004). Measuring empathy – Reliability and validity of the empathy quotient. *Psychological Medicine, 34,* 911–919.

Lehto, J. (1996). Are executive function tests dependent on working memory capacity? *The Quarterly Journal of Experimental Psychology, 49A,* 29–50.

Leslie, A. M. (1987). Pretense and representation: The origins of "theory of mind." *Psychological Review, 94*, 412–426.

Leslie, A. M., & Thaisse, L. (1992). Domain specificity in conceptual development. *Cognition, 43,* 225–251.

Levin, H. S., Goldstein, F. C, Williams, D. H., & Eisenberg, H. M. (1991). The contribution of frontal lobe lesions to the neurobehavioral outcome of closed head injury. In H. S. Levin, H. M. Eisenberg, & A. I. Benton (Eds.). *Frontal lobe function and dysfunction* (pp. 318–338). New York, NY: Oxford University Press.

Levine, B., Robertson, I. H., Clare, L., Carter, G., Hong, H., Wilson, B. A., . . . Stuss, D. T. (2000). Rehabilitation of executive functioning: An experimental-clinical validation of goal management training. *Journal of the International Neuropsychological Society, 6*, 299–312.

Lundgren, K., Brownell, H., Cayer-Meade, C., & Spitzer, J. (2007). Training theory of mind following right hemisphere damage: A pilot study. *Brain and Language, 103*, 209–210.

Lundgren, K., Brownell, H., Roy, S., & Cayer-Meade, C. (2006). A metaphor comprehension intervention for patients with right hemisphere brain damage: A pilot study. *Brain and Language, 99*, 69–70.

Lundgren, K., Moya, K. L., & Benowitz, L. I. (1984). Perception of nonverbal cues after right brain damage (Abstract). In R. H. Brookshire (Ed.), *Clinical aphasiology: Conference proceedings* (p. 282). Minneapolis, MN: BRK Publishers.

Martin, I., & McDonald, S. (2005). Evaluating the causes of impaired irony comprehension following traumatic brain injury. *Aphasiology, 19*(8), 712–730.

McDonald, S. (1993). Viewing the brain sideways? Frontal versus right hemisphere explanations of non-aphasic language disorders. *Aphasiology, 7,* 535–549.

McDonald, S. (1999). Exploring the process of inference generation in sarcasm: A review of normal and clinical studies. *Brain and Language, 68*, 486–506.

McKnight, D. D., McKean, J. W., & Huitema, B. E. (2000). A double bootstrap method to analyze linear models with autoregressive error terms. *Psychological Methods, 5*, 87–101.

Murdoch, B. E., & Theodoros, D. G. (2001). *Traumatic brain injury: Associated speech, language, and swallowing disorders.* San Diego, CA: Singular Publishing Group.

Myers, P. S. (1999). *Right hemisphere damage: Disorders of communication and cognition.* San Diego, CA: Singular Publishing Group.

Olswang, L. B., Thompson, C. K., Warren, S. F., & Minghetti, N. J. (Eds.). (1990). *Treatment efficacy research in communication disorders.* Rockville, MD: American Speech-Language-Hearing Foundation.

Ownsworth, T. L., & McFarland, K. (1999). Memory remediation in long-term acquired brain injury: Two approaches in diary training. *Brain Injury, 13*, 605–626.

Premack, D., & Woodruff, G. (1978). Does the chimpanzee have a theory of mind? *The Behavioral and Brain Sciences, 1*, 515–526.

Prutting, C.A., & Kirchner, D. M. (1987). A clinical appraisal of the pragmatic aspects of language. *Journal of Speech and Hearing Disorders, 52,* 105–119.

Qualls, C. E., Bliwise, N. G., & Stringer, A. Y. (2000). Short forms of benton judgment of line orientation test: Development and psychometric properties. *Archives of Clinical Neuropsychology, 15*, 159–163.

Rath, J. F., Simon, D., Langenbahn, D. M., Sherr, R. L., & Diller, L. (2003). Group treatment of problem-solving deficits in outpatients with traumatic brain injury: A randomized outcome study. *Neuropsychological Rehabilitation, 13,* 461–488.

Rizzo, M., & Robin, D. A. (1996). Bilateral effects of unilateral visual cortex lesions. *Brain, 119*, 951–963.

Robey, R. R., & Schultz, M. C. (1998). A model for conducting clinical-outcome research: An adaptation of the standard protocol for use in aphasiology. *Aphasiology, 12,* 787–810.

Roth, D., & Leslie, A. M. (1998). Solving belief problems: Toward a task analysis. *Cognition, 66,* 1–31.

Saxe, R., Carey, S., & Kanwisher, N. (2004). Understanding other minds: Linking developmental psychology and functional imaging. *Annual Reviews of Psychology, 55,* 87–124.

Saxe, R., & Kanwisher, N. (2003). People thinking about people. The role of the temporoparietal junction in "theory of mind." *NeuroImage, 19,* 1835–1842.

Smith, E. E., & Jonides, J. (1999). Storage and executive processes in the frontal lobes. *Science, 283,* 1657–1661.

Sohlberg, M. M., Avery, J., Kennedy, M., Ylvisaker, M., Coelho, C., Turkstra, L.S., & Yorkston, K. (2003). Practice guidelines for attention training. *Journal of Medical Speech Language Pathology, 11*(3), xix–xxxix.

Sohlberg, M. M., & Mateer, C. A. (1987). Effectiveness of an attention-training program. *Journal of Clinical and Experimental Neuropsychology, 9,* 117–130.

Spreen, O., & Strauss, E. (1998). *A compendium of neuropsychological tests: Administration, norms, and commentary* (2nd ed.). New York, NY: Oxford University Press.

Stone, V., Baron-Cohen, S., & Knight, R. (1998). Frontal lobe contributions to theory of mind. *Journal of Cognitive Neuroscience, 10,* 640–656.

Stuss, D., Gallup, G., Jr., & Alexander, M. (2001). The frontal lobes are necessary for "theory of mind." *Brain, 124,* 279–286.

Tompkins, C. A. (1990). Knowledge and strategies for processing lexical metaphor after right or left hemisphere brain damage. *Journal of Speech and Hearing Research, 33,* 307–316.

Tompkins, C. A. (1995). *Right hemisphere communication disorders: Theory and management.* San Diego, CA: Singular Publishing Group.

Tompkins, C. A., Bloise, C. G. R., Timko, M. L., & Baumgaertner, A. (1994). Working memory and inference revision in brain-damaged and normally aging adults. *Journal of Speech and Hearing Research, 37,* 896–912.

Tompkins, C. A., Boada, R, & McGarry, K. (1992). The access and processing of familiar idioms by brain-damaged and normally aging adults. *Journal of Speech and Hearing Research, 35,* 626–637.

Von Cramon, D. Y., Matthes-von Cramon, G., & Mai, N. (1991). Problem solving deficits in brain injured patients. A therapeutic approach. *Neuropsychological Rehabilitation, 1,* 45–64.

Wellman, H. M. (1990). *Children's theories of mind.* Cambridge, MA: Bradford Books, MIT Press.

Wellman, H. M., Baron-Cohen, S., Caswell, R., Gomez, J. C., Swettenham, J., Toyer, E., & Lagattuta, K. (2002). Thought-bubbles help children with autism acquire an alternative to a theory of mind. *Autism, 6,* 343–363.

Wimmer, H., & Perner, J. (1983). Beliefs about beliefs: Representation and constraining function of wrong beliefs in young children's understanding of deception. *Cognition, 13,* 103–128.

Winner, E., Brownell, H., Happé, F., Blum, A., & Pincus, D. (1998). Distinguishing lies from jokes: Theory of mind deficits in right hemisphere brain-damaged patients. *Brain and Language, 62,* 89–106.

Ylvisaker, M., Turkstra, L. S., & Coelho, C. (2005). Behavior and social intervention for individuals with traumatic brain injury: A summary of the research with clinical implications. *Seminars in Speech and Language, 4*(26), 256–267.

Zaitchik, D. (1990). When representations conflict with reality: The preschooler's problem with false beliefs and "false" photographs. *Cognition, 35*, 41–68.

Zelazo, P. D., Jacques, S., Burack, J., & Frye, D. (2002). The relation between theory of mind and rule use: Evidence from persons with autism-spectrum disorders. *Infant and Child Development, 11*, 171–195.

APPENDIX: DETAILED DESCRIPTION OF THE THEORY OF MIND TRAINING PROGRAM

The tasks in this training protocol are ordered to move a patient along a conceptually and empirically defined performance continuum from easier to more difficult. Also, some tasks build directly on other tasks, as detailed below. The program begins with a "Warm-Up Phase," which is then followed by Phases I and II. On the basis of testing completed to date, we anticipate that Phases I and II will consistently be easier and should be presented first in order to engage patients. Phases III and IV require more effort and call on a number of skills (i.e., second-order beliefs) that are often at risk in brain-damaged patients. Phases III and IV are roughly comparable to each other in difficulty except that Phase IV requires a patient to recognize elements of motivation and deception in one of the characters. For this reason, Phase III precedes Phase IV. While the ordering of difficulty of Phases III and IV varied among the pilot patients who have already completed the protocol, these two tasks were the most difficult of the program.

Criterion For Initiating Training: Stable baseline performance should be documented in cartoon interpretation, spatial orientation, and quality of life (as measured by the SAQOL-39) before training is started. Baseline assessment is repeated 10 times (twice per week during the 5 week training period).

ToM Training: The training program is designed to provide multiple opportunities for a patient to practice, correct, and learn skills necessary to progress from one phase of the training program to another. Training begins with the Warm-Up Phase and is followed by four distinct training phases (Phases I–IV).

Warm-Up Phase—Generating words.

Overview: The patient is provided multiple items in each task (Tasks I–III) in order to practice generating associations for printed and pictured nouns. Five trials of 10 items each are presented for each task. (See Figure 28.2.)

Task I—Generate five associations about a printed word (a typical, pictureable noun, such as red apple or ordinary dog).

Task II—Generate five associations about a pictured noun (an atypical noun, such as a green apple or very small dog). Get the patient to shift what is most relevant about the object; that is, using the perceptual information as a basis for the atypical associations.

Task III—Generate five associations about a pictured noun (same as used for Task II) with changes (broken vase, flat tire, spilled drink, cooked spaghetti, tipped over chair, broken window, bitten apple).

Scoring: The warm-up phase is not scored.

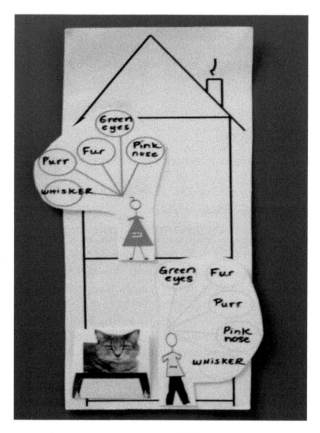

FIGURE 28.2   Visual support for the Theory of Mind training protocol.

Phase I—Changes in Beliefs.

Overview: During Phase I the patient is told that he or she will be asked to help tell a number of stories. Each story involves two characters, Alice and Greg. The patient is told that both Alice and Greg have ideas or beliefs about what is happening in each story, and that sometimes the characters' beliefs stay the same over several turns of events, and that sometimes they change. The patient is instructed to observe each situation to help decide when the characters' beliefs change and when they do not. (Please refer to the figure to see an example of the training materials.)

Instructions:

Part A.

Task I—The patient is told to notice that Alice is looking at an [object]. The patient is asked to think of five things that Alice might think about the [object].

Task II—The patient is told to notice that Alice goes upstairs in the two-family house, and that Alice is thinking about the [object]. The patient is asked to think of five things that Alice might think about the [object].

Part B.

Task I—The patient is told to notice that Alice sees the [object]. The patient is asked to review previous responses from Part A.

Task II—The patient is told to notice that Alice goes upstairs and that she is still thinking about the [object]. The patient is asked to review previous responses from Part A.

Task III—The patient is told to notice that Alice is back downstairs and is again looking at the [object] with Greg, who has changed the [object]. The patient is asked to think of five things that Alice might think about the changed [object].

Task IV—The patient is told to notice that Alice is upstairs talking on the phone about the [object]. Alice's beliefs about the [object] are reviewed. The patient is then asked to choose the response (from a set of three alternatives) that represents what Alice says to her friend about the [object].

Part C.

Task I—The patient is told to notice that Alice is looking at an [object]. The patient is asked to review previous responses.

Task II—The patient is told to notice that Alice goes upstairs and is still thinking about the [object]. The patient is asked to review previous responses.

Task III—The patient is told to notice that Alice comes back downstairs and meets Greg, who changes the [object] while both Alice and Greg are present. The patient is asked to review previous responses.

Task IV—The patient is told to notice that Alice is upstairs talking on the phone about the [object]. Alice's beliefs about the [object] are reviewed. The patient is asked to choose the response (from a set of three alternatives) that represents what Alice says to her friend about the [object].

Task V—The patient is told to notice that Greg can either change or not change the [object] while Alice is upstairs talking on the phone. The patient is asked to choose the response (from a set of three alternatives) that represents what Alice says to her friend about the [object] now.

Scoring: Responses to each task are scored as correct (1 point), delayed correct (.5), or incorrect (0). A patient can progress to the next task after achieving 90% accuracy on five trials of 10 items or 100% accuracy on three trials of 10 items.

Phase II—Word knowledge/perceptual access for two characters.

Overview: During Phase II, the patient is told that he or she will be asked to help tell a number of stories. Each story involves two characters: Alice and Greg. The patient is told that both Alice and Greg think they know what is happening in each story. Sometimes Alice's and Greg's beliefs will stay the same over several turns of events, and sometimes they will change. In addition, in some stories one person will know something that the other person does not know. This knowledge can change what one person thinks, but may not change what the other person thinks. The patient is instructed to look at each situation and to decide when Alice's and Greg's thinking changes and when their thinking does not.

Part A.

Task I—Alice and Greg look at an [object]. The patient is asked to generate five possible thoughts about the [object] that will be used for both Alice and Greg.

Task II—Alice goes upstairs and is still thinking about the [object], and Greg remains downstairs thinking about the object; the patient generates five possible thoughts for each character.

Task III—The patient identifies the common elements in Alice's and Greg's thoughts about the [object], by viewing a bubble transparency.

Part B.

Task I—Alice and Greg look at an [object]. The patient reviews previous responses.

Task II—Alice goes upstairs and thinks about the [object]. The patient reviews previous responses.

Task III—Alice is upstairs thinking about the [object], and Greg remains downstairs. The [object] downstairs is changed by Greg. The patient generates five possible thoughts about the [object] for Alice and for Greg, and identifies the similarities and differences between Alice and Greg's beliefs about the object.

Part C.

Task I—Alice and Greg view an [object]. The patient reviews previous responses.

Task II—Alice goes upstairs and thinks about the [object]. The patient reviews previous responses.

Task III—Alice is upstairs thinking about the [object] and Greg remains downstairs. The [object] downstairs is changed by Greg. The patient generates five possible thoughts about the [object] for Alice and for Greg, and identifies the similarities and differences between Alice and Greg's beliefs about the [object]. The patient reviews previous responses.

Task IV—Alice is talking to her friend on the phone about the [object]. The patient is asked to choose the response (from a set of three alternatives) that represents what Alice says to her friend about the [object] now.

Task V—Alice is talking on the phone about the [object]. The patient is asked what does Alice say to her friend about the [object]. Greg can either alter the [object] or keep it the same while Alice is talking to her friend. The patient is asked to choose the response (from a set of three alternatives) that represents what Alice says to her friend about the [object] now.

Scoring: Responses to each task are scored as correct (1 point), delayed correct (.5), or incorrect (0). A patient can progress to the next task after receiving 90% accuracy on five trials of 10 items or 100% accuracy on three trials of 10 items.

Phase III—Second-Order Beliefs.

Overview: During Phase III, the patient is told that he or she will be asked to help tell a number of stories. Each story involves two characters, Alice and Greg. The patient is told that both Alice and Greg have ideas or beliefs about what is happening in each story. Sometimes their beliefs will stay the same over several turns of events, and sometimes their beliefs will change. In addition, in some stories one person, either Alice or Greg, will know something that the other person does not know, and in some stories one of the characters will lie to the other one. This knowing or not knowing what is really going on will change one person's beliefs but will not change what the other person believes. The patient is instructed to observe each situation and to decide when each person's beliefs change and when they do not.

Task I—Alice and Greg view an [object]. The patient generates five possible thoughts about the [object] for each character.

Task II—Alice goes upstairs and thinks about the [object]. The patient generates five possible thoughts about the [object] for each character.

Task III—Alice is upstairs thinking about the [object], and Greg remains downstairs. The [object] downstairs is changed by Greg. The patient generates five possible ideas about the [object] that Alice might have, and then five ideas that Greg might have. Next, the patient identifies one idea that is the same for both Alice and Greg, and one idea that is different for Alice than for Greg.

Task IV—Alice is upstairs talking on the phone to Greg about [object]. The patient is reminded that these are accurate beliefs about the [object]. The patient is told that Greg says [. . .] about the [object]. The patient is asked whether what Greg says is accurate or not accurate according to Greg's understanding.

Task V—Alice is upstairs talking on the phone to Greg about the [object]. Greg lies about the [object] and says [. . .]. The patient is asked to choose the response (from a set of three alternatives) that represents what Greg says about the [object].

Scoring: Responses to this task are scored as correct (1 point), delayed correct (.5), or incorrect (0). A patient can progress to the next task after receiving 90% accuracy on five trials of 10 items or 100% accuracy on three trials of 10 items.

Phase IV—Second-Order Belief (motivation/deception)

Overview: During Phase IV, the patient is told that he or she will be asked to help tell a number of stories. Each story involves two characters, Alice and Greg. The patient is told that, of course, Alice and Greg both have some understanding of what is happening in each story. Sometimes one person's understanding will stay the same over several turns of events, but sometimes their ideas about what is going on will change. In addition, in some stories one person will know something that the other person does not know, and in some stories one of the characters will play a joke on the other one. This knowing or not knowing what is really going on might affect one person's understanding but not the other person's. The patient is instructed to observe each situation to help decide when Alice's and Greg's beliefs change and when they do not.

Task I—Alice and Greg view an [object] while Greg is changing the [object]. The patient generates five possible thoughts about the [object] for Alice and five for Greg.

Task II—Alice goes upstairs and thinks about the [object]. The patient generates five possible ideas about the [object] for Alice and five for Greg.

Task III—Alice is upstairs thinking about the [object], and Greg remains downstairs. Have their ideas changed? (Y/N)

Task IV—Greg is downstairs with the [object]. He remembers that Alice said, "Please do not change the [object] again while I am upstairs." Greg changes the [object] just as the phone rings. It is Alice and she is checking on the [object]. [Show Alice upstairs talking on the phone to Greg.] Greg does not want Alice to know that he touched the [object]. Greg tells Alice [. . .]. The patient is asked to choose the response (from a set of three alternatives) that represents what Greg tells Alice.

Task IV—Greg is downstairs with the [object]. Alice is upstairs on the phone to Greg. Greg follows Alice's instructions and does not change the [object]. Greg wants to play a joke on Alice to make her think he changed the [object]. Greg tells Alice [. . .]. The patient is asked to choose the response (from a set of three alternatives) that represents what Greg tells Alice about the [object].

Scoring: Responses to each task are scored as correct (1 point), delayed correct (.5), or incorrect (0). A patient can progress to the next task after receiving 90% accuracy on five trials of 10 items or 100% accuracy on three trials of 10 items.

Posttraining testing

Overview: The purpose is to assess generalization and maintenance of gains achieved during training, and, in addition, to provide a preliminary basis for interpreting any gains. Of course, cartoon interpretation and judgment of line orientation will be assessed immediately posttraining. Other tests administered immediately after completion of training include: (1) Empathy Quotient, (2) The Delis-Kaplan Executive Function System (3) Florida Affect Battery, (4) Working memory test, (5) Pragmatic Assessment, and (6) Quality of Life measure.

Maintenance Phase. (Eight sessions, once per week) cartoon interpretation assessment. Half of the patients (randomly selected) will also receive a "booster" consisting of two to three cartoons that the patient can accurately explain to family and friends.

Long-Term Follow-Up. (One session, 3–4 months after end of training). Cartoon interpretation assessment and line orientation judgment.

Scores (i.e., percentage of possible points obtained and time to completion) will be recorded for individual task. Performance on tasks, and progression from one task to the next, will be matched with performance on the cartoon assessments administered each session. We will examine the data for evidence of any discontinuity in cartoon interpretation performance that will corroborate the importance of mastering a particular phase of training for overcoming a patient's individual cognitive limitations.

29 Cognitive Communication Disorders After Traumatic Brain Injury

Leanne Togher

TRAUMATIC BRAIN INJURY: DEMOGRAPHIC/EPIDEMIOLOGY

According to the World Health Organization (WHO), traumatic brain injury (TBI) will surpass many diseases as the major cause of death and disability by the year 2020 (Hyder, Wunderlich, Puvanachandra, Guraj, & Kobusingye, 2007). It is estimated that 10 million people are affected worldwide annually leading to a significant pressure on health and medical resources. TBI most often affects young adults who suffer devastating life-long disabilities; however, there is also a higher incidence in early childhood and the elderly (Bruns & Hauser, 2003). The majority of TBIs in young adults are the result of motor vehicle accidents, while typically children and the elderly sustain injuries as a result of falls. There has also been an increase in the number of injuries resulting from violence and war, particularly in low and middle income countries (Hyder et al., 2007). The disabilities resulting from TBI span both physical and psychological domains of function. Communication problems may be a consequence of disabilities within and across these domains and represent a unique challenge for clinicians and researchers alike. The past four decades have seen an evolution in the description of these communication disorders, with advances in the fields of pragmatics, social cognition, sociolinguistic applications to disordered language, and neuroimaging, and these will be outlined in this chapter.

The term traumatic brain injury refers to brain injury caused by trauma rather than disease, vascular accidents, alcohol, and so on. Traumatic brain injury is a consequence of a head injury of sufficient severity to cause damage to the brain beneath and can be either penetrating or blunt. Penetrating or open head injuries are an uncommon cause of TBI, with the exception of war-wounds. These occur when a missile, such as a bullet, pierces the skull and traverses the brain tissue. High velocity missile wounds cause catastrophic focal and diffuse damage and are usually fatal while low velocity missiles or missile fragments produce focal lesions restricted to the area of direct damage (Grafman & Salazar, 1987). The more common mechanism of injury is an acceleration–deceleration movement that impacts on the brain in a number of ways causing both localized damage at the site of impact and at distant points in the brain due to the ricocheting movement of the brain, but also a series of catastrophic sequelae at the cellular level including diffuse axonal injury, where the nerve fibers are twisted and stretched by the force of the injury. Secondary injuries can exacerbate the initial insult such as edema or swelling, hypoxic damage to due lack of oxygen after the injury, metabolic disturbances, hypothermia, and hypotension (McHugh et al., 2007).

COMMUNICATION AND TBI

Communication problems following a TBI are distinctly different to those subsequent to a more focal lesion such as occurs in a cerebrovascular accident (or a penetrating head injury) requiring different approaches to assessment and remediation. This has come from the recognition that, due to the multifocal nature of TBI, there is a complex interplay of cognitive, linguistic, physical, behavioral, and organic psychosocial factors that may contribute to the communication difficulties experienced. While traditional communication impairments can result from TBI, such as aphasia that has been reported to occur in up to 30% of cases, and dysarthria, which typically affects about one third of cases (Sarno & Levita, 1986), it is the social communication difficulties that predominate. These have posed researchers with a conundrum for the past 30 years, leading to the development of new theories of social communication, and thus, new methods of standardized and nonstandardized assessment. It is interesting to examine the evolution of current views of cognitive communication disorders after TBI.

Descriptions of the unique nature of communication deficits after TBI did not emerge until the 1980s. Prior to this time, reports of communication difficulties after TBI focused on aphasic deficits resulting from war injuries (e.g., Goldstein, 1942; Luria, 1970). Such descriptions did not reflect the true nature of closed traumatic head injuries, and debate commenced in the early 1980s about ways of describing communication after TBI. Holland (1982) asked the question "when is aphasia aphasia?" raising the idea that if people with TBI were labeled as aphasic they would, in turn, receive inappropriate treatment that would fail to take their cognitive impairments into account. Other researchers recognized this interplay between cognition and language leading to the introduction of the term *cognitive-language disorder* (Hagen, 1984; Kennedy & DeRuyter, 1991). Researchers began to investigate the relationship between the cognitive disturbances that frequently follow TBI and psycholinguistic aspects of language. Hagen (1984) described the relationship between the commonly occurring cognitive impairments following TBI and their effects on language processing. For example, the impairments of attention, memory, sequencing, categorization, and associative abilities are seen to result in an impaired capacity to organize and structure incoming information, emotional reactions, and the flow of thought. Such impairments, Hagen argued, caused a disorganization of language processes. Cognitive disorganization is reflected through language use, which is characterized by irrelevant utterances that may not make sense, difficulty inhibiting inappropriate utterances, word-finding difficulties, and problems ordering words and propositions. Prigatano, Roueche, and Fordyce (1985) described nonaphasic language disturbances following TBI including the problems of talkativeness, tangentiality, and fragmented thought processes.

In the 1990s, the term *cognitive-communication disorder* emerged (Hartley, 1995) in recognition of the relationship between impaired cognition and its wider ramifications for everyday communication skills. The focus on cognition arose from an examination of the underlying pathophysiology of TBI that commonly results in multifocal cerebral damage with a preponderance of injury to the frontal lobes. Cognition can be broadly described as "mental activities or operations involved in taking in, interpreting, encoding, storing, retrieving and making use of knowledge or information and generating a response" (Ylvisaker & Szekeres, 1994, p. 548). Examples of cognitive processes attributed to the frontal lobes include ability to focus attention to stimuli, remembering and learning, organizing information, reasoning, and problem solving. In addition to specific cognitive processes, the frontal lobes appear to mediate executive control of thought and behavior. Such executive functions include goal setting, behavior planning and sequencing, goal oriented behavior, initiation, and evaluation of behavior (Lezak, 1993). It became increasingly obvious to researchers that it was impossible to assess language functioning without taking neuropsychological functioning into account.

The debate regarding the definition of "cognitive-linguistic" disorders continues with the proposition that the term lacks terminological clarity, which undermines the assessment of complex communication functioning (Body & Perkins, 2006). Nonetheless, it is now widely accepted that the communication difficulties following TBI are mostly the result of a combination of cognitive and linguistic impairments. In addition, it is also recognized that executive functioning impairments in the domains of attention, memory, organization, planning, flexible problem solving, and self-awareness are consistently seen in people after TBI (Anderson, Bigler, & Blatter, 1995; Levin, Goldstein, Williams & Eisenberg, 1991). These types of difficulties can have a significant deleterious impact on a person's day to day interactions leading to social communication impairments. It is these social communication difficulties that will be described in further detail in the next section.

SOCIAL COMMUNICATION DEFICITS AFTER TBI

Many people with severe TBI have difficulty in everyday social situations, making participation in activities such as conversation with family and friends, shopping at a local shopping center or engaging with colleagues in a work interaction awkward and in some cases, impossible. These social communication impairments often result in difficulty for the person with a TBI in making and maintaining relationships with consequent social isolation and loss of leisure activities. This is particularly apparent when the long-term outcomes of individuals with TBI are examined.

While the majority of people with TBI achieve independence in areas of activities of daily living (Tate, Lulham, Broe, Strettles, & Pfaff, 1989) they experience poor outcomes in their psychosocial functioning. For example, almost 50% of people with a severe TBI were found to have no social contacts and few leisure interests one year or more after the injury (Tate et al., 1989), with a greater reliance on family for emotional support following the injury (Olver, Ponsford, & Curran, 1996). A TBI can deleteriously affect vocational outcomes, and the ability to form new relationships (Olver, Ponsford, & Curran, 1996). Communication underlies these outcomes, and promoting the best communication recovery possible is the goal of speech pathology intervention throughout the recovery process.

The challenge for those working with these people and their social networks is describing their impairments in such a way that treatments can be developed to target the difficulties. The complexity of the underlying deficits has led to a wide array of approaches to examining this problem. Given the demonstrated relationship between the typical sites of brain damage and impairments in executive functioning some researchers have sought to find a relationship between these impairments and measures of communication. For example, Godfrey, Knight, Marsh, Moroney, and Bishara (1989) evaluated the relationship between speed of information processing and global ratings of social interaction with a null finding. Coelho, Liles, and Duffy (1995) found a significant correlation between a factor score on the Wisconsin Card Sort Test reflecting perseverative responses and a measure of narrative story structure (i.e., percentage of incomplete story episodes), the latter of which Coelho et al., suggested was more "cognitive" than some of the other variables they studied such as measures of sentence production or cohesion, which were more "linguistically" based.

Difficulty achieving significant correlation between measures of executive functioning and measures of communication has been limited by the nature of the available measures. However, as tests have become more sophisticated, and better targeted to the specific problems affecting people with TBI, it has become possible to find relationships between these variables. For example, Struchen, Sander, Mills, Evans, and Kurtz (2008) found that performance on measures of executive functioning and social communication ability was significantly related to occupational and social integration outcomes. These findings were probably made possible by the assessment measures Struchen and colleagues used in the study, which, among others, included the La Trobe Communication Questionnaire (LCQ) (Douglas, O'Flaherty, & Snow, 2000), a measure of perceived communication ability; and the Florida Affect Battery, a test of perception and identification of nonverbal communicative signals of emotion (Bowers, Blonder, & Heilman, 1991).

One of the challenges in measuring communication in people with TBI has been finding assessment tools that will detect the unique communication deficits in this population. Early attempts at measuring everyday communication were based in the theory of pragmatics (Levinson, 1983) and Grice's (1975) Cooperative Principle of conversation encompassing four maxims of conversation including Quality, Quantity, Relation, and Manner. Penn and Cleary (1988) were one of the first to publish a profile of communicative appropriateness that took the following pragmatic parameters into account: nonverbal communication, sociolinguistic sensitivity, fluency, cohesion, control of semantic content, and responsiveness to the interlocutor. Prutting and Kirchner (1987) published a seminal work with the Pragmatic Protocol that was based on the tenets of Levinson's (1983) treatise that the range of pragmatic aspects of interaction exists on a continuum and includes both context-dependent aspects of language structure (e.g., cohesion) in addition to those relying on principles of language use, such as physical proximity of communication partners and use of eye gaze. It was recommended that individuals be observed for a 15 minute spontaneous unstructured conversation with a communicative partner and then the rater completed the protocol with ratings of appropriateness. The Pragmatic Protocol was subsequently used widely in clinical contexts and as a research tool (Penn & Cleary, 1988), and fostered continued interest in studying language use of people with TBI (rather than language performance; Turkstra, McDonald, & Kaufmann, 1995).

Pragmatic theory underpins two distinct approaches to the assessment of communication after TBI (Body, Perkins, & McDonald, 1999). One approach has led to a proliferation of checklists or profiles of communication (Linscott, Knight, & Godfrey, 1996; Milton, Prutting, & Binder, 1984; Snow, Douglas, & Ponsford, 1998). The Profile of Functional Impairment in Communication (PFIC; Linscott et al., 1996), based on Grice's theories, includes feature summary scales that assess communication skills on a six-point scale from normative (0) to very severely impaired (5), with lower scores indicating better performance. These summary scales include logical content, general participation, quantity, quality, internal relation, external relation, clarity of expression, social style, subject matter, and aesthetics. There are 84 specific behavior items that assess the frequency of communication impairments from "not at all" to "almost always/always." Dahlberg and colleagues (2007) used this scale as their primary outcome measure in a randomized controlled trial of social skills treatment, finding that their treated group of 26 participants with chronic TBI improved on seven of the 10 summary scales after 12 weeks of treatment, with no significant changes in a deferred treatment group. The authors concluded that the PFIC was an appropriate outcome measure to evaluate the social communication of people with TBI.

At about the same time that Prutting and Kirchner were publishing the Pragmatic Protocol, Damico (1985) published the Clinical Discourse Analysis, an observational communication measure also based on Grice's maxims and that eventually influenced the development of the LCQ. The LCQ is an excellent example of a response to the quandary of assessing the communication of a person with TBI and represents a significant and important advance. Rather than relying on a standardized test of communication, it investigates the perception of communication skills from the perspective of the person with TBI and also their significant other. It is designed to assess social communication skills by asking the person with TBI and a significant other a total of 30 questions, 22 of which are based on Damico's Clinical Discourse Analysis (Damico, 1985) and eight that were based on commonly reported communication problems after TBI such as tangentiality and disinhibition. The person is asked a question such as "When talking to others do you go over and over the same ground in conversation?" and then given a Likert scale that ranges from 1 (Never or rarely) to 4 (Usually or Always). While the use of self-report can be limited if the person with TBI has impairments in insight, the use of an "other report" enables the clinician to determine whether communicative competence has been compromised by the brain injury and also gain an insight into the level of awareness of the person with TBI.

Another approach that has evolved from the early proponents of pragmatics is a focus on specific aspects of interpersonal communication including the ability to make inferences as exemplified by the body of work by McDonald and colleagues (McDonald, 1992, 1993; McDonald & Pearce, 1996, 1998; Pearce, McDonald, & Coltheart, 1998; Turkstra et al., 1995). This research has shown that a proportion of TBI adults misinterpret conversational inferences generated by discrete speech acts. Given that linguistic performance is relatively normal in these people, it is thought that they have difficulty utilizing the contextual information necessary to generate these inferences. However, the nature of the contextual cues involved and whether any particular sources of contextual cues are more poorly processed is not well understood (McDonald, 2000).

Studying the effect of how indirect contextual information is detected by conversational speakers has led to advances in the study of sarcasm (McDonald, 2007; McDonald & Pearce, 1996), use of hints (McDonald & van Sommers, 1993) and, more recently, theory of mind investigations with people with TBI (Bibby & McDonald, 2005; Martin & McDonald, 2005). It is thought that the ability to detect sarcasm is impaired because the frontal lobes, which are commonly damaged in TBI, control the executive processes that enable us to respond adaptively to novel stimuli by overriding routine, habit-driven responses. It is thought that damage to these processes may lead to more automatic responses, which are either stimulus-bound or habit driven. This therefore leads to a reduced appreciation of inferential meanings in language because they are stimulus-bound to the most concrete aspects of the information given and are not able to suppress their tendency to respond in a routine way to such attributes. They are therefore unable to appreciate alternative meanings or associations (McDonald & Pearce, 1996). In McDonald and Pearce's (1996) study of 10 people with TBI it was determined that this group could interpret consistent verbal exchanges but had difficulty with literally contradictory (sarcastic) verbal exchanges. They found that the literal meaning of a sarcastic comment needed to be rejected in order for the inference to be detected.

Theory of mind concerns the ability to make judgments about the mental states of others. It is thought that this skill underpins the ability to interpret and predict how others will behave. The traditional approach to evaluating this skill is through the use of "false belief" and complex story tasks that examine how participants use conceptual or pictorial information about the beliefs of those depicted in the story. While this has been a tantalizing line of inquiry in the study of the unique frontal deficits that are associated with TBI, it seems that theory of mind is not a singular ability, and that the judgments made in these traditional story tasks could involve nontheory of mind inferential reasoning (Bibby & McDonald, 2005) and cognitive flexibility (Henry, Phillips, Crawford, Ietswaart, & Summers, 2006). Nonetheless, people with severe TBI demonstrate specific impairments on tasks requiring them to make inferences about others' mental states when compared to control participants (Bibby & McDonald, 2005). Given the complexity of the underlying processes thought to mediate theory of mind, such as inferential ability, language comprehension, working memory capacity, theory of mind ability, and perhaps even humor comprehension, it is difficult to translate the findings of this work into clinical practice.

Another promising avenue of research in the field of social cognition after TBI is the investigation of the role of emotion in cognition. The ability to recognize emotions is obviously critical to our ability to respond appropriately to communication partners in conversational interactions. People with TBI can present with difficulties in emotional control, with poor frustration tolerance, temper outbursts, disinhibition, and irritability. Clearly, such behavior is likely to penalize the person in their everyday interactions. Acknowledgement of this difficulty was first made by Prigatano and Pribram (1982) who showed people with brain injury a series of pictures depicting happy, sad, fearful, and angry faces and asking them to identify verbally the facial emotion and later freely recall the affect when shown some of the faces having neutral expressions. People with unilateral and bilateral lesions were reported to have greater difficulty, particularly with the memory component of this task. There has since been a plethora of studies that report deficits in emotion recognition across a range of visual and auditory media including photographs, videoed portrayals of emotion, and audio tapes of emotionally charged voices (Green, Turner, & Thompson, 2004; Hopkins, Dywan, & Segalowitz, 2002; Milders, Fuchs, & Crawford, 2003; Spell & Frank, 2000). It is now well established that people with TBI have difficulty with this task, as emotion processing is mediated in the frontal lobes, and is therefore frequently impaired after injury. Specifically, animal, neuroimaging, and human lesion studies have consistently attributed impaired emotion recognition to dysfunction within a frontolimbic circuit that entails the striatum and anterior cingulate gyrus, ventromedial prefrontal cortex, and dorsomedial nucleus of the thalamus. Of particular importance to the identification of emotional stimuli are the amygdala and anterior insula (Phillips, 2003).

The task in the future is to develop treatments to remediate emotion recognition. While this area of research is in its infancy there has been a promising first study that aimed to teach people with TBI to attend to salient features of various emotions. Bornhofen and McDonald (2008) employed a randomized controlled trial to evaluate the treatment of a group of 12 individuals with TBI using a program specifically designed to address the perception of static and dynamic emotion cues. They found that the TBI participants who received the treatment showed improved accuracy when judging dynamic cues related to basic emotions (happiness, surprise, disgust, sadness, anger, and anxiety) and that participants improved on distinguishing these from a neutral emotional presentation. The treatment group also improved in their ability to draw inferences on the basis of emotional cues in order to judge whether a speaker was being sarcastic, sincere, or deceptive. The authors suggested that participants may have been better able to monitor multiple simultaneously occurring dynamic cues such as eye contact, facial expression, voice tone and body language, and to integrate these carefully to make higher order judgments about a speaker's attitude, intentions, and opinions. Clearly, much more needs to be done in this area, and ideally, emotion perception training could be combined with conversational skills treatment programs to facilitate social interactions. The following section will focus on a wider perspective of communication skills of people with TBI, with an emphasis on their ability to produce extended discourse.

DISCOURSE AND TBI

At the same time that pragmatics was being taken up as a basis for examining the communication of people with TBI there was a corollary growth in discourse studies (e.g., Mentis & Prutting, 1987; Milton et al., 1984; Penn & Cleary, 1988). Discourse is described by Ulatowska and Bond-Chapman (1989) as a unit of language that conveys a message. There are different types of discourse tasks that have also been referred to as different discourse *genres*. A genre is a particular text-type, which has its own structure and sequence. Some types of discourse genres include narrative (or recounting a story), procedural (a set of instructions for doing something), expository (giving an opinion or discussing a topic in detail), and conversation.

Developments in discourse analysis were related to a proliferation of interest across a number of disciplines including sociology (e.g., Hymes, 1986; Labov, 1970), psychology (e.g., Mandler & Johnson, 1977), artificial intelligence (e.g., Schank & Abelson, 1977), and linguistics (e.g., Grimes, 1975; van Dijk, 1977). Particular techniques in discourse analyses have been derived from both the psycholinguistic and sociolinguistic perspectives. The psycholinguistic analyses include measures of syntax (Chapman et al., 1992; Ellis & Peach, 2009; Ewing-Cobbs, Brookshire, Scott, & Fletcher, 1998; Glosser & Deser, 1990; Liles, Coelho, Duffy, & Zalagens, 1989), productivity (Hartley & Jensen, 1991; Mentis & Prutting, 1987), and content (Hartley & Jensen, 1991) including propositional analysis (Coelho, Grela, Corso, Gamble, & Feinn, 2005). On the other hand, sociolinguistic techniques include cohesion analysis (Coelho, 2002; Coelho et al., 1991; Davis & Coelho, 2004; Hartley & Jensen, 1991; McDonald, 1993; Mentis & Prutting, 1987), analysis of coherence (Chapman et al., 1992; Ehrlich & Barry, 1989; McDonald, 1993), story grammar (Cannizaro & Coelho, 2002; Coelho, 2002), analysis of topic (Mentis & Prutting, 1991), and compensatory strategies (Penn & Cleary, 1988). The practical application of these new methodologies to individuals with TBI has proven to be fruitful as a means to exemplify communication disorders not apparent in traditional testing.

COMMUNICATION IN EVERYDAY CONTEXTS

People with TBI are typically described as showing little to no impairment on conventional language tests (confrontation naming, syntactical comprehension, fluency), although there has been some recent evidence to the contrary (Ellis & Peach, 2009). Nonetheless, people with TBI are clearly impaired when required to use language appropriately in social contexts. The most commonly used interaction type in the daily life of people with TBI is a "chat" or a "conversation" (Larkins, Worrall, & Hickson, 2004). Typically, this chat occurs with people in the person with TBI's everyday life, such as their wife, mother, children, or friends. However, until the mid-1990s, there was little research investigating the nature of these everyday interactions, as the focus had primarily been on the manner in which the person with TBI interacted in a clinical interaction. The work that follows is from my own lab, where I have studied everyday interactions using the work of Halliday (1994) as my theoretical guide.

SYSTEMIC FUNCTIONAL LINGUISTICS AND COMMUNICATION AFTER TBI

The analytic framework of Systemic Functional Linguistics (Halliday, 1994), and specifically, Generic Structure Potential (GSP), has been useful in measuring the interactions of people with TBI (Togher & Hand, 1999; Togher, Hand, & Code, 1997b) and revealing areas of difficulty that can be targeted in remediation. The GSP analysis examines oral texts as *genre* (Hasan, 1985). Genres in literary terms describe typical realizations of particular types of texts. Some examples of genres include telling a joke, engaging in gossip, making an appointment, and engaging in a service encounter where you are asking for goods and services (such as in a shop). In each of these, the content varies according to the activity (known as field) and the participants involved (known as tenor), however, there is a common core of structural elements for each genre. Therefore each genre has a unique common set of elements, so that for example, a shopping encounter genre has a different structure to a casual conversation genre (Ventola, 1987). We can use this basic structure to analyze the interactions of people with TBI and thus establish areas of strength and weakness within the interaction. Examining interactions in this way can then enable the development of new treatments that focus on the person with TBI and their communication partners within specific everyday interactions.

Generic structure analysis provides specific information about the extent to which communication partners can improve or inhibit the communication opportunities available to a person with TBI. Togher, Hand, and Code (1997a) studied five participants with TBI and five matched control participants, who were brothers of the people with TBI in four out of the five cases, in information requesting telephone interactions. They spoke with a range of communication partners including their mothers, therapists, the bus timetable information service providers, and the police (Togher, Hand, & Code, 1996;

Togher et al., 1997a, 1997b). A scenario was set up prior to each data collection to facilitate the ecological validity of the call. In the case of the police, for example, subjects were engaged in a discussion about their (or their brother's) driving license, which had been suspended as a result of the injury. Participants were asked about the process of regaining a driver's license after brain injury. All participants answered that they did not know the details of this process and were therefore prompted to contact a member of the NSW Police Service to make a request for this information. Transcripts of these interactions were analyzed using exchange structure analysis (Togher et al., 1997a), use of politeness markers (Togher & Hand, 1998), and GSP analysis (Togher et al., 1997b).

The generic structure of the service encounter texts in Togher et al. (1997b) was derived from Hasan (1985). In Togher et al. (1997b) transcripts were divided into moves, which are units of information similar to a T-unit. The texts were then divided into component structural elements that typically occur during a service encounter. The percentage of moves that made up each element could then be computed. Results indicated that people with TBI were disadvantaged in their interactions on the telephone particularly with the police during information seeking interactions when compared with those of the matched control participants. People with TBI were more frequently questioned regarding the accuracy of their contributions, asked to repeat information more often, and their contributions were followed up less often. Police officers gave less information, used patronizing comments, flat voice tone, and slowed speech production when talking to people with TBI. This was in contrast to the control interactions, where participants were asked for unknown information, encouraged to elaborate, did not have their contributions checked frequently, and had their contributions followed up. In contrast, the bus timetable interactions were similar for both people with TBI and control participants, possibly suggesting that the power of the context, with the person with TBI being a customer resulted in a more equivalent interaction.

In a subsequent study, we found that communicative effectiveness can be improved by manipulating the speaking situation for the person with TBI. For example, when people with TBI were placed in a powerful information-giving role, for example, as a guest speaker invited to interact with high school students about the experience of having a serious injury, their communication approximated matched control participants (who had a spinal injury; Togher & Hand, 1998). Thus, when provided with a facilitative context, such as an equal communicative opportunity, TBI participants were primed to match the performance of control participants.

IMPLICATIONS FOR TREATMENT OF SOCIAL COMMUNICATION DIFFICULTIES

Two approaches have been shown to improve the communication of those with TBI. Training in social skills is helpful, as is training partners to deal with difficult communication behaviors. Both these approaches will be addressed in turn, with a focus on those studies addressing the social communication skills of people with TBI.

TRAINING THE PERSON WITH TBI

Since the 1980s there have been only a handful of empirical studies conducted that have evaluated social skills remediation with TBI individuals. These have been aimed at overall social interaction deficits, or specific elements of such deficits (e.g., excessive talkativeness or inappropriate remarks; Braunling-McMorrow, Lloyd, & Fralish, 1986; Brotherton, Thomas, Wisotzek, & Milan, 1988; Flanagan, McDonald, & Togher, 1995; Gajar, Schloss, Schloss, & Thompson, 1984; Helffenstein & Wechsler, 1982; Johnson & Newton, 1987; McDonald et al., 2008; Schloss, Thompson, Gajar, & Schloss, 1985). The reader is referred to Coelho, DeRuyter, and Stein, 1996; Godfrey and Shum, 2000; and Marsh, 1999 for reviews.

Traditionally, communication training has focused on improving the social skills and interpersonal abilities of the person with TBI. Training programs have been in the form of games (Braunling-McMorrow et al., 1986), individual programs (Gajar et al., 1984; Schloss et al., 1985) or small group activities (Flanagan et al., 1995). In general the gains, if any, are few, despite the amount of resources required. Although this may suggest that such interventions are unsupportable, it needs to be emphasized that even a small improvement in problem behavior can sometimes make a large difference in the social opportunities that are available to individuals with TBI (Lewis, Nelson, Nelson, & Reusink, 1988). Nevertheless, an inherent limitation to social skills and communication training with people with TBI, is that these individuals usually experience a range of severe and disabling cognitive deficits that limit the extent to which they are able to compensate for their impairments or learn and apply new knowledge and skills. As an indication, a systematic review of cognitive rehabilitation following TBI found very few interventions in this group to have demonstrable effectiveness (Carney et al., 1999). Nonetheless, in our most recent randomized controlled trial of 39 participants (McDonald, Tate, Togher et al., 2008), those receiving a 12 week program of social skills intervention improved on one measure of social behavior, the Partner Directed Behaviour Scale of the Behaviourally Referenced Rating System of Intermediary Social Skills-Revised (BRISS-R; Farrell, Rabinowitz, Wallander, & Curran, 1985; Wallander, Conger, & Conger, 1985). The scale focuses on the ability to adapt to the social requirements of others. The self-centered behavior and partner involvement behavior subscales, in particular, showed improvement, indicating that participants with social skills training were less inclined to talk about themselves and more inclined to encourage their conversational partner to contribute to the conversation. Improving these interpersonal skills has clear implications for those situations where the person is meeting a new person at a social gathering or in a work context. Therefore, we found it very encouraging that poor social skills that clearly relate to poor executive function appeared amenable to treatment.

TRAINING COMMUNICATION PARTNERS OF PEOPLE WITH TBI

Given the inherent limits to training people with TBI, an alternative way of dealing with the problem of communication difficulties following TBI is to work with communication partners. We have found that the behavior of a conversational partner is important; facilitating, or diminishing opportunities for the individual with brain injury to continue the conversation in a successful manner. We therefore asked the question of whether training communication partners could have an impact on the interactions of people with TBI. The move toward training communication partners in a variety of clinical groups has been increasingly investigated over the past decade. It has been the product of a number of ideological and economic forces including:

1. Recognition that people with communication problems have inherent competence that can be facilitated by their communication partners (Kagan, Black, Felson-Duchan, Simmons-Mackie, & Square, 2001; Simmons-Mackie & Kagan, 1999).
2. Recognition that both the person with a neurogenic communication disorder and their immediate social network are the "client" in the therapy process.
3. A shift from a narrow focus on the impairment to a broader emphasis on the person's ability to participate in their social network (WHO, 2001).
4. The economic reality of the pursuit of productivity savings and an emphasis on rapid discharge. Speech pathologists are pressured to provide limited services in the acute phase of treatment declining to a relative absence of service in the long-term.

Despite the need for research in this area, there has been a paucity of intervention studies with communication partners of people with TBI. However, some research has been undertaken with communication partners of other communicatively disordered populations, with the majority of work completed with the partners of people with aphasia. Aphasia is a communication disorder that most commonly follows stroke. The following section briefly summarizes those studies aiming to improve the communication partner's proficiency in interacting with people with aphasia.

THEORETICAL APPROACHES TO TRAINING COMMUNICATION PARTNERS WITH APHASIA

Studies investigating the issue of training communication partners of people with neurogenic communication disorders have used a range of perspectives including Conversational Analysis (CA; Booth & Perkins, 1999; Wilkinson et al., 1998), functional perspectives (Lyon et al., 1997; Worrall & Yiu, 2000), pragmatic models of communication (Newhoff, Bugbee, & Ferreira, 1981), behavioral approaches (Simmons, Kearns, & Potechin, 1987), and social models of disability (Byng, Pound, & Parr, 2000; Kagan et al., 2001; Simmons-Mackie, 2000). The core principles of these approaches are similar. They all focus on improving conversational interaction by training the communication partner and/or the communication interaction rather than the person with communication problems. There have been considerable advances in the training of communication partners of people with aphasia over the past two decades, ranging from a focus on the minutiae of conversation through to the social contexts of language use.

Functional perspectives have also been used in designing training studies for communication partners (Lyon et al., 1997; Worrall & Yiu, 2000). The functional approach has developed partly in response to financial pressures (Frattali, 1993), a belief within the speech pathology profession that functional outcomes are important (Smith & Parr, 1986), and a recognition of the WHO (2001) guidelines that differentiate between the dimensions of Impairment, Activity, and Participation (WHO, 2001). Worrall and Yiu (2000) incorporated these underlying tenets into a training program for volunteers called "Speaking Out." This program focused on 10 general communication domains such as banking and using a telephone. Scripted modules consisted of a "trigger" to raise awareness of participants regarding the topic of the module. For example, in the banking module, participants engaged in a discussion around electronic banking and the possible benefits of this for a person with aphasia. A discussion ensued with the volunteer regarding ways a person with aphasia could remain involved in managing their finances and a plan was set up for the volunteer to assist the person with aphasia during the following week. This planning was accompanied by practical information handouts, which gave general strategies for the volunteers. The training continued over a 10-week training period. Functional measures showed small changes posttraining; however, the authors point out that these changes were nonetheless clinically significant. It was also suggested that a more individualized training approach may have further increased the effects of training.

The social approach to disability is a more recent movement in the way intervention is viewed in relation to people with aphasia (Pound, Parr, Lindsay, & Woolf, 2000). This approach takes the broader view that therapy should identify social barriers for people with aphasia including the way communication partners may interact. The Conversation Partners program described by Pound et al. (2000) is a scheme where student speech pathologists and some members of the community commit to spending 2 hours per 14 days for at least 6 months with a person with aphasia. Volunteers attend group training sessions before meeting their aphasic partner. Training is focused on information giving about aphasia, its communicative and social consequences and basic communication techniques. While this program has not been evaluated empirically, Pound et al. (2000) presented a case study demonstrating the value of regular visits by a student speech pathologist with regard to increased communicative opportunities for a person with aphasia.

The value of these partner-focused treatment regimes is that communication partners, when suitably skilled, can reveal the inherent competence of the person with brain injury by providing communicative opportunity (Kagan et al., 2001; Ylvisaker, Feeney, & Urbanczyk, 1993). In other words, when provided with the opportunity, people with acquired communication problems can capitalize on their preserved cognitive and social abilities to participate in conversation. Kagan et al. (2001) reported empirical evidence of the positive communication and social outcomes of training communication partners of people with severe aphasia. In a randomized controlled trial, 20 communication partners were trained how to keep talk as natural as possible, avoid being patronizing and explicitly letting the person know that his/her competence was not in question. Partners were also trained to improve the exchange of information. Results provided experimental support for the efficacy of communication partner training in improving the communication skills of conversation partners. Their brain impaired partners also improved significantly even though they did not receive specific training.

Communication partners of a range of participants with communication problems have taken part in training programs. These include volunteers talking with people with aphasia (Kagan et al., 2001; Lyon et al., 1997), nursing staff who were trained to use memory aids as an augmentative and alternative communication device with people with Alzheimer's disease (Bourgeois, Dijkstra, Burgio, & Allen-Burge, 2001; Burgio et al., 2001) and caregivers who underwent communication training to facilitate communication with people with Alzheimer's disease (Ripich, Ziol, Fritsch, & Durand, 1999). The type and amount of training has also varied across studies, ranging from a one hour in-service to nursing staff (Bourgeois et al., 2001), a one and a half day workshop format to volunteers (Kagan et al., 2001), a four week training program for nursing staff on memory book use and general communication skills (Burgio et al., 2001), a small group training format where four carers of adults with aphasia attended 2 hour sessions once a week for six consecutive weeks (Booth & Perkins, 1999; Booth & Swabey, 1999), and up to a 10-week training program for volunteers (Worrall & Yiu, 2000). The length of training programs for communication partners that is required for effective communication modification has not been specifically investigated to date.

Training programs are now beginning to emerge to help families and other caregivers deal with the ongoing problems that can follow TBI (Carnevale, 1996; Holland & Shigaki, 1998; Ylvisaker et al., 1993). Ylvisaker et al. (1993) describe the importance of providing a positive communication culture within the rehabilitation context. They suggest that role-playing and modeling combined with ongoing coaching and support in vivo are appropriate methods to facilitate communication training for communication partners of people with TBI. Further work is needed, however, to develop such training programs to address individual communication profiles in collaboration with the family and peer network of the person with TBI. Importantly, there has been no description of training programs that may be appropriate for community groups who interact with people with TBI. Thus, although community reintegration is frequently suggested as the primary objective of TBI rehabilitation (Coelho et al., 1996; Ylvisaker, Sellars, & Edelman,

1998), there are few documented cases where community agencies have been assisted to encourage more appropriate participation for these clients and none where the efficacy of such an approach has been demonstrated. This is despite the fact that there are now a number of studies that have clearly documented the nature of social interaction difficulties that commonly occur when people with TBI communicate in everyday settings.

To examine the effect of training communication partners we developed a training program for carers, which was piloted with a single case in 2000 (Togher & Grant, 2001). We trained a paid attendant care-giver who supported the daily activities of a 28-year-old man with TBI. The main communication problems reported separately by the care-giver and the person with TBI were keeping conversations going and staying on topic. After identifying target speaking situations (e.g., lunch at the shopping center), we taught the structure of casual conversation (Ventola, 1979) in combination with the conversational strategies of collaboration and elaboration (Ylvisaker et al., 1998). Pilot data indicated that the care-giver improved his ability to facilitate communication by using collaborative statements, explicitly acknowledging difficulty in the interaction, confirming his partner's contribution, and asking questions in a supportive manner.

We subsequently expanded this approach by developing and evaluating a communication-training program for police officers, as members of a service industry who are likely to encounter people with TBI. We trained a group of police officers to manage specific service encounters with people with TBI who they had not previously met. This approach was evaluated in an RCT (Togher & Grant, 1998; Togher, McDonald, Code, & Grant, 2004). The TBI speakers rang the police to ask their advice both before and after the police had been trained. Training resulted in more efficient, focused interactions. In other words, this study confirmed that training communication partners improved the competence of people with TBI. What is unknown is whether this approach is better than, or equal to the efficacy of direct remediation work with the person with TBI or whether a combined approach is more effective still.

FUTURE DIRECTIONS

The social communication difficulties that typically follow severe TBI are complex, multilayered, and therefore difficult to describe and treat. This chapter has outlined some of the approaches that have investigated this area including a focus on pragmatics, with an expanding literature in the fields of theory of mind, emotion perception and social cognition, on discourse, and on everyday interactions of people with TBI. Given the vastly different underlying theoretical approaches that have been taken, it is impossible to reconcile them all neatly into a composite. Perhaps, this merely reflects the heterogenous nature of communication breakdown after TBI, which is in concert with the complexity of the interplay between cognitive and language processes interacting with the fast moving everyday environments where communication occurs. It is heartening, however, that theoretical advances have been made that are now translating into novel treatment approaches. It is reasonable to say that no one treatment is the panacea to communication difficulties and that a combination of approaches is needed to assist the person and their families re-engage with their lives and society after the chaos that TBI can bring. Nonetheless, there are some exciting new directions on the horizon for studying and therefore treating the intricacies of interactions of people with TBI that can only lead to improved integration into everyday life, and enhanced quality of life.

REFERENCES

Anderson, C.V., Bigler, E.D. & Blatter, D.D. (1995). Frontal lobe lesions, diffuse damage, and neuropsychological functioning in traumatic brain-injured patients. *Journal of Clinical and Experimental Neuropsychology, 17*, 900–908.

Bibby, H., & McDonald, S. (2005). Theory of mind after traumatic brain injury. *Neuropsychologia, 43*(1), 99–114.

Body, R., & Perkins, M. (2006). Terminology and methodology in the assessment of cognitive-linguistic disorders. *Brain Impairment, 7*(3), 212–222.

Body, R., Perkins, M., & McDonald, S. (1999). Pragmatics, cognition, and communication in traumatic brain injury. In S. McDonald, L. Togher, & C. Code (Eds.), *Communication disorders following traumatic brain injury* (pp. 81–112). Hove, England: Psychology Press/Taylor & Francis (UK).

Booth, S., & Perkins, L. (1999). The use of conversation analysis to guide individualized advice to carers and evaluate change in aphasia: A case study. *Aphasiology, 13*(4–5), 283–303.

Booth, S., & Swabey, D. (1999). Group training in communication skills for carers of adults with aphasia. *International Journal of Language and Communication Disorders, 34*(3), 291–309.

Bornhofen, C., & McDonald, S. (2008). Treating deficits in emotion perception following traumatic brain injury. *Neuropsychological Rehabilitation, 18*(1), 22–44.

Bourgeois, M. S., Dijkstra, K., Burgio, L., & Allen-Burge, R. (2001). Memory aids as an alternative and augmentative communication strategy for nursing home residents with dementia. *Alternative and Augmentative Communication, 17*(3), 196–210.

Bowers, D., Blonder, L. X., & Heilman, K. M. (1991). *The Florida affect battery*. Gainesville, Center for Neuropsychological Studies-University of Florida.

Braunling-McMorrow, D., Lloyd, K., & Fralish, K. (1986). Teaching social skills to head injured adults. *Journal of Rehabilitation, 52*, 39–44.

Brotherton, F. A., Thomas, L. L., Wisotzek, I. E., & Milan, M. A. (1988). Social skills training in the rehabilitation of patients with traumatic closed head injury. *Archives of Physical Medicine and Rehabilitation, 69*, 827–832.

Bruns, J. J., & Hauser, W. (2003). The epidemiology of traumatic brain injury: A review. *Epilepsia, 44*(Suppl. 10), 2–10.

Burgio, L., Allen-Burge, R., Roth, D. L., Bourgeois, M. S., Dijkstra, K., Gerstle, J., . . . Bankester, L. (2001). Come talk with me: Improving communication between nursing assistants and nursing home residents during care routines. *The Gerontologist, 41*(4), 449–460.

Byng, S., Pound, C., & Parr, S. (2000). Living with aphasia: A framework for therapy interventions. In I. Papathanasiou (Ed.), *Acquired neurological communication disorders: A clinical perspective*. London, UK: Whurr.

Cannizzaro, M. S., & Coelho, C. A. (2002). Treatment of story grammar following trau-matic brain injury: A pilot study. *Brain Injury, 16*(12), 1065–1073.

Carnevale, G. (1996). Natural-setting behavior management for individuals with traumatic brain injury: Results of a three-year caregiver training program. *Journal of Head Trauma Rehabilitation, 11*(1), 27–38.

Carney, N., Chesnut, R., Maynard, H., Mann, N. C., Patterson, P., & Helfand, M. (1999). Effect of cognitive rehabilitation on outcomes for persons with traumatic brain injury: A systematic review. *Journal of Head Trauma Rehabilitation, 14*(3), 277–307.

Chapman, S. B., Culhane, K. A., Levin, H. S., Harward, H., Mendelsohn, D., Ewing-Cobbs, L., . . . Bruce, D.(1992). Narrative discourse after closed head injury in children and adolescents. *Brain and Language, 43*, 42–65.

Coelho, C. A. (2002). Story narratives of adults with closed head injury and non-brain-injured adults: Influence of socioeconomic status, elicitation task, and executive functioning. *Journal of Speech, Language, & Hearing Research, 45*(6), 1232–1248.

Coelho, C. A., DeRuyter, F., & Stein, M. (1996). Treatment Efficacy: Cognitive-communicative disorders resulting from traumatic brain injury. *Journal of Speech and Hearing Research, 39*(5), S5–S17.

Coelho, C., Grela, B., Corso, M., Gamble, A., & Feinn, R. (2005). Microlinguistic deficits in the narrative discourse of adults with traumatic brain injury. *Brain Injury, 19*(13), 1139–1145.

Coelho, C. A., Liles, B. Z. & Duffy, R. J. (1991). Discourse analysis with closed head injured adults: Evidence for differing patterns of deficits, *Archives of Physical Medicine and Rehabilitation, 72,* 465–468.

Coelho, C. A., Liles, B. Z., & Duffy, R. J. (1995). Impairments of discourse abilities and executive functions in traumatically brain-injured adults. *Brain Injury, 9*(5), 471–477.

Dahlberg, C. A., Cusick, C. P., Hawley, L. A., Newman, J. K., Morey, C. E., Harrison-Felix, C. L., & Whiteneck, G. G. (2007). Treatment efficacy of social communica-tion skills training after traumatic brain injury: A randomized treatment and deferred treatment controlled trial. *Archives of Physical Medicine & Rehabilitation, 88*(12), 1561–1573.

Damico, J. S. (1985). Clinical discourse analysis: A functional approach to language assessment. In C. S. Simon (Ed.), *Communication skills and classroom success* (pp. 165–203). London, UK: Taylor & Francis.

Davis, G. A., & Coelho, C. A. (2004). Referential cohesion and logical coherence of narra-tion after closed head injury. *Brain and Language, 89*(3), 508–523.

Douglas, J., O'Flaherty, C., & Snow, P. (2000). Measuring perception of communica-tive ability: The development and evaluation of the La Trabe communication questionnaire. *Aphasiology, 14*(3), 251–268.

Ehrlich, J., & Barry, P. (1989). Rating communication behaviours in the head-injured adult. *Brain Injury, 3*(2), 193–198.

Ellis, C., & Peach, R. K. (2009). Sentence planning following traumatic brain injury. *NeuroRehabilitation, 24*(3), 255–266.

Ewing-Cobbs, L., Brookshire, B., Scott, M.A., Fletcher, J.M. (1998). Children's narratives following traumatic brain injury: Linguistic structure, cohesion and thematic recall, *Brain and Language, 61,* 395–419.

Farrell, A. D., Rabinowitz, J. A., Wallander, J. L., & Curran, J. P. (1985). An evaluation of two formats for the intermediate-level assessment of social skills. *Behavioural Assessment, 7,* 155–171.

Flanagan, S., McDonald, S., & Togher, L. (1995). Evaluating social skills following trau-matic brain injury: The BRISS as a clinical tool. *Brain Injury, 9*(4), 321–338.

Frattali, C. (1993). Perspectives on functional assessment: Its use for policy making. *Disability and Rehabilitation, 15*, 1–9.

Gajar, A., Schloss, P. J., Schloss, C. N., & Thompson, C. K. (1984). Effects of feedback and self-monitoring on head trauma youth's conversation skills. *Journal of Applied Behavior Analysis, 17*, 353–358.

Glosser, G., & Deser, T. (1990). Patterns of discourse production among neurological patients with fluent language disorders. *Brain and Language, 40*, 67–88.

Godfrey, H. P. D., Knight, R. G., Marsh, N. V., Moroney, B., & Bishara, S. N. (1989). Social interaction and speed of information processing following very severe head injury. *Psychological Medicine, 19*, 175–182.

Godfrey, H., & Shum, D. (2000). Executive functioning and the application of social skills following traumatic brain injury. *Aphasiology, 14*(4), 433–444.

Goldstein, K. (1942). *After-effects of brain injuries in war.* New York, NY: Grune & Stratton.

Grafman, J., & Salazar, A. (1987). Methodological considerations relevant to the comparison of recovery from penetrating and closed head injuries. In H. S. Levin, J. Grafman, & H. M. Eisenberg (Eds.), *Neurobehavioral recovery from head injury* (pp. 44–54). New York, NY: Oxford University Press.

Green, R. E. A., Turner, G. R., & Thompson, W. F. (2004). Deficits in facial emotion perception in adults with recent traumatic brain injury. *Neuropsychologia, 42*(2), 133–141.

Grice, H. P. (1975). Logic and conversation. In P. Cole & J. L. Morgan (Eds.), *Syntax and semantics, Vol. 3, Speech Acts* (pp. 41–58). New York, NY: Academic Press.

Grimes, J. (1975). *The thread of discourse. The Hague: Mouton.*

Hagen, C. (1984). Language disorders in head trauma. In A. Holland (Ed.), *Language disorders in adults* (pp. 245–281). San Diego, CA: College Hill Press.

Halliday, M. A. K. (1994). *An introduction to functional grammar.* London, UK: Edward Arnold.

Hartley, L. L. (1995). *Cognitive-communicative abilities following brain injury: A functional approach.* San Diego, CA: Singular.

Hartley, L. L., & Jensen, P. J. (1991). Narrative and procedural discourse after closed head injury. *Brain Injury, 5*(3), 267–285.

Hasan, R. (1985). *Language, context, and text: Aspects of language in a social-semiotic perspective.* Victoria, Australia: Deakin University Press.

Helffenstein, D. A., & Wechsler, F. S. (1982). The use of Interpersonal Process Recall (IPR) in the remediation of interpersonal and communication skill deficits in the newly brain-injured. *Clinical Neuropsychology, 4*, 139–143.

Henry, J. D., Phillips, L. H., Crawford, J. R., Ietswaart, M., & Summers, F. (2006). Theory of mind following traumatic brain injury: The role of emotion recognition and executive dysfunction. *Neuropsychologia, 44*(10), 1623–1628.

Holland, A. L. (1982). When is aphasia aphasia? The problem of closed head injury. In R. H. Brookshire (Ed.), *Clinical aphasiology conference proceedings* (pp. 345–349). Minneapolis, MN: BRK Publishers.

Holland, D., & Shigaki, C. (1998). Educating families and caretakers of traumatically brain injured patients in the new health care environment: A three phase model and bibliography. *Brain Injury, 12*(12), 993–1009.

Hopkins, M. J., Dywan, J., & Segalowitz, S. J. (2002). Altered electrodermal response to facial expression after closed head injury. *Brain Injury, 16*(3), 245–257.

Hyder, A. A., Wunderlich, C. A., Puvanachandre, P., Gururaj, G., & Kobusingye, O. C. (2007). The impact of traumatic brain injuries: A global perspective. *NeuroRehabilitation, 22*(5), 341–353.

Hymes, D. (1986). Models of the interaction of language and social life. In J. J. Gumperz & D. Hymes (Eds.), *Directions in sociolinguistics. The ethnography of communication* (pp. 35-71). Oxford, UK: Basil Blackwell.

Johnson, D., & Newton, A. (1987). Social adjustment and interaction after severe head injury: II. Rationale and bases for intervention. *British Journal of Clinical Psychology, 26,* 289–298.

Kagan, A., Black, S., Felson-Duchan, J., Simmons-Mackie, N., & Square, P. (2001). Training volunteers as conversational partners using supported conversation with adults with aphasia (SCA): A controlled trial. *Journal of Speech, Language and Hearing Research, 44,* 624–638.

Kennedy, M. R. T., & DeRuyter, F. (1991). Cognitive and language bases for communication disorders. In D. R. Beukelman & K. M. Yorkston (Eds.), *Communication disorders following traumatic brain injury: Management of cognitive, language and motor impairments* (pp. 123–190). Austin, TX: Pro-Ed.

Labov, W. (1970). The study of language in its social context. *Studium Generale, 23,* 30–87.

Larkins, B. M., Worrall, L. E., & Hickson, L. M. (2004). Stakeholder opinion of functional communication activities following traumatic brain injury. *Brain Injury, 18*(7), 691–706.

Levin, H. S., Goldstein, F. C., Williams, D. H., & Eisenberg, H. M. (1991). The contribution of frontal lobe lesions to the neurobehavioural outcome of closed head injury. In H. Levin, H. Eisenberg, & A. Benton (Eds.), *Frontal lobe function and dysfunction* (pp. 318–338). New York, NY: Oxford University Press.

Levinson, S. C. (1983). *Pragmatics.* London, UK: Cambridge University Press.

Lewis, F. D., Nelson, J., Nelson, C., & Reusink, P. (1988). Effect of three feedback contingencies on the socially inappropriate talk of a brain-injured adult. *Behavior Therapy, 19,* 203–211.

Lezak, M. D. (1993). Newer contributions to the neuropsychological assessment of executive functions. *Journal of Head Trauma Rehabilitation, 8*(1), 24–31.

Liles, B. Z., Coelho, C. A., Duffy, R. J., & Zalagens, M. R. (1989). Effects of elicitation procedures on the narratives of normal and closed head-injured adults. *Journal of Speech and Hearing Disorders, 54,* 356–366.

Linscott, R. J., Knight, R. G., & Godfrey, H. P. D. (1996). The profile of functional impairment of communication (PFIC): A measure of communication impairment for clinical use. *Brain Injury, 10*(6), 397–412.

Luria, A. R. (1970). *Traumatic aphasia.* The Hague, The Netherlands: Mouton.

Lyon, J. G., Cariski, D., Keisler, L., Rosenbek, J., Levine, R., Kumpula, J., . . . Blanc, M. (1997). Communication partners: Enhancing participation in life and communication for adults with aphasia in natural settings. *Aphasiology, 11,* 693–708.

Mandler, J. A., & Johnson, N. S. (1977). Remembrance of things parsed: Story structure and recall. *Cognitive Psychology, 9,* 111–151.

Marsh, N. (1999). Social skills deficits following traumatic brain injury: Assessment and treatment. In S. McDonald, L. Togher, & C. Code (Eds.), *Communication disorders following traumatic brain injury* (pp. 175–210). Hove, UK: Psychology Press.

Martin, I., & McDonald, S. (2005). Evaluating the causes of impaired irony comprehension following traumatic brain injury. *Aphasiology, 19*(8), 712–730.

McDonald, S. (1992). Communication disorders following closed head injury: New approaches to assessment and rehabilitation. *Brain Injury, 6,* 283–292.

McDonald, S. (1993). Pragmatic skills after closed head injury: Ability to meet the informational needs of the listener. *Brain and Language, 44*(1), 28–46.

McDonald, S. (2000). Neuropsychological studies of sarcasm. *Metaphor and Symbol, 15*(1–2), 85–98.

McDonald, S. (2007). Neuropsychological studies of sarcasm. In R. W. J. Gibbs (Ed.), *Irony in language and thought: A cognitive science reader* (pp. 217–230). Mahwah, NJ: Lawrence Erlbaum Associates Publishers.

McDonald, S., & Pearce, S. (1996). Clinical insights into pragmatic theory: Frontal lobe deficits and sarcasm. *Brain and Language, 53*(1), 81–104.

McDonald, S., & Pearce, S. (1998). Requests that overcome listener reluctance: Impairment associated with executive dysfunction in brain injury. *Brain and Language, 61*, 88–104.

McDonald, S., Tate, R. L., Togher, L., Bornhofen, C., Long, E., Gertler, P., & Bowen, R. (2008). Social skills treatment for people with severe, chronic acquired brain injuries: A multicenter trial. *Archives of Physical Medicine & Rehabilitation, 89*, 1648–1659.

McDonald, S. & van Sommers, P. (1993). Differential pragmatic language loss following closed head injury: Ability to negotiate requests. *Cognitive Neuropsychology, 10*, 297–315.

McHugh, G. S., Engel, D. C., Butcher, I., Steyerberg, E. W., Lu, J., Mushkudiani, N., . . . Murray, G. D. (2007). Prognostic value of secondary insults in traumatic brain injury: Results from the IMPACT study. *Journal of Neurotrauma, 24*(2), 287–293.

Mentis, M., & Prutting, C. A. (1987). Cohesion in the discourse of normal and head-injured adults. *Journal of Speech and Hearing Research, 30*, 88–98.

Mentis, M. & Prutting, C. A. (1991). Analysis of topic as illustrated in a head-injured and a normal adult, *Journal of Speech and Hearing Research, 34,* 583–595.

Milders, M., Fuchs, S., & Crawford, J. R. (2003). Neuropsychological impairments and changes in emotional and social behaviour following severe traumatic brain injury. *Journal of Clinical and Experimental Neuropsychology, 25*(2), 157–172.

Milton, S. B., Prutting, C. A., & Binder, G. M. (1984). Appraisal of communicative competence in head injured adults. In R. H. Brookshire (Ed.), *Clinical aphasiology conference proceedings.* Minneapolis, MN: BRK Publishers.

Newhoff, M., Bugbee, J. K., & Ferreira, A. (1981). A change of PACE: Spouses as treatment targets. In R. H. Brookshire (Ed.), *Clinical aphasiology* (Vol. 11, pp. 234–243). Minneapolis, MN: BRK Publishers.

Olver, J. H., Ponsford, J. L. & Curran, C. A. (1996). Outcome following traumatic brain injury: a comparison between 2 and 5 years after injury, *Brain Injury, 10* (11), 841–848.

Pearce, S., McDonald, S., & Coltheart, M. (1998). Interpreting ambiguous advertisements: The effect of frontal lobe damage. *Brain and Cognition, 38*(2), 150–164.

Penn, C., & Cleary, J. (1988). Compensatory strategies in the language of closed head injured patients. *Brain Injury, 2*(1), 3–17.

Phillips, M. L. (2003). Understanding the neurobiology of emotion perception: Implications for psychiatry. *British Journal of Psychiatry, 182*(3), 190–192.

Pound, C., Parr, S., Lindsay, J., & Woolf, C. (2000). *Beyond aphasia: Therapies for living with communication disability.* Oxon, UK: Speechmark.

Prigatano, G. P., & Pribram, K. H. (1982). Perception and memory of facial affect following brain injury. *Perceptual and Motor Skills, 54*(3, Pt 1), 859–869.

Prigatano, G. P., Roueche, J. R., & Fordyce, D. J. (1985). Nonaphasic language disturbances after closed head injury. *Language Sciences, 7*, 217–229.

Prutting, C. A., & Kirchner, D. M. (1987). A clinical appraisal of the pragmatic aspects of language. *Journal of Speech and Hearing Disorders, 52*, 105–119.

Ripich, D. N., Ziol, E., Fritsch, T., & Durand, E. J. (1999). Training Alzheimer's Disease caregivers for successful communication. *Clinical Gerontologist, 21*(1), 37–53.

Sarno, M. T., & Levita, E. (1986). Characteristics of verbal impairment in closed head injured patients. *Archives of Physical Medicine and Rehabilitation, 67*, 400–405.

Schank, R., & Abelson, R. (1977). *Scripts, plans, goals and understanding*. Hillsdale, NJ: Lawrence Erlbaum.

Schloss, P. J., Thompson, C. K., Gajar, A. H., & Schloss, C. N. (1985). Influence of self-monitoring on heterosexual conversational behaviours of head trauma youth. *Applied Research in Mental Retardation, 6,* 269–282.

Simmons, N. N., Kearns, K. P., & Potechin, G. (1987). Treatment of aphasia through family member training. In R. H. Brookshire (Ed.), *Clinical aphasiology* (Vol. 17, 106–116). Minneapolis, MN: BRK Publishers.

Simmons-Mackie, N. (2000). Social approaches to the management of aphasia. In L. Worrall & C. Frattali (Eds.), *Neurogenic communication disorders: A functional approach* (pp. 162–187). New York, NY: Thieme.

Simmons-Mackie, N., & Kagan, A. (1999). Communication strategies used by "good" versus "poor" speaking partners of individuals with aphasia. *Aphasiology, 13*(9–11), 807–820.

Smith, L., & Parr, S. (1986). Therapists' assessment of functional communication in aphasia. *Bulletin of the College of Speech Therapists, 409,* 10–11.

Snow, P. C., Douglas, J., & Ponsford, J. (1998). Conversational discourse abilities following severe traumatic brain injury: A follow up study. *Brain Injury, 12*(11), 911–935.

Spell, L. A., & Frank, E. (2000). Recognition of nonverbal communication of affect following traumatic brain injury. *Journal of Nonverbal Behavior, 24*(4), 285–300.

Struchen, M. A., Clark, A. N., Sander, A. M., Mills, M. R., Evans, G., & Kurtz, D. (2008). Relation of executive functioning and social communication measures to functional outcomes following traumatic brain injury. *NeuroRehabilitation, 23,* 185–198.

Tate, R. L., Lulham, J. M., Broe, G. A., Strettles, B., & Pfaff, A. (1989). Psychosocial outcome for the survivors of severe blunt head injury: The results from a consecutive series of 100 patients. *Journal of Neurology, Neurosurgery, and Psychiatry, 52,* 1128–1134.

Togher, L., & Grant, S. (1998). *Community policing: A training program for police in how to communicate with people with traumatic brain injury,* Unpublished manuscript.

Togher, L., & Grant, S. (2001). *Communication training program for carers.* Sydney, Australia: University of Sydney.

Togher, L., & Hand, L. (1998). Use of politeness markers with different communication partners: An investigation of five subjects with traumatic brain injury. *Aphasiology, 12*(7/8), 491–504.

Togher, L., & Hand, L. (1999). The macrostructure of the interview: Are traumatic brain injury interactions structured differently to control interactions? *Aphasiology, 13*(9–11), 709–723.

Togher, L., Hand, L., & Code, C. (1996). A new perspective in the relationship between communication impairment and disempowerment following head injury in information exchanges. *Disability and Rehabilitation, 18*(11), 559–566.

Togher, L., Hand, L., & Code, C. (1997a). Analysing discourse in the traumatic brain injury population: Telephone interactions with different communication partners. *Brain Injury, 11*(3), 169–189.

Togher, L., Hand, L., & Code, C. (1997b). Measuring service encounters in the traumatic brain injury population. *Aphasiology, 11*(4/5), 491–504.

Togher, L., McDonald, S., Code, C., & Grant, S. (2004). Training communication partners of people with traumatic brain injury: A randomised controlled trial. *Aphasiology, 18*(4), 313–335.

Turkstra, L. S., McDonald, S., & Kaufmann, P. M. (1995). Assessment of pragmatic skills in adolescents after traumatic brain injury. *Brain Injury, 10*(5), 329–345.

Ulatowska, H. K., & Bond Chapman, S. (1989). Discourse considerations for aphasia management. *Seminars in Speech and Language, 10* (4), 298–314.

van Dijk, T. A. (1977). *Text and context: Explorations in the semantics and pragmatics of discourse.* London, UK: Longman.

Ventola, E. (1979). The structure of casual conversation in English. *Journal of Pragmatics, 3,* 267–298.

Ventola, E. (1987). *The structure of social interaction: A systemic approach to the semiotics of service encounters.* London, UK: Pinter.

Wallander, J. L., Conger, A. J., & Conger, J. C. (1985). Development and evaluation of a behaviourally referenced rating system for heterosocial skills. *Behavioural Assessment, 7,* 137–153.

Wilkinson, R., Bryan, K., Lock, S., Bayley, K., Maxim, J., Bruce, C., . . . Moir, D. (1998). Therapy using conversation analysis: Helping couples adapt to aphasia in conversation. *International Journal of Language & Communication Disorders, 33*(Suppl), 144–149.

World Health Organization. (2001). *The international classification of functioning, disability and health—ICF.* Geneva, Switzerland: WHO.

Worrall, L., & Yiu, E. (2000). Effectiveness of functional communication therapy by volunteers for people with aphasia following stroke. *Aphasiology, 14*(9), 911–924.

Ylvisaker, M., Feeney, T. J., & Urbanczyk, B. (1993). Developing a positive communication culture for rehabilitation: Communication training for staff and family members. In C. J. Durgin, N. D. Schmidt, & L. J. Fryer (Eds.). *Staff development and clinical intervention in brain injury rehabilitation* (pp. 57–81). Gaithersburg, MD: Aspen.

Ylvisaker, M., Sellars, C., & Edelman, L. (1998). Rehabilitation after traumatic brain injury in preschoolers. In M. Ylvisaker (Ed.), *Traumatic brain injury rehabilitation. Children and adolescents* (pp. 303–329). Newton, MA: Butterworth-Heinemann.

Ylvisaker, M., & Szekeres, S. F. (1994). Communication disorders associated with closed head injury. In R. Chapey (Ed.), *Language intervention strategies in adult aphasia* (pp. 546–568). Baltimore, MD: Williams & Wilkins.

30 Breakdown of Semantics in Aphasia and Dementia: A Role for Attention?

John Shelley-Tremblay

INTRODUCTION

In Chapter 10 in this volume, I reviewed the semantic memory system, and suggested that an understanding of semantic memory may help us to understand the nature of language breakdown in a number of disorders that involve difficulties with communication. In this chapter I address two of the most commonly diagnosed disorders of adulthood, aphasia, and Alzheimer's dementia (AD), and examine how problems with semantic memory may be contributing to the clinical communication problems. I try to provide support for the hypothesis that what is going on in both of these disorders may be partially explained not only by problems with representation of semantic information, but also by problems with the allocation of attention to the concepts.

I begin with a brief presentation of a Center-Surround Model (CSM) to account for attentional selection of semantic concepts, followed by some evidence about the nature of the language disturbance in aphasia, and whether or not it can be classified as semantic. I then discuss how the CSM may be used to explain aphasic language behavior. Following the review of the issues in aphasia, we will continue with a discussion on the nature of the semantic deficit in AD. We end by reviewing some event-related potential studies of AD, and propose that these results can also be partially explained by the action of an attentional center-surround mechanism.

AN ATTENTIONAL CENTER-SURROUND MODEL

Dagenbach and Carr (1994) proposed a model where individuals would facilitate access to word meanings in semantic memory by directing their attention selectively to different parts of their spreading activation network. The attentional center-surround theory draws on the work of Hubel and Weisel (1962) on the structure and function of visual interneurons. In summary, it is established that the action of one visual interneuron inhibits that of its neighbors that fall along a sort of inhibitory border (surround). At the *cytoarchitectural* level, this border seems to be comprised of microcolumns of like-functioning neurons. These functional groups are structured to amplify the summed activity of their own group and dampen the activity of neighboring groups. Those neurons falling within the center of the structural group and the edge of its surround may not be inhibited, or even mildly facilitated, while those neurons slightly farther away, but falling on the border of this surround, may be dampened. Neurons beyond the center-surround field should not be directly affected, but may be indirectly affected by the action of a mutually connected interneuron.

Dagenbach, Carr, and Wilhelmsen (1989) first proposed a CSM as a possible mechanism to explain unexpected results in a masked behavioral semantic priming paradigm. Subjects were required to make lexical decisions to targets following masked primes, and their performance varied as a function of the threshold setting task used. In the key condition, participants performed a semantic similarity judgment task in the threshold setting phase, which lead to related words being responded to less quickly than words from an unrelated baseline condition. This finding lead Carr and Dagenbach (1990) to replicate and extend these findings using both semantic and repetition priming in the same task. In the first phase of this study, subjects made either detection, or semantic similarity judgments under the assumption that the later would encourage subjects to continue to use primarily semantic information to complete the lexical decision task in phase two. The prediction was that when subjects encountered a masked prime it would produce relatively little activation, and they would subsequently focus their attention on the prime. This attentional allocation would take the form of increased activation for the weak prime, in conjunction with a decrement in activation for associated words (CSM). Results indicated that subjects in the semantic decision condition showed facilitation for responses to repeats, and inhibition for semantic associates. I shall attempt to present a case that this type of mechanism may play a role in the language problems seen in aphasia and AD.

APHASIA

Many individuals suffering from brain damage can be classified as aphasic. A common symptom associated with many subtypes of aphasia is semantic paraphasia, and related paralexias. There exists some debate about the nature of this semantic deficit, with some researchers arguing for a qualitative difference in aphasic semantic processing (Zurif, Caramazza, Myerson, & Galvin, 1974) that manifests itself as a disorganization of the structure of the semantic store (Fromkin, Unpublished; Goodglass & Baker, 1976). The other position views the semantic difficulties exhibited by aphasics as quantitatively different from normals (Chenery, Ingram, & Murdoch, 1990; Milberg & Blumstein, 1981).

Blumstein, Milberg, and Shrier (1982) performed a study using a variety of aphasic patients with naming and comprehension deficits ranging from moderate to severe, as assessed by performance on the *Token Test*, and multiple confrontation naming tasks. However, these same patients showed evidence of semantic priming for semantic level relation judgments, regardless of level of severity of their naming deficits. These authors interpreted this striking dissociation of explicit and implicit processes as evidence that the lexicon of even profound aphasics is intact, but that conscious access to that lexicon is impaired. Other studies were conducted (Zurif et al., 1974) that were designed to measure the intactness of aphasics semantic lexicon. Wernicke's and Broca's aphasics and normal controls were presented with triplets of words and the task of grouping them according to "what goes best together." The words varied along multiple semantic dimensions, including: human–nonhuman, male–female, and so on. The normals and Broca's aphasics clustered according to category or functional relationship. Wernicke's aphasics showed no systematic pattern of grouping. These results were taken as evidence that the structure of the lexicon is significantly affected in Wernicke's aphasics.

In a related experiment, Fromkin (unpublished) used a hierarchical grouping technique to test the degree of cohesion in the lexicon of aphasics. For this particular group of patients with language disorders due to subcortical pathology, normals were found to place related words together in much the same way across subjects. For example, if presented with the triplet "husband, chair, wife" normals would place husband and wife together over 85% of the time, and move chair to join the category of furniture and its associates. Aphasics showed much greater variability in the way they arranged the words, often ignoring traditional category boundaries, confirming the notion of a lexicon with marked differences from normal. Similar conclusions were drawn by Goodglass and Baker (1976), who required that aphasics judge whether a target word paired to particular types of semantic associates were related to each other.

Milberg and Blumstein (1981) point out that even though the (Wernicke's) aphasics demonstrated significant deficits, there may be alternate explanations for their poor performance. One such explanation is that these subjects have an intact lexicon, but that they cannot consciously access that lexicon to the degree that normals can. In addition, all of the above tasks required the overt classification of words into overtly demarcated lexical categories. A failure to complete this kind of task along normal parameters could reflect the altered operation of classification mechanisms, or of any number of metalinguistic processes.

Chenery et al. (1990) sought to replicate and extend these results by carrying out further behavioral semantic priming studies. Their studies classified aphasics as low comprehension (LC) or high comprehension (HC) based on their performance above or below 50% on the Neurosensory Center Comprehensive Examination for Aphasics (NCCEA). These subjects were matched with normal and nonaphasic brain injured controls. The subjects were required to complete the RT task to targets preceded by nonwords, real word unrelated primes, real word functionally associated primes, and real word superordinate categorically related primes. They were required to listen to pairs of words and make a lexical decision about the target. In a secondary task, the subjects were required to judge the pictures of the target stimuli according to their relatedness to real word targets from the lexical decision stimulus set. Subjects were also asked to name the target during this phase of the experiment.

The results of this experiment were complex: (1) All brain damaged patients showed slowed reaction times compared to normals; (2) marked differences appeared in the ability of LC aphasics to perform accurate semantic judgments, as compared to normal and HC controls; (3) normal and HC controls showed normal semantic facilitation of RT, regardless of accuracy rate of their responses; but (4) LC aphasics showed a pattern of results in their association judgments contingent upon their ability to name the targets, but performed equivalently (even slightly better than nonaphasic brain damaged controls) to HC aphasics. In particular, LCs showed no difficulty with one task that HC and normals did have trouble with. When asked to respond to stimuli that seemed to be related by means of a super-ordinate category, LC subjects showed no slowing in reaction, while normals did. This suggests LC subjects, who did not have access to the normal judgment mechanisms, were left with simple association mediated by spreading activation (Meyer & Schvaneveldt, 1971).

It appears that LC aphasics can make relatedness judgments, but that they may use different, more simplified strategies than normals and less impaired aphasics. Chenery et al. (1990) explain that LC aphasics "base their relatedness decisions on a global comparison of perceived referential similarity." For example, a response linking "chair" to "knife" or "fence" to "sheep" would tend to suggest a global comparison of referential similarity rather than a conscious, critical evaluation of shared features. Luria explains this phenomenon by hypothesizing that when effected by a lesion the cerebral cortex has its inhibitory mechanisms disrupted, and therefore has trouble distinguishing important connections from less important connections, and therefore that a more relevant feature will fail to override irrelevant or more abstract features.

RELATIONSHIP TO THE CENTER-SURROUND MODEL (CSM)

Chiarello (1985) proposed a model of left (LH) and right hemisphere (RH) language function that ascribes different levels of automaticity and control in lexical access to each hemisphere. Specifically, she showed that priming based on phonological relatedness was equal between the hemispheres, but that priming was greater for categorically and associatively related words in the LH, and orthographically similar words produced greater priming in the RH. This suggests significantly different approaches to lexical access between hemispheres. It may be that the differences seen in aphasic relationship judgment tasks, and similarly, in semantic paraphasias, are due to the continued functioning of automatic processes in intact RH structures. Some of the representational lexicon may indeed be intact in aphasics, but the processes available for the inspection and manipulation of that lexicon are largely those found in normal RH language operation.

Recently, researchers have begun to propose mechanisms for how the left hemisphere uses attention to achieve selective activation and inhibition of the lexicon

(Barnhardt, Glisky, Polster, & Elam, 1996; Burgess & Simpson, 1988). It may be that anomias due to competition between related targets, and accompanying paraphasia can best be ascribed to the failure of an attentional inhibition mechanism found primarily in the left hemisphere, in the case of language. Building on the model of the attentional center-surround mechanism of Dagenbach and Carr (1994) described above, Barhardt et al. (1996) sought to directly test the prediction that synonyms would be facilitated while associated would be inhibited for weakly represented words. After learning a list of rare words to criterion (50% recall), subjects performed a lexical decision task with the newly learned rare words as primes. When targets were weakly associatively related to the primes lexical decisions were speeded only for correctly recalled words. But, following synonyms of the rare word responses were speeded regardless of their being remembered or not remembered. They interpreted this finding to support a model in which very closely related words have a facilitatory relationship, due to their proximity in semantic space. On the other hand, those words that are weakly associated are inhibited so as to better differentiate them from the weakly associated concept. Unrelated words would fall beyond the edge of this "surround" mechanism, and hence would be unaffected.

This is particularly relevant to the current review in that Chenery et al. (1990) suggest that aphasics may base their semantic decisions more heavily on postlexical information, because normal, controlled lexical strategies are less available. If this is true, then perhaps other disorders involving a disruption of language will evidence a relatively normal semantic network, but show evidence of a reliance on postlexical processes as a means of compensatory mechanism. It is proposed next that at least the earlier stages of AD provide an example of such a situation, and that the operation of the CSM mechanism has been the source of some of the disparate results obtained thus far.

ALZHEIMER'S DEMENTIA (AD)

It is well agreed upon that a high percentage of dementia patients suffer from a decline in language that appears to be correlated with the severity of their impairment in memory and cognitive functioning (Bayles & Tomoeda, 1983; Heilman & Valenstein, 1993). What is unclear is the precise nature of this language impairment. In light of the prevalence and severity of AD, it is important to attempt to understand as much as possible about the nature of the language disturbance, and also to attempt to create theories that can explain how the general decline in cognitive functioning interacts with the language problems.

First, articles arguing that there is a true degradation of the semantic lexical network itself will be discussed, followed by studies advocating for a disruption in the organization of the semantic system that may not imply any loss of content. It is suggested that the center-surround mechanism introduced earlier may reside primarily in the LH, and may contribute to the disordered performance of patients with AD. Finally, we discuss several neuroimaging studies utilizing Event-Related Potentials (ERPs) to support the LH CSM hypothesis. It is argued that the disparate pattern of priming results may be explained reasonably well by positing the action of a CSM on a degraded semantic network.

Huff, Corkin, and Growdon (1986) describe a study of object naming that examines the high incidence of semantic paraphasias in the language of AD. These authors report that of the five major language function categories measured by the *Western Aphasia Battery*, naming was the most severely impaired ability in those persons with probable AD (PAD). The study reportedly set out to test competing hypothesis about the nature of the naming deficit: (1) the naming deficit reflects an inability to establish the correct "set" in a naming task (the proper category is never identified, or cannot be maintained); (2) naming problems reflect impaired visual perception; or (3) an underlying semantic decrement. Several researchers provided evidence that PAD patients were more sensitive to the effects of degraded, or abstracted stimuli than normal controls, and that moderate patients showed greater naming deficits than mild patients as a function of the degree of visual degradation (Kirshner, Webb, & Kelly, 1984). Prompted by the work of Warrington (1975), Schwartz, Marin, and Saffran (1979), and Benson (1979) who all showed specific semantic problems in AD patients, Huff, Corkin and Growdon employed measures of confrontation naming, visual form discrimination, differentiation of items by semantic category, and lexical-semantic word retrieval tasks.

Using the Battig and Montague (1969) norms, the authors prepared a list of common words and their frequent associates, as well as a group of line drawings depicting the associates, for example: corn, bus, drill, and pants. In the first experiment, subjects with PAD performed dramatically worse on a word fluency test with category names as prompts (52.6 for normals, 23.9 for PAD). When the authors used form discrimination scores as the covariant, and naming ability as the dependant variable, differences in naming ability were highly significant. The authors suggest that this is strong evidence that impaired confrontation naming is independent of any visual processing decline. In a second experiment, the authors provided evidence that while AD patients were able to reject incorrect category designations on a category recognition test, they were impaired in rejecting incorrect names from within the same category. This was accomplished by using the same stimuli in two separate tasks. First, subjects were shown an item (in picture, and later in word form) and asked if it was a kind of "X," like a vegetable, vehicle, tool, or clothing. Then subjects were shown the same items as stimuli, but asked, "Is this called an 'X'?" where X was either the correct name or a foil from the same category.

Several aspects are remarkable in this study, the first of which is that subjects' results on a category fluency task were the same regardless of dementia severity. Many authors have made the point that, similarly to aphasia, the semantic difficulties associated with dementia seem to show distinctive patterns based on severity (Nicholas, Obler, Au, & Albert, 1996). Second, in contrast to Huff et al. (1986), they showed that subjects' difficulty with naming at the moderate stages of AD and beyond may be exacerbated by, if not largely due to, failure to get a clean perceptual activation of concepts as a result of perceptual impairment. This is particularly germane to an abstract debate such as this one, in that it reminds us to keep lower level deficits in mind at all times when trying to interpret cognitive level ones.

The previous study was not alone in finding evidence for semantic degeneration in PAD with pictorial stimuli. Margolin, Pate, and Friedrich (1996) employed a priming task with combinations of visually presented word targets and pictorial primes in the form of line drawings. The subjects experienced one of four types of trials: (1) identity, where prime and target represented the same semantic information (picture of dog-word dog); (2) semantically related, in which prime and target were exemplars from within the same category; (3) nonrelated, where prime and target were from different categories with no obvious relationship; and (4) nonsense, where the prime was a nonobject shape. As an aside, the study could be criticized for not adequately controlling possible aspects of the prime-target relationship. For example, the authors list the example of bed-dog as being "unrelated," when both often have four legs. It would perhaps be better if they referred to this category of relationship as "noncategorically related."

The results of their first experiment were partitioned according to subject type, with normal elderly, very mild PAD, and mild PAD showing some differences. First, it must be noted that these authors failed to achieve significant semantic priming in the normal and very mild PAD groups, so all of their findings must be interpreted with caution. Margolin et al. (1996) did find a significant amount of identity priming in the normals and very mild PAD patients, but no effect of identity priming in mild PAD. They interpreted this to signify a serious deterioration in the semantic network, even relatively early in the disease course. Specifically, when pictures were used as primes, the mild PAD subjects showed significantly slower reaction times compared to nonsense primes. These authors ask us to imagine a semantic network that has been degraded such that normal spreading activation may occur automatically (Meyer & Schvaneveldt, 1971), but inhibition is faulty.

In this conceptualization, semantically related information actually served to inhibit processing for mild PADs, possibly because the eroded category boundaries allow for multiple exemplars to become activated, but with no reliable way of determining the correct target. If this were so, then the delayed RT may reflect the use of postlexical processes to try to sharpen the distinction between concepts—a process that would normally happen automatically. It is also possible that the CSM becomes activated at inappropriate times in AD patients because words that are normally strongly represented are difficult to access, or have damaged representations. If this is the case, then the identity primes that would normally produce facilitation may be treated as associates, because the degraded semantic network may result in increased semantic distances between normally close concepts. As reviewed above, concepts that fall outside of the immediate surround of the currently activated representation may be inhibited to reduce noise in the recognition process.

Their second experiment, using word-word pairs, produced initially unintuitive results. As would be expected, RTs slowed as a function of subject group, with mild PAD being the slowest. Similarly, word primes were faster than non-word across the board. However, significant priming was produced by both identical and semantically related words in the mild PAD group only, but neither type of prime was effective for normals and very mild PAD groups. This phenomenon, termed "hyperpriming" has been seen in tasks involving degraded stimuli.

Margolin et al. (1996) attempt to form a connection between visually degraded stimuli, and possible internal degradation of the semantic network. This idea explains how mild AD subjects could initially appear to be more "sensitive" to the relationships between words than normals. While responding more slowly overall, mild AD subjects may benefit from information that normals would not; normals may perceive this information but their system has already made the necessary lexical selection by the time the additional information reaches their decision mechanism. They refer to this idea as a "cognitive crutch." Alternately, it may not be a question of time-to-decision being effected directly by AD, but perhaps the threshold for decision is higher, and semantic relatedness decisions not much utilized in normals becomes needed in the lexical selection process of ADs.

On the other hand, a more parsimonious explanation for this effect can be seen if we interpret Margolin et al.'s (1996) results in light of Huff et al.'s (1986) finding that the quality of the perceptual information available to the AD subject is significantly degraded as their disease progresses. The blurring, addition of noise, or attention fluctuations, or reduction in contrast and luminance done experimentally by some authors (Schvaneveldt, Meyer, & Becker, 1976; Stanovich & West, 1983) may happen internally in more severe AD patients. It does not follow that we must look to a detriment in the content of the patient's semantic network at all; instead, we may postulate that an intact network is receiving an inferior quality of information from perception. In summary, these authors findings are consistent with the proposition that more detailed semantic information is eroded first, thereby blurring distinctions within categories, then progressing to a pervasive difficulty that is reflected in anomia. It is not clear, as they claim, that this pattern necessarily reflects information loss within the semantic network.

Goldstein, Green, Presley, and Green (1992) performed a study consistent with the notion of a semantic processing deficit in PAD. Their patients were classified as having a verbal, visual, or global type of dementia. This subdivision is not typically observed in studies of the language of dementia, may prove to be as important as subtyping based on severity. Shuttleworth and Huber (1988) stated that:

> Attempting to average patient scores may tend to confuse rather than to clarify the nature of their naming disorder. In fact, at any given time, there may well be several possible anomic syndromes in DAT, varying over a continuum from mostly verbal to mostly visual. (p. 309)

This statement is compatible with the distinction cited previously by Huff et al. (1986) in which patients difficulties with word naming tasks could be due to the poor quality of their perceptual input. Subjects were presented with a group of normed line drawings selected from the Boston Naming Task (BNT; Van Gorp, Satz, Kiersch, & Henry, 1986) that were grouped according to two variables: complexity and frequency (high and low levels for both). Subjects were to name the pictures as quickly as possible.

The results of this study indicated that there was no difference in naming performance between any AD group and normals for high frequency words. This may be related to the findings cited earlier that mild AD patients were highly accurate at simple tasks with common English words. However, in the low frequency word condition, normals were significantly better at naming than all AD subtypes. These results were taken to signify the presence of a semantic deficit in AD. The authors found support for their subtyping system because their visual type AD patients showed more visually based errors, and their semantic subtype patients showed more semantic errors, according to the Bayles and Tomoeda (1983) coding scheme. This scheme has face validity in that errors that resemble surface alexias, such as mistaking "dog" for "log" are seen as visually based, while mistaking "dog" for "cat" would be a semantic error, like that seen in deep dyslexia. In conclusion, this paper showed classic effects of frequency in naming for AD, such that low frequency words were harder to name. However, this paper is open to the criticism that no semantic content deficit is necessary to account for these findings; a lexical access problem could just as well be the culprit.

One possible explanation of PAD patients poor language performance relates to their primary short-term memory deficit. While short-term memory is usually assessed for episodic memory, as in the Weschler Memory Scale story memory task, there may be an equivalent decline in semantic memory. One author, Kopelman (1986) explored the relationship between global memory loss and semantic decline. Subjects included normal controls, depressed patients, Korsakoff's amnesics, and mildly demented PAD patients. These people were told to repeat eight sentences exactly as they were read to them, with the sentences falling into four types: two semantically/syntactically normal (The team of workers built the bridge), four syntactically legal/semantically aberrant (Colorless green ideas sleep furiously), one semantically reversible, and one random word string.

Results showed that all subjects were able to recall the normal sentences without difficulty, and that all subjects experienced a drop in recall for the anomalous sentences. However, PAD subjects scored more than three times worse than normals and clinical controls on the semantically anomalous sentences. The explanation offered for this phenomenon is that Alzheimer's patients rely more heavily on semantic cues in the verbal environment as a way of compensating for their semantic difficulties. This is germane both to the claims of postlexical dependence cited above, as well as to the auditory ERP studies discussed below. In an analysis of error types made by all subjects, it was found that PAD patients made a large proportion of "normalizing" semantic errors, suggesting that semantic processors were functioning enough to automatically regularize semantically anomalous sentences. This performance was drastically limited by impaired verbal short-term memory. The conclusion of this author is that the presence of a semantic deficit is indicated, but that it must be viewed in interaction with the inability to maintain internal semantic mediation for any length of time.

Several studies emphasize the nature of the language deficit in AD is not in the content of the semantic network, but in its organization, or in impaired access to this network. Similarly, they point out that methodological errors may lead to erroneous conclusions. The first of these papers (Nicholas et al., 1996) investigated the nature of naming errors produced in response to Boston Naming Test stimuli using an experimental scoring system. This system divides error types into misperceptions and nonmisperceptions. The misperceptions were excluded from the analysis, and included responses like, "Some kind of bottle," for whistle, or "Needle to give a shot," for dart. This might appear to create a bias in the results right away, creating a percentage error analysis in favor of non-PAD controls. In actuality, older controls produced more errors overall (218) than mild (130) and moderate PAD (206) subjects. Similarly, blind raters judged the number of misperception errors to be greater in older controls (19) than in mild AD patients (13). Moderate AD patients did produce the most misperception errors (38).

An analysis of the remaining errors was completed in which new, blind raters with significant experience in the field of dementia rated each response according to its degree of semantic relatedness to the target. It was found that no significant differences existed between groups in the degree of semantic relatedness of their single word errors. It seems as if PAD patients, even moderate ones, are no "more wrong" than normal controls. For multiword responses, a significant effect of group was obtained, but the significantly highest group was the mild AD, not the moderate AD. In fact, Moderate PAD patients and older controls performed equivalently in this regard. This study did find significant evidence of gross naming defects, prior to semantic cuing, in AD subjects, but the further analysis of these errors is incompatible with a semantic deterioration hypothesis. The authors suggest that much of the evidence showing that a specific semantic deficit exists in AD may be an artifact of the dichotomous nature of the testing tasks imposed by researchers.

Particularly relevant to this question is the research report of Bayles, Tomoeda, & Rein (1996) who state that their results failed to confirm a performance pattern consistent with semantic memory loss theory. Their study exposed subjects (PAD and matched controls) to sentences of six or nine syllables that were meaningful, improbable, or meaningless. For all subjects, meaningless nine syllable sentences were significantly more difficult to remember correctly. For mild PAD subjects, nine syllable improbable phrases were more difficult than nine syllable meaningful and six syllable improbable phrases. The results were similar for moderate AD patients. In general, the effect of stimulus meaningfulness did not diminish as a function of disease severity, as would be the case if a pure semantic loss theory were true. It is argued that semantic information is not lost, but that for mild and moderate PAD patients it becomes difficult to work with this information, and to make fine grained distinctions between semantic exemplars. This inability to discriminate is consistent with the working hypothesis of this review that AD involves the abnormal action of a CSM that would ordinarily function to aid in fine comparisons by boosting signal to noise ratios for semantic decisions.

Grober, Buschke, Kawas, and Fuld (1985) explored the loss of semantic attributes that is said to occur in dementia. These authors also view the deterioration in language ability that accompanies dementia as being due to a problem with semantic organization more than of a loss of semantic organization. They performed three experiments attempting to demonstrate that under certain conditions, the semantic content of their concepts was relatively well preserved. The first study assessed the extent to which attributes have been eroded from common words like "airplane" and "car."

In selecting this kind of task, Grober et al. (1985) make an assumption that may not be well founded, namely that one can assess the intactness of a concept's representation by examining the number of appropriate associates that the subject judges to be related to it. This technique may be susceptible to the intrusion of nonsemantic attributes, such as mere frequency of association, as well as post semantic processes, such as attentional mediation. This problem is addressed somewhat in their second and third experiments.

Experiment one asked subjects to complete a checklist that contained words that were closely related to, or foils to, a common English word. Subjects were normal controls, those with MID, PAD, normal pressure hydrocephalus, or dementia of a mixed etiology. Normal subjects were 98% accurate at identifying the words that had been previously determined to be highly related to the target. Remarkably, the demented subjects were 95% accurate on the same task. It appears as if even moderately demented subjects (as assessed by the Blessed Mental Status Test) knew what words "go with" another common English word, at this basic level. In experiment two, subjects were presented a target word and a dichotomous forced choice task with a related word and a foil. Again, there was no significant difference between normals and subjects with dementia. This surprising lack of deficit can be contrasted with the results of experiment three. Experiment three provided subjects with a list of words related to a target by various degrees, and had them rank order these words according to degree of relation. Here, demented subjects had great difficulty.

In experiments one and two, demented subjects were equally as likely to miss a highly related word as they were to miss a distant associate. Combined with experiment three, these results suggest that a significant amount of semantic information (if not 95%) is intact in the patient group, but that it is difficult for the subjects to differentiate its relative importance. Grober et al. (1985) cite the work of Smith and Medin (1981) as a framework to interpret these results. Smith and Medin describe semantic networks in terms of weights on the links between concepts, such that a normal semantic network would contain a high value for the link between "dog" and "cat," but a lower weight for "dog" and "dish." This type of theory is also compatible with parallel distributed processing models of cognition, which have the advantage of a structure that is analogous to actual neural structures. It may be that if the neurochemical milieu of the cortex is compromised by plaques and abnormal transmitter levels, this would appear as an equalizing of the strengths of associations.

As an analogy, imagine an ice cube tray with different amounts of water in each compartment. This tray becomes old and cracked from freezing and warming, and develops cracks in its structure, thereby permitting the gradual flow of water from section to section. If this analogy is extended, it would follow that structural changes would result in changes in semantic informational content (water level changes). This may be helpful in reconciling the dichotomy that exists between the "structure" and "content" theorists, in that what begins as a structural problem directly effects content. It is important not to allow ourselves to slip backward to the 1950s and view human memory as a "warehouse," but instead to realize that information concepts are represented by distinctive patterns of neurochemical activity.

Much evidence has been accumulated both for and against a semantic loss theory of language deterioration in AD. One way to reconcile these accounts is to posit that semantic information is actually not lost, but appears as if it is lost on many of the classic tests of confrontation naming, and other explicit measures. In addition to overt responses, ERPs may offer converging evidence about the functioning of semantic processes in AD, and also allow us to make some guesses about the underlying neural substrates that may accompany the language deficits.

EVENT-RELATED POTENTIALS (ERPS) IN THE STUDY OF ALZHEIMER'S DISEASE

ERPs reflect the action of populations of synchronously firing neurons that are continuously recorded, and then averaged according to the occurrence of time-locked stimuli. One particular ERP, the N400, has been shown to reliably covary with the magnitude of semantic discrepancy between a target word and its preceding prime (Holcomb, 1993; see Kutas, Van Petten, & Gernsbacher, 1994 for a review; Otten, Rugg, & Doyle, 1993). The amplitude of the N400 decreases with word frequency, repetition, orthographic, phonological, and most commonly, with semantic priming (Ganis, Kutas, & Sereno, 1996). The N400 may be particularly well-suited to probe the nature of the language deficit in AD because it can provide evidence for intact semantic processing, if it exists, even in patients who may have difficulty with an overt response. The N400 has also been shown to be strongly correlated with paper-and-pencil measures of semantic knowledge, such as the Dementia Rating Scale (Ford et al., 2001). In the case of AD patients, who are often confused and significantly slowed during task administration, it may be a more sensitive tool than RT for demonstrating a differential response to primed and unprimed targets.

Only a handful of studies thus far have employed the N400 in a semantic priming task with an AD population (Castaneda, Ostrosky-Solis, Perez, Bobes, & Rangel, 1997; Ford et al., 2001; Hamberger, Friedman, Ritter, & Rosen, 1995; Revonsuo, Portin, Juottonen, & Rinne, 1998; Schwartz, Kutas, Butters, Paulsen, & Salmon,

1996). Of these studies, some have reported reduced or nonexistent N400 priming, while others have reported normal priming (Ford et al., 2001; Hamberger et al., 1995; Schwartz et al., 1996). While all of these studies used AD patients who were mild to moderate in disease severity, and long SOAs (1000 msec or more), many other factors differ among them. While some use auditorially presented category names as primes, others use pictures, and still others use words. I propose that the large discrepancy in the results of these studies may best be explained by differences in materials, specifically the semantic distance between the prime and target and the amount of context provided in single stimulus versus sentence priming paradigms.

Hamburger et al. (1995) presented AD patients and normal elderly controls with sentences that had either congruent or incongruent final words in a variation of the first N400 studies performed by Kutas and Hillyard (1980). They found that while the controls showed evidence of reduced efficiency of semantic processing in the form of smaller and later N400 priming effects, the AD group, surprisingly showed no evidence of a smaller N400 effect than younger adults. The N400 response (not the effect produced by subtracting primed from unprimed waves) for unprimed words was larger for AD patients than age-matched controls, which may indicate that in the absence of facilitating context, AD patients have greater difficulty in accessing the word's meaning. The presence of significant priming, coupled with the long SOA, could suggest the action of the type of "crutch" mechanism discussed above in behavioral studies.

To my knowledge, the only other studies to report significant N400 priming in AD patients were both reported by Ford et al. (1996, 2001), and Schwartz et al. (1996). Ford et al. (1996) used similar sentences to Hamburger et al. (1995) as primes, but presented them in the auditory modality in an attempt to reduce the confounding influence of education level and reading ability that may have influenced the above results. They found that the N400 priming effect was significantly smaller for AD patients than for elderly controls, but that it was still significant in a pair-wise comparison for the AD group. An inspection of their waves reveals that the amplitude of this effect is about half of that seen in elderly controls, and about one-quarter of the amplitude of young adults' N400 effect.

Interestingly, these authors also reported that when all subjects were required to engage in a phoneme monitoring task that was designed to draw their attention away from actively processing the meaning of the task, their N400 amplitudes did not decrease. This would seem to indicate that even AD patients can perform automatic semantic analysis on sentence level stimuli, or perhaps only lexical analysis on each item in the sentence without concomitant integration. Unfortunately, the phoneme task may not have imposed a very high attentional load on the subjects, and so the common criticism of attention switching between tasks raised in Holender's (1986) criticism of automatic semantic processing studies may be leveled against this study as well, and leaves the implications of this finding unclear.

The next study to test AD patients using the N400 was Schwartz et al. (1996) who used auditorially presented category names as primes, and visually presented words that were judged to be either related or unrelated to these categories as targets. The category names were either superordinate (living, nonliving), ordinate (animal, musical instrument, etc.), or subordinate (land animals, wind instruments, etc.). In addition to demonstrating N400 priming in AD patients, this study had the goal of showing that N400 priming effect amplitude would be sensitive to the degree of category constraint imposed by the level of the category name. Behavioral studies had indicated a deficit in lower level category priming for AD patients with relatively normal superordinate level priming. While the category level manipulation was for the most part successful, with N400 amplitude inversely related to specificity, AD patients did not show significant N400 priming at any level. This study can be criticized for failing to report, and most likely to control for the associative strength of the primes and targets adequately. This may be important, because the lower level category primes may not have effectively limited the set size for semantic search, but may have produced smaller N400 effects simply because they were less associated to the targets.

Castaneda et al. (1997) used pictures of common objects and animals as a stimuli, with related primes defined as pictures belonging to the same category, and unrelated primes being from different categories. The subjects performed a category discrimination task. As in the previous study, the level of association was not strictly controlled for. These authors also found no significant N400 priming, but performed an additional comparison to illuminate the nature of their N400 effect. AD patients had the same N400 response to congruent trials as normals, but the N400 for incongruent trials was significantly more positive. Two explanations are offered for this result, one that supposes that the N400 is an indicator of lexical level activation (Deacon, Dynowska, Ritter, & Grose-Fifer, 2004; Kutas & Hillyard, 1984) and a second that supposes that it indexes postlexical processes (Brown & Hagoort, 1993; Halgren, Scheibel, & Wechsler, 1990). Because the preponderance of evidence to date argues for the first interpretation, we will discuss this option more thoroughly (Deacon & Shelley-Tremblay, 2000).

Castaneda et al. (1997) suggest that this finding tells us that less priming is produced by incongruent stimuli, "since the amount of negativity should be inversely related to the amount of contextual preactivation." A normal congruent response combined with a diminished incongruent response again could suggest that while abnormal activation often occurs, subjects are able to benefit enough from the presence of congruent information (priming) to effectively over-come some of the processing deficit. This should not be possible if the semantic representations were truly impaired. Instead, a degradation of the associative links may occur that results in a shifting of the semantic space. This is consistent with Castaneda et al.'s (1997) comment that AD is known as a "neocortical disconnection syndrome," in which the associative network is deteriorated perhaps due to the accumulation of neurofibrillary plaques and tangles.

Revonsuo et al. (1998) reported greatly diminished N400 responses for AD patients compared to controls in a spoken sentence priming paradigm.

However, they included an analysis of another ERP component, the phonological mismatch negativity, which is purported to be a measure of early lexical selection. For this component, peaking at about 300 msec, AD patients showed normal responses. Analyses of congruent and incongruent words were also carried out separately in this study and indicated that while congruous responses were equivalent between the mild AD patients and elderly controls, the incongruent responses were greatly reduced. Revonsuo et al. suggest that their study, which uses spoken sentences as well, supports the position of a relatively well-preserved lexicon.

The most recent study to test the effects of priming on N400 in AD is Ford et al. (2001). Unlike Revonsuo et al. (1998) and Castaneda et al. (1997), they reported significant N400 priming effects for AD patients. Their stimuli deserve special notice, as they are a (serendipitously) critical test of a CSM account of semantic priming in AD. While most of the ERP studies cited here used stimuli with varying degrees of associative strength and found reduced or eliminated N400 effects in AD, these authors defined their congruent condition as a picture prime, followed a word that *named* the picture. This is effectively a synonym. Their incongruent condition was defined simply as a word, from the *same category* that did not name the picture. Common words that are categorically related are likely to share at least some features, and will often be associatively related. Thus this study provides an approximate test of the Barnhardt et al. (1996) behavioral study described above that used synonyms and associates. As in Barnhardt et al. (1996), the present study showed facilitation for synonyms, and a lack of priming for associates.

Ford et al. (2001) offer that their results are evidence of spared semantic knowledge in AD, and I tend to agree. To this could be added the idea that under conditions where individuals have difficulty accessing the semantic representation, then a normally adaptive signal-to-noise enhancement mechanism may serve to interfere with normal processing. Further studies should be conducted to test for the action of an inhibitory CSM using ERPs in both normal and AD populations. Preliminary data from my own study suggests that such a mechanism is in effect, and that it is localized to the LH. If such a mechanism were operating in AD, then it could help to understand the seemingly discordant body of research.

An obvious problem for this hypothesis is the finding of normal priming in the studies using auditory and visual sentences as primes. For these studies, the CSM may activate, but its effects are reduced by the buildup of evidence from the sentence. To say that the N400 is sensitive to the accumulation of the rich sources of evidence in a sentence does not necessitate that it is indexing a postlexical integrative process. Instead, as suggested by Deacon (personal communication), the semantic information gleaned from each word in the sentence may act to reset the level of activation in the target word's representation before its meaning is processed. Thus, the AD patient may benefit greatly from context, because they must in order to approach normal performance to any degree, but still battle against a normally beneficial center-surround mechanism.

SUMMARY OF CLINICAL EVIDENCE

We have reviewed evidence that a CSM may be at work in both aphasia, and AD. In aphasia, the CSM that normally facilitates word recognition and subsequent naming may go awry when confronted with a damaged LH. The preserved priming seen in some studies of aphasics was suggested to be due in part to the intact functioning of the RH that, when unchecked by the LH, may contribute to semantic paraphasias. In AD, it has been suggested that priming should be found when (1) there is a high degree of semantic support, in the form of sentence context; and/or (2) when the prime and target are synonymous, and thus cannot activate the CSM. What remains to be discussed is the final topic outlined in the introduction; namely, how can we conceptualize the format of the semantic system in a way that is compatible with evidence from the study of the functional anatomy and physiology of the brain? If we are to posit the action of a general cognitive mechanism, such as the CSM, in modulating semantic processing in AD, then we must at least attempt to specify in what format the information is likely to be stored *in cortex*.

SUGGESTED READING

Bayles, K., & Tomoeda, C. (2007). *Cognitive-communication disorders of dementia*. San Diego, CA US: Plural Publishing.

Bayles, K., Kim, E., Azuma, T., Chapman, S., Cleary, S., Hopper, T., et al. (2005). Developing evidence-based practice guidelines for speech-language pathologists serving individuals with Alzheimer's dementia. *Journal of Medical Speech-Language Pathology, 13*(4), xiii-xxv.

Mathalon, D., Roach, B., & Ford, J. (2010). Automatic semantic priming abnormalities in schizophrenia. *International Journal of Psychophysiology, 75*(2), 157–166.

REFERENCES

Barnhardt, T. M., Glisky, E. L., Polster, M. R., & Elam, L. (1996). *Memory & Cognition, 24*, 60–69.

Battig, W. F., & Montague, W. E. (1969). Category norms of verbal items in 56 categories: A replication and extension of the Connecticut category norms. *Journal of Experimental Psychology: General, 80*, 1–46.

Bayles, K. A., & Tomoeda, C. K. (1983). Confrontation naming impairment in dementia. *Brain and Language, 19*(1), 98–114.

Bayles, K., Tomoeda, C., & Rein, J. (1996). Phrase repetition in Alzheimer's disease: Effect of meaning and length. *Brain and Language, 54*, 246–261.

Benson, D. F. (1979). Neurologic correlates of anomia. In H. W. H. A. Whitaker (Ed.), *Studies in Neurolinguistics* (Vol. 4, pp. 293–328). New York, NY: Academic Press.

Blumstein, S. E., Milberg, W., & Shrier, R. (1982). Semantic processing in aphasia: Evidence from an auditory lexical decision task. *Brain and Language, 17*, 301–316.

Brown, C., & Hagoort, P. (1993). The processing nature of the N400: Evidence from masked priming. *Journal of Cognitive Neuroscience, 5*(1), 34–44.

Burgess, C., & Simpson, G. B. (1988). Cerebral mechanisms in the retrieval of ambiguous word meanings. *Brain and Language, 33*, 86–103.

Carr, T. H., & Dagenbach, D. (1990). Semantic priming and repetition priming from masked words: Evidence for a center-surround attentional mechanism in perceptual recognition. *Journal of Experimental Psychology: Learning, Memory, and Cognition, 16*(2), 341–350.

Castaneda, M., Ostrosky-Solis, F., Perez, M., Bobes, M. A., & Rangel, L. E. (1997). ERP assessment of semantic memory impairment in Alzheimer's disease. *International Journal of Psychophysiology, 27*, 201–214.

Chenery, H. J., Ingram, J. C., & Murdoch, B. E. (1990). Automatic and volitional semantic processing in aphasia. *Brain and Language, 38*(2), 215–232.

Chiarello, C. (1985). Hemisphere dynamics in lexical access: Automatic and controlled priming. *Brain and Language, 26*(1), 146–172.

Dagenbach, D., & Carr, T. H. (1994). Inhibitory processes in perceptual recognition: Evidence for a center-surround attentional mechanism. In D. Dagenbach & T. H. Carr (Eds.), *Inhibitory processes in attention, memory, and language* (pp. 327–358). San Diego, CA: Academic Press.

Dagenbach, D., Carr, T. H., & Wilhelmsen, A. (1989). Task-induced strategies and near-threshold priming: Conscious influences on unconscious perception. *Journal of Memory & Language, 28*, 412–443.

Deacon, D., & Shelley-Tremblay, J. F. (2000). How automatically is meaning accessed: A review of the effects of attention on semantic processing. *Frontiers in Bioscience, 5*, e82–94.

Deacon, D., Dynowska, A., Ritter, W., & Grose-Fifer, J. (2004). Repetition and semantic priming of nonwords: Implications for theories of N400 and word recognition. *Psychophysiology, 41*, 60–74.

Ford, J. M., Askari, N., Gabrieli, J. D. E., Mathalon, D. H., Tinklenberg, J. R., Menon, V., & Yesavage, J. (2001). Event-related potential evidence of spared knowledge in Alzheimer's disease. *Psychology and Aging, 16*, 161–176.

Ford, J. M., Woodward, S. H., Sullivan, E., Isaacks, B. G., Tinklenberg, J., Yesavage, J., & Roth, W. T. (1996). N400 evidence of abnormal responses to speech in Alzheimer's disease. *Electroencephalography and Clinical Neurophysiology, 99*, 235–246.

Fromkin, R. (Unpublished). Category sorting responses in normal and language disordered subjects. City University of New York.

Ganis, G., Kutas, M., & Sereno, M. I. (1996). The search for "common sense": An electrophysiological study of the comprehension of words and pictures in reading. *Journal of Cognitive Neuroscience, 8*(2), 89–106.

Goldstein, F. C., Green, J., Presley, R., & Green, R. C. (1992). Dysnomia in Alzheimer's Disease: An evaluation of neurobehavioral subtypes. *Brain & Language, 43*, 308–322.

Goodglass, H., & Baker, E. (1976). Semantic field, naming, and auditory comprehension in aphasia. *Brain and Language, 3*(3), 359–374.

Grober, E., Buschke, H., Kawas, C., & Fuld, P. (1985). Impaired ranking of semantic attributes in dementia. *Brain and Language, 26*, 276–286.

Halgren, E., Scheibel, A. B., & Wechsler, A. F. (1990). Insights from evoked potentials into the neuropsychological mechanisms of reading. In *Neurobiology of higher cognitive function.* (pp. 103–150). New York, NY: Guilford Press.

Hamberger, M., Friedman, D., Ritter, W., & Rosen, J. (1995). Event-related potential and behavioral correlates of semantic processing in Alzheimer's patients and controls. *Brain and Language, 48*, 33–68.

Heilman, K., & Valenstein, E. (Eds.). (1993). *Clinical Neuropsychology* (3rd ed.). New York, NY: Oxford University Press.

Holcomb, P. J. (1993). Semantic priming and stimulus degradation: Implications for the role of the N400 in language processing. *Psychophysiology, 30*, 47–61.

Holender, D. (1986). Semantic activation without conscious identification in dichotic listening, parafoveal vision, and visual masking: A survey and appraisal. *Behavioral and Brain Sciences, 9*(1), 1–66.

Hubel, T. H., & Weisel, D. N. (1962). Receptive fields, binocular interaction and functional architecture in the cat's visual cortex. *Journal of Physiology, 160*, 106–154.

Huff, J. F., Corkin, S., & Growdon, J. H. (1986). Semantic impairment and anomia in Alzheimer's Disease. *Brain & Language, 28*, 235–249.

Kirshner, H. S., Webb, W. G., & Kelly, M. P. (1984). The naming disorder of dementia. *Neuropsychologia, 22*, 23–30.

Kopelman, M. D. (1986). Recall of anomalous sentences in dementia and amnesia. *Brain & Language, 29*, 154–170.

Kutas, M., & Hillyard, S. A. (1980). Event-related brain potentials to semantically inappropriate and surprisingly large words. *Biological Psychology, 11*, 99–116.

Kutas, M., & Hillyard, S. A. (1984). Event-related brain potentials (ERPs) elicited by novel stimuli during sentence processing. *Annals of the New York Academy of Sciences, 425*, 236–241.

Kutas, M., Van Petten, C. K., & Gernsbacher, M. A. (1994). Psycholinguistics electrified: Event-related brain potential investigations. In *Handbook of psycholinguistics.* (pp. 83–143). San Diego, CA: Academic Press.

Margolin, D. I., Pate, D. S., & Friedrich, F. J. (1996). Lexical priming by pictures and words in normal aging and in dementia of the Alzheimer's type. *Brain and Language, 54*, 275–301.

Meyer, D. E., & Schvaneveldt, R. W. (1971). Facilitation in recognizing pairs of words: Evidence of a dependence between retrieval operations. *Journal of Experimental Psychology, 90*, 227–234.

Milberg, W., & Blumstein, S. E. (1981). Lexical decision and aphasia: Evidence for semantic processing. *Brain and Language, 14*, 371–385.

Nicholas, M., Obler, L. K., Au, R., & Albert, M. L. (1996). On the nature of naming errors in aging and dementia: A study of semantic relatedness. *Brain & Language, 54*, 184–195.

Otten, L. J., Rugg, M. D., & Doyle, M. C. (1993). Modulation of event-related potentials by word repetition: The role of selective attention. *Psychophysiology, 30*, 559–571.

Revonsuo, A., Portin, R., Juottonen, K., & Rinne, J. O. (1998). Semantic processing of spoken words in Alzheimer's disease: An electrophysiological study. *Journal of Cognitive Neuroscience, 10*(3), 408–420.

Schvaneveldt, R. W., Meyer, D. E., & Becker, C. A. (1976). Lexical ambiguity, semantic context, and visual word recognition. *Journal of Experimental Psychology: Human Perception and Performance, 2*, 243–256.

Schwartz, T. J., Kutas, M., Butters, N., Paulsen, J. S., & Salmon, D. P. (1996). Electrophysiological insights into the nature of the semantic deficit in Alzheimer's disease. *Neuropsychologia, 34*, 827–841.

Schwartz, M. F., Marin, O. S. M., & Saffran, E. M. (1979). Dissociations of language function in dementia: A case study. *Brain and Language, 7*, 277–306.

Shuttleworth, E. C., & Huber, S. J. (1988). A longitudinal study of the naming disorder of dementia of the Alzheimer type. *Neuropsychiatry, Neuropsychology, & Behavioral Neurology, 1*(4), 267–282.

Smith, E. E., & Medin, D. L. (1981). *Categories and concepts.* Cambridge, MA: Harvard University Press.

Stanovich, K. E., & West, R. F. (1983). On priming in a sentence context. *Journal of Experimental Psychology: General, 112*, 1–36.

Van Gorp, W. P., Satz, P., Kiersch, M. E., & Henry, R. (1986). Normative data on the Boston naming test for a group of normal older adults. *Journal of Clinical and Experimental Neuropsychology, 8,* 702–705.

Warrington, E. K. (1975). The selective impairment of semantic memory. *Quarterly Journal of Experimental Psychology, 27,* 635–657.

Zurif, E. B., Caramazza, A., Myerson, R., & Galvin, J. (1974). Semantic feature representations for normal and aphasic language. *Brain and Language, 1,* 167–187.

31 Neurolinguistic and Neurocognitive Considerations of Language Processing in Bilingual Individuals

José G. Centeno

Bilingualism and multilingualism are a common occurrence in today's world. Many bilinguals (speakers of two languages) and multilinguals or polyglots (speakers of more than two languages) in multilingual population centers receive speech therapy for acquired language problems or aphasia resulting from neurological damage. Interpretation of the heterogenous clinical language profiles exhibited by bilingual and multilingual speakers with aphasia has stimulated the examination of the neurological correlates of language processing in these individuals. Aphasic bilingual and multilingual persons generally show the same extent of impairment in both languages after a neurological insult (*parallel recovery pattern*). Yet, a considerable number of bilinguals may demonstrate a variety of poststroke language restitution profiles in which there is uneven recovery of the two languages (*nonparallel recovery patterns*). For example, both languages may be affected, though one more than the other (*differential recovery*); both languages may be alternatively affected over periods of time (*antagonistic recovery*); or only one language may be available after the stroke (*selective recovery*; Paradis, 2004).

To explore the neurological underpinnings of such variability, investigators have attempted to elucidate whether the bilingual brain is organized differently from the monolingual brain, whether neural organization for the first (L1) language is similar to or contrasts with that for the second (L2) language, whether some important factors in bilingual development, such as age of L2 acquisition and L2 proficiency, have an effect on neural distribution, and whether typical skills in unimpaired bilingual discourse, such as language selection and translation, impact on neural organization.

In this chapter, we will provide an overview of the research conducted to address the preceding queries. Throughout our discussion, the terms bilingual, multilingual, and polyglot will be used interchangeably as the multilingual stroke population may include persons that speak two (bilinguals) or more than two languages (multilinguals or polyglots), as mentioned earlier. Though content chiefly focuses on bilinguals, the most investigated group, specific information on multilingual speakers will be highlighted wherever pertinent.

We will start with important information on bilingualism relevant to the understanding of the studies and theoretical constructs to review and will follow with a summary of valuable investigations that have attempted to explicate cerebral language organization and processing in multiple language users. We will end with a discussion on future directions in this research and some possible implications of the presented findings in aphasia therapy with bilinguals. For the sake of length, this chapter summarizes studies and highlights the merits, limitations, and trends in the reported evidence. This chapter does not provide an in-depth discussion of each study or the anatomical areas involved. Readers, rather, are advised to refer to the cited works for further reading. For neuro-anatomical descriptions and assessment tools, excellent publications similarly are provided (e.g., Bhatnagar, 2008; Dougherty, Rauch, & Rosenbaum, 2004; Patestas & Gartner, 2006).

IMPORTANT ACQUISITIONAL AND DISCOURSE FACTORS IN NEUROLINGUISTIC RESEARCH WITH BILINGUAL SPEAKERS

Language acquisition in multilingual environments, be it bilingual or multilingual learners, is a complex phenomenon. In this section, while we focus on bilingual speakers, acquisitional and discourse factors similarly apply to the linguistic development and communication contexts of multilinguals and polyglots.

Bilingual acquisition and ultimate linguistic proficiency are highly variable. Multiple terms have been proposed to describe the numerous bilingual learning contexts and the considerable diversity in the linguistic abilities of bilingual speakers (see Centeno, 2007a; Centeno & Obler, 2001, for review). In general, bilingual communication environments and their learners may be classified as *simultaneous* or *sequential (successive)*. Simultaneous bilinguals refer to young language learners regularly exposed to two languages since a very early age whereas sequential bilinguals are introduced to L2 from late childhood onward (Centeno, 2007a). In both acquisitional contexts, mastery in each language and concomitant processing operations depend on individual communication circumstances shaping exposure and practice in L1 and L2 along the oral–literate–metalinguistic continuum of language experiences (Bialystok, 2001).

Age additionally has an important role in bilingual development. Maturational age-related constraints in bilingual development were initially described as a time-restricted *critical period* for language development that lasted from birth to puberty, reflecting progressive lateralization of cerebral language sites (see Centeno, 2007a, for review). However, the evidence for child and adult L2 learners suggest a more flexible maturational situation. While most research suggests that younger learners have better results than older learners, it also shows less rigid time-windows for L2 acquisition that may extend beyond puberty. Some postpubertal L2 learners may show L2 native-like performance in several linguistic areas, such as grammaticality judgment and pronunciation (Johnson & Newport, 1989; Yavaş, 1996). Age-related acquisitional restrictions may thus be viewed as a gradual decrease in cerebral plasticity resulting in separate *sensitive periods* or *multiple critical periods* for different linguistic skills (Johnson & Newport, 1989; Seliger, 1978).

Expressive patterns in bilingual discourse similarly have cognitive implications. Depending on their monolingual or bilingual interlocutor, bilingual speakers routinely have to monitor for appropriate language choice during conversation. In addition, expressive features of bilingual speakers may include language mixing or switching (using both languages in an utterance either as a lexical item [mixing] or a longer syntactic structure [switching]), borrowing (using phonologically adapted words from one language into another), transfer effects (using an L1 syntactic or phonetic feature in L2 utterances), or attrition (L1 expressive limitations due to loss of L1 mastery; Centeno, 2007a). Particularly, neurocognitive accounts of translation and language mixing and selection have been proposed, as these expressive skills may impose certain processing demands with valuable insights on language representation in bilinguals (Ansaldo & Marcotte, 2007; Green, 2005; Paradis, 2004).

Hence, understanding L1 and L2 proficiency and pertinent cognitive strategies would require knowledge about the complex interactions among linguistic experiences, age of acquisition, and cognitive challenges for each language in each individual learner. Given the different language modalities (i.e., reading, listening, writing, and speaking), the different linguistic levels (i.e., vocabulary, sentence comprehension, and production, etc.), and the different contexts of language use (i.e., formal [academic/literary] vs. informal [social/conversational], etc.), linguistic mastery and processing in each language would depend on the extent of input and practice each bilingual person has had in each language in the preceding domains (modality, skill, and context) throughout life (Centeno, 2007a, 2007b; Centeno & Obler, 2001). Clearly, because no two bilinguals have experienced each language equally over time, bilingual speakers are linguistically and cognitively heterogenous. Such variability is critical in bilingualism research because it impacts on participant selection, experimental task design and administration, and data interpretation (Centeno, 2007a; Grosjean, 2004; Marian, 2008).

NEUROLOGICAL BASES OF LANGUAGE PROCESSING IN BILINGUAL SPEAKERS

Understanding language lateralization (specific hemisphere) and localization (specific hemispheric site) in the bilingual brain has been possible through the insights provided by the symptomatology of aphasia cases and experimental results from laterality studies, electro-cortical stimulation investigations, and neuroimaging research. As mentioned earlier, the main questions driving these investigations have attempted to explain whether the bilingual brain is organized differently from the monolingual brain, whether neural organization for L1 is similar to or contrasts with that for L2, whether some important factors in bilingual development, such as age of L2 acquisition and L2 proficiency, have an effect on neural distribution, and whether typical skills in unimpaired bilingual discourse, such as language selection and translation, impact on neural organization. Exhaustive reviews of the available evidence and theoretical proposals have been published (e.g., Abutalebi, Cappa, & Perani, 2005; Fabbro, 1999; Goral, Levy, & Obler, 2002; Hull & Vaid, 2005; Paradis, 2004; Vaid, 2008). In this section, we provide an overview of the evolution of this research and summarize important clinical and experimental evidence to highlight merits, limitations, and trends in the reported data.

Interest in the study of brain-language relationships dates back to the mid-eighteenth century. At that time, phrenologists, such as Gall and Sperzheim, claimed that human moral, intellectual, and spiritual faculties were stored in discrete brain organs, whose individual sizes reflected the extent of activity in the organ and, in turn, the size of the skull area just above the organ. Speech abilities, according to phrenologists, were in the frontal lobe, just above the eye socket (Caplan, 1987). Next, Paul Broca's and Carl Wernicke's careful analysis of aphasic symptoms paved the way to view language abilities and complex thinking as being associated with specific brain convolutions. Specifically, Broca identified the inferior frontal convolution as the area responsible to articulate language. Wernicke suggested that the posterior part of the first temporal gyrus was the site for the sensory image of words or language comprehension. Wernicke additionally provided a theoretical framework consisting of motor and sensory speech areas, interconnected by fibers, to account for many aphasic symptoms (see Caplan, 1987; Ijalba, Obler, & Chengappa, 2004, for historical discussion).

The multilingual European context in which these early discussions on brain-language relationships were taking place soon provided the clinical cases that stimulated thinking about language localization in the bilingual or polyglot brain. Reacting to claims suggesting separate cerebral areas for the languages known by a bilingual, Albert Pitres (1895; as cited in Abutalebi et al., 2005; Ijalba et al., 2004) proposed that it would be very unlikely for lesions to affect all of the proposed independent cerebral centers (sensory centers [for auditory and visual images] and motor centers [for graphic and phonetic images]) for each language. Rather, an initial disruption after the stroke would affect all of the language centers followed by a gradual recovery of both comprehension and expression in the most familiar language (known as Pitres's principle to language restitution).

In the following sections, we turn to the clinical and experimental evidence that have shaped the ongoing discussion on language localization and processing in the brain of multiple language users.

CLINICAL EVIDENCE

Aphasia cases of bilingual and multilingual speakers have provided symptomatology to generate accounts on the possible neuroanatomical sites for language localization in bilinguals. As mentioned earlier, parallel language recovery is the most frequent poststroke language restitution profile in aphasic bilinguals. Such a pattern would prompt us to think that language foci in multiple language users may be represented in close proximity in cortical areas. This observation, however, is challenged by the nonparallel profiles that no theoretical principle can uniformly explain.

Several claims to account for the stronger poststroke language have been posited. These proposals included the language most familiar to the patient at the time of the stroke (Pitres's principle), discussed above; the language first acquired because it involves the oldest memories, most resistant to impairment (Ribot's principle), the language associated with the strongest affective experiences (Minkowski's account), and the language most useful to the patient at the time of the cerebral insult (Goldstein's account; Paradis, 2004). Very often, however, clinical literature on multilingual aphasia reports the unusual cases. Review of unselected cases suggest that, most often, the languages known by a multilingual speaker premorbidly are recovered proportionally to their prestroke proficiency, consistent with reports of parallel recovery as the most frequent pattern. Interestingly, when nonparallel recovery occurs, the language most frequently used by the patient at the time of the stroke is the most likely to be restituted hence supporting Pitres's principle (Albert & Obler, 1978; Goral et al., 2002).

Crossed aphasia in bilinguals and polyglots (aphasia resulting from damage in the right hemisphere, the nondominant hemisphere for language) has similarly provided observational grounds for speculation. Prompted by a tendency to report unusual bilingual aphasic patients in the literature, as mentioned above, some early cases suggested a possible higher incidence of crossed aphasia in bilinguals and polyglots hence encouraging the claim of right-sided language processing in these speakers. However, the overwhelming occurrence of aphasia in bilinguals after left-sided lesions strongly supports the left hemisphere to be dominant for both languages (Goral et al., 2002).

More recently, selective language loss or recovery in polyglots with aphasia has been described in terms of language representations or neurocognitive operations. The representational account posits that selective language impairments reflect damage to specialized neural networks for each language that may be housed in the same or different areas of the left or right hemisphere (Vaid, 2008). Neurocognitive accounts suggest that procedural-declarative memory processes or control mechanisms are involved in nonparallel language restitution. Paradis (2004, 2009) advances the notion that language recovery in bilinguals with aphasia appears to depend on the possible interaction between each bilingual speaker's acquisitional context (simultaneous vs. sequential bilingualism) and its concomitant memory strategies. A first language or two simultaneously learned languages since a young age, mostly in informal communication environments, rely on implicit/procedural memory strategies, dependent on subcortical neural regions. Languages successively learned later in life, often in structured instructional contexts, rely on declarative/explicit memory strategies (emphasizing metalinguistic knowledge), housed in cortical areas. Thus, in this perspective, nonparallel recovery may reflect the neurofunctional modularity (separation) of the languages known by the multilingual speaker; the language recovered in a nonparallel pattern would reflect the interplay of acquisitional factors, procedural/declarative memory traces affected, and the extent of subcortical–cortical damage (see also Ullman, 2001). In more cognitive terms, Green (2005) proposes that, rather than neuroanatomical cerebral regions being affected by the stroke, what might be impaired is the temporary or permanent control mechanisms that regulate the activation or deactivation of the linguistic systems or part of those systems in a particular language.

Hence, clinical evidence has provided important information on the heterogeneity and complexity in the recovery patterns in aphasic bilinguals that has served to formulate theoretical accounts on the bilingual brain. Experimental data, based on the assessment of brain activity in bilinguals, have yielded critical complementary data on the inter- and intrahemispheric processing sites and the possible variables impacting on neural language distribution in bilinguals. Though there are numerous techniques to study brain-language relationships (see Bhatnagar, 2008), we discuss the most frequently used tools in the study of cerebral language processing in multilingual individuals, particularly laterality measures and electrophysiological and neuroimaging research.

LATERALITY STUDIES

Hemispheric language processing has been examined using the presentation of auditory (dichotic listening) or visual stimuli (tachitoscopic viewing). These techniques rely on the contralateral (opposite side) sensory organization of the brain. For example, auditory or visual stimuli presented to the left ear or left visual field will be processed in the right hemisphere. By assessing processing differences between stimuli presented contralaterally or ipsilaterally (same side), for example, in terms of stimulus recognition speed, researchers may gauge the extent of specific hemispheric involvement. For monolinguals, a right ear advantage (REA) or right visual field advantage (RFVA) generally are reported for verbal information (i.e., words, syllables, etc.) thus suggesting faster language recognition when linguistic items arrive in the left hemisphere auditorily or visually, respectively (Fabbro, 1999; Vaid, 2008).

Extensive reviews of the laterality evidence revealed no difference between L1 and L2 or between bilinguals and monolinguals for left hemispheric language localization (Goral et al., 2002; Hull & Vaid, 2005; Vaid, 2008). Some studies suggest the possibility of bilateral hemispheric representation in early simultaneous bilinguals, apparently due to semantic (meaning-based) processing compared to syntactic (form-based) processing in late, sequential bilinguals. Yet, some methodological issues, concerning language pairs examined, limited bilingualism history of the participants, linguistic level studied, and so forth, raise interpretive issues about this research (see Hull & Vaid, 2005, for discussion). Findings, however, overwhemingly support the dominant role of the left hemisphere in language representation for both monolingual and bilingual persons and for both languages known by the bilingual speaker, including the possibility of bilateral involvement in early stages of bilingualism (Goral et al., 2002; Vaid, 2008).

Hence, laterality measures have shed light into interhemispheric language organization. For intrahemispheric localization, electrophysiological, and neuroimaging studies have yielded important evidence, as summarized next.

ELECTRO-CORTICAL STIMULATION INVESTIGATIONS

The study of language organization in the bilingual brain was stimulated by the use of electro-cortical stimulation to map out cortical language areas in epileptic patients undergoing surgical removal of epileptogenic brain sites. This technique applies electricity to cortical language sites thus causing temporary aphasia when the electrical current briefly inhibits the stimulated area from functioning. Identification of the cerebral language regions before surgery prevents them from damage during the surgical intervention. Because the brain has no pain receptors, testing language functions under cortical stimulation can be carried out in the conscious patient once the craniotomy has exposed the target brain areas and the patient is fully awake (Fabbro, 1999; Lucas, McKhann, & Ojemann, 2004).

Ojemann and Whitaker (1978) and Rapport, Tan, and Whitaker (1983) conducted the first electro-cortical studies on bilingual and multilingual individuals, respectively. Based on naming tasks, results suggested that naming could be impaired in either language in some cortical sites, could be more impaired in one language than in the other in other areas, or could be simultaneously impaired in both languages in other areas. The regions of language disruption, however, were not the same for all the bilinguals or multilinguals tested. Essential areas for naming in the later-acquired, less-fluent language were more dispersed than those areas in the earlier-acquired, more-fluent language. All of the naming regions detected were within the frontal and temporoparietal cortex (Ojemann, 1991; Ojemann & Whitaker, 1978).

Later cortical mapping studies further highlight the variability in language localization in bilinguals. For example, Roux and Trémoulet (2002) investigated 12 French-speaking bilinguals of various L2 backgrounds on three different tasks (counting, naming, and reading) in each language. These patients were classified in terms of age of acquisition and proficiency as early-acquisition/high-proficiency, late-acquisition/high-proficiency, and late-acquisition/low-proficiency. The age of 7 years was chosen as the cutoff date to identify a patient as early or late L2 learner. Results showed a heterogenous localization pattern with five patients having overlapping language regions (for all language tasks) and the remaining seven patients having at least one area that was language-specific and, sometimes, task-specific. In terms of age of acquisition and proficiency, results similarly differed among participants. The authors found that three out of four early bilinguals exhibited naming difficulty in one language under electrical stimulation, which suggests separate foci. Regarding proficiency level, only one patient demonstrated more cortical sites dedicated to the less-fluent language. Like earlier studies, all language areas were found in the temporoparietal regions and in frontal regions of the brain.

Lucas et al. (2004) set out to examine language representation in 22 bilingual patients by assessing naming. They aimed to answer whether multiple languages are functionally separated within the brain, whether these languages are similarly organized, and whether language organization in bilinguals mirror that in monolinguals. The authors found that the most common pattern of language representation in bilinguals was one of discrete language-specific sites (either for L1 or L2) coexisting with shared (S) sites. However, eight patients had no S sites. The number of essential sites for L1, L2, and S did not differ thus suggesting a similar extent of site distribution. Neither L1 or L2 proficiency scores predicted the number of L1, L2, or S regions. In terms of anatomical distribution, the L2-specific sites were located exclusively in the posterior temporal and parietal regions, whereas the L1-specific sites and S could be found throughout the mapped regions. When comparing language areas in both monolingual and bilingual brains, L1 representation was indistinguishable hence suggesting that L2 acquisition does not alter L1 organization. However, L2 sites were distributed differently from L1 sites in the bilingual brain, clustered around the receptive language areas and in significantly smaller proportions of L2 sites relative to language sites in monolinguals. This finding led the authors to argue that, once cortical regions are dedicated to L1 processing, they may inhibit the establishment of new language sites (for L2) in their vicinity.

The preceding studies advance the descriptive symptomatology reported by clinical cases and laterality studies. Specifically, there seems to be left-hemispheric representational dominance for both languages whose individual distribution may depend on age of acquisition, proficiency, and linguistic task. The evidence generated by electro-cortical research, however, is largely variable and based on the assessment of naming skills. It also is limited by the extent and site of the craniotomy. Stimulation only is applied on the surface of the exposed areas in the left hemisphere, a frequent site of epileptic foci. Therefore, we do not know about the patterns of language organization in the areas deeper in the brain, beyond the craniotomy, or in the nondominant right hemisphere (see Goral, Levy, & Obler, 2002; Vaid, 2008, for discussion).

EVOKED RESPONSE POTENTIAL MEASURES

Evoked response potential (ERP) studies measure the normal electrical activity that takes place in the brain under the effect of specific and controlled sensory stimulation. In this technique, signal averaging is employed to extract stimulus-relevant ERP activity from nonstimulus related background signals. The resulting ERP, representing a summation and average of the activity of multiple neurons, allow researchers to infer the extent and timing of neuronal activation upon a presented task (Bhatnagar, 2008; Hull & Vaid, 2005). This unobtrusive technique only employs electrodes on the participant's scalp thus allowing the examination of real-time (online) brain activity while, for example, the person is engaged in a reading or listening task.

ERP measures of both semantic and syntactic processing support the role of age of L2 acquisition and proficiency in neural language organization in bilinguals. Late and fluent (high-proficiency) bilinguals and monolinguals show similar left hemispheric patterns of language organization whereas early and nonfluent (low-proficiency) bilinguals tend to be less lateralized, demonstrating more bilateral involvement, consistent with the laterality findings reported above. For example, Meuter, Donald, and Ardal (1987) assessed the ERP (N400 effect) responses of French–English bilinguals to semantically congruent and incongruent sentences. A response approximately 400 ms after presentation of an incongruent sentence suggests the participant has recognized the anomaly. Meuter et al. (1987) found larger ERP effects for left parietal areas in late French–English bilinguals reading semantically incongruent sentences, particularly in their L2 (English) hence supporting more L2-related brain activity. Likewise, ERP measures in late bilinguals and monolinguals detecting semantic anomalies (Weber-Fox & Neville, 2001) and late fluent and nonfluent bilinguals processing syntactic violations (Friederici, Steinhauer, & Pfeifer, 2002) further supported that late, fluent L2 learners show lateralization patterns similar to those in monolingual persons (see also Hull & Vaid, 2005). Indeed, exhaustive meta-analysis of laterality, in which fluent bilinguals are subdivided by age of acquisition, robustly reveal that late bilinguals are more left-hemisphere dominant relative to early bilinguals, who show more bilateral hemispheric participation overall (Hull & Vaid, 2005).

The ERP evidence, however, warrants caution in view of the small data sets reported and the need for further research along different lines. Specifically, ERP data would be enhanced by examining multilingual speakers from a larger group of contrasting language pairs (i.e., inflectionally rich [Spanish] vs. inflectionally limited [English], alphabetic [Spanish] vs. ideographic scripts [Chinese], etc.) in a larger variety of semantic and syntactic tasks in the various language modalities (see also Goral et al., 2002; Hull & Vaid, 2005).

NEUROIMAGING RESEARCH

Advances in neuroimaging techniques, particularly positron emission tomography (PET) and functional magnetic resonance imaging (fMRI) have contributed to the study of intrahemispheric language organization in bilingual speakers. These hemodynamic techniques are based on the changes in regional cerebral blood flow (rCBF) resulting from synaptic activity. As neuronal functioning increases, this physiological event results in increased metabolic rate and rCBF. Hence, both PET and fMRI allow us to capture in vivo images of brain functioning as neuronal activation, in response to the online (real-time) execution of a cognitive task, results in changes in local cerebral blood flow, and concomitant metabolic activity.

PET images, collected through the use of radiopharmaceuticals (radioactive labeled molecules, such as water or glucose), show strong signals in radioactive-rich areas as high neuronal activation stimulates high blood flow and increased radiopharmaceutical consumption relative to other less-activated cortical areas.

In contrast, fMRI, which gives better temporal and spatial resolution than PET imaging, is based on metabolic oxygen use. Images captured through fMRI scanning reflect blood oxygen levels in response to the extent of cortical-neuronal activity (Bhatnagar, 2008; Dougherty et al., 2004; Vaid, 2008).

Neuroimaging investigations of the multilingual brain have examined both production (e.g., word repetition and word generation) and comprehension abilities (e.g., grammatical and semantic judgment) as well as language selection and translation in bilingual speakers (see Abutalebi et al., 2005, for exhaustive review). Language imaging research assessing production areas in bilinguals and multilinguals suggest a dominant pattern of left-sided language organization in the multilingual brain similar to that reported for monolinguals, namely, the most brain activation occurs in the left perisylvian area, accompanied by lesser activation in some regions away from the left perisylvian area and in some regions of the right hemisphere (Abutalebi et al., 2005; Vaid, 2008). Yet, the distribution of language foci in the multilingual brain appears to primarily include overlapping language-processing sites, whose distribution may depend on certain variables, such as language proficiency, age of acquisition, and language exposure.

Regarding proficiency, early evidence from PET studies by Klein and colleagues (Klein, Milner, Zatorre, Meyer, & Evans, 1995; Klein, Zatorre, Milner, Meyer, & Evans, 1994) suggested that late, fluent English–French bilinguals engaged very similar areas of the left frontal lobe during word repetition and word generation tasks (e.g., rhyming, synonyms, and translation) in each language. Based on a word generation activity administered to trilinguals, Yetkin, Yetzkin, Haughton, and Cox (1996) provided fMRI results that supported a widespread organization of the foci for the less-fluent language, actively involving the left prefrontal cortex. Hence, high-proficiency may result in a tighter left-sided representational frontal area for lexical foci.

In terms of age of acquisition, Kim, Relkin, Lee, and Hirsch (1997) conducted fMRI scannings of early and late bilingual speakers of different language backgrounds as they silently produced sentences in each language. In Broca's area, patterns of brain activity included common areas of activation, if the languages were learned early, and segregated areas, if L2 was learned late, at a mean age of 11.2 years for the participants. In Wernicke's area, there was minimal or no separation of foci for both early and late bilinguals. However, Chee, Tan, and Thiel (1999b) found considerable left-sided activation involving minimal differences in the fMRI readings of early and late Mandarin–English bilinguals of similar fluency levels in a stem-based word completion task. Likewise, in another study controlling the degree of proficiency, Illes et al. (1999) showed that high-fluency may be associated with common left-hemisphere language foci independent of age of acquisition, as supported by fMRI patterns of early and late fluent English–Spanish bilinguals performing semantic judgment tasks. Substantial activation was observed in the left inferior frontal gyrus in the participants with minimal activation in homologous right-sided sites in a few participants. Thus, proficiency, rather than age, appears to be critical in the distribution of language foci (high-proficiency/common sites) in the dominant left hemisphere, as supported by different bilingual groups (Mandarin–English and English–Spanish) and different tasks (word completion and semantic decision).

Environmental language exposure seems to be an additional variable. Perani et al. (2003) examined fMRI imaging in early, fluent Spanish–Catalan bilinguals who were dominant in either Spanish or Catalan, and who lived in a Catalan environment. Perani and colleagues found that the dominant language (which coincided with the L1 in these bilinguals) engaged fewer cerebral areas in a word generation task. Additionally, for speakers producing words in the language with the least daily exposure, namely, Spanish in the Catalan-dominant bilingual cohort, there was more widespread brain activation (in the left dorsolateral frontal region) when these speakers generated words in Spanish, relative to Spanish-dominant bilinguals generating words in Catalan, the language of the community. Hence, according to these findings, the brain engages fewer neural networks when processing the dominant language or the more frequently used language.

Imaging studies examining cerebral foci for comprehension in bilingual speakers further support the important role of proficiency in language localization. Perani et al. (1996) investigated PET activation in late, low-proficiency Italian–English bilinguals while listening to stories in each language. Results showed minimal overlap for the two languages; L1 (Italian) activation was concentrated in the left perisylvian regions with participation of some homologous right-sided areas and, for the low-proficient language (L2, English), activation was considerably more reduced in both left and right hemispheres, mainly involving the temporal area. In contrast, for both early and late high-proficiency bilinguals of Spanish–Catalan and Italian–English backgrounds, respectively, Perani et al. (1998) found a different PET pattern. Both groups listened to stories in each language. The Italian–English group listened to a story in an additional unknown language (Japanese). Activation showed in similar left temporal regions for both languages in both groups and, only for the late bilinguals, in the unknown language. Activation also included some right areas for both languages in both groups.

Support to the critical role of fluency in language organization comes from studies of bilingual speakers of languages of contrasting orthographies such as English (alphabetic orthography) and Mandarin (ideographic orthography). Chee et al. (1999a) examined fMRI scannings of early, high-fluency English–Mandarin bilinguals in a printed sentence comprehension task to assess sentence meaning. The investigators found a similar brain activation pattern for both languages involving an extensive portion of the left fronto-temporal region and, to a lesser extent, bilateral parieto-occipital areas.

Despite left-sided dominance, the preceding evidence, nonetheless, suggests the possible recruitment of the right hemisphere in language processing in cases of low L2 proficiency. Similarly, based on fMRI readings, Dehaene and colleagues (1997) found that late, low-proficiency French–English bilinguals engaged a considerably larger portion of the left frontal area when listening to stories in L1 (French) relative to a much larger right-sided fronto-temporal participation in their less-fluent L2 (English). Interestingly, Dehaene et al.'s (1997) findings suggested that, while L1 is localized in the left frontal lobe, there was large intersubject variability for the organization of the less-fluent L2, involving both left and right frontal and temporal areas and, in some participants, an exclusive right-sided activation pattern.

In sum, the preceding findings thus suggest that, regardless of acquisition age, high-proficiency may be associated with a main left-sided overlapping of L1 and L2 in the perisylvian region for both aural and written comprehension. Right-sided involvement seems to be related to low L2 proficiency.

Translation and language switching and selection, two typical expressive features of bilingual discourse, have also been examined using neuroimaging tools for their valuable insights into language representation in the bilingual brain (Ansaldo & Marcotte, 2007; Paradis, 2004). For example, Price, Green, and von Studnitz (1999) used PET to explore neural activation during word reading and word translation in late, fluent German–English bilinguals. Results showed contrasting PET patterns for both tasks. For reading, considerable activity was seen in the left Broca's area and bilateral supramarginal gyri. For translation, extensive engagement outside the typical left perisylvian language zone, including bilateral subcortical regions, was observed. The authors claim that activation differences may be related to mapping orthography to phonology (reading) and semantic processing (translation).

Hernández, Dapretto, Mazziotta, and Bookheimer (2001) found active participation of the left dorsolateral prefrontal cortex when examining language switching in early, high-proficiency Spanish–English speakers, based on fMRI readings. Further, Rodriguez-Fornells, Rotte, Heinze, Nösselt, and Münte's (2002) ERP and fMRI data suggested considerable involvement of the left anterior prefrontal region when early, high-proficiency Catalan–Spanish bilinguals had to inhibit either language for target language selection in a lexical access task. Hence, these three studies provide emerging evidence on translation, language switching, and language selection that support the possible participation of different neural areas for contrasting tasks (reading vs. translation) and the dominant role of the left hemisphere across linguistic tasks in both languages.

FUTURE DIRECTIONS

The preceding overview provided a brief snapshot of important research that has attempted to explicate language lateralization and localization in bilingual and multilingual speakers. While the evidence is far from conclusive, findings support the dominant role of the left hemisphere in bilinguals, particularly its perisylvian regions, just like in monolinguals; the possible recruitment of the right hemisphere in early stages of bilingualism and in low L2 proficiency, and the possible impact of proficiency, rather than acquisition age and exposure, on bilingual representation. The clinical and experimental data seem to coincide as the larger number of parallel aphasia cases in bilinguals relative to nonparallel cases is consistent with the reported higher incidence of overlapping L1–L2 sites over separate sites. Evidence on typical expressive features in bilinguals, such as translation and language switching and selection, despite being small, further support the strong role of left foci in language representation in bilinguals.

Evidence is still emerging. Inconsistencies and intersubject variability still persist, as our discussion showed. Similarly, there are methodological concerns. Studies largely do not acknowledge the complexities in bilingual acquisition and discourse and their cognitive consequences, or possible cross-language processing differences. Chief concerns include minimal or no information on the bilingualism history of the participants, focus on naming and the spoken modality for experimental tasks, and a small number of contrasting language pairs.

There is, however, reason for excitement and for further inquiry. Applying neurocognitive accounts of translation and language switching and cognitive stimulation to aphasia therapy with bilinguals shows promise (Ansaldo & Marcotte, 2007; Kohnert, 2008; see also Centeno, 2007b; Paradis, 2004). In fact, because language therapy may positively impact on post-stroke neurological reorganization (e.g., Centeno & Ansaldo, 2010; Cherney & Small, 2006; Gonzalez-Rothi & Barrett, 2006), coupling neurocognitive and psycholinguistic principles of bilingualism to aphasia intervention in multilinguals support further exploration. Our understanding of the bilingual brain and its clinical implications may be enhanced by integrating neuroimaging advances with sound theoretical accounts of bilingualism and bilingual psycholinguistic processing, and using tasks that assess both individual speakers and groups of bilinguals of multiple language pairs in different semantic and syntactic tasks across language modalities.

REFERENCES

Abutalebi, J., Cappa, S. F., & Perani, D. (2005). What can functional neuroimaging tell us about the bilingual brain. In J. F. Kroll & A. M. B. de Groot (Eds.), *Handbook of bilingualism: Psycholinguistic approaches* (pp. 497–515). New York, NY: Oxford University Press.

Albert, M., & Obler, L. K. (1978). *The bilingual brain.* New York, NY: Academic Press.

Ansaldo, A. I., & Marcotte, K. (2007). Language switching in the context of Spanish-English bilingual aphasia. In J. G. Centeno, R. T. Anderson, & L. K. Obler (Eds.), *Communication disorders in Spanish speakers: Theoretical, research, and clinical aspects* (pp. 214–230). Clevedon, UK: Multilingual Matters.

Bhatnagar, S. C. (2008). *Neuroscience for the study of communicative disorders* (3rd ed.). Philadelphia, PA: Lippincott Williams and Wilkins.

Bialystok, E. (2001). *Bilingualism in development: Language, literacy, and cognition.* Cambridge, UK: Cambridge University Press.

Caplan, D. (1987). *Neurolinguistics and linguistic aphasiology.* Cambridge, UK: Cambridge University Press.

Centeno, J. G. (2007a). Bilingual development and communication: Implications for clinical language studies. In J. G. Centeno, R. T. Anderson, & L. K. Obler (Eds.), *Communication disorders in Spanish speakers: Theoretical, research, and clinical aspects* (pp. 46–56). Clevedon, UK: Multilingual Matters.

Centeno, J. G. (2007b). Considerations for an ethnopsycholinguistic framework for aphasia intervention. In A. Ardila & E. Ramos (Eds.), *Speech and language disorders in bilingual adults* (pp. 195–212). New York, NY: Nova Science.

Centeno, J. G., & Ansaldo, A. I. (2010). Neurobiological treatment of bilinguals with aphasia. Manuscript in preparation.

Centeno, J. G., & Obler, L. K. (2001). Principles of bilingualism. In M. Pontón & J. L. Carrión (Eds.), *Neuropsychology and the Hispanic patient: A clinical handbook* (pp.75–86). Mahwah, NJ: Lawrence Erlbaum.

Chee, M., Caplan, D., Soon, C. S., Sriram, N., Tan, E. W., Thiel, T., & Weekes, B. (1999a). Processing of visually presented sentences in Mandarin and English studied with fMRI. *Neuron, 23*, 127–137.

Chee, M. W., Tan, E. W., & Thiel, T. (1999b). Mandarin and English single word processing studied with functional magnetic resonance imaging. *Journal of Neuroscience, 19*, 3050–3056.

Cherney, L. R., & Small, S. L. (2006). Task-dependent changes in brain activation following therapy for nonfluent aphasia: Discussion of two individual cases. *Journal of the International Neuropsychological Society, 12*, 828–842.

Dehaene, S., Dupoux, E., Mehler, J., Cohen, L., Paulesu, E., Perani, D., . . . Le Bihan, D. (1997). Anatomical variability in the cortical representation of first and second languages. *Neuroreport, 8*, 3809–3815.

Dougherty, D. D., Rauch, S. L., & Rosenbaum, J. F. (Eds.). (2004). *Essentials of neuroimaging for clinical practice*. Washington, DC: American Psychiatric Publishing.

Fabbro, F. (1999). *The neurolinguistics of bilingualism: An introduction*. East Sussex, UK: Psychology Press.

Friederici, A., Steinhauer, K., & Pfeifer, E. (2002). Brain signatures of artificial language processing: Evidence challenging the critical period hypothesis. *Proceedings of the National Academy of Sciences, 99*, 529–534.

Gonzalez-Rothi, L., & Barrett, A. M. (2006). The changing view of neurorehabilitation: A new era of optimism. *Journal of the International Neuropsychological Society, 12*, 812–815.

Goral, M., Levy, E., & Obler, L. K. (2002). Neurolinguistic aspects of bilingualism. *International Journal of Bilingualism, 6*, 411–440.

Green, D. (2005). The neurocognition of recovery patterns in bilingual aphasics. In J. F. Kroll & A. M. B. de Groot (Eds.), *Handbook of bilingualism: Psycholinguistic approaches* (pp. 516–530). New York, NY: Oxford University Press.

Grosjean, F. (2004). Studying bilinguals: Methodological and conceptual issues. In T. K. Bhatia & W. C. Ritchie (Eds.), *The handbook of bilingualism* (pp. 32–63). Malden, MA: Blackwell.

Hernández, A., Dapretto, M., Mazziotta, J., & Bookheimer, S. (2001). Language switching and language representation in Spanish-English bilinguals: An fMRI study. *Neuroimage, 14*, 510–520.

Hull, R., & Vaid, J. (2005). Clearing the cobwebs from the study of the bilingual brain: Converging evidence from laterality and electrophysiological research. In J. F. Kroll & A. M. B. de Groot (Eds.), *Handbook of bilingualism: Psycholinguistic approaches* (pp. 480–496). New York, NY: Oxford University Press.

Ijalba, E., Obler, L. K., & Chengappa, S. (2004). Bilingual aphasia. In T. K. Bhatia & W. C. Ritchie (Eds.), *The handbook of bilingualism* (pp. 32–63). Malden, MA: Blackwell.

Illes, J., Francis, W., Desmond, J., Gabrieli, J., Glover, G., Poldrack, R., . . . Wagner, A. D. (1999). Convergent cortical representation of semantic processing in bilinguals. *Brain and Language, 70*, 347–363.

Johnson, J. S., & Newport, E. L. (1989). Critical periods effects in second language learning: The influence of maturational state on the acquisition of English as a second language. *Cognitive Psychology, 21*, 60–99.

Kim, K. H. S., Relkin, N. R., Lee, K. M., & Hirsch, J. (1997). Distinct cortical areas associated with native and second languages. *Nature, 388,* 171–174.

Klein, D., Milner, B., Zatorre, R., Meyer, E., & Evans, A. (1995). The neural substrates underlying word generation: A bilingual functional-imaging study. *Proceedings of the National Academy of Sciences USA, 92,* 2899–2903.

Klein, D., Zatorre, R., Milner, B., Meyer, E., & Evans, A. (1994). Left putaminal activation when speaking a second language: Evidence from PET. *Neuroreport, 5,* 2295–2297.

Kohnert, K. (2008). *Language disorders in bilingual children and adults.* San Diego, CA: Plural.

Lucas, T. H., McKhann, G. M., & Ojemann, G. A. (2004). Functional separation of languages in the bilingual brain: A comparison of electrical stimulation language mapping in 25 bilingual patients and 117 monolingual control patients. *Journal of Neurosurgery, 101,* 449–457.

Marian, V. (2008). Bilingual research methods. In J. Altarriba & R. R. Heredia (Eds.), *An introduction to bilingualism: Principles and processes* (pp. 13–38). New York, NY: Lawrence Erlbaum.

Meuter, R., Donald, M., & Ardal, S. (1987). A comparison of first- and second-language ERPs in bilinguals. *Current Trends in Event-Related Potential Research, Supplement 40,* 412–416.

Ojemann, G. A. (1991). Cortical organization of language. *Journal of Neuroscience, 11,* 2281–2287.

Ojemann, G. A., & Whitaker, H. (1978). The bilingual brain. *Archives of Neurology, 35,* 409–412.

Paradis, M. (2004). *A neurolinguistic theory of bilingualism.* Amsterdam, The Netherlands: John Benjamins.

Paradis, M. (2009). *Declarative and procedural determinants of second languages.* Philadelphia, PA: John Benjamins.

Patestas, M. A., & Gartner, L. P. (2006). *A textbook of neuroanatomy.* Malden, MA: Blackwell.

Perani, D., Abutalebi, J., Paulesu, E., Brambati, S., Scifo, P., Cappa, S. F., & Fazio, F. (2003). The role of age of acquisition and language usage in early, high-proficient bilinguals: An fMRI study during verbal fluency. *Human Brain Mapping, 19,* 179–182.

Perani, D., Dehaene, S., Grassi, F., Cohen, L., Cappa, S. F., Dupoux, E., . . . Mehler, J. (1996). Brain processing of native and foreign languages. *Neuroreport, 7,* 2439–2444.

Perani, D., Paulesu, E., Sebastian Galles, N., Dupoux, E., Dehaene, S., Bettinerdi, . . . Mehler, J. (1998). The bilingual brain: Proficiency and age of acquisition of the second language. *Brain, 121,* 1841–1852.

Price, C. J., Green, D. W., & von Studnitz, R. (1999). A functional imaging study of translation and language switching. *Brain, 122,* 2221–2235.

Rapport, R. L., Tan, C. T., & Whitaker, H. (1983). Language function and dysfunction among Chinese- and English-speaking polyglots: Cortical stimulation, Wada testing, and clinical studies. *Brain and Language, 18,* 342–366.

Rodriguez-Fornells, A., Rotte, M., Heinze, H. J., Nösselt, T., & Münte, T. F. (2002). Brain potential and functional MRI evidence for how to handle two languages with one brain. *Nature, 415,* 1026–1029.

Roux, F. E., & Trémoulet, M. (2002). Organization of language areas in bilingual patients: A cortical stimulation study. *Journal of Neurosurgery, 97,* 857–864.

Seliger, H. (1978). Implications of a multiple critical period hypothesis for second language learning. In W. C. Ritchie (Ed.), *Second language acquisition research: Issues and implications* (pp. 11–19). San Diego, CA: Academic Press.

Ullman, M. T. (2001). The neural basis of lexicon and grammar in first and second language: The declarative/procedural model. *Bilingualism: Language and Cognition, 4*, 105–122.

Vaid, J. (2008). The bilingual brain: What is right and what is left? In J. Altarriba & R. R. Heredia (Eds.), *An introduction to bilingualism: Principles and processes* (pp. 129– 146). New York, NY: Lawrence Erlbaum.

Weber-Fox, C., & Neville, H. J. (2001). Sensitive periods differentiate processing of open- and closed-class words: An ERP study of bilinguals. *Journal of Speech, Language, and Hearing Research, 44*, 1338–1353.

Yavaş, M. (1996). Differences in voice onset time in early and late Spanish-English bilinguals. In J. Jensen & A. Roca (Eds.), *Spanish in contact: Issues in bilingualism* (pp. 131–141). Sommerville, MA: Cascadilla Press.

Yetkin, O., Yetzkin, F. Z., Haughton, V., & Cox, R. W. (1996). Use of functional MR to map language in multilingual volunteers. *American Journal of Neuroradiology, 17*, 473–477.

Section IV

Language and Other Modalities

32 Gestures and Growth Points in Language Disorders

David McNeill and Susan Duncan

INTRODUCTION

Gestures shed light on thinking-for-(and while)-speaking. They do this because they are components of speaking, not accompaniments but actually integral parts of it. Much evidence supports this idea, but its full implications have not always been recognized. Consider modular-style modeling of the relationship between gesture and speech, for example, De Ruiter (2000) and Kita and Özyürek (2003), based on the theory of speech production in Levelt (1989). Modular theory and its spin-offs are incompatible, we have argued, with the facts of integration of gesture into speaking (McNeill, 2000; McNeill & Duncan, 2000). Such models require a fundamental separation of speech and gesture; the "modules" exchange signals but cannot combine into a unit. The growth point (GP) hypothesis, which we describe here, is designed in contrast to explicate the integral linkage of gesture and speech in natural language production. In a GP, speaking and gesture are never separated, and do not occupy different brain processes that must in turn then be linked (cf. the brain model, below). A key insight is that speech on the one hand and gesture (or, more broadly speaking, global-imagistic thinking), on the other, jointly forming a GP, bring together semiotically opposite modes of cognition at the same moment. This opposition, and the processes that speakers undergo to resolve it, propels thought and speech forward. Semiotic contrasts are a key component in the dynamic dimension of language. It is in this mechanism that we seek insights into language disorders. We explore four situations—disfluent (agrammatic) aphasia, Down syndrome (DS), Williams syndrome (WS), and autism. Each can be seen to stem from a breakdown, interruption, or inaccessibility of a different part of the GP, and from a disturbance of the dynamic dimension of language in general. Considered together, they manifest—by interruption—aspects of the processes of thinking-for/while-speaking itself. In this chapter we do not attempt to review the field of gesture studies, the psycholinguistics of speech production, or language disorders, but we do provide a brief exposition of the GP hypothesis and spell out some implications of a new paradigm in which language and cognition are embodied (cf. Johnson, 1987) and dynamic, and show how a theory within this paradigm, the GP theory, leads to new insights into four language disorders.

THE GROWTH POINT

The GP is so named because it is a distillation of a growth process—an ontogenetic-like process but vastly sped up and made functional in online thinking-for-speaking. While we are not addressing language acquisition as such we regard it as a general model of cognitive change valid across many time scales. According to this framework, the GP is the initial unit of thinking-for/while-speaking (from Slobin, 1987, elaborated to include thinking online, during speech) out of which a dynamic process of utterance-level and discourse-level organization emerges. Imagery and spoken form are mutually influencing. It is not that imagery is the input to spoken form or spoken form is the input to imagery. The GP is fundamentally both. The following exposition of the GP covers essential points for the purpose of elucidating language abnormalities. More thorough presentations are in McNeill (2005, 2002), McNeill and Duncan (2000), and, with a language origins slant, in McNeill, Duncan, Cole, Gallagher, and Bertenthal (2008).

A MINIMAL UNIT OF IMAGERY-LANGUAGE DIALECTIC

The GP is an irreducible, "minimal unit"* of imagery-language code combination. It is the smallest packet of an idea unit encompassing the unlike semiotic modes of imagery and linguistic encoding. A GP is empirically recoverable, inferred from speech-gesture synchrony and co-expressiveness.[†] Even when the information (the "semantic content") in speech and gesture is similar, it is formed according to contrasting semiotic modes. Simultaneous unlike modes create instability. Instability fuels thinking-for-speaking as it seeks resolution (McNeill & Duncan, 2000).[‡] The result is an idea unit in which holistic imagery and discrete code are combined, and this drives thinking-for/while-speaking.

EXAMPLE

The temporal and semantic synchronies represented in Figure 32.1 imply a GP built on the idea of rising interiority. We infer the simultaneous presence of the

---

* The concept of a "minimal unit" with the property of being a whole is from Vygotsky (1987, pp. 4–5), concisely stated in this passage: "By a unit we mean a product of analysis which, in distinction from elements, possesses all the basic properties of a whole. Further, these properties must be a living portion of the unified whole which cannot be broken down further. ..." (Vygotsky, *Thinking and Speech* [Russian, 1934], p. 9, quoted in Zinchenko, 1985, p. 97).

† A growth point is inferred (not "operationally defined") from: (a) gesture form; (b) coincident linguistic segment(s); (c) co-expression of the same idea unit; and (d) what Vygotsky (1987, p. 243) termed a "psychological predicate" in the immediate context of speaking.

‡ The reasons why semiotic opposition creates instability and initiates change include:
  a *conflict* (between semiotic modes: analog imagery/analytic categorical); and
  b *resolution* (through change: fueling thinking-for-speaking, seeking stability).
  Simultaneous semiotic modes comprise an inherently dynamic psycholinguistic model.

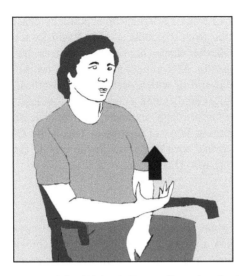

FIGURE 32.1   Gesture embodying "rising hollowness" synchronized with "up thróugh."

idea of ascent inside the pipe in two unlike semiotic modes.* The speaker was describing a cartoon episode in which one character (a cat named Sylvester) tries to reach another character (a bird named Tweety) by climbing up inside a drainpipe. The speaker is saying, "and he tries going **up thróugh** it this time," with the gesture occurring during the boldfaced portion (the illustration captures the moment when the speaker says the vowel of "thróugh"). Co-expressively with "up" her hand rose upward and co-expressively with "thróugh" her fingers spread outward to create an interior space. These took place together, and were synchronized with the entirety of "up thróugh," the linguistic package that carries the same meanings.

The GP pairs linguistic segments with a uniquely gestural way of packaging meaning—something like "rising hollowness," which does not exist as a semantic package of English at all. Speech and gesture, at the moment of their synchronization, were co-expressive, yet embodied this shared idea in contrasting semiotic modes. The very fact that there is a shared reference to the character's climbing up inside the pipe makes clear that it is being represented by the speaker simultaneously in two ways—analytic/combinatoric in speech and global/synthetic in gesture.

AND CONTEXT

An important point is that we can fully understand what motivates any gesture-speech combination only with reference to how a GP relates to its context of

---

* Computer art from video by Fey Parrill, now at the Department of Cognitive Science, Case-Western University. All figures, except Figure 32.4, are from McNeill (2005). Used with permission.

occurrence. The GP-to-context relationship is mutually constitutive. The GP is a point of differentiation from the context, what Vygotsky termed a "psychological predicate." The speaker shapes her representation of the context, or "field of oppositions," to make this differentiation possible. A robust phenomenon is that the gesture form and its timing with speech embody just those features that differentiate the psychological predicate in a context that is at least partly the speaker's own creation. In the "up through" example, interiority is newsworthy in a field of oppositions concerning Ways of Getting at Tweety By Climbing Up A Pipe; a previous description had been that it was on the outside, now it is on the inside (see McNeill 2005, pp. 108–112).

THE CATCHMENT

The effective contextual background can often be discovered by finding the catchment(s) of which a target gesture is a part. Catchments are when space, trajectory, hand shapes, and so on, recur in two or more (not necessarily consecutive) gestures. The recurring imagery embodies the discourse theme (the metaphor relates to the geophysical domain, referring to the land area—"the theme"—that drains—"the significant oppositions"—into a body of water—"the GP"). For both climbing up the outside and climbing up the inside of the pipe the same space and trajectory occurred (iconically depicting Sylvester's entrance at the bottom of the pipe)—verbally, too, the full expression, "he goes up thróugh it this time," indexes the catchment theme in that the inside ascent was a recurrent attempt. Newsworthy content appears as a modification of the catchment, relating itself to the theme while also adding new contrast. For the inside ascent the speaker's hand rose at the lower periphery, as before, but now also created the open space seen in Figure 32.1—not only a shape change but also, to the up-the-pipe theme, adding the newsworthy content that it was on the inside this time. Jointly with co-expressive "thróugh," prosodic emphasis also highlighting interiority, the gesture was part of a fresh psychological predicate in this context.

Catchments, if they are present or absent and if present how they are formed, and what restrictions if any they impose on potential discourse themes (cf. Furuyama and Sekine, 2007), are important variables that we can conceptualize systematically by applying the GP theory to the three language disorders. We are unaware of other approaches that frame these questions.

UNPACKING THE GROWTH PIONT (GP)

Unpacking is the process that creates the structures with which to stabilize the combination of unlike cognitive modes in the GP. It is "unpacking" the GP into a grammatical construction (or viable approximation thereto) that preserves the core significance of the GP while cradling it in a stable grammatical format. Achieving this often takes additional meaning formulation. The process is regulated by the speaker's linguistic intuitions—called intuitions-1 (a sense of

well-formedness and contextual appropriateness of the linked semantic frame).*
The construction also supplies a "stop-order" for the impulse to change initiated by the imagery-linguistic code instability. In Figure 32.1, "up thróugh" is
analytic: up-ness and interiority are separated and combined grammatically.
The linguistic encoding has meaning because it combines meaningful parts.
The synchronous gestural image embodies similar information without combining separately meaningful parts—"Sylvester as rising hollowness"; the gesture's parts are meaningful only because of the gesture as a whole. Unpacking
resolves the tension of the semiotic modes. The full construction, "(he) goes up
thróugh it this time," its co-expressive elements exactly synchronizing with the
gesture stroke, preserves the GP, does not dim the highlighted interiority, and
adds indexing of the catchment value—that it was a second ascent—which was
also in the gesture.†

At times, of course, unpacking fails. A construction may not be found; or one
is found but its semantic pattern conflicts with the GP on some dimension; or
the conflict is with the field of oppositions, the context of the GP. It is important
to keep these possibilities in mind, for they appear in different language disorders. To illustrate one case, not a chronic disorder but a momentary interruption
of normally fluent speech, we offer an example from a paper with Nancy Dray
(Dray & McNeill, 1990)—the "nurturing" example: a speaker (having a conversation with a friend) was attempting to convey a delicately nuanced idea that a
third person she was describing was given to performing nurturing acts, but these
good deeds were also intrusive, cloying, and unwelcome. Initial false starts were
based on the use of "nurture" as a transitive verb (she would "nurture" someone)
and were repeatedly rejected as inappropriate. Ultimately the right construction
was found. The field of oppositions was initially something like, Things This
Woman Would Do, and "nurture" was an appropriate significant opposition. The
direct object construction the speaker first attempted ("she's . . . she's nu-uh")
means that, roughly, the woman described has a direct transformative impact via
nurturing on the recipient of her action. However, this meaning distorted the idea
the speaker intended to convey—an oblique reference that separated effect from
act. A slight updating of the field of oppositions to something like *Otiose Things
This Woman Would Do* yielded the final construction, which could differentiate it
appropriately with a meaning of doing something without implying transformative efficacy ("she's done this nurturing thing"). This example illustrates a subtle
but far from uncommon occurrence of GP differentiation, context shaping, and
unpacking going awry.

---

* To be distinguished from "intuitions-2" with which a linguist tests possible analyses, often evoked
  with purpose-constructed forms designed to violate some rule under test.
† When gesture and speech synchronize, the two modes are in direct contact. If there is less than
  perfect synchrony, the GP can still urge unpacking. The ultimate criterion is whether an idea is
  embodied in two forms (with or without different aspects of the idea) and this creates instability.
  However, incomplete synchrony can also open the process to error, as we see next.

FURTHER COMMENTS[*]

Some additional comments to fill out the GP picture:

- First, the following question may come to mind: If gesture is "part of language," how could it and language be "semiotically unalike"? We admit a certain polysemy in the word "language." When we say gesture is part of language, we mean language in the sense of Saussure's *langage*. When we say that gesture contrasts to language we mean it in the sense of *langue*. We are analyzing *parole*/speaking but we believe in a way broader than this concept is usually understood (Saussure himself, in his recently discovered notes, seems to have had the aim of combining *parole* and *langue*—here we rely on Roy Harris's 2003, interpretation).
- By "gesture" most centrally we mean a kind of semiosis that is both "global" and "synthetic."[†] By "global" we mean that the significance of the gesture's parts (= the hands/fingers/trajectory/space/orientation/ movement details of it) is dependent upon the meaning of the gesture as a whole. The parts do not have their own separate meanings, and the meaning of the whole is not composed out of the parts; rather, meaning moves downward, whole to parts. This is the reverse of the linguistic semiotic mode, where the meaning of the whole is composed of the parts, which, for this to work, must have their own separate meanings. By "synthetic" we mean that the gesture has a meaning as a whole that may be analytically separated into different linguistic segments in the speech counterpart.
- Another contrast is that gestures (and imagery more broadly) lack so-called duality of patterning. The form of the gesture-signifier is a nonarbitrary product of the signified content (including, via metaphor, abstract "nonimagistic" meanings), so its form doesn't need or get its own level of structure (= "patterning" in the Hockett, 1960 phraseology). Speech again contrasts: it has this duality of patterning—meaning and sound are each structured by schemes at their own levels, and are paired arbitrarily.
- This has to do with the role of convention and where it intrudes. There are conventions of good-form for speech, but none for gesture (apart from the well-known emblem vocabularies in every culture; also general kinesic conventions for how much space you can use, whether you can enter the space of an interlocutor with a gesture, and the many kinds of metaphor that constrain forms in their gesture versions. These however are not specific gesture conventions in parallel with the sound-system conventions of speech).

---

[*] Originally written as replies to questions raised by Liesbet Quaeghebeur in an exchange of emails. We thank her for a most engaging back and forth.

[†] "Gesture" in this sense is realized in the manual, bodily, and vocal (prosody) modalities.

- Even constructions, like "up through it," while they are macro-units, don't negate the possibility of decomposing them into separately meaningful subunits (up, through, it). Also, the meaning of "up through it," as a construction, is still something traceable to lexical atoms. The gesture, on the other hand, does not admit any decomposition, since there are no subunits with independent meanings, no repeatable significances to the outspread fingers, upward palm and motion upward (arguably, there is upward motion and it independently means upward, but there are exceptions to this seeming transparency as well, gestures where up-down signifies the vertical dimension as a whole, and up actually means down in some cases). Significance exists only in the whole gesture. Also, we think the gesture is more a unified whole than just the combination of up and through. We have tried to convey the unification with the expression "rising hollowness" but whatever the phrase, the gesture has interiority, entity, and upward motion in one undecomposable symbolic form.
- In a GP, then, two semiotic modes, contrasting in the ways listed above, combine to embody the same underlying idea. The instability of having one idea in two "unlike" modes fuels thought and is the dynamic dimension of language viewed psycholinguistically.
- In the verbal modality, as in the manual modality, the meaning of the first part ("up" or the spread fingers) remains, as Liesbet Quaeghebeur (personal communication, 2008) wrote, "alive," "present," or "active" while the second part is being produced ("thróugh" or the upward movement). There is this kind of continuation in both cases, but the explanation differs—a construction in the verbal case; a global image in the gesture case. The continuities differ as well—sequential in the linguistic form, simultaneous in the gesture. Between the two means of attaining continuation the difference comes down to whether symbolic actions are organized by syntactic patterns or by imagery.

FOUR LANGUAGE DISORDERS

We now make use of the GP hypothesis to elucidate aspects of four forms of language disorder. The four are disfluent (agrammatic) aphasia, DS, WS, and autism. To develop our analyses, we begin by proposing the necessary aspects of a brain model.

A Brain Model

Based on what we currently understand of gesture-speech semiosis a neurogesture system involves both the right and left sides of the brain in a choreographed operation with the following parts (see McNeill, 2005, for supporting references). The left posterior temporal speech region of Wernicke's area supplies categorial content, not only for comprehension but for the creative production of verbal thought. This content becomes available to the right hemisphere, which seems particularly adept at creating imagery and to capture discourse content. The right hemisphere must also play a role in the creation of GPs. This is plausible since GPs depend on the differentiation of newsworthy content from context and require the simultaneous presence of linguistic categorial content and imagery, both of which seem to be activated in the right hemisphere. The frontal cortex may also play a role in constructing fields of oppositions and psychological predicates, and supply these contrasts to the right hemisphere, there to be embodied in GPs. Underlying the rhythmicity of speech "pulses" (cf. Duncan, 2006) and interactional entrainment (cf. Gill, 2007) we assume a continuous circulation of cerebellum inputs or feedback. Finally, the right hemisphere and the prefrontal cortex are almost certainly involved in metaphor. The results of processing (right hemisphere, left posterior hemisphere, frontal cortex, cerebellum) converge on the left anterior hemisphere, specifically Broca's area, and the circuits specialized there for action orchestration (cf. McNeill et al., 2008, for a brain mechanism, "Mead's Loop," to account for how GP units orchestrate/synchronize movements of the articulators, manual and vocal). Broca's area may also be the location of two other aspects of the imagery-language dialectic—the generation of further meanings in constructions and their semantic frames, and intuitions of formal completeness to provide "stop orders" to this dialectic. All of these—left, right, cerebellar, frontal—thus may be called language areas of the brain.

The language centers of the brain have classically been regarded as just two, Wernicke's and Broca's areas, but if we are on the right track in our sketch of a brain model, contextual background information must be present to activate the broader spectrum of brain regions that the model describes. Typical item-recognition and production tests, inspired by modular-type conceptions in which language is regarded as encapsulated, would not tap these other brain regions but discourse, conversation, play, work, and the exigencies of language in daily life would.

DISFLUENT (AGRAMMATIC) APHASIA

The "verb problem" in Broca's aphasia is the tendency to omit or nominalize verbs in utterances (Miceli, Silveri, Villa, & Caramazza, 1984; Zingester & Berndt, 1990). On the assumption that verbs are the core syntactic constituents of utterances, this symptom has been studied and interpreted by some as evidence in support of a neurologically grounded grammar "module." However, depending upon discourse context, verb salience varies within-language and across languages, depending on facts about verb behavior in each language. Conceptualized in the GP framework, Broca's aphasia arises from a more or less severe disruption of the unpacking cycle, but the GP itself (formed, we hypothesize, by the uninjured right hemisphere with inputs from the prefrontal cortex and the posterior left hemisphere language area) is unimpaired. A Broca's aphasic speaker differentiates psychological predicates in reasonably constituted fields of oppositions, but is unable to unpack the GP. The following excerpt (Duncan & Pedelty, 2007, p. 271) is a person with Broca aphasia's description of Sylvester trying to reach Tweety by climbing the drainpipe and the sequel in which Tweety drops a bowling ball into it. There are only two identifiable verbs, "is" and "shows." In contrast, six noun tokens were uttered generally clearly and forcefully (Table 32.1).

The speaker performed two well-synchronized, co-expressive gestures. With speech they constituted a likely (repeated) psychological predicate:

[a- and **down**] [(pause) **t- d- down** (breath)]

(Boldface font indicates a gesture "stroke." This is the meaningful phase of a gesture. Brackets indicate the larger gesture phrase. This is the period including preparation before and retraction after the stroke). The strokes in this instance were downward thrusts of the right hand synchronized closely with the two occurrences of the co-expressive path particle, "down," the second stammered. Figure 32.2 illustrates these downward strokes.

In the context of the cartoon story that we, as observers, independently recognize, plus her own fragments of speech in advance of the two instantiations of the gesture, we can identify the gesture plus the synchronous particle, "down," as the single piece of newsworthy information in the excerpt. The speech–gesture pairings thus suggest an intact GP (repeated). Equally important, no verbs occur at all as the linguistic components of the GPs and the verbs that did occur were utterly nonnewsworthy; one a copula coupling nothing, the other "shows" showing nothing.

TABLE 32.1
Agrammatic Aphasic's Description of a Cartoon Event

(1) the (pause) vlk- (pause) uh (breath) bird? (pause) and c- (breath) cat

(2) (pause) and uh (breath) ss- uh (pause) she ss- (breath) (pause) apartment

(3) and uh- (pause) the (pause) uh (pause) old (pause) my (breath) ss- uh (pause) woman (pause)

(4) and uh (pause) she ss- (pause) like (pause) uh ae- f- f-fas-t (breath)

(5) cat (pause) and uh (pause) bird is-ss-ss (pause) (breath)

(6) I uh (pause)

(7) (breath) sh-sho- shows t- (pause)

(8) a- an' down (pause) t- d- down (breath)

Transcription from Duncan & Pedelty (2007: 271).

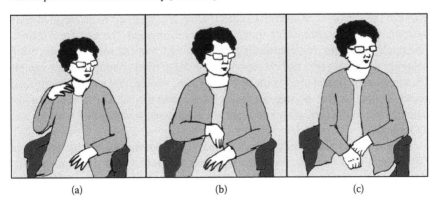

FIGURE 32.2   Gesture by a disfluent (agrammatic) speaker timed with (a) and (b) "an' down," and (c) "t- d- down."

This lack of participation by verbs may be no accident. Duncan and Pedelty propose that in English and some other languages (they refer to Chinese as well), "sentential main verbs are often not the information-loaded, discourse-focal utterance constituents that our usual ways of thinking about them would suggest" (Duncan & Pedelty, 2007, p. 280). The omission or nominalization of verbs in Broca's aphasic speech (whatever the role of their internal semantic complexity in causing an absence from picture-naming and other nondiscourse tasks) is also a predictable result of how GPs embody newsworthy content in the context of speaking. Verb absence would accordingly be, at best, ambiguous evidence for support of modular brain models of language.

Verb absence in Broca's discourse (as opposed to naming) can be explained by a lack of ready access to constructions. In normal speech, noninformation-laden verbs enter utterances riding on these kinds of structures. Nonetheless, agrammatic speakers can formulate and differentiate contexts to obtain GPs. Thus our first illustration of language abnormality demonstrates a separation of GP formation and unpacking, normally two seamlessly fused (while analytically distinct) steps of utterance formation.

The lack of construction-access in Broca's aphasia, nonetheless, is far from absolute. With time and catchment support constructions can be accessed by even highly agrammatic aphasic speakers. A case described in McNeill (2005, p. 217) demonstrates the phenomenon: a patient began his description with single nouns but after more than 2 minutes of gradual expansion, accompanied by appropriate spatial gesture mappings, came out eventually with a two-clause, embedded sentence including appropriate verbs—slow speech indeed but far from "agrammatic." Figure 32.3 depicts the stages in this gradual unpacking.

The speaker begins by referring to a trolley as the "el," which is the local way of referring to Chicago's elevated train system. The important feature of the example is his repeated indicating of the upper gesture space—first raising his left arm at the elbow, and then lifting his arm overhead. This recurrent indexing is a source of gestural cohesion. Verbally, speech was initially limited to just "el" (with and without an article). Then it expanded to "on the tracks" (which, like the trolley wires in the cartoon episode he was describing, are overhead in an elevated train system). A full sentence with a single clause then emerged ("he saw the el train"), and finally, dramatically, considering the depth of his initial agrammatism, a full sentence with two verbs and clauses ("he saw the el train comin' "). The example illustrates a catchment (the overhead wires/tracks, no apparent metaphoricity) and under its spell a step-by-step accessing of a construction. The duration of the catchment and the time it took to reach the final construction was 2 minutes and 17 seconds.

In terms of our brain model, Broca's aphasia, true to its name, is a breakdown of GP unpacking in Broca's area. The area normally orchestrates vocal and manual actions with significances other than those of the actions themselves. Consistent with such a breakdown, recent reports state that Broca's aphasics have difficulty recognizing other people's actions (Fadiga, 2007). This can be regarded as the perceptual equivalent of impaired orchestrating capabilities. On the other hand,

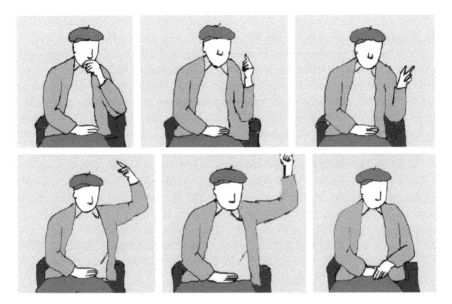

FIGURE 32.3 Catchment from a disfluent (agrammatic) speaker made of repeated gestures in upper space.

processes said in the model to be carried out elsewhere in the brain, the posterior left hemisphere, the right hemisphere, and the prefrontal cortex—imagery, the combination of imagery with linguistically encoded categories, and the relating of all this to tailor-made fields of oppositions, as well as prosodic emphasis on the linguistic realization (cf. Goodglass, 1993)—appear intact, evidenced in the continuing ability by agrammatic speakers to synchronize co-expressive speech and gesture, and to differentiate contextually newsworthy information with them.

DOWN SYNDROME

Down syndrome is characterized by a linguistic disability beyond what an also-present cognitive disability would predict. The DS children lag in language but are relatively spared in visuospatial and visuomotor abilities (Stefanini, Caselli, & Volterra, 2007). It is not surprising therefore that DS children show a "gesture advantage" (also called gesture enhancement)—a preference for and receptivity to gesture over vocal speech, a phenomenon first noted by Abrahamsen, Cavallo, and McCluer (1985) with taught signs and words. A gesture advantage has also been observed with spontaneous gestures during naming tests in recent studies at the Institute of Cognitive Science and Technology (ISTC), in Rome, part of the CNR. However, in this situation, unlike Abrahamsen et al.'s (1985) findings with signs, DS children do not show gesture enhancement at the one-word stage; enhancement emerges only after the children reach the two-word threshold. DS, the ISTC finds, display a significantly smaller repertoire of representational gestures but produce them with a frequency equaling that of typically developing

(TD) children (Stefanini et al., 2007). In picture naming, DS gestures are semantically related to meaning in the picture, and so can convey information even if there is nothing corresponding to them in speech. These "unimodal" messages suggest a mode of information processing fundamentally unlike that of the typical GP. Ultimately, according to Abrahamsen et al. (1985), the gesture advantage weakens and disappears with the emergence of syntax. So it is a transient phenomenon of development, emerging earlier with taught signs than with spontaneous gestures, and eventually disappearing or reducing in size with the establishment of some kind of syntax.

Typically developing children also show a gesture advantage at early ages, but with two crucial differences: unlike DS, the gestures of TD combine with words to encode semantic relations, whereas for DS the word-gesture combinations tend to be redundant. Secondly, the gesture advantage with TD occurs *before* the two-word threshold, and in fact, reliably predicts when and with what semantic relations this threshold will be crossed (Butcher & Goldin-Meadow, 2000; Goldin-Meadow & Butcher, 2003). These differences, when examined, shed light on the nature of the DS linguistic deficit itself.

What is impressive about DS, revealed by work at the Rome Institute, is that DS gestures are often "unimodal," as noted, and, further, when they occur with speech they are mostly *semantically redundant* with the accompanying speech. What does this imply for GPs? The chart in Figure 32.4, from Iverson, Longobardi, and Caselli (2003), shows that the predominant gesture-speech combination in DS (white bars) is "equivalent" ("redundant"), in contrast to TD (dark bars). Volterra, Caselli, Capirici, and Pizzuto (2005, p. 29) say of this:

> [w]hen children with DS combined gestures and words, they did so primarily in an informationally redundant fashion. The vast majority of combinations produced by these children were in fact equivalent combinations in which the two representational elements referred to the same referent and conveyed the same meaning (e.g., headshake for no = "no").

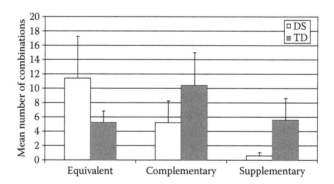

FIGURE 32.4 Information conveyed in gesture plus word combinations by Down's Syndrome and mental age matched typically developing children (Iverson, J. M., Longobardi, E., and Caselli, M. C. *International Journal of Language and Communicative Disorders, 38*, 179–197, 2003. With permission.)

In TD, on the other hand, early speech-gesture combinations are "complementary" (partially redundant gesture and speech referring to the same object but different aspects of it, which DS also create, though far less than "equivalent") and "supplementary" (nonredundant, gesture and speech referring to different entities in some kind of semantic relation, like POINT AT CHAIR + "daddy" = "daddy's chair," possessive, which DS create virtually not at all).

Goldin-Meadow and Butcher (2003), with TD children, classified the semantic relationships in speech and gesture combinations, and found that speech-gesture combinations foreshadowed the child's first word-word combinations, these appearing a few weeks later with the same semantic relationships. A child who pointed at an object and said "go" would, a couple of weeks later, produce word-word combinations with "go" plus object names. The early gesture-word combinations cover a range of semantic relations: "open" + points at drawer, "out" + holds up toy bag, "hot" + points at furnace, "no" + points at box, "monster" + two vertical palms spread apart (= big; Goldin-Meadow & Butcher, 2003, Table 3). Kelly (2006) observed an earlier step, in which the first pairings involve gestures and speech that denote the same elements; it is only slightly later that different speech and gesture elements synchronize to form the semantic units described by Goldin-Meadow and Butcher (2003).

Thus TD children begin with a gesture advantage, first with redundant gestures and speech, then with semantic combinations of gesture and speech foreshadowing the same semantic combinations a few weeks later in speech-speech. DS in contrast appear to take only the first step. Even their "complementary" gesture-speech combinations are a species of redundant combination. It is only "supplementary" combinations that combine semantic elements into structures that foreshadow combinations of words, and DS lack these almost totally.

To understand these differences in GP terms, we note that redundancy and the exclusion of semantic connections between gesture and speech suggest that DS GPs, in whatever form they exist, are narrowly constrained. The opposition of semiotic modes within these narrow limits would give them little traction. The type of example in Figure32.1, in which the underlying idea of Sylvester moving up inside a pipe is symbolized in two semiotically opposite forms, may be beyond their reach. Imagining them recounting this episode, they may say "pipe" and gesture its shape; or "sidewalk" (where Sylvester paced before going up the pipe) and gesture a flat surface; or "ball" and make a circle; but not "rising hollowness" or even "down" if, as we suppose, the Figure 32.2 aphasic speaker was differentiating the idea of downward force in a context of things that Tweety and Sylvester were doing. In DS, this apparent narrowness in turn could impact the dependence of the GP on fields of oppositions. DS GPs, redundantly welded, would differentiate only equally narrow contexts where synonymy of gesture and speech is meaningful. Verbalized thought, for DS, would then be confined in at least two ways—GPs with little dynamic push, and contexts cramped to make minimal differentiation significant: in this way coming up short on the dynamic dimension of language. Their dynamic shortfall joins the deficits on the static dimension of factual linguistic competence (where naming and syntactic deficits are noted). The aphasic speaker who after two arduous minutes reached a two-clause, embedded sentence was sustained throughout by his spatially configured catchment (observable in gesture), and this kind of achievement, and any benefit of catchment formations in general, may be largely out of reach for a DS speaker. Finally, a lack of GP semiotic opposition could impair the unpacking step, limiting access to constructions, even if they have been acquired. So the picture is of limited GP potential, lessened dynamism of thinking-for/while-speaking, limited contextual scope, and limited potential to form gestural (catchment) discourse segments. Bellugi, Wang, and Jernigan (1994) describe older DS responses to vocabulary tests as often involving perseverations or category errors (e.g., "horsie, dog, ice cream" to one picture), which also seem to be manifestations of cognitive narrowness.

Given that DS speakers have comparatively good visuo-spatial and visuo-motor cognition, the shortcomings we describe refer specifically to GP formation. Our suggestion is that DS start out with gestures preferentially. In this they are not unlike TD children in the second year. But they differ in that, when they add speech, the speech-gesture combinations are redundant, totally, or partially. As such, speech-gesture combinations fail to carry the DS over the language threshold. So if normal development involves certain types of gesture-speech combinations as way stations toward language, DS development seems excessively stuck at the level of redundant gestures. It is telling that the gestures they do produce, after considerable experience, are also not ones likely to foster semiotic oppositions with linguistic encodings. Volterra et al. (2005) offer an interesting suggestion:

> children with DS may be able to make use of actions produced in the context of object-related activities and social routines as communicative gestures. Once this happens, they may begin to develop relatively large repertoires of gestures and make enhanced use of gesture to compensate for poor productive language. (p. 32)

These kinds of compensatory gestures are the not co-equal participants with encoded language with which to create the semiotic oppositions a GP demands; in fact, such gestures are substitutes, and doubly so—not only for deficient language, but also for deficient gestures (cf. Chan & Iacono, 2001).

WILLIAMS SYNDROME

Williams syndrome (WS) is often pictured as the mirror image of DS. WS children have cognitive deficits, IQs in the 50–70 range, yet seem to have *greater* language skills than the cognitive deficits would predict. They are also highly socially engaged, musical, and lively. Social engagement and musicality we think are the keys to their language as well.

WS poses an interesting challenge to the GP theory: how, given the theory, can language go beyond cognition's offerings? The seeming sparing of language has made WS the poster child of purported language modules. However, from a nonmodular, GP perspective, another interpretation seems possible. We shall answer the challenge in the following way. Although it may seem perverse to refer to better-than-predicted language as a "disorder" we shall in fact conclude that, in the WS case, good language arises from disruption of the GP, namely a disconnect between the social framing of thinking-for-speaking, of which WS clearly are capable, and what Vygotsky (1987) termed "pure thought." Gesture mimicry and other forms of "mind-merging" (Franklin, 2007; Kimbara, 2006, 2007; McNeill et al., 2010) participate in constructing social interactions (Kimbara, 2006), and we believe that WS children have similar capabilities. In effect, WS speakers maintain the connection of idea units, GPs, to the social context of speaking, via what is sometimes called hypersociability (Bellugi, Lichtenberger, Mills, Galaburda, & Korenberg, 1999), creating joint GPs with interlocutors (as unimpaired speakers also do), but are unable to shape thought outside the social fabric, and this is their disorder. Vygotsky visualized thought and speech as overlapping circles, one for thought, one for speech, and the overlap was inner speech; the GP is a theory about this overlap, and what we propose for WS is truncation or inaccessibility of the thought circle from the overlap. An important factor in this flattening could be a WS weakness at global organization in the visual domain (Bellugi et al., 1999). If WS are unable to create visual global wholes they would gain little from the global-synthetic imagery created in GPs as part of the speaking process. The result leaves little room for the GP to shape cognition—the reverse of trying to explain how cognition affects language: it is cognition in WS that is not shaped by the ongoing thinking-for-speaking process.

If this is on the right track, WS is thus a disorder of the dynamic dimension of language *par excellence*. Language is weak at shaping cognition, while it retains what is also usually integrated with thought, the social-interactive fabric. There is a distinctive gesture profile of WS (Bello et al., 2004), in which only certain kinds of imagery take part: iconic gestures and a plenitude of socially constituted "emblems," if available in the culture, both of which are engaged in social interactions, but also an absence of gesture metaphor with metadiscourse resonances. An interpretation of WS in terms of our proposed brain model is far from certain, and we do not attempt it, other than to suggest that among the unique qualities of WS, GP formation is an energetic rhythmicity that can underlie both their fluency of speaking as well as the other quality of the syndrome, musicality. The role of the cerebellum in organizing rhythmic pulses of speech (Duncan, 2006) is echoed by the discovery of hyperdevelopment of the cerebellar vermis of WS. The vermis is thought to play a role in human rhythmic sense and movement (Schmitt, Eliez, Warsofsky, Bellugi, & Reiss, 2001).* These rhythmic pulses are also obviously engaged in the musical lives of WS individuals (cf. Bellugi et al., 1999), and also, we hypothesize, play into sociability, underlying the entrainments of the children with social others during interactions (cf. Gill, 2007).

It has been said that WS are slow to develop gestures (Volterra et al. citing Bertrand, Mervis, & Neustat, 1998), and that their gestures, when started, are not frequent (Laing et al., 2002), but other studies at the ISTC in Rome have observed

---

* Interestingly, children with infantile autism show the reverse, reduction in posterior cerebellar vermis volume (Courchesne, Townsend, & Saitoh, 1994).

no difference between TD and WS matched for developmental age (Volterra et al., 2005). In their recent work, with 9–12-year-old WS children, researchers at the Rome Institute find WS perform gestures in picture-naming and Frog Story narrations at a *higher* rate than TD children of comparable developmental ages, have *more iconic gestures* and *more pointing gestures*, and *combine gestures to a greater extent with "social evaluation devices,"* such as character speech, sound effects, exclamations, and rhetorical questions that function to capture the listener's attention (Bello, Capirci, & Volterra, 2004; Capirci, 2007). More precisely, they found a significant correlation between total spoken social evaluation devices and the use of gestures only for WS children ($p = 0.0078$). A significant correlation was found in particular with iconic gestures ($p = 0.0001$) and beat gestures ($p = 0.004$). Those children with WS who produced more gestures (in particular more iconic gestures and more beat gestures) were also the children who produced more spoken social evaluation devices.[*]

We get a picture of WS children as socially interactive, with gesture a well-established modality for human interaction. Their "enhanced language" we propose, stems from this lively social engagement, as described above. This implicates the GP in the following way. Vygotsky, in his reanalysis of egocentric speech, argued that a child's development is from the outside, the social context, to the inside—the once-social becoming thought. This ontogenetic process has an echo on the much tighter time scale of GP microgenesis, in that the field of oppositions includes, among other information, social interaction variables and the GP itself can be shared interpsychically (cf. McNeill et al., 2010, for descriptions of "mind-merging" in normal adult conversations). We suggest that WS have GPs of this kind. This is not only mimicry; speaking can be self-generated but depend for sustenance on continuing social interactions; closed off is self-directed thought carried by language, including metaphor. Distinctive about WS thinking-for-speaking is its dominant social frame assisted by rhythmic entrainment. Cognitive deficits, including relative inability to access the semantic values of words (Karmiloff-Smith, Brown, Grice, & Paterson, 2003), may deflate the thought circle, but sociability is the key to their language. In this sense, the skill of WS children in language is an aspect of the disability.

However, the facts of actual WS language ability are less than totally clear. In keeping with their sociability and rhythmicity, speech flow is impressively fluent. But the depth of WS language skill is debated. On the one hand are those who argue for near-normal language abilities. Zukowski (2001), for example, compared WS and neurotypical children's language production data on noun-noun compounds, embedded relative clauses, and yes/no questions; also grammaticality judgments of uses of expressions with "any" and "some." She found performance in the two groups to be similar, concluding, "WS is indeed highly relevant to the modularity debate. The findings also suggest that imperfect levels of language performance in WS may reflect an exaggerated influence of normal processing factors" (from the abstract). On the other hand, Karmiloff-Smith et al.

---

[*] We thank Virginia Volterra and Olga Capirci for emphasizing these points.

(2003) summarize numerous tests of WS, concluding that "... the WS language system is not only delayed but also develops along a different trajectory compared to controls, with individuals with WS placing relatively more weight on phonological information and relatively less weight on semantic information" (p. 230). Karmiloff-Smith et al. (2003) are emphatic in their rejection of innateness linguistic "modularity" claims based on spared WS language skills in the absence of general cognitive ability (cf. Pinker, 1999), citing both the relative inaccessibility of semantic content to WS, and also tests of sentence comprehension, which show "findings inconsistent with the view that WS syntax is intact" (p. 231). In thinking about the modularity issue, it is important to recognize that no general principle relating a given level of cognitive ability or inability to a specific grammatical form presence or absence has ever been defined; so an ability to produce relative clause responses in experiments, for example, may or may not count as evidence of a syntax module, particularly if [as Karmiloff-Smith et al. (2003) propose] WS children reach these abilities over different developmental routes (which may include tracks, not seen in typical development, linked to their hypersociability). And again, in general, sociocentric inputs may create an illusion of structure.

Social framing can also create an appearance of narrative cohesion. Bellugi et al. (1994) observed an abundance of "paralinguistic and linguistic devices for expressive purposes and to maintain audience interest" (p. 16); that is, a cohesion based, not on thematic linkages in discourse, but on the continuation of purposes in social interactions. We can predict that, despite their better than expected language and gesture output, gesture catchments from WS will tend to emphasize this kind of sociocentric cohesion, with few if any catchments built out of recurring gesture references, as we saw created for example by the agrammatic speaker in Figure 32.3.* Social but nonreferential catchments may thus be another aspect of the WS syndrome. It is possible that in WS there is an absence of discourse awareness itself (cf. Sullivan, Winner, & Tager-Flushberg, 2003, for WS inability to distinguish lies from irony, where doing so required relating verbal uses to context in comprehension).

To summarize, using Vygotsky's image of overlapping circles, the WS thought-circle is flattened (Figure 32.5).

CHILDHOOD AUTISM

Elena Levy (2007, 2008; Levy & Fowler, 2005) has developed a method by which to observe the emergence of spoken discourse cohesion over short intervals—short, but extended enough to permit observation of emergence. A child is shown a classic film, *The Red Balloon*, and tells the story to a listener. Specific to the method is that the child tells the story repeatedly, over several days (sometimes on the same day), to the same or different listeners. In this way, changes,

---

* This refers to catchments, not mere gesture repetition; that is, recurring gesture features that mark off a discourse theme (we have found no information bearing on whether WS do or do not repeat gestures).

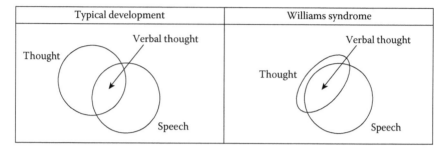

FIGURE 32.5 Representations in the manner of Vygotsky (1987) of the relationship between thought, speech, and verbal thought, in typically developing and Williams syndrome children.

which typically are consolidations that enhance cohesion, can be tracked as they emerge. The method can be employed with speakers of all sorts and has been used by Levy with autistic children. We concentrate on a case study of a 13-year-old boy (Levy, 2008). While many differences from TD children are found with autistics, we focus, following Levy, on the catchment and its theoretical role in creating fields of oppositions. In his first attempts at retelling the story, speech was fragmented and gestures few, responses were "single utterances or utterance fragments, usually in the absence of focused enactment, and often accompanied by diffuse body motion, for example, shifting position, swaying back and forth, rocking, and fidgeting" (p. 5 ms.).

Levy documents that from this point fully encoded descriptions gradually emerged and—equally striking—also gestures that look typical for such speech; in other words, GPs in what appear to be appropriate fields of oppositions. Coherence increased via catchments: "As D. combined speech with enactment ... he created a sequence that was more temporally coherent than the first: All utterances were accurate descriptions of events, and all occurred in accurate temporal sequence" (p. 11). An example analyzed in detail by Levy involves two catchments at early points in the child's narrative attempts—*flying* gestures, and *holding* gestures—that resulted eventually, after several retellings, in a correctly narrated sequence of events (corresponding to the film's sequence). As fields of oppositions, we can see in these catchments how the narrative order was finally straightened out. Initially, the boy first described flying with balloons, then, immediately following, holding onto the balloons (while reversing the film order, the order of D's utterances is the same as by the adults when first prompting the scene). Then the following (Table 32.2, compiled from Levy, p. 23).

Although starting out with an airborne reference, again out of sequence, he had the holding gesture in the correct narrative sequence (holding first). The GP at this point would be something like that suggested in the table: differentiating what could happen while the boy was holding—floating. The child continued with the correct sequence: holding followed by flying. Achieving temporal coherence

TABLE 32.2

Achieving Discourse Cohesion by an Autistic Adolescent

Narrative order	Speech	Gesture	Fields of Oppositions (possible):
1	he floated	start of holding gesture	What Happened While Holding: Floating
2	he hanged on tight	continuation of holding gesture	Still What Happened While Holding: Holding Tight
3	[no speech]	flying gesture	The Thing That Happened: Flying

Source: Based on Levy, 2008.

thus stemmed from catchments and the realization that, eventually, the holding and flying catchments interrelate, one continuing what the other began. This is a kind of imagery-enactment version of the logical relationship of an enabling cause/resultant, which the boy could achieve in this form even if not with a clear vision of the logical connections themselves.

From a GP point of view, as exhibited in this case study, autism seems to involve an imbalance between enactment and speech that was overcome with repeated telling. Like the aphasic in Figure 32.3, a catchment emerged accompanied by coherence (they differ of course in that the autistic child recycles entire descriptions, whereas the aphasic took time to create a single description). In the brain, we speculate, the imbalance focuses on the prefrontal and motor cortexes, with the latter at first flooding the former. Eventually, an awakened prefrontal area is energized and creates something like a normal field of oppositions. In cyclic retelling there is something that activates and/or restores balance across brain regions and leads the autistic speaker toward the realm of the typical. We can imagine that autistic children might seek this kind of cyclic activation on their own—some of the repetitious behavior often remarked upon in the disorder may be an effort to overcome enactment imbalance. At the same time, however, such an effort is a recipe for impaired social communication. What, for an autistic child, may be an effort for eventual enhancement is limited if not actually counterproductive as a kind of social foray. Thus the child would be denied the propulsion from socially engaged cognition that carries WS children so far.

SUMMARY AND CONCLUSIONS: WHAT THE GP SHOWS

We began this chapter saying that the four language disorders—agrammatic aphasia, DS, WS, and autism—disrupt different aspects of the GP. We conclude by summarizing the disruptions and what they reveal about human speech and its points of possible breakdown. We suggest that a GP view of language shows the disorders in new light. For this reason, we believe, it is worthy of consideration by clinicians and researchers who deal directly with communication disorders.

Disfluent (agrammatic) aphasia preserves the psychological predicate charac-ter of the GP, the point of newsworthy information differentiated from context. Context and catchments are accessible. Broca's aphasia concentrates specifically on the unpacking of GPs via constructions or other syntax. Constructions may also be intact, in part, but are hard to access due to shallow level motor impedi-ments interacting with the vocal articulators. The evidence for this is that, with catchment support and sufficient time, agrammatic aphasics can develop even multiclause unpackings. It is accordingly easy to understand the frustration some-times shown by agrammatic aphasics, since they experience basically the whole process of thinking-for-speaking but cannot execute it in action. Autism reveals an imbalance of enactment and catchment formation that, with repetition, can be overcome; so the disorder is one of balance, not specifically a breakdown of the GP. In contrast to the aphasic, once balance is reached, speech and discourse appear to function with something like normalcy. Down syndrome speakers, children at least, may not experience thinking-for-speaking in anything like the form it is encountered by normal speakers, the autistic child, or the agrammatic aphasic. The elements opposed semiotically in their GPs are redundant, there is little scope for cognitive movement, and the contexts from which these rigid GPs are differentiated are comparably narrow. The impression one gets of DS speech therefore is of stasis, immobility, and little potential for fueling thinking-for-speaking. Williams speakers unusually seem to have half the normal complement of thinking-for-speaking, missing the other half. Their GPs are socially engaged but do not pass into thought, possibly because their cognitive deficits prevent it. Down and Williams syndrome speakers are mirror images in respect to thinking as well; both are unable to use language as an enriching element of cognition but for opposite reasons—Down cannot break out of limited GPs; Williams cannot translate GPs structured as lively social interactions into cognition.

A further dimension of comparison involves the place of the catchment in the four disorders. Disfluent aphasia retains at least the capability of thematic link-ages with spatial, deictically established catchments, as we see in both Figure 32.2 (correct deictic placement of the bowling ball placement) and Figure 32.3 (the overhead locus). Autistics initially cannot form catchments but attain them with appropriate enactments, as in the flying example. This may limit their dis-course cohesion to the enactable, just as the aphasic's, with no or little potential in either case to extend imagery metaphorically. Children with DS, because of the near-total redundancy of imagery and speech, possibly cannot form catch-ments at all. Each image is tied to a specific lexical form. Finally, in Williams, we may find catchments (if sought) based on social interaction, and these catchments could be the richest of all, since interaction can lead the child into complex and enduring forms of cohesive discourse. In respect to catchments, WS and autism differ diametrically. Autistic social catchments may never be reached if recycling is the route, since it is so disruptive to the normal parameters of social interaction, whereas, in WS, where hypersociability is the style, such catchments might be the starting point of almost all of their speech.

ACKNOWLEDGMENTS

Preparation supported by research grants from NSF and NIH to the University of Chicago, and award number NIH NIDCD 5R01DC001150-14 to the University of colorado. We are grateful to Elena Levy and Virginia Volterra for very helpful comments.

REFERENCES

Abrahamsen, A., Cavallo, M. M., & McCluer, J. A. (1985). Is the sign advantage a robust phenomenon? From gesture to language in two modalities. *Merrill-Palmer Quarterly, 31*, 177–209.

Bello, A., Capirci, O., & Volterra, V. (2004). Lexical production in children with Williams syndrome: Spontaneous use of gesture in a naming task. *Neuropsychologia, 42*, 201–213.

Bellugi, U., Lichtenberger, L., Mills, D., Galaburda, A., & Korenberg, J. R. (1999). Bridging cognition, the brain and molecular genetics: Evidence from Williams syndrome. *Trends in Neuroscience, 22*, 197–207.

Bellugi, U., Wang, P. P., & Jernigan, T. L. (1994). Williams syndrome: An unusual neuropsychological profile. In S. Broman & J. Grafman (Eds.), *Atypical cognitive deficits in developmental disorders: Implications for brain function* (pp 23–56). Hillsdale, NJ: Lawrence Erlbaum Associates.

Bertrand, J., Mervis, C. B., & Neustat, I. (1998). Communicative gesture use by preschoolers with Williams syndrome: A longitudinal study. *Presentation at the International Conference of Infant Studies*, Atlanta, GA.

Butcher, C., & Goldin-Meadow, S. (2000). Gesture and the transition from one- to two-word speech: When hand and mouth come together. In D. McNeill (Ed.), *Language and gesture* (pp. 235–257). Cambridge, UK: Cambridge University Press.

Capirci, O. (2007, December). Gesture and language in children with Williams syndrome. *Presentation at the 2007 ESF Exploratory Workshop/ESRC Workshop,* Sign language vs. gesture: Where is the boundary, and how can we know more? (pp. 6–7). Rome, Italy: Institute of Cognitive Sciences & Technologies.

Chan, J. B., & Iacono, T. (2001). Gesture and word production in children with Down Syndrome. *AAC Augmentative and Attentive Communication, 17*, 73–87.

Courchesne, F., Townsend, J., & Saitoh, O. (1994). The brain in infantile autism: Posterior fossa structures are abnormal. *Neurology, 44*, 214–223.

De Ruiter, J.-P. (2000). The production of gesture and speech. In D. McNeill (Ed.), *Language and gesture* (pp. 285–311). Cambridge, UK: Cambridge University Press.

Dray, N. L., & McNeill, D. (1990). Gestures during discourse: The contextual structuring of thought. In S. L. Tsohatzidis (Ed.), *Meanings and prototypes: Studies in linguistic categorization* (pp. 465–487). London, UK: Routledge.

Duncan, S. (2006). Co-expressivity of speech and gesture: Manner of motion in Spanish, English, and Chinese. In *Proceedings of the 27th Berkeley Linguistic Society Annual Meeting* (pp. 353–370). [Meeting in 2001.] Berkeley, CA: Berkeley Linguistics Society, University of California, Berkeley, Department of Linguistics.

Duncan, S., & Pedelty, L. (2007). Discourse focus, gesture, and disfluent aphasia. In S. D. Duncan, J. Cassell, & E. T. Levy (Eds.), *Gesture and the dynamic dimension of language* (pp. 269–283). Amsterdam/Philadelphia, PA: John Benjamins.

Fadiga, L. (2007, December). Report in *OMLL (Origin of Man, Language and Languages),* *ESF EUROCORES Program Highlights* (p. 13). Online: http://www.esf.org/activities/eurocores/programmes/omll.html

Franklin, A. (2007). Blending in deception: Tracing output back to its source. In S. D. Duncan, J. Cassell, & E. T. Levy (Eds.), *Gesture and the dynamic dimension of language* (pp. 99–108). Amsterdam/Philadelphia, PA: John Benjamins.

Furuyama, N. & Sekine, K. 2007. Forgetful or strategic? The mystery of the systematic avoidance of reference in the cartoon story narrative. In S. D. Duncan, J. Cassell & E. T. Levy (Eds.), *Gesture and the dynamic dimension of language* (pp. 75–81). Amsterdam and Philadelphia: Benjamins.

Gill, S. (2007). Entrainment and musicality in the human system interface. *AI & Society, 21,* 567–605.

Goldin-Meadow, S., & Butcher, C. (2003). Pointing toward two-word speech in young children. In S. Kita (Ed.), *Pointing: Where language, culture, and cognition meet* (pp. 85–107). Mahwah, NJ: Erlbaum Associates.

Goodglass, H. (1993). *Understanding aphasia.* San Diego, CA: Academic Press.

Harris, R. (2003). *Saussure and his interpreters* (2nd ed.). Edinburgh, Scotland: Edinburgh University Press.

Hockett, C. F. (1960). The origin of speech. *Scientific American, 203,* 88–96.

Iverson, J. M., Longobardi, E., & Caselli, M. C. (2003). Relationship between gestures and words in children with Down's syndrome and typically developing children in the early stages of communicative development. *International Journal of Language and Communicative Disorders, 38,* 179–197.

Johnson, M. (1987). *The body in the mind: The bodily basis of meaning, imagination, and reason.* Chicago, IL: University of Chicago Press.

Karmiloff-Smith, A., Brown, J. H., Grice, S., & Paterson, S. (2003). Dethroning the myth: Cognitive dissociations and innate modularity in Williams syndrome. *Developmental Neuropsychology, 23,* 227–242.

Kelly, B. F. (2006). The development of constructions through gesture. In E. V. Clark & B. F. Kelly (Eds.), *Constructions in acquisition* (pp. 11–25). Palo Alto, CA: CSLI.

Kimbara, I. (2006). On gestural mimicry. *Gesture, 6,* 39–61.

Kimbara, I. (2007). Indexing locations in gesture: Recalled stimulus image and interspeaker coordination as factors influencing gesture form. In S. D. Duncan, J. Cassell, & E. T. Levy (Eds.), *Gesture and the dynamic dimension of language* (pp. 213–220). Amsterdam/Philadelphia, PA: John Benjamins.

Kita, S., & Özyürek, A. (2003). What does cross-linguistic variation in semantic coordination of speech and gesture reveal? Evidence for an interface representation of spatial thinking and speaking. *Journal of Memory and Language, 48,* 16–32.

Laing, E., Butterworth, G., Ansari, D., Gsodl, M., Longhi, E., Paterson, S., & Karmiloff-Smith, A. (2002). Atypical development of language and social communication in toddlers with Williams syndrome. *Developmental Science, 5,* 233–246.

Levelt, W. J. M. (1989). *Speaking: From intention to articulation.* Cambridge, MA: MIT Press/Bradford Books.

Levy, E. (2007). The construction of temporally coherent narrative by an autistic adolescent: Co-construction of speech, enactment and gesture. In S. D. Duncan, J. Cassell, & E. T. Levy (Eds.), *Gesture and the dynamic dimension of language* (pp. 285–301). Amsterdam/Philadelphia, PA: Benjamins.

Levy, E. T. (2008). The mediation of coherent discourse by kinesthetic reenactment: A case study of an autistic adolescent, Part II. Manuscript. Department of Psychology, University of Connecticut at Stamford.

Levy, E. T., & Fowler, C. A. (2005). How autistic children may use narrative discourse to scaffold coherent interpretations of events: A case study. *Imagination Cognition and Personality, 24*(3), 207–244.

McNeill, D. (1992). *Hand and mind: What gestures reveal about thought.* Chicago, IL: University of Chicago Press.

McNeill, D. (2000). Catchments and contexts: Non-modular factors in speech and gesture production. In D. McNeill (Ed.), *Language and gesture* (pp. 312–328). Cambridge, UK: Cambridge University Press.

McNeill, D. (2005). *Gesture and thought.* Chicago, IL: University of Chicago Press.

McNeill, D., & Duncan, S. D. (2000). Growth points in thinking for speaking. In D. McNeill (Ed.), *Language and gesture* (pp. 141–161). Cambridge, UK: Cambridge University Press.

McNeill, D., Duncan, S., Cole, J., Gallagher, S., & Bertenthal, B. (2008). Growth points from the very beginning. *Interaction Studies, 9,* 117–132.

McNeill, D., Duncan, S., Franklin, A., Goss, J., Kimbara, I., Parrill, F., Welji, H., Chen, L., Harper, M., Quek, F. and Tuttle, R. (2010) Mind-merging. In E. Morsella (Ed.), *Expressing oneself/Expressing one's self: Communication, language, cognition, and identity: A Festschrift in honor of Robert M. Krauss* (pp. 141–164). New York, NY: Taylor & Francis.

Miceli, G., Silveri, M. C., Villa, G., & Caramazza, A. (1984). On the basis of the agrammatic's difficulty in producing main verbs. *Cortex, 20,* 207–220.

Pinker, S. (1999). *Words and rules: The ingredients of language.* New York, NY: Basic Books.

Schmitt, J. E., Eliez, S., Warsofsky, I. S., Bellugi, U., & Reiss, A. L. (2001). Enlarged cerebellar vermis in Williams syndrome. *Journal of Psychiatric Research, 35,* 225–229.

Slobin, D. I. (1987). Thinking for speaking. In J. Aske, N. Beery, L. Michaelis, & H. Filip (Eds.), *Proceedings of the thirteenth annual meeting of the Berkeley Linguistic Society* (pp. 435–445). Berkeley, CA: Berkeley Linguistic Society.

Stefanini, S., Caselli, M. C., & Volterra, V. (2007). Spoken and gestural production in a naming task by young children with Down's syndrome. *Brain and Language, 101,* 208–221.

Sullivan, K., Winner, E., & Tager-Flushberg, H. (2003). Can adolescents with Williams syndrome tell the difference between lies and jokes? *Developmental Neuropsychology, 23,* 85–103.

Volterra, V., Caselli, M. C., Capirici, O., & Pizzuto, E. (2005). Gesture and the emergence and development of language. In M. Tomasello & D. I. Slobin (Eds.), *Beyond nature-nurture: Essays in honor of Elizabeth Bates* (pp. 3–40). Mahwah, NJ: Lawrence Erlbaum.

Vygotsky, L. S. (1987). *Thought and language.* Edited and translated by E. Hanfmann & G. Vakar (revised and edited by A. Kozulin). Cambridge, MA: MIT Press.

Zinchenko, V. P. (1985). Vygotsky's ideas about units for the analysis of mind. In J. V. Wertsch (Ed.), *Culture communication, and cognition: Vygotskian perspectives* (pp. 94–118). Cambridge, UK: Cambridge University Press.

Zingester, L. B., & Berndt, R. S. (1990). Retrieval of nouns and verbs in agrammatism and anomia. *Brain and Language, 39,* 14–32.

Zukowski, A. (2001). *Uncovering grammatical competence in children with Williams Syndrome.* PhD dissertation, Boston University.

33 Neural Organization of Language: Clues From Sign Language Aphasia

Gregory Hickok and Ursula Bellugi

A central issue in understanding the neural organization of language is the extent to which this organization is dependent on the sensory and motor modalities through which language is perceived and produced. There are many reasons to think that the neural organization of language should be profoundly influenced by extrinsic factors in development such as sensory and motor experience. The temporal processing demands imposed by the auditory system have been argued to favor left hemisphere systems (Tallal, Miller, & Fitch, 1993), which could, in turn, determine aspects of the lateralization pattern of auditory-mediated language. Superior temporal lobe regions thought to be important for language comprehension are situated in and around auditory cortices—a natural location given auditory sensory input of language. Likewise, Broca's area, which is classically thought to play a role in speech production, is situated just anterior to motor cortex controlling the speech articulators. Thus, it would not be unreasonable to hypothesize that the neural organization of language—including its lateralization and within hemisphere organization—is determined in large part by the particular demands imposed by the sensory and motor interface systems.

By studying the functional neuroanatomy of the signed languages of the deaf, we can test this hypothesis in a straightforward manner. It has been shown that signed languages share much of the formal linguistic structure found in spoken languages, but differ radically in the sensory and motor systems through which language is transmitted (Bellugi, Poizner, & Klima, 1989; Emmorey, 2002; Klima & Bellugi, 1979). In essence, signed language offers a kind of natural experimental manipulation: central linguistic structure and function are held constant, while peripheral sensory and motor experience is varied. Thus, a comparison of the neural organization of signed versus spoken language will provide clues concerning the factors that drive the development of the functional neuroanatomy of language. Here we provide a summary of the findings from studies of the neural organization of the signed languages of the deaf.

687

HEMISPHERIC ASYMMETRIES FOR SIGN LANGUAGE PROCESSING

Left hemisphere damage (LHD) in hearing/speaking individuals is associated with deficits at sublexical ("phonetic/phonemic"), lexical, and sentence levels, both in production and in comprehension to some degree (Damasio, 1992; Goodglass, 1993; Hillis, 2007). Right hemisphere damage (RHD), on the other hand, has been associated with supra-sentential (e.g., discourse) deficits (Brownell, Potter, Bihrle, & Gardner, 1986). Given the radical differences in modality of perception and production of sign language, one might expect sign language to differ dramatically in hemispheric asymmetries. But instead our studies have found very strong evidence of highly similar patterns of hemispheric asymmetries in the deaf signing population compared to hearing/speaking individuals.

SUBLEXICAL-, LEXICAL-, AND SENTENCE-LEVEL PROCESSES

A variety of sublexical-, lexical-, and sentence-level deficits have been found in individual LHD deaf signers (Bellugi et al., 1989; Hickok & Bellugi, 2001; Hickok, Kritchevsky, Bellugi, & Klima, 1996b; Poizner, Klima, & Bellugi, 1987). These deficits have been noted both in production, and to varying degrees in comprehension. In production, a range of paraphasic error types have been identified in LHD signers, including "phonemic," morphological, and semantic subtypes, demonstrating the breakdown of these various levels of computation. Some examples of phonemic paraphasias are shown in Figure 33.1. Disorders in sign language sentence formation in LHD signers have emerged both in the form of agrammatism, a tendency to omit grammatical markers, and in the form of paragrammatism, a tendency toward grammatically rich but error prone utterances, showing that sentence-level computations can also be disrupted following LHD in deaf signers (Hickok & Bellugi, 2001; Hickok, Bellugi, & Klima, 1998a). Production errors at all these levels are fairly common in LHD signers, but occur relatively rarely in RHD signers. In our sample of over 50 unilateral brain injured signers, we have found only one RHD signer who was in fact aphasic on standard clinical-type assessment; this individual was left handed and had evidence of a reversed dominance pattern (Pickell et al., 2005). As for comprehension, we have documented deficits at the word (i.e., sign) and sentence level (Hickok, Klima, & Bellugi, 1996a; Hickok, Love-Geffen, & Klima, 2002). At the word level, comprehension deficits have been observed only following LHD, not RHD. These deficits are relatively mild and appear to result from breakdowns primarily at the postphonemic level (Hickok, Klima, Kritchevsky, & Bellugi, 1995). At the sentence level, the most severe deficits occur following LHD, but, consistent with findings in the hearing/speaking population, some difficulties in sentence comprehension can be found in RHD signers, particularly as sentence complexity increases (Hickok et al., 2002).

Group studies confirmed the generalizability of these case study observations. In an analysis of 13 LHD and 10 RHD signers, one study (Hickok et al.,

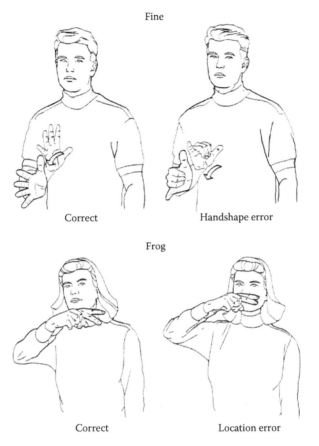

FIGURE 33.1   Examples of sign paraphasic errors in left hemisphere damaged deaf signers.

1996a) found that LHD signers performed significantly worse than RHD signers on a range of standard language measures, including production, comprehension, naming, and repetition (Figure 33.2). These differences between LHD and RHD signers could not be attributed to variables such as: (a) age at test; (b) onset of deafness; or (c) age of exposure to ASL, as these variables did not correlate with any of the language behaviors tested. Further reinforcing this finding, it was found that LHD versus RHD group differences showed the same patterns if only native signers were included in the analysis (Figure 33.2; Hickok et al., 2002). This is not to say that these variables have no impact on sign language organization or language ability, because surely they do at some level of detail (Neville et al., 1997; Newport & Meier, 1985), only that the dominant factor that predicts performance on these aphasia assessment measures is whether the left or right hemisphere is damaged.

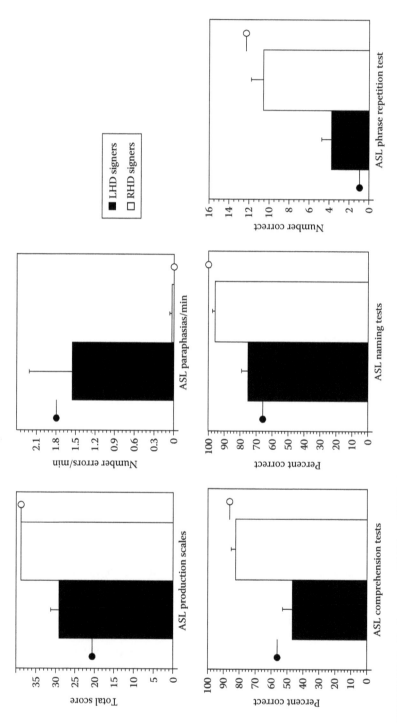

FIGURE 33.2 Performance of LHD and RHD signers on a range of standard aphasia assessments including production, naming, repetition, and comprehension. Circles indicate average values for the subset of the lesion population that includes only native deaf signers.

Supra-Sentential (Discourse) Deficits

One linguistic deficit associated with RHD in hearing/speaking individuals involves discourse-level processes, for example, the ability to appropriately link (in production and comprehension) discourse referents across multiple sentences (Brownell et al., 1986; Wapner et al., 1981). These deficits manifest as failures to integrate information across sentences, including impairments in understanding jokes, in making inferences, and in adhering to the story line when producing a narrative. In contrast, phonological and syntactic processes in these hearing/speaking individuals appear to be intact. Using a story narration task given to two deaf RHD signers, two distinct types of discourse deficits have been documented (Hickok et al., 1999). The first involves a failure to adhere to the story line, evidenced by confabulatory or tangential utterances. The second type of deficit involves errors in the use of the spatialized discourse of ASL. Discourse organization in ASL is unique in that discourse referents are established, referred to, and manipulated in a plane of signing space, and it was the ability to use this spatial mechanism in a discourse that was disrupted in one of the patients studied. These results suggest: (a) the right hemisphere is involved in discourse processing in ASL, as it is in spoken language; and (b) there are dissociable subcomponents of discourse processes in ASL.

Classifier Constructions

American Sign Language contains an interesting type of construction, classifier signs, which is not typically assessed on standard aphasia exams in signed or spoken language. Classifier signs are complex forms that can be used to specify a range of spatial information, relative location, movement path, movement manner, object size and shape (see Emmorey, 2002 for a review). These forms are typically comprised of two parts: (1) a handshape configuration, where different handshapes can correspond to different semantic classes of object referents (e.g., people, vehicles, etc.), or to object shape-related properties (e.g., flat, narrow, etc.); and (2) a specification of the location or movement of the referent, denoted by the location/movement of the hand(s) in signing space. The linguistic status of classifier forms is a matter of debate, but what is clear is that they differ from canonical lexical signs in that they can encode information, for example spatial information, non-categorically. Whereas a lexical sign like DRIVE-TO can indicate that a vehicle was driven from one place to another, a classifier sign can convey more detailed information about the route traversed (e.g., it was curvy and uphill; Figure 33.3).

It has been suggested that the right hemisphere may be more involved in processing classifier signs than in processing canonical lexical signs (Hickok, Bellugi, & Klima, 1998b; Poizner et al., 1987), and a handful of recent functional imaging studies have provided some evidence supporting this idea. For example, a PET study by Emmorey et al. (2002), found that deaf native signers activated parietal regions bilaterally when describing spatial relations using ASL classifier signs (compared to naming objects). See Campbell and Woll (2003), for additional discussion.

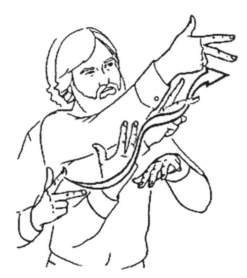

FIGURE 33.3   An example of classifier form use showing a "vehicle" handshape moving upward along a curvy path. (From Hickok, G., et al., *Neuropsychologia, 47*, 382–387, 2009. Reprinted with permission.)

A study of ASL production using a narrative task in 21 unilateral brain injured signers (13 LHD) reported that RHD signers made relatively few lexical errors but a substantial number of classifier errors. LHD signers made both lexical and classifier errors in roughly equal proportions. The source of the classifier errors is not clear. For example, it could be that classifier errors in RHD patients are caused by a fundamentally different deficit (e.g., some nonlinguistic spatial deficit) than those in LHD patients (e.g., linguistic form selection). What is clear is that the production of ASL classifier forms is supported to some extent both by the left and right hemispheres, whereas lexical sign production is under the control of predominantly left hemisphere systems.

HEMISPHERIC ASYMMETRIES FOR SPATIAL COGNITION

It appears that language functions have a similar hemispheric organization in deaf signers compared to hearing/speaking individuals. But what about nonlinguistic spatial functions? Might these abilities be differently organized in the brain of deaf signers? Available evidence suggests that the answer is no and that the lateralization pattern of nonlinguistic spatial functions is also similar between deaf and hearing people.

Gross Visuospatial Deficits in RHD Signers

RHD in hearing people often leads to substantial visuospatial deficits evidenced, in the most severe cases, by grossly distorted productions in drawing tasks and

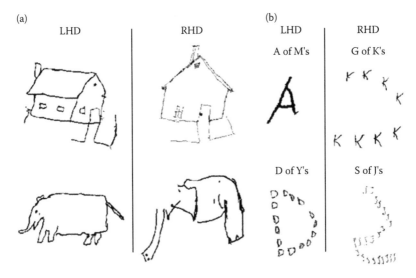

FIGURE 33.4   Example copy-from-sample drawings by LHD and RHD signers. Note that LHD signers are able to reproduce the basic configuration of the figures but may omit details, whereas the RHD signers often fail to reproduce the configural structure but include many details. Evidence of hemispatial neglect is also apparent in the RHD drawings. (From Hickok, G., et al., *Brain and Language, 65*, 276–286, 1998. Reprinted with permission.)

block arrangement tasks (Kirk & Kertesz, 1994). Deaf RHD signers can have similar kinds of deficits (Figure 33.4). Despite sometimes severe nonlinguistic visuospatial impairments, none of the RHD signers had aphasia (Bellugi et al., 1989; Hickok et al., 1998a, 1996a; Poizner et al., 1987).

Local/Global Differences

While gross visuospatial deficits may more commonly occur with RHD (both in deaf and hearing populations), it has been reported that some visuospatial deficits can be reliably observed in LHD hearing individuals (Delis, Kiefner, & Fridlund, 1988; Kirk & Kertesz, 1994). When LHD individuals have visuospatial deficits, they typically involve difficulties in attending to and/or reproducing the local-level details of a visuospatial stimulus, while global-configuration aspects are correctly identified/reproduced. RHD individuals tend to show the opposite pattern. Thus, it has been suggested that the left hemisphere is important for local-level visuospatial processes, whereas the right hemisphere is important for global-level processes (Delis et al., 1988). Does a similar asymmetry hold for the deaf signing population? To answer this question a group of left or right lesioned deaf signers were asked to reproduce: (1) two line drawings (a house and an elephant); and (2) four hierarchical figures (e.g., the letter 'D' composed of small 'Y's). Drawings were scored separately for the presence of local versus global features. Consistent with data from hearing patients, the LHD deaf subjects were significantly better at reproducing global-level features, whereas the RHD deaf subjects were significantly better at reproducing local-level features (Figure 33.4; Hickok, Kirk, & Bellugi, 1998).

Overall, available evidence suggests a similar pattern of hemispheric asymmetries for nonlinguistic spatial cognitive function in the deaf signer population.

WITHIN HEMISPHERE ORGANIZATION

FUNCTIONAL ASPECTS: SYNDROMES AND SYMPTOMS

To the extent that the types and patterns of deficits found in sign language aphasia are similar to those found in spoken language aphasia, it would suggest a common functional organization for the two forms of language. There are many commonalities in individual language deficits found; many of the aphasic symptom clusters that have been observed in LHD deaf signers fall within the bounds of classical clinical syndromes defined on the basis of hearing aphasics (Damasio, 1992; Goodglass, 1993; Goodglass & Kaplan, 1983). For example: (a) nonfluent aphasic signers have lesions involving anterior language regions; and (b) fluent aphasic signers have lesions involving posterior language regions. In addition, the range of common deficit types that have been reported in hearing aphasics have been observed regularly in sign language aphasia. Examples of these include the presence of word (i.e., sign) finding problems in most cases of aphasia, paraphasic errors, agrammatism, and the tendency for comprehension deficits to be more closely associated with fluent aphasia than with nonfluent aphasia. In addition, the brain lesions producing these patterns of deficits in LHD signers are roughly consistent with clinical-anatomic correlations in hearing people (Hickok, 1992; Hickok & Bellugi, 2001; Hickok et al., 1998a; Poizner et al., 1987). To a first approximation, the within hemisphere organization of signed and spoken language appear to be remarkably similar.

ROLE OF BROCA'S AREA

Broca's area has figured prominently in attempts to determine the anatomy of speech production. We had the opportunity to investigate the role of Broca's area in sign language production through an in-depth case study of LHD-130, a congenitally deaf, native user of ASL, who suffered an ischemic infarct involving the frontal operculum and inferior portion of the primary motor cortex (Figure 33.5, top; Hickok et al., 1996b). Acutely, she presented with sign "mutism," consistent with what one might expect in a hearing/speaking individual. Chronically, she had good comprehension, fluent production with occasional sign finding problems, semantic paraphasias, and what appeared to be a deficit involving the ability to control bimanual movements during sign production. That deficit showed up: (a) in her tendency on one-handed signs, to "shadow," with her nondominant

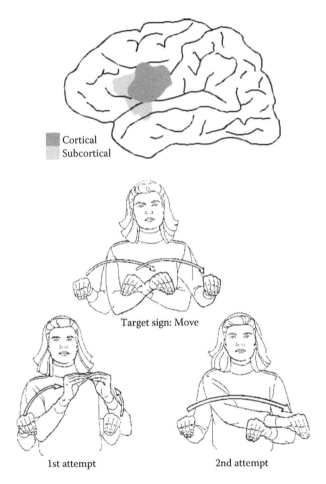

Cortical
Subcortical

Target sign: Move

1st attempt   2nd attempt

FIGURE 33.5 Reconstructed brain lesion in a native deaf signer with damage to Broca's region (top), and an example of her bimanual coordination deficit (bottom). (From Hickok, G., et al., *Neurocase, 2*, 373–380, 1996. Reprinted with permission.)

hand, sign-articulatory gestures carried out by her dominant hand; (b) in her tendency on two-handed signs, to assimilate the handshape and/or movement of the nondominant hand with that of the dominant hand; and (c) in her occasional failure to complete the movement of a two-handed sign when the movement's endpoint involved contact between the two hands (Figure 33.5, bottom). We were not able to find any evidence of a bimanual control deficit in nonlinguistic tasks. Blumstein (1995) has suggested that speech production errors in anterior aphasia reflect a breakdown at the phonetic (not phonemic) level caused by a loss of the ability to coordinate independent speech articulators (e.g., larynx, tongue, lips). For a signer, the two hands are independent articulators that are often required to perform independent (i.e., nonsymmetric) movements. The deficit observed in

LHD-130 may represent the sign analogue of a phonetic-level breakdown. This case suggests that Broca's area plays an important role in sign production.

A CASE OF SIGN BLINDNESS

"Pure Word Blindness" or "Alexia without Agraphia" has been well-documented in the literature (Friedman & Albert, 1985). Hearing/speaking patients with this disorder are typically blind in the right visual field (right homonymous hemianopia), have normal auditory-verbal language capacity, are able to write, but cannot read. The lesion typically involves left occipito-temporal cortex (explaining the visual field defect) and splenium of the corpus callosum. Language areas are thus preserved, allowing normal production, auditory comprehension, and writing, but according to the classical disconnection analysis of the syndrome (Geschwind, 1965), these areas are isolated from visual input (because of cortical blindness in the right visual field and deafferentation of information coming from the left visual field through the splenium). An alternative possibility is that the occipito-temporal lesion damages a visual word form area that directly affects perceptual reading centers (Beversdorf, Ratcliffe, Rhodes, & Reeves, 1997). Either way, one wonders what effects such a lesion would have on sign language comprehension in a deaf signer.

We had the opportunity to study such a case (Hickok et al., 1995). LHD-111 had a lesion involving all of the left primary visual cortex, most of area 18, with some extension into medial aspects of the temporal lobe (area 37); this lesion also clearly involved white matter fibers lateral to the splenium (Figure 33.6, top). Consistent with the neurological effects of such a lesion in hearing subjects, the deaf patient had a right visual field blindness and was alexic (i.e., she couldn't read written English). Her sign language comprehension was profoundly impaired; she could not follow even simple one-step (ASL) commands such as "point to the floor" (Figure 33.6, bottom). Her single-sign comprehension was also significantly impaired although to a lesser extent than her sentence comprehension, and virtually all of her comprehension errors were semantic in nature. Her visual object recognition, however, was unimpaired: she had no problem naming line-drawings of objects presented to her visually. Her sign production was fluent and grammatical, although she did make occasional paraphasic errors. This case provides strong evidence favoring the view that the left hemisphere is dominant for the comprehension of ASL sentences in deaf individuals because it demonstrates that the right hemisphere by itself is severely constrained in its ability to process signed language. However, the case also suggests a more bilateral organization for early stages of processing in single sign recognition in that her comprehension errors seemed to indicate a semantically underspecified representation rather than a disruption of sign phonological information. A similar pattern of bilateral organization at early stages of spoken word recognition has been reported (Hickok & Poeppel, 2000, 2004, 2007). Finally, this case shows a dramatic difference in the within hemisphere organization of signed versus spoken language processing resulting from differences in the input modality between the two language systems.

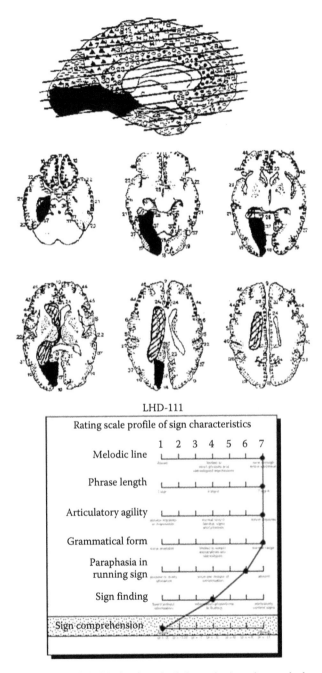

FIGURE 33.6   A left occipital lesion in a deaf signer (top), and a graph showing her rating profile of sign characteristics. Note the patient's production scales are in the normal or near normal range, whereas her sign comprehension is at floor (From Hickok, G., et al., *Neuropsychologia, 33,* 1597–1606, 1995. Reprinted with permission.)

NEUROLOGY OF SIGN COMPREHENSION

Auditory comprehension deficits in aphasia in hearing/speaking individuals are most closely associated with left temporal lobe damage (Bates et al., 2003; Dronkers, Wilkins, Van Valin, Redfern, & Jaeger, 2004). We investigated the relative role of the left versus right temporal lobe in the comprehension of ASL (Hickok et al., 2002). Nineteen life-long signers with unilateral brain lesions (11 LHD, 8 RHD) performed three tasks, an isolated single-sign comprehension task, a sentence-level comprehension task involving one-step commands, and a sentence-level comprehension task involving more complex multiclause/multistep commands. Performance was examined in relation to two factors: whether the lesion was in the right or left hemisphere and whether the temporal lobe was involved or not. The LHD group performed significantly worse than the RHD group on all three tasks confirming left hemisphere dominance for sign language comprehension. The group with left temporal lobe involvement was significantly impaired on all tasks, although minimally so on the single-sign task, whereas the other three groups performed at better than 95% correct on the single sign and simple sentence comprehension tasks, with performance falling off only on the complex sentence comprehension items. A comparison with previously published data (Swisher & Sarno, 1969) suggests that the degree of difficulty exhibited by the deaf RHD group on the complex sentences is comparable to that observed in hearing RHD subjects. This result suggests that language comprehension, particularly at the lexical-semantic and sentence level, depends primarily on the integrity of the left temporal lobe, independent of modality.

DISSOCIATIONS

The functional divisions within the neural systems supporting language and other cognitive abilities have been highlighted by several dissociations observed in deaf signers.

DISSOCIATIONS BETWEEN LINGUISTIC AND NONLINGUISTIC SPATIAL ABILITIES

It was noted above that LHD, but not RHD, frequently produces aphasia in deaf signers whereas RHD, but not LHD, frequently produces gross visuospatial deficits. This pattern of deficits constitutes a double dissociation between sublexical-, lexical-, and sentence-level aspects of spatialized linguistic ability on the one hand, and gross nonlinguistic spatial cognitive ability on the other. Additional dissociations between sign language abilities and nonlinguistic spatial abilities have been demonstrated both within the left hemisphere and within the right hemisphere. Within the left hemisphere we examined the relation between local-level visuospatial deficits evident on a drawing copy task and several measures of sign language ability, including rate of paraphasias in running sign, single sign comprehension, and sentence-level comprehension (Hickok et al., 1998). No significant correlations were found between the hit rate for local features in the drawing copy task and any of the sign language performance measures. In fact, cases were identified in which local-level scores were near perfect, yet scores on tests of sign language ability were among the worst in the sample. This suggests that aphasic deficits cannot be reduced to a more general deficit in local-level visuospatial processing. Within the right hemisphere, two case studies have provided evidence that the ability to use the spatialized referential system in ASL discourse does not depend substantially on nonlinguistic visuospatial abilities of the right hemisphere (Hickok et al., 1999). Case RHD-221 had severe visuospatial deficits following a large right perisylvian stroke, yet was not impaired in his ability to set up and utilize spatial loci for referential purposes. Case RHD-207, showed the reverse pattern. Her performance on standard visuospatial tasks was quite good, yet she had difficulty with spatialized aspects of ASL discourse. This finding hints at the possibility that there are nonidentical neural systems within the right hemisphere supporting spatialized discourse functions versus nonlinguistic spatial abilities.

DISSOCIATIONS BETWEEN SIGN AND GESTURE

Evidence supporting the view that deficits in sign language are qualitatively different from deficits in the ability to produce and understand pantomimic gesture comes from a case study of an LHD signer (Corina et al., 1992). Following an ischemic infarct involving both anterior and posterior perisylvian regions, LHD-108 became aphasic for sign language. His comprehension was poor and his sign production was characterized by frequent paraphasias, reduced grammatical structure, and a tendency to substitute pantomime for ASL signs—a tendency not present prior to his stroke. These pantomimic gestures were used even in cases in which the gesture involved similar or more elaborate sequences of movements arguing against a complexity-based explanation of his performance. LHD-108 showed a similar dissociation in his comprehension of signs versus pantomime where he had more trouble matching a sign to a picture than matching a pantomimed gesture to picture. This case makes the point that disruptions in sign language ability are not merely the result of more general disruptions in the ability to communicate through symbolic gesture. Since this initial report, we have seen several additional patients who show a similar tendency to use gesture in place of lexical signs.

EVIDENCE FROM FUNCTIONAL NEUROIMAGING

Lesion evidence has indicated clearly that hemispheric asymmetries for signed and spoken language are similar, and has provided some indication that the within hemisphere organization of signed language is similar in some ways to that of spoken language, but perhaps different in others. But the spatial resolution of the lesion method is relatively poor, particularly in a rare population, limiting the amount of information one can derive from lesion studies alone. Recent functional imaging studies have provided additional insights into the within hemisphere organization of sign language processing and has highlighted both similarities and differences.

Neural Systems Underlying Signed Language Production

One of the first questions that neuroimaging studies of signed language sought to address was whether Broca's area—a putative *speech* production region—was involved in signed language production. Lesion evidence has suggested it was (see above) but functional imaging promised to shed additional light on the question and further to assess whether the same degree of left lateralization might be found in sign versus speech production. This was an open question because of the bimanual nature of signed language production. Several studies of signed language production have now been published using PET as well as fMRI methodologies (Corina, San Jose-Robertson, Guillemin, High, & Braun, 2003; Emmorey, Mehta, & Grabowski, 2007; Kassubek, Hickok, & Erhard, 2004; McGuire et al., 1997; Pa, Wilson, Pickell, Bellugi, & Hickok, 2008; Petitto et al., 2000). A consistent finding is that indeed Broca's area *is* involved in signed language production, and this activity is strongly left dominant; this is true even when the sign articulation involved one-handed signs produced with the nondominant hand (Corina et al., 2003). Such a result could be interpreted in one of two ways. Either a canonical "speech area," Broca's region, has been recruited to support manual language production in deaf signers, or Broca's area is not a speech-dedicated region. Given that Broca's area has been implicated in a range of nonspeech, even nonlanguage functions in the last several years (Fink et al., 2006; Schubotz & von Cramon, 2004), the latter possibility seems likely. More research is needed to sort out the functional organization of this brain region.

Language production is not merely a function of the frontal lobe. Regions of the posterior temporal lobe also play an important role in speech production (Hickok & Poeppel, 2007; Indefrey & Levelt, 2004). Signed language production also involves nonfrontal structures including some areas in the posterior inferior temporal lobe that appear to be shared with spoken language production (Emmorey et al., 2007). Signed language production also seems to recruit structures in the posterior parietal lobe that are unique to sign (Buchsbaum et al., 2005; Corina et al., 2003; Emmorey et al., 2007). The involvement of these regions may reflect sensory–motor functions that are specific to manual gestures (Buchsbaum et al., 2005; Emmorey et al., 2007).

Neural Systems Underlying Sign Language Perception/Comprehension

A number of studies of signed language perception have found activation of superior temporal regions; that is, regions that are also typically implicated in spoken language perception (Binder et al., 2000; Hickok & Poeppel, 2007). One of the early fMRI studies hinted that sign perception may involve a more bilateral network than processing spoken language (studied via written presentation; Neville et al., 1998), but subsequent work has shown similar lateralization patterns when sign perception is compared to audio-visually presented speech (MacSweeney et al., 2002). There are differences, however, in the within hemisphere activation pattern for the perception of signed and spoken language. Pa et al. (2008) presented ASL nonsigns and English nonwords (forms that are phonotactically permissible in their respective languages but do not correspond to a word) to bilingual hearing signers who had native-level proficiency in both languages (they were hearing offspring of deaf signing adults). This allowed the direct comparison of activation patterns for sign and speech perception within the same individual's brain. Sign perception activated large regions of occipito-temporal cortex, portions of the posterior superior temporal lobe bilaterally, posterior parietal cortex, and posterior frontal regions. Speech perception activated most of the superior temporal lobe and posterior frontal regions. Overlap between the two language forms was found in the posterior superior temporal cortex and in the posterior frontal lobe (Figure 33.7). Thus speech activated auditory-related areas in the superior middle and anterior temporal lobe greater than sign (consistent with the input modality for speech), and sign activated visual-related areas in the ventral occipito-temporal lobe greater than speech (consistent with the input modality for speech). Sign also activated posterior parietal areas whereas speech did not, possibly reflecting visual-manual sensory–motor mechanisms.

One fMRI study attempted to identify regions that are specifically activated during sign perception above and beyond perception of nonlinguistic gestures (MacSweeney et al., 2004). These investigators showed videos of British Sign Language (BSL) or videos of a non–BSL gestural communication system ("TicTac," a gestural code used by racetrack bookmakers) to hearing nonsigners and deaf native signers of BSL. Deaf BSL signers showed greater activation in the left posterior superior temporal sulcus and temporal-parietal boundary during the perception of BSL compared to TicTac. Hearing nonsigners showed no differences in their brain response within this region (although there were differences elsewhere). It is unclear from these findings exactly what this brain region is doing with respect to sign language processing, however, it is interesting that in the study described above a very similar region showed responsivity to both speech and sign in hearing bilingual (English and ASL) signers. This hints that the region supports some type of linguistic specific function.

NEURAL SUBSTRATE FOR WORKING MEMORY FOR SIGNS

The neural basis of sign language working memory is an area that has not received extensive attention, but one that has the potential for shedding light on some fundamental questions regarding short-term memory generally. For example, the nature of the representations maintained in verbal working memory is still open to debate. Some authors argue for sensory–motor based codes

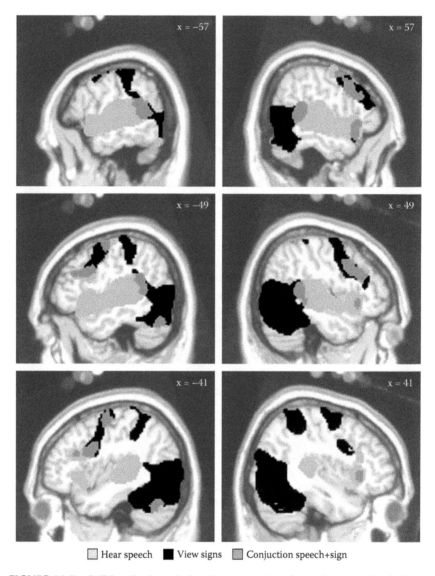

☐ Hear speech   ■ View signs   ▨ Conjuction speech+sign

FIGURE 33.7   fMRI activations during the *perception of speech versus sign* in hearing bilingual (English and ASL) participants. (From Pa, J., et al., *Journal of Cognitive Neuroscience, 20,* 2198–2210, 2008. Reprinted with permission.)

(modality-dependant; Buchsbaum & D'Esposito, 2008; Hickok, Buchsbaum, Humphries, & Muftuler, 2003; Wilson, 2001) while others promote a modality-independent model (Baddeley, 1992; Jones & Macken, 1996). Sign language provides a unique perspective on this issue because it is possible to manipulate the sensory–motor modality, while keeping the linguistic nature of the stimuli effectively constant. One can then ask, is the neural organization of working memory for a acoustic-vocal language different from that for a visual-manual language?

One study examined working memory for sign language in deaf native signers using fMRI (Buchsbaum et al., 2005) and compared its findings to a similar published study involving speech and hearing nonsigner subjects (Hickok et al., 2003). This study used a design with a several second delay period between encoding and recall, which allowed for the measurement of storage-related activity. The pattern of activation during the retention phase was substantially different from what had been found in hearing participants performing a similar task with speech. Short-term maintenance of sign language stimuli produced prominent activations in the posterior parietal lobe, which were not found in the speech study. This parietal activation was interpreted as a reflection of visual–motor integration processes. Posterior parietal regions have been implicated in visual–motor integration in both human and nonhuman primates (Andersen, 1997; Milner & Goodale, 1995), and studies of gesture-imitation in hearing subjects report parietal activation (Chaminade, Meltzoff, & Decety, 2005). It seems likely therefore, that parietal activation in an STM task for sign language does not reflect activity of a sensory store, but instead results from sensory–motor processes underlying the interaction of storage and manual articulatory rehearsal. Additional maintenance activity was found in the posterior superior temporal lobe, as well as in posterior frontal regions, both of which have been shown to activate during maintenance of speech information, suggestive of some form of common process. However, because cross-modality comparisons could only be made between subjects and studies, it is difficult to make solid inferences about patterns of overlap and dissociation. No maintenance activity was found in visual-related areas in that study, such as the ventral temporal–occipital regions that are so strongly activated during sign perception. Activation in these regions would provide more convincing support for sensory-dependent working memory storage systems.

A follow-up study directly compared working memory for signed and spoken language using hearing bilinguals (native in English and ASL; Pa et al., 2008). This study clearly demonstrated sensory modality-specific activity in working memory. Delay activity was found in left ventral occipito-temporal (i.e., visual) areas during sign maintenance but not for speech maintenance, whereas delay activity was found in left superior temporal (i.e., auditory) areas for speech maintenance but not sign maintenance. However, regions of overlap were also noted in both lateral frontal lobe regions as well as a small focus in the posterior superior temporal lobe (Figure 33.8). These findings indicate there may be both modality dependent and modality independent components to working memory for linguistic stimuli.

SUMMARY

The lateralization pattern of neural systems supporting sign language processing are remarkably similar to that found for spoken language. Likewise, the patterns of

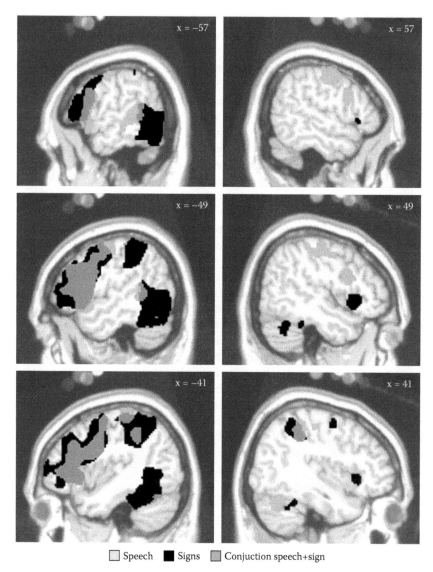

☐ Speech ■ Signs ▨ Conjuction speech+sign

FIGURE 33.8 fMRI activations during the *short-term maintenance of speech versus sign* in hearing bilingual (English and ASL) participants. (From Pa, J., et al., *Journal of Cognitive Neuroscience, 20,* 2198–2210, 2008. Reprinted with permission.)

aphasic deficits found among brain injured deaf signers are quite recognizable in the context of aphasiological research on hearing individuals with acquired language disorders. However, differences in the neural organization of signed and spoken language processing have emerged in recent years. These differences appear to be tied to the unique sensory–motor demands of the two language forms.

REFERENCES

Andersen, R. (1997). Multimodal integration for the representation of space in the posterior parietal cortex. *Philosophical Transactions of the Royal Society of London B: Biological Sciences, 352*, 1421–1428.

Baddeley, A. D. (1992). Working memory. *Science, 255*, 556–559.

Bates, E., Wilson, S. M., Saygin, A. P., Dick, F., Sereno, M. I., Knight, R. T., & Dronkers, N. F. (2003). Voxel-based lesion-symptom mapping. *Nature Neuroscience, 6*(5), 448–450.

Bellugi, U., Poizner, H., & Klima, E. (1989). Language, modality, and the brain. *Trends in Neurosciences, 10*, 380–388.

Beversdorf, D. Q., Ratcliffe, N. R., Rhodes, C. H., & Reeves, A. G. (1997). Pure alexia: Clinical-pathologic evidence for a lateralized visual language association cortex. *Clinical Neuropathology, 16*(6), 328–331.

Binder, J. R., Frost, J. A., Hammeke, T. A., Bellgowan, P. S., Springer, J. A., Kaufman, J. N., & Possing, E. T. (2000). Human temporal lobe activation by speech and non-speech sounds. *Cerebral Cortex, 10*, 512–528.

Blumstein, S. (1995). The neurobiology of the sound structure of language. In M. S. Gazzaniga (Ed.), *The cognitive neurosciences* (pp. 913–929). Cambridge, MA: MIT Press.

Brownell, H. H., Potter, H. H., Bihrle, A. M., & Gardner, H. (1986). Inference deficits in right brain-damaged patients. *Brain and Language, 27*, 310–321.

Buchsbaum, B. R., & D'Esposito, M. (2008). The search for the phonological store: From loop to convolution. *Journal of Cognitive Neuroscience, 20*(5), 762–778.

Buchsbaum, B., Pickell, B., Love, T., Hatrak, M., Bellugi, U., & Hickok, G. (2005). Neural substrates for verbal working memory in deaf signers: fMRI study and lesion case report. *Brain Lang, 95*(2), 265–272.

Campbell, R., & Woll, B. (2003). Space is special in sign. *Trends in Cognitive Sciences, 7*, 5–7.

Chaminade, T., Meltzoff, A. N., & Decety, J. (2005). An fMRI study of imitation: Action representation and body schema. *Neuropsychologia, 43*(1), 115–127.

Corina, D., Poizner, H., Bellugi, U., Feinberg, T., Dowd, D., & O'Grady-Batch, L. (1992). Dissociation between linguistic and non-linguistic gestural systems: A case for compositionality. *Brain and Language, 43*, 414–447.

Corina, D. P., San Jose-Robertson, L., Guillemin, A., High, J., & Braun, A. R. (2003). Language lateralization in a bimanual language. *Journal of Cognitive Neuroscience, 15*(5), 718–730.

Damasio, A. R. (1992). Aphasia. *New England Journal of Medicine, 326*, 531–539.

Delis, D. C., Kiefner, M. G., & Fridlund, A. J. (1988). Visuospatial dysfunction following unilateral brain damage: Dissociations in hierarchical and hemispatial analysis. *Journal of Clinical and Experimental Neuropsychology, 10*, 421–431.

Dronkers, N. F., Wilkins, D. P., Van Valin, Jr., R. D., Redfern, B. B., & Jaeger, J. J. (2004). Lesion analysis of brain regions involved in language comprehension. In *Cognition, 92*(1–2), 145–177. (special issue entitled, " The New Functional Anatomy of Language", eds., G. Hickok & D. Poeppel).

Emmorey, K. (2002). *Language, cognition, and the brain: Insights from sign language research.* Mahwah, NJ: Lawrence Erlbaum and Associates.

Emmorey, K., Damasio, H., McCullough, S., Grabowski, T., Ponto, L. L., Hichwa, R. D., & Bellugi, U. (2002). Neural systems underlying spatial language in American Sign Language. *Neuroimage, 17*(2), 812–824.

Emmorey, K., Mehta, S., & Grabowski, T. J. (2007). The neural correlates of sign versus word production. *Neuroimage, 36*, 202–208.

Fink, G. R., Manjaly, Z. M., Stephan, K. E., Gurd, J. M., Zilles, K., Amunts, K., & Marshal, J. C. (2006). A role for Broca's area beyond language processing: Evidence from neuropsychology and fMRI. In Y. Grodzinsky & K. Amunts (Eds.), *Broca's region* (pp. 254–268). Oxford, UK: Oxford University Press.

Friedman, R. B., & Albert, M. L. (1985). Alexia. In K. M. Heilman & E. Valenstein (Eds.), *Clinical neuropsychology*. New York, NY: Oxford University Press.

Geschwind, N. (1965). Disconnexion syndromes in animals and man. *Brain, 88*, 237–294, 585–644.

Goodglass, H. (1993). *Understanding aphasia*. San Diego, CA: Academic Press.

Goodglass, H., & Kaplan, E. (1983). *The assessment of aphasia and related disorders* (2nd ed.). Philadelphia, PA: Lea & Febiger.

Hickok, G. (1992). *Agrammatic comprehension and the trace-deletion hypothesis* (Occasional Paper 45), Cambridge, MA: MIT Center for Cognitive Science.

Hickok, G., & Bellugi, U. (2001). The signs of aphasia. In R. S. Berndt (Ed.), *Handbook of neuropsychology,* (2nd edition., Vol. 3, pp. 31–50). New York, NY: Elsevier.

Hickok, G., Bellugi, U., & Klima, E. S. (1998a). The neural organization of language: Evidence from sign language aphasia. *Trends in Cognitive Sciences, 2*, 129–136.

Hickok, G., Bellugi, U., & Klima, E. S. (1998b). What's right about the neural organization of sign language? A perspective on recent neuroimaging results. *Trends in Cognitive Science, 2*, 465–468.

Hickok, G., Buchsbaum, B., Humphries, C., & Muftuler, T. (2003). Auditory-motor interaction revealed by fMRI: Speech, music, and working memory in area Spt. *Journal of Cognitive Neuroscience, 15*, 673–682.

Hickok, G., Kirk, K., & Bellugi, U. (1998). Hemispheric organization of local- and global-level visuospatial processes in deaf signers and its relation to sign language aphasia. *Brain and Language, 65*, 276–286.

Hickok, G., Klima, E. S., & Bellugi, U. (1996a). The neurobiology of signed language and its implications for the neural basis of language. *Nature, 381*, 699–702.

Hickok, G., Klima, E., Kritchevsky, M., & Bellugi, U. (1995). A case of "sign blindness" following left occipital damage in a deaf signer. *Neuropsychologia, 33*, 1597–1606.

Hickok, G., Kritchevsky, M., Bellugi, U., & Klima, E. S. (1996b). The role of the left frontal operculum in sign language aphasia. *Neurocase, 2*, 373–380.

Hickok, G., Love-Geffen, T., & Klima, E. S. (2002). Role of the left hemisphere in sign language comprehension. *Brain and Language, 82*, 167–178.

Hickok, G., Pickell, H., Klima, E. S., & Bellugi, U. (2009). Neural dissociation in the production of lexical versus classifiers signs in ASL: Distinct patterns of hemispheric asymmetry. *Neuropsychologia, 47*, 382–387.

Hickok, G., & Poeppel, D. (2000). Towards a functional neuroanatomy of speech perception. *Trends in Cognitive Sciences, 4*, 131–138.

Hickok, G., & Poeppel, D. (2004). Dorsal and ventral streams: A framework for understanding aspects of the functional anatomy of language. *Cognition, 92*, 67–99.

Hickok, G., & Poeppel, D. (2007). The cortical organization of speech processing. *Nature Reviews Neuroscience, 8*(5), 393–402.

Hickok, G., Wilson, M., Clark, K., Klima, E. S., Kritchevsky, M., & Bellugi, U. (1999). Discourse deficits following right hemisphere damage in deaf signers. *Brain and Language, 66*, 233–248.

Hillis, A. E. (2007). Aphasia: Progress in the last quarter of a century. *Neurology, 69*(2), 200–213.

Indefrey, P., & Levelt, W. J. (2004). The spatial and temporal signatures of word production components. *Cognition, 92*(1–2), 101–144.

Jones, D. M., & Macken, W. J. (1996). Irrelevant tones produce an irrelevant speech effect: Implications for phonological coding in working memory. *Journal of Experimental Psychology: Learning, Memory, and Cognition, 19*, 369–381.

Kassubek, J., Hickok, G., & Erhard, P. (2004). Involvement of classical anterior and posterior language areas in sign language production, as investigated by 4 T functional magnetic resonance imaging. *Neuroscience Letters, 364*(3), 168–172.

Kirk, A., & Kertesz, A. (1994). Localization of lesions in constructional impairment. In A. Kertesz (Ed.), *Localization and neuroimaging in neuropsychology* (pp. 525–544). San Diego, CA: Academic Press.

Klima, E., & Bellugi, U. (1979). *The signs of language.* Cambridge, MA: Harvard University Press.

MacSweeney, M., Campbell, R., Woll, B., Giampietro, V., David, A. S., McGuire, P. K., . . . Brammer, M. J. (2004). Dissociating linguistic and nonlinguistic gestural communication in the brain. *Neuroimage, 22*(4), 1605–1618.

MacSweeney, M., Woll, B., Campbell, R., McGuire, P. K., David, A. S., Williams, S. C., . . . Brammer, M. J. (2002). Neural systems underlying British Sign Language and audio-visual English processing in native users. *Brain, 125*(Pt 7), 1583–1593.

McGuire, P. K., Robertson, D., Thacker, A., David, A. S., Kitson, N., Frackowiak, R. S., & Frith, C. D. (1997). Neural correlates of thinking in sign language. *Neuroreport, 8*, 695–698.

Milner, A. D., & Goodale, M. A. (1995). *The visual brain in action.* Oxford, UK: Oxford University Press.

Neville, H., Bavelier, D., Corina, D., Rauschecker, J., Karni, A., Lalwani, A., . . . Turner, R. (1998). Cerebral organization for language in deaf and hearing subjects: Biological constraints and effects of experience. *Proceedings of the National Academy of Sciences, 95*, 922–929.

Neville, H. J., Coffey, S. A., Lawson, D. S., Fischer, A., Emmorey, K., & Bellugi, U. (1997). Neural systems mediating American Sign Language: Effects of sensory experience and age of acquisition. *Brain and Language, 57*, 285–308.

Newport, E., & Meier, R. (1985). The acquisition of American Sign Language. In D. I. Slobin (Ed.), *The crosslinguistic study of language acquisition: Volume 1: The data* (pp. 881–938). Hillsdale, NJ: LEA.

Pa, J., Wilson, S. M., Pickell, B., Bellugi, U., & Hickok, G. (2008). Neural organization of linguistic short-term memory is sensory modality-dependent: Evidence from signed and spoken language. *Journal of Cognitive Neuroscience, 20*, 2198–2210.

Petitto, L. A., Zatorre, R. J., Gauna, K., Nikelski, E. J., Dostie, D., & Evans, A. C. (2000). Speech-like cerebral activity in profoundly deaf people processing signed languages: Implications for the neural basis of human language. *Proceedings of the National Academy of Sciences, 97*(25), 13961–13966.

Pickell, H., Klima, E., Love, T., Kritchevsky, M., Bellugi, U., & Hickok, G. (2005). Sign language aphasia following right hemisphere damage in a left-hander: A case of reversed cerebral dominance in a deaf signer? *Neurocase, 11*(3), 194–203.

Poizner, H., Klima, E. S., & Bellugi, U. (1987). *What the hands reveal about the brain.* Cambridge, MA: MIT Press.

Schubotz, R. I., & von Cramon, D. Y. (2004). Sequences of abstract nonbiological stimuli share ventral premotor cortex with action observation and imagery. *Journal of Neuroscience, 24*(24), 5467–5474.

Swisher, L. P., & Sarno, M. T. (1969). Token Test scores of three matched patient groups: Left brain-damaged with aphasia, right brain-damaged without aphasia, non-brain damaged. *Cortex, 5*, 264–273.

Tallal, P., Miller, S., & Fitch, R. H. (1993). Neurobiological basis of speech: A case for the preeminence of temporal processing. *Annals of the New York Academy of Sciences, 682*, 27–47.

Wapner, W., Hamby, S., & Gardner, H. 1981. The role of the right hemisphere in the apprehension of complex linguistic materials. *Brain and Language, 14*, 15–33.

Wilson, M. (2001). The case for sensorimotor coding in working memory. *Psychonomic Bulletin & Review, 8*, 44–57.

34 Sign Languages and Sign Language Research

Myriam Vermeerbergen and
Mieke Van Herreweghe

THE LINGUISTIC STATUS OF SIGN LANGUAGES

In the past, sign languages were generally ignored, not only in mainstream society, but also in linguistic research. The main reason for this indifference was that sign languages were not considered to be genuine natural languages. Before the start of modern sign linguistics, it was often assumed that all deaf people across the world used a kind of universal, primitive system of gestures and pantomime. At the same time, many people seemed (and some still seem) to believe that "sign language" is nothing but a word for word transliteration of the local spoken language in which the signs are produced simultaneously with the spoken (content) words. Neither assumption is correct and these false beliefs only gradually started to change after the publication of the book *Sign Language Structure* by the American linguist William Stokoe in 1960. One of the effects of the publication was that interest into sign linguistics was steadily aroused, and today, even though still not all linguists and nonlinguists are equally convinced of the linguistic status of sign languages, linguistic research into sign languages has conquered a solid position in various linguistic subdisciplines. Among other things, Stokoe maintained in this book that the signs used in American Sign Language (or ASL) should not be considered unanalyzable wholes but should be regarded as consisting of various smaller meaning-distinguishing component parts. As such he was the first to show that a sign language exhibits *duality of patterning*, exactly as is the case for spoken languages.[*] ASL could be considered a genuine human language as in mainstream linguistics duality of patterning is considered to be a:

> defining property of human language, which sees language as structurally organized into two abstract levels; also called double articulation. At one level, language is analysed into combinations of meaningful units (such as words and sentences); at the other level, it is analysed as a sequence of phonological segments which lack meaning. (Crystal, 1999, p. 94)

---

[*] However, the focus on duality of patterning in sign languages only started later (Padden, 1988b; Siple, 1982).

Stokoe's (1960) first modern linguistic analysis of a sign language[*] received a great deal of attention and particularly during the 1970s, other researchers began to express an interest in the linguistic structure of signs and sign languages, first mainly in the USA, and from the 1980s onward also in other countries. This has led to detailed analyses of ASL and other sign languages in various linguistic domains. Providing a survey of all of this research lies outside the scope of this paper, but to give some idea, attention has been paid to various aspects in phonetics/phonology (Loncke, 1983 and Demey, 2005 for Flemish Sign Language; Van der Kooij, 2002 and Crasborn, 2001 for Sign Language of the Netherlands), morphology (Bergman, 1983 for Swedish Sign Language; Pizzuto, 1986 for Italian Sign Language; Engberg-Pedersen, 1993 for Danish Sign Language; Brennan, 1990 for British Sign Language), syntax (Deuchar, 1984 for British Sign Language; Vermeerbergen, 1996 and 1997 for Flemish Sign Language; Rissanen, 1986 for Finnish Sign Language), and lexicography/lexicology (Johnston, 1989 for Australian Sign Language; De Weerdt, Vanhecke, Van Herreweghe, & Vermeerbergen for Flemish Sign Language, 2003), and so on.[†]

Early modern sign linguistics often emphasized the differences between sign languages. Publications from the 1970s and 1980s regularly begin by stating that there is not one universal sign language but instead many different, mutually unintelligible sign languages.[‡] At that time, cross-linguistic sign language studies were rare and the limited amount of comparative research mainly concentrated on the lexicon, more specifically on signs belonging to the established lexicon. Toward and in the 1990s, there was an increase in the number of sign languages being studied (although this evolution remained mostly limited to North America, Australia, and Western Europe). Johnston (1989, p. 208) noted in his doctoral dissertation on Auslan or ASL:

> Overall, fragmentary studies of parts of the grammar of a number of natural sign languages do nonetheless contribute to an impression of shared syntactic patterning across sign languages. The lexical diversity among sign languages—long established and recognised—remains a valid observation. Only now, as studies such as the present are being made of other sign languages, is the degree of commonality among sign languages on the grammatical level coming to light.

Apart from such *explicit* references to the similarities between the grammars of different sign languages, it seemed to be common practice for researchers to compare their own interpretation of a specific grammatical mechanism in sign

---

[*] In fact, Stokoe was not the first to study a sign language. In 1953 the Dutch linguist Tervoort had presented a doctoral dissertation on the use of signs by deaf children, but his work remained largely unknown for quite some time, and what's more, he didn't present his work as research on a "sign language" but talked about an "esoteric language" of deaf children.

[†] For a fuller bibliography we would like to refer the reader to the International Bibliography of Sign Language at http://www.sign-lang.uni-hamburg.de/bibweb/Bibliography.html

[‡] Woll (2003, p. 20) mentions the following studies: Baker & Cokely, 1980; Fischer, 1974; Klima & Bellugi, 1979; Kyle & Woll, 1985; Lane, 1977; Stokoe, 1972.

language A to the interpretation of another researcher studying the same mecha-nism in sign language B as if both researchers were dealing with one and the same language—or at least with one and the same mechanism across the sign languages (e.g., Van Herreweghe, 1995). From this, it seemed that a high degree of similarity was at least implicitly assumed. And indeed, the overall picture one obtains from the body of sign language literature available at that time was that sign languages are typologically more similar than spoken languages.

However, with the increasing number of cross-linguistic analyses and typolog-ical studies and the addition of previously unstudied or understudied languages the field has moved on again. Some of the current cross-linguistic studies seem to confirm the high degree of similarity between sign languages (which may lead scholars to comment on this issue, e.g., Liddell, Vogt-Svendsen, & Bergman, 2007) whereas other studies, often involving more "exotic" sign languages (e.g., Nyst, 2007), seem to point at more variation than previously assumed. There is clearly a need for much more comparative work—and for yet more sign languages to be documented—before more conclusive answers can be given. Nevertheless, the similarities that were found between different sign languages have been attrib-uted to a number of different reasons, both internally linguistic and sociolinguis-tic. Johnston (1989, p. 211) discusses

> four major constraints on grammatical organization to show how they variously contribute to produce particular characteristics of Auslan and other sign languages. The four constraints are: (1) the visual-gestural nature of sign languages, (2) the absence of a written form for sign languages, (3) the unique contact features of sign languages and their host languages, and (4) the patterns of acquisition of sign languages by their speakers.

Woll (2003, p. 25) adds a number of mutually compatible and to some extent overlapping reasons of which (a) iconicity and (b) a link between sign languages and gesture are most relevant here.

Since these characteristics seem to be defining factors for many (or maybe even all?) sign languages, we shall briefly discuss them in the following section.

SOME SALIENT CHARACTERISTICS OF SIGN LANGUAGES

A VISUAL–GESTURAL MODALITY

Sign languages make use of the visual–gestural modality and this opens up struc-tural possibilities that are not—or to a (much) lesser extent—available for spoken languages, which are oral–aural languages. These possibilities are: (1) the use of three dimensional space for linguistic expression; and (2) the availability of a range of articulators, including both hands and arms, the torso, the mouth and the eyes, as well as other parts of the face. As a result, rather than showing a primarily linear patterning similar to that of spoken languages, sign languages

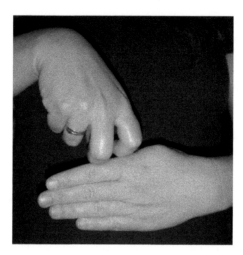

FIGURE 34.1 "Classifier construction" in VGT referring to a cat sitting on a fence.

exhibit a highly simultaneous organization.* In the VGT-utterance the construction illustrated in Figure 34.1. Is taken from, the signer expresses the actions of a cat sitting on a fence looking from left to right. The dominant hand refers to the figure (the cat) while the nondominant hand represents the ground (the fence). The way these manual articulators are positioned in signing space is meaningful; the spatial arrangement not only reflects the locative relation between figure and ground but also expresses the position of the fence relative to other parts of the scene (e.g., the house from which the narrator witnesses the event).† In order to further refer to the cat's activities and emotional state the signer moves her head and uses her eye-gaze and facial expressions, which results in an even higher level of simultaneous organization.

The utterance discussed here is an example of *multichannel simultaneity involving nonmanual articulators other than the mouth*. This type of simultaneity is often related to the simultaneous expression of different elements of a multifaceted event or to the simultaneous expression of different points of view (Leeson & Saeed, 2007; Perniss, 2007; Sallandre, 2007). It can also occur with nonmanual sentence type marking; in order to "transfer" a positive declarative sentence into a negative one, users of a wide range of sign languages may simply combine the manual part of the sentence (in the same word—or sign—order)

---

* We want to point out here that with regard to the linear/sequential versus simultaneous organization the difference between sign languages and spoken languages is one of degree: spoken languages too show simultaneous patterning, for example, tones in tone languages and intonation in other languages. More recently co-speech gesture is also increasingly considered to be an integrated part of spoken language communication. And of course, not all elements of a signed utterance are produced at the same time.

† The locative relation between the cat and the fence is expressed by the position of the hands with respect to each other, while the relation between the fence and the house is expressed by the position of the hands with respect to the body of the signer (and this is not clearly visible on the photograph: the hands are in a horizontal plane on the left side of the signer).

with a headshake. Furthermore, the same utterance can become a (negative) polar question by adding a nonmanual marker to the same sequence of signs. The non-manual marker typically consists of "a combination of several features, including raised eyebrows, wide open eyes, eye contact with the addressee, and a forward head and/or body position" (Zeshan, 2006b, p. 40).

Many examples of simultaneity described in the literature involve *manual simultaneity* where each hand is used to convey different information. This may take the form of one hand holding a sign in a stationary configuration while the other hand produces one or more other signs. In an example from Flemish Sign Language, the signer narrates a scene from an animated movie. The signer first explains that the two main characters are driving in one car and are being followed by two men in a second car. The final sign in this utterance is FOLLOW, which is produced with two "fist-with-thumb-up" hand configurations, each representing one car. After the production of this sign, one hand remains in place, still showing the "fist-with-thumb-up" configuration, while the dominant hand produces the following signs:[*]

EXAMPLE 34.1

Right hand: FOLLOW // Ps KNOW NOTHING BEHIND FOLLOW // Ps STOP
Left hand:　FOLLOW_____

"They (i.e., the men in the first car) don't know they are being followed. They stop."

Thus the sign FOLLOW is "held" by the left hand, while the other hand continues to sign the rest of the story (Vermeerbergen & Demey, 2007, p. 269).

Examples as the one above contrast with cases of "full manual simultaneity"; that is the simultaneous production of two different full lexical items. With full manual simultaneity, one of the two signs that are simultaneously produced often shows a relatively simple form, for example, a pointing sign (PS) or a numeral (handshape). In the following example, again taken from Flemish Sign Language, the sign simultaneously produced by the nondominant hand is a Ps directed toward a locus previously associated with a specific boy (Vermeerbergen & Demey, 2007, p. 270):

EXAMPLE 34.2

Right hand: GRAND^PARENTS　DEAF　　GRAND^PARENTS
Left hand:　　　　　　　　　　　Ps_____

"His grandparents are deaf." or "He has deaf grandparents."

---

[*] Manual signs are represented here as English "glosses": words (more or less closely) representing the meaning of the sign. Pointing signs are glossed "Ps." The lengthened production of a sign is indicates by a line following its gloss. // indicate a clause boundary.

Finally, *manual–oral simultaneity* occurs when the oral and manual channels are used at the same time, for example, when a manual sign is combined with the (silent) production of a spoken word (so-called mouthings, see also further down). Often the meaning of the mouthing and the manual sign is related, for example, when a signer signs SIT and produces the mouthing "sit", but in some cases the mouthing is combined with a sign that is morphologically and/or lexically unrelated, for example, when a Flemish signer produces SIT and simultaneously (silently) articulates the Dutch word "op" (on) resulting in the meaning "sit on". Other examples of manual–oral simultaneity involve "mouth gestures": activities of the mouth that are unrelated to spoken languages, such as the use of a fff-sound when manually signing the meaning "fill-with-water-from-tap" (Vermeerbergen & Demey, 2007, p. 261).*

With regard to the use of space in sign languages, it should be noted that space is not only used to convey spatial information, for example, to express the locative relationship between different referents as in Figure 34.1, but also to encode grammatical information. In most—if not all—of the sign languages described so far, space is used as a medium to express agreement with a certain group of verbs. In order to indicate the relationship between the verb and its argument(s), the signer may alter the movement, orientation or place of articulation of the verb with respect to the location of the argument(s). An example of a spatially modified verb in Flemish Sign Language is the verb sign INVITE. The production of this sign always involves a linear horizontal movement of the hand, but the signer can relocate the beginning and end points of the movement. If the arguments of the verb are actually present, the movement begins close to (or in the direction of) the body of the "invited referent" and the end point relates to the actual location of the "inviting referent." If a referent is not present, the signer may decide to establish a "locus"; that is, s/he may relate the nonpresent referent to a certain area in space. In order to talk about her nonpresent colleague, for example, a signer can produce the signs MY and COLLEAGUE and consequently point at a certain area or "locus" in signing space. This area now "represents" the colleague. The choice of a locus is often motivated, for example, when that particular colleague was in the room before, the signer will most probably choose a locus in relation to the place where s/he was actually standing, sitting, ... while s/he was present. Or the locus is related to his/her now empty chair/desk/office. After having established the loci for two referents, for example, "colleague" and "son," INVITE can be produced with a movement away from the locus for "son" and toward the locus for "colleague," meaning "the/my colleague invited his/her son" (or: "the son was invited by my colleague"). Loci can also be pointed at by means of a PS sign, for example, for the purpose of anaphoric reference, another example of nonlocative use of signing space.

---

* We would like to refer the reader to Vermeerbergen, Leeson, and Crasborn (2007a) for a recent collection of papers dealing with different aspects of simultaneity across a wide range of sign languages.

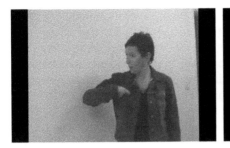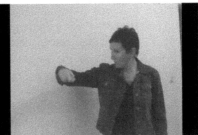

FIGURE 34.2   VGT-sentence meaning "Don't/Didn't you invite me?"

The example shown in Figure 34.2 from Flemish Sign Language illustrates both the use of space and the simultaneous use of a range of manual and nonmanual articulators. The sentence contains only one single manual sign: the verb sign INVITE, but its spatial configuration results in the "incorporation" of the patient "I/me" and the agent "You": "you invite me" (or: "I am invited by you"). The manual production is combined with a headshake to add a negative reading and there is also nonmanual polar question marking (see Figure 34.2). This whole combination results in the expression of the utterance "Don't/Didn't you invite me?"

AN ATYPICAL ACQUISITION PROCESS

In most Western countries it is maintained that 90–95% of deaf children have hearing parents (Schein, 1989), so that only 5–10% of deaf children have deaf parents and are as such potential "native signers." The majority of deaf children are born to hearing parents who are not likely to know any sign language. Most of these children start acquiring the local sign language only when beginning (pre) school. In some (Western) countries this can be quite early in life, for example, in Flanders, Belgium normally at the age of 2; 6 (i.e. 2 years and 6 months),* but in other countries the first contact with (a form of) the local sign language is sometimes much later, for example, in South Africa some (mainly black) children occasionally only start attending school at age 11 or 12 (Van Herreweghe & Vermeerbergen, 2010, p.129), either because their deafness was only detected later and/or because schooling is not deemed important by or simply not possible for the parents. Sometimes such children develop a form of what is called "home signing" in the literature, which is a form of gestural communication "invented" by deaf children, together with one or more of their hearing relatives, when these children are not able to spontaneously acquire a spoken language and at the same time are not exposed to a conventional sign language (Goldin-Meadow, 2003; Mylander & Goldin-Meadow, 1991).† It is possible that these early home sign systems have a certain influence on an individual's later sign language acquisition

---

* And thanks to early intervention programs contact with the local sign language can be even earlier.
† When at a later age there is still no or insufficiently accessible linguistic input these home sign systems continue to develop and become "emerging sign languages" (Fusellier-Souza, 2004, 2006).

and usage, and also on the language itself. Especially in deaf communities where a good number of the signers have gone through a similar pattern of development and where many of them did not come into contact with the conventional sign language until later in life, the impact of home sign systems on the community sign language may be far-reaching. Following Labov's "Uniformitarian Principle" (Labov, 1972), what happens now may have happened in the past as well. It may well be that for sign languages such as Flemish Sign Language or ASL, which are used in a community in which today (most) deaf children have access to an adequate language model relatively early in life (so that the use of home sign systems may be more limited, at least in length of time), there once was a time when there was more home signing and possibly also more contact between home sign systems and the community sign language. Hence the structure of the sign language as we know it today, may have been influenced by home sign systems in the past. It will be clear to the reader that many questions regarding the impact of home sign systems on the structure of sign languages remain to be explored, including questions related to the significance of home signing in communities where usable language models are available relatively early in the lives of deaf children.

Moreover, because of the atypical acquisition process, schools for the deaf, especially if they are residential schools, play an important role in the development of sign languages. In most countries sign languages are still not widely used as a medium of instruction in deaf education. Until recently, in may cases the language of instruction in the deaf classroom was, and often still is, not a sign language but a spoken language (possibly in its written form) and/or a "signed spoken language"; that is, a (simplified form of the) spoken language combined with signs (Loncke, 1990). This is also known as "sign supported speech" or "simultaneous communication," but does not reflect the typical spatial and simultaneous characteristics of fully fledged sign languages. Consequently in the (residential) deaf schools, significant deaf peers function as linguistic role models rather than significant hearing adults. Nevertheless, in the last decade(s) there have been important changes in this respect. On the one hand, in some (residential) deaf schools there has been a movement toward bilingual–bicultural education with more and more deaf adults being active in deaf education and as such also functioning as linguistic role models. At the same time, especially in Western countries, there has been a movement toward mainstream education, so that deaf adults/peers are not or no longer present as linguistic role models in the lives of many young deaf mainstreamed pupils, especially in those countries where the degree of cochlear implantation is high. In the latter countries in particular, many deaf adults are concerned about the survival of their deaf communities (Johnston, 2004).

THE UNIQUE CONTACT FEATURES WITH THE SURROUNDING SPOKEN LANGUAGE

One of the factors by which all sign languages seem to be influenced is/are the surrounding spoken language(s), especially in their written form. Since sign languages have only recently begun to be written down, there is no tradition of literacy in any sign language to date. That means that

> literacy in any signing community is, strictly speaking, always literacy of another language (usually the host spoken language) rather than knowledge of a written form of sign. It is possible for this knowledge of the host spoken language to interfere with and influence the sign language of the community lexically and grammatically. (Johnston, 1989, p. 234)

This also means that sign languages and spoken languages have a different function: the sign language will be the preferred language for face-to-face communication with other signers, whereas the spoken language will mostly be used in written forms of communication and in interactions with hearing people, since most hearing people do not sign and interpreters are not always available. Moreover, sign languages are not as prestigious as spoken languages. The result is a situation of diglossia with the surrounding spoken language(s) as the "high language(s)" and the sign language as the "low language," since many people— both deaf and hearing—do not consider sign languages as bona fide languages to be used in society, but as a form of in-crowd code. Signers' knowledge and use of (the written form of) a spoken language may leave its mark on their sign language:

> For example, in Flanders, the northern part of Belgium, the influence from spoken Dutch can be seen in the lexicon and possibly also the grammar of VGT (Vlaamse Gebarentaal or Flemish Sign Language; cf. Van Herreweghe & Vermeerbergen, 2004; Vermeerbergen, 2006). One example from the lexicon is the parallelism between Dutch compounds and VGT compounds; often Dutch compounds such as *schoonbroer* (meaning *brother-in-law* but in fact a compound consisting of *beautiful* and *brother*) are also compounds in VGT consisting of the same component parts (SCHOON^BROER). [...] It should be noted here that the influence from a spoken language on a signed language may be the result of "direct import" from the oral language (i.e., the language in its spoken/written form), or may be related to the knowledge and use of a signed spoken language (i.e., the "signed version" of the spoken language). (Akach, Demey, Matabane, Van Herreweghe, & Vermeerbergen, 2009, p. 337)

Other direct influences from the surrounding spoken language can be seen in finger spelling (which constitutes direct borrowing from the spoken language into the sign language) and the fact that a sign, especially a sign from the established or "frozen" lexicon, can be accompanied by a "mouthing" that refers to a mouth pattern derived from the equivalent word in the surrounding spoken language (Boyes Braem & Sutton-Spence, 2001). As already mentioned, mouthing leads to manual–oral simultaneity. However, mouthing can sometimes be misleading, in that people seem to think that the lexical properties of the spoken word are automatically transferred to the lexical properties of the sign. Needless to say that this is not necessarily the case. A clear example is the verb "to have" in Dutch that can be used as a full lexical verb with a possessive meaning, but also as an auxiliary of aspect. In Flemish Sign Language the equivalent verb, usually glossed as HAS and with the mouthing "heeft" (= "has"), can also be used as a full lexical verb of possession (and of existence) but not as an aspectual auxiliary.

SIGN LANGUAGES AS ORAL OR FACE-TO-FACE LANGUAGES

Sign languages are in essence "oral" or "face-to-face" languages and as such they are more comparable to spoken languages in nonliterate communities than to spoken languages with a tradition of literacy. One of the characteristics that sign language communities have in common with nonliterate spoken language communities is that "they have a much wider and tolerant concept of acceptability that takes into account innovation and improvisation with no clear idea of 'right' or 'wrong' or even of what is 'grammatical' in sign language" (Johnston, 1989, p. 232). This lack of codification and the fact that these oral tradition languages are not used in education seem to have led to more variation and a greater instability in the lexicon and maybe also in the grammar "and there is no reason why the characteristics known to result from the lack of a written form in spoken languages should not be there for sign languages" (Vermeerbergen, 2006, p. 179). The influence of a "strictly oral tradition" on language structure has been well documented (Ong, 1982; Givón, 1979). Johnston (1989, p. 233) gives the following example:

> In particular, both parataxis and topicalization seem to be strongly encouraged by the face to face, unplanned nature of communications in sign language which are always rooted in a shared communicative context between signer and addressee (e.g., Ochs, 1979). Topic-prominence can thus be seen to stem from both (a) conversational face to face discourse patterning of oral cultures and (b) the need to locate in space the agreement point[...].

ICONICITY

Another intrinsically linguistic characteristic that all sign languages have in common is iconicity that can be found at different levels of linguistic organization. Taub defines "pure iconicity" as follows:

> Let me give a strict definition of those items which I consider purely iconic. In iconic items, some aspect of the item's physical form (shape, sound, temporal structure, etc.) resembles a concrete sensory image. That is, a linguistic item that involves only iconicity can represent only a concrete, physical referent (...). Thus, ASL tree (...), whose form resembles the shape of a prototypical tree, is purely iconic: Its form directly resembles its meaning. (Taub, 2001, pp. 20–21)

In sign languages iconicity is far more pervasive than in spoken languages since "objects in the external world tend to have more visual than auditory associations.

Many entities and actions have salient visual characteristics. It is difficult [...] to imagine any characteristic sounds that might be associated with any of these meanings" (Deuchar, 1984, p. 12). Still, iconicity does not lead to complete transparency and thus to complete similarity between sign languages in the world, since also culture, conventionalization, and conceptualization need to be taken into account. In certain sign languages, WATER is signed by means of a sign referring to the sea, in other sign languages the sign refers to a tap, in yet other sign languages, the sign mirrors a drinking action. All these signs can be considered iconic, yet they are clearly different from each other:

> Iconicity is not an objective relationship between image and referent; rather, it is a relationship between our mental models of image and referent. These models are partially motivated by our embodied experiences common to all humans and partially by our experiences in particular cultures and societies. (Taub, 2001, pp. 19–20)

One of the central questions in sign phonology today is whether iconicity plays a part in the linguistic structure of sign languages. Put more simply: *Do sublexical elements carry meaning?* This is an important question with respect to the phonological or morphological status of sublexical elements (i.e., the elements signs are composed of). Traditionally sublexical elements have been characterized in terms of place of articulation, movement, handshape, and orientation and as such they have been identified as phonemes (i.e., meaningless elements). However, take for instance the handshape featuring an extended index-finger (the handshape often used to point at things), with the finger pointing upward. In some signs, for example, MEET in Flemish Sign Language and a number of other sign languages, the form of this handshape can be associated with an upright person and as such it can be said to carry meaning. A second, related, question is: when signers use the handshape just mentioned as part of a sign (e.g., MEET in Flemish Sign Language), are they aware of the form-meaning association? Do they only use this handshape to refer to one upright person and not to a bent one for instance, or to two people meeting two other people, or is this irrelevant? If sublexical elements do carry meaning that conflicts with the idea that signs—like words—are composed of phonemes (i.e., meaningless but meaning-distinguishing sublexical elements) and as such with duality of patterning (see the first section of this chapter). Demey (2005) tries to resolve this enigma by proposing that the sublexical form elements have potential meaningfulness, but this meaningfulness need not be accessed. The sign language user has the possibility to step into

> an iconic superstructure that can remotivate the sublexical form-meaning relations. This superstructure offers the language user the possibility—either productively or receptively—to relate a phonetic form element directly with a meaning. Nevertheless, as stated before, the *potential* meaningfulness of sublexical form elements does not indicate a modality difference between sign languages and spoken languages. Iconic—or otherwise motivated—relations between form and meaning can be found in both signed and spoken languages. However, the enormous potentiality of the

visual-gestural signal for iconic motivation, and specifically for image iconicity, is a modality consequence. (Demey, Van Herreweghe, & Vermeerbergen, 2008, p. 212)

Iconicity is an undeniable characteristic of sign languages, present at all levels of organization. Iconicity does also exist in spoken languages. It cannot only be found in onomatopoeia, but also in intonation, in sound symbolism, and so on. The two modalities (sign and speech) "do not produce differences in kind, but only in degree" (Demey et al., 2008, p.212).

A Link Between Sign Languages and Gesture?

Because in the early stages of sign linguistic research the linguistic status of sign languages was emphasized, attention for the presence of gesture in sign language usage was obscured. However, in the last decade that has clearly changed. Some of the more recent analyses seem to provide support for a model of sign language structure that incorporates both linguistic and gestural elements (e.g., Liddell, 2003a; Schembri, 2001; Schembri, Jones, & Burnham, 2005; Vermeerbergen & Demey, 2007, among others). From our own cross-linguistic study of aspects of the grammar of Flemish Sign Language and South African Sign Language (Vermeerbergen, Van Herreweghe, Akach, & Matabane, 2007b; Van Herreweghe & Vermeerbergen, 2008) it has become clear that a different choice of data can lead to very different results. Narratives resulting from a description of picture stories are a completely different set of data when compared to elicited sentences produced in isolation. "Visual imagery" for instance, is much more prominent in the narratives than in the isolated sentences and it is exactly in the domain of visual imagery that there is overlap with gesture. A clear example is "constructed action"; that is, the narrator's construction of another person's actions (Metzger, 1995), which seems to be similar in sign languages and in gesture (Liddell & Metzger, 1998). As part of the study just mentioned both a Flemish signer and a South African signer use constructed action to personify a pigeon which comfortably sits down on a nest with three eggs to start brooding. This construction is similar in both signed stories. However, the exact nature of the link between gesture and sign languages needs to be explored further.

TWO IMPORTANT DEVELOPMENTS IN SIGN LINGUISTICS[*]

Moving Away From a Description of Sign Languages as Essentially Analogous to Spoken Languages

The early days of modern sign linguistics showed the desire to emphasize the equivalence of the linguistic status of sign languages and spoken languages. Characteristics that seem to be more typical of sign languages were often ignored, minimized, or interpreted as being comparable to certain spoken language

---

[*] Obviously the picture of the development of sign language research sketched in this chapter is very much simplified and generalized.

mechanisms (see e.g., Johnston, 1989, for a discussion of the minimization of the importance of iconicity). Moreover, the theories, categories, terminology, and so on, developed and used for spoken language research were considered appropriate for the analysis and description of sign languages as well.[*] Since the 1990s, in part because the status of sign languages has become established, there is a growing interest in the properties typical of (although not always unique to) sign languages. It is also less taken for granted that spoken language research tools automatically "fit" sign language research. This evolution will be briefly illustrated here with regard to: (1) the use of space in verb agreement; and (2) the analysis of classifiers and classifier constructions (see also Vermeerbergen, 2006).

The Use of Space in Verb Agreement

As already explained, in many sign languages the form of certain verb signs may be adapted in order to spatially refer to one or more of the arguments of the verb, whether they are present or nonpresent referents. For nonpresent referents, signers may establish loci, which can also be used for pronominal reference.

In the (earlier) literature (especially on ASL, e.g., Padden, 1988a; Poizner, Klima, & Bellugi, 1987), the use of space in such spatialized grammatical mechanisms is differentiated from "spatial mapping techniques." The latter are said to occur in "topographical space," in which very detailed representations of locative relations can be visualized. The "syntactic space" on the other hand is used to express syntactic or semantic nonlocative information mostly through the use of loci. A locus in this type of space is described as an "arbitrary, abstract point" in space "referring" to a certain referent, but its actual location in signing space is considered to be irrelevant. In the 1970s and 1980s we generally see similar interpretations of the use of syntactic space for agreement verbs (also called "inflecting verbs") and—in connection with this—the use of loci. These interpretations are expressed in grammatical terminology that is regarded as analogous to "agreement" in spoken language, for example, morpheme, cliticization, pronoun, agreement in person and number, and so forth.

In the 1990s the clear-cut distinction between "spatial mapping" and "spatialized syntax" is being questioned [e.g., Bos (1990) for Sign Language of the Netherlands, Johnston (1991) for Australian Sign Language, Engberg-Pedersen (1993) for Danish Sign Language and Vermeerbergen (1998) for Flemish Sign Language]:

> It is argued that the spatialised representation is, for at least part of the syntactical mechanisms, not based on "abstract linguistic properties" (Poizner et al., 1987, p. 211) but on the inherent locative relationships among real world people, objects and places. At the same time Engberg-Pedersen (1993) and Liddell (1990) challenge the interpretation of a locus as an arbitrary, abstract point in space. They argue that instead a locus should be seen as a "referent projection" (Engberg-Pedersen, 1993, p. 18) or as being based on the real-world location and extension of imagined referents (Liddell, 1990). (Vermeerbergen, 2006, p. 176)

---

[*] It may be pointed out that, however, in his 1960 book on ASL, Stokoe did propose some sign language specific terminology such as chereme and cherology instead of phoneme and phonology. However, his attempt did not meet with much approval.

Liddell (2003a) moves even further on this path and considers the directionality in ASL verb signs such as GIVE[*] to be gestural in nature. He analyses these spatially modified signs as being composed of a linguistic part, expressed by the handshape, type of movement and certain aspects of the hand's orientation, and a gestural part relating the sign to a locus. (Vermeerbergen, 2006, pp. 176–177). Agreement verbs (or indicating verbs as Liddell calls them) are thus considered to be heterogeneous elements, partly linguistic and partly gestural.

The Analysis of Classifiers and Classifier Constructions

In many sign languages, signers may "represent" referents by means of a handshape or a combination of a handshape and a specific orientation of the hand. This is illustrated in Figure 34.1 in this chapter, where one hand refers to a (sitting) cat and the other hand to a fence. Such handshapes are generally called "classifiers", a notion introduced in the sign language literature by Frishberg (1975) in a paper on historical change in ASL. As can be seen from the example in this chapter, aspects of the form or dimensions of the referent (usually) play an important part in the choice of a certain (classifier) handshape. In some earlier descriptions (e.g., McDonald, 1982; Supalla, 1978), sign languages are compared to predicate classifier languages, such as the Athapaskan languages, which represent one of the four types in Allan's (1977) typology of spoken classifier languages (Engberg-Pedersen, 1993). This parallel between classifiers and classifier constructions in sign languages on the one hand and classificatory verbs in Athapaskan languages, especially in Navaho, on the other hand, often quoted in (earlier) sign language publications, was (later) shown to be problematic (Engberg-Pedersen, 1993; Schembri, 2003). This, among other reasons, has led a number of sign linguists to argue against an analysis of the handshape in these so-called classifier constructions as classifiers (see Schembri, 2003, for an elaborate discussion of this issue). The idea that all component parts of these constructions are discrete, listable, and specified in the grammar of individual sign languages, each having morphemic status (e.g., Supalla, 1982) has also been questioned.[†] Some sign linguists consider the possibility of dealing with mixed forms; that is, structures

---

[*] As is the case for INVITE in Flemish Sign Language (as well as for GIVE in Flemish Sign Language), ASL GIVE includes a linear movement that may be altered to relate the verb to one or more of its arguments.

[†] Already in 1977, DeMatteo argued in favor of an analysis of classifier constructions as visual analog reconstructions of an actual scene. However, as noted by Liddell (2003b, pp. 202–203):

DeMatteo's (1977) analysis appeared at a time when linguists were demonstrating remarkable parallels between signed and spoken language grammars. By doing so, they were amassing evidence that ASL should be treated as a real human language. Given this progress in finding linguistic structure underlying ASL utterances, DeMatteo's proposal did not receive a welcome reception. After all, his claim was that the underlying representation of a classifier predicate cannot be analyzed as one would analyze a spoken language utterance (i.e., as combinations of morphemes). It would follow, then that ASL was different in an important way from spoken languages.

involving both linguistic and "nonlinguistic components"* (e.g., Liddell, 2003a; Schembri et al., 2005), which is closer to the view of Cogill-Koez (2000), who argues that a "classifier construction" may be a visual representation of an action, event, or spatial relationship rather than a lexical or a productive sign.

A GROWING NUMBER OF SIGN LANGUAGES STUDIED

A second important development in the field of sign linguistics relates to the number of sign languages studied. In the early stages of sign linguistics most of the research concerned ASL with little cross-linguistic research. According to Perniss, Pfau, and Steinbach (2007) this last issue remained unchanged in the "postmodern area starting in the 1980s" when sign language researchers continued to focus on a comparison of sign languages to spoken languages. Since the turn of the century, however, there has been a growing interest in the cross-linguistic comparison of sign languages. Whereas most cross-linguistic analyses involve a limited number of sign languages (often two or three), there are also some larger scale typological projects (Zeshan & Perniss, 2008; Zeshan, 2006a). At the same time, the number of sign languages being studied is increasing and now also includes (more) non-Western sign languages as well as previously un(der)studied Eastern European sign languages (e.g., Indo-Pakistan Sign Language, Adamorobe Sign Language, Jordanian Sign Language, Croatian Sign Language).

SIGN LANGUAGE RESEARCH TODAY

It is now generally accepted that sign languages are fully fledged natural languages, independent of—and on a par with—spoken languages. Rather than stressing the structural similarities between sign languages and spoken languages, current sign language research prefers to focus on the cross-linguistic comparison and typological study of a number of different sign languages, including previously un(der)studied sign languages.

As already discussed earlier in this chapter, some of the more recent analyses seem to provide support for a model of sign language structure that incorporates both linguistic and gestural elements. A growing number of researchers propose to analyze sign languages as "essentially heterogeneous systems in which meanings are conveyed using a combination of elements, including gesture (Schembri, 2001)" (Johnston, Vermeerbergen, Schembri, & Leeson, 2007, p. 198). According to Schembri (2001, p. 257) support for such views is coming

> not only from new analyses of signed language grammar (Liddell, 1990, 2000a, 2000b) and grammaticalization (Zeshan, 2000), but from the study of signed language pidginization and creolization (Morford & Kegl, 2000), historical change (Wilcox et al., 2000), signed language acquisition (Slobin et al., 2000),

---

* Nonlinguistic" meaning "traditionally regarded as not being linguistic in nature" here.

psycholinguistics (Emmorey & Herzig, 2000), neurolinguistics (Corina, 1999), and new theories about the origins of human language (Armstrong, Stokoe, & Wilcox, 1995).

Related to this, a number of researchers argue that when the communication of signers and speakers is being compared, it is speech in combination with (co-speech) gesture—and not speech by itself—that constitutes the appropriate level for cross-linguistic analysis (e.g., Enfield, 2004; Taub, Pinar, & Galvan, 2002; Vermeerbergen & Demey, 2007). Schembri (2001, p. 257) suggests that a paradigm shift is underway in sign language research, "with new developments in sign linguistics at the vanguard of a much broader shift in the study of human communication generally."

Whereas not even 50 years ago sign language researchers often felt they needed to explain and prove that studying a sign language is indeed genuine linguistics, today it is clear—and accepted—that a better understanding of various aspects of the structure and use of sign languages constitutes an important contribution to a better understanding of human language in general/the field of general linguistics.

REFERENCES

Akach, P., Demey, E., Matabane, E., Van Herreweghe, M., & Vermeerbergen, M. (2009). What is South African sign language? What is the South African deaf community? In B. Brock-Utne & I. Skattum (Eds). *Languages and education in Africa. A comparative and transdisciplinary analysis* (pp. 333–347). Oxford, UK: Symposium Books.

Allan, K. (1977). Classifiers. *Language, 53,* 285–311.

Armstrong, D. F., Stokoe, W. C., & Wilcox, S. E. (1995). *Gesture and the nature of language.* Cambridge, UK: Cambridge University Press.

Baker, C., & Cokely, D. (1980). *American Sign Language: A teacher's resource text on grammar and culture.* Silver Spring, MD: T.J. Publishers.

Bergman, B. (1983). Verbs and adjectives: Morphological processes in Swedish sign language. In J. Kyle & B. Woll (Eds.). *Language in sign: An international perspective on sign language* (pp. 3–9). London, UK: Croom Helm.

Bos, H. (1990). Person and location marking in SLN: Some implications of a spatially expressed syntactic system. In S. Prillwitz & T. Vollhaber (Eds.), *Current trends in European sign language research: Proceedings of the third European congress on sign language research* (pp. 231–248). Hamburg, Germany: Signum Press.

Boyes Braem, P., & Sutton-Spence, R. (Eds.). (2001). *The hands are the head of the mouth: The mouth as articulator in sign languages.* Hamburg, Germany: Signum Press.

Brennan, M. (1990). *Word formation in British Sign Language.* Stockholm, Sweden: University of Stockholm.

Cogill-Koez, D. (2000). Signed language classifier predicates: Linguistic structures or schematic visual representation? *Sign Language and Linguistics, 3*(2), 153–207.

Corina, D. P. (1999). Neural disorders of language and movement: Evidence from American Sign Language. In L. S. Messing & R. Campbell (Eds.), *Gesture, speech, and sign* (pp. 27–44). New York, NY: Oxford University Press.

Crasborn, O. (2001). *Phonetic implementation of phonological categories in sign language of the Netherlands.* Utrecht, The Netherlands: LOT.

Crystal, D. (1999). *The Penguin dictionary of language.* London, UK: Penguin.

DeMatteo, A. (1977). Visual imagery and visual analogues. In L. Friedman (Ed.), *On the other hand: Recent perspectives on American Sign Language* (pp. 109–136). New York, NY: Academic Press.

Demey, E. (2005). *Fonologie van de Vlaamse Gebarentaal: distinctiviteit en iconiciteit* [Phonology of Flemish Sign Language: Distinctivity and iconicity]. Unpublished doctoral dissertation, Ghent University.

Demey, E., Van Herreweghe, M., & Vermeerbergen, M. (2008). Iconicity in sign languages. In K. Willems & L. De Cuypere (Eds.), *Naturalness and iconicity in linguistics* (pp. 189–214) [Iconicity in Language and Literature Series, Vol. 7]. Amsterdam, The Netherlands: Benjamins.

Deuchar, M. (1984). *British Sign Language.* London, UK: Routledge & Kegan Paul.

De Weerdt, K., Vanhecke, E., Van Herreweghe, M., & Vermeerbergen, M. (2003). *Op (onder)zoek naar de Vlaamse gebaren-schat.* [In search of a Flemish sign lexicon] Gent, Belgium: Cultuur voor Doven.

Emmorey, K., & Herzig, M. (2000). *Categorical versus analogue properties of classifier constructions in American Sign Language.* Poster presented at the Seventh international conference on Theoretical Issues in Sign Language Research, Amsterdam, The Netherlands.

Enfield, N. J. (2004). On linear segmentation and combinatorics in co-speech gesture: A symmetry-dominance construction in Lao fish trap descriptions. *Semiotica, 149*(1–4), 57–123.

Engberg-Pedersen, E. (1993). *Space in Danish Sign Language.* Hamburg, Germany: Signum-Verlag.

Fischer, S. (1974). Sign language and linguistic universals. In *Actes du Colloque Franco-Allemand de Grammaire Transformationelle* (pp. 187–204). Tubingen, Germany: Niemeyer.

Frishberg, N. (1975). Arbitrariness and iconicity: Historical change in American Sign Language. *Language, 51*, 676–710.

Fusellier-Souza, I. (2004). *Sémiogenèse des langues des signes : Étude de langues des signes primaires (LSP) pratiquées par des sourds brésiliens* [Semiogenesis of sign languages: Study of primary sign languages used by Brazilian deaf people]. Unpublished doctoral dissertation, Université Paris 8, Saint-Denis.

Fusellier-Souza, I. (2006). Emergence and development of signed languages: From diachronic ontogenesis to diachronic phylogenesis. *Sign Language Studies, 7*(1), 30–56.

Givón, T. (1979). From discourse to syntax: Grammar as a processing strategy. In T. Givón (Ed.), *Syntax and semantics. Vol. 12 Discourse and syntax* (pp. 81–109). New York, NY: Academic Press.

Goldin-Meadow, S. (2003). *The resilience of language. What gesture creation in deaf children can tell us about how all children learn language.* New York, NY: Psychology Press.

Johnston, T. (1989). *Auslan: The sign language of the Australian deaf community.* Doctoral dissertation, University of Sydney, Sydney. Retrieved, from http://homepage.mac.com/trevor.a.johnston/dissertation.htm

Johnston, T. (1991). Spatial syntax and spatial semantics in the inflection of signs for the marking of person and location in Auslan. *International Journal of Sign Linguistics, 2*(1), 29–62.

Johnston, T. (2004). W(h)ither the deaf community? Population, genetics, and the future of Australian Sign Language. *American Annals of the Deaf, 148*(5), 358–375.

Johnston, T., Vermeerbergen, M., Schembri, A., & Leeson, L. (2007). "Real data are messy": Considering cross-linguistic analysis of constituent ordering in Auslan, VGT, and ISL. In P. Perniss, R. Pfau, & M. Steinbach (Eds.) *Sign languages: A cross-linguistic perspective* (pp. 163–205). Berlin, Germany: Mouton de Gruyter.

Klima, E. S., & Bellugi, U. (1979). *The signs of language*. Cambridge, MA: Harvard University Press.

Kyle, J. G., & Woll, B. (1985). *Sign language. The study of deaf people and their language*. Cambridge, UK: Cambridge University Press.

Labov, W. (1972). *Sociolinguistic patterns*. Philadelphia, PA: University of Pennsylvania Press.

Lane, H. (1977). *The wild boy of Aveyron*. London, UK: Allen & Unwin.

Leeson, L., & Saeed, J. I. (2007). Conceptual blending and the windowing of attention in simultaneous constructions in Irish Sign Language. In M. Vermeerbergen, L. Leeson, & O. Crasborn (Eds.), *Simultaneity in signed languages: Form and function* (pp. 55–72). Amsterdam, The Netherlands: John Benjamins.

Liddell, S. (1990). Four functions of a locus: Reexamining the structure of space in ASL. In C. Lucas (Ed.), *Sign language research: Theoretical issues* (pp. 176–198). Washington, DC: Gallaudet University Press.

Liddell, S. K. (2000a). Indicating verbs and pronouns: Pointing away from agreement. In K. Emmorey & H. Lane (Eds.), *The signs of language revisited: An anthology to honor Ursula Bellugi and Edward Klima* (pp. 303–320). Mahwah, NJ: Lawrence Erlbaum Associates.

Liddell, S. K. (2000b). Blended spaces and deixis in sign language discourse. In D. McNeill (Ed.), *Language and gesture* (pp. 331–357). Cambridge, UK: Cambridge University Press.

Liddell, S. K. (2003a). *Grammar, gesture, and meaning in American Sign Language*. Cambridge, UK: Cambridge University Press.

Liddell, S. K. (2003b) Sources of meaning in ASL classifier predicates. In K. Emmorey (Ed.), *Perspectives on classifier constructions in sign languages* (pp. 199–220). Mahwah, NJ: Lawrence Erlbaum Associates.

Liddell, S. K., & Metzger, M. (1998). Gesture in sign language discourse. *Journal of Pragmatics, 30*(6), 657–697.

Liddell, S. K., Vogt-Svendsen, M., & Bergman, B. (2007). A crosslinguistic comparison of buoys. Evidence from American, Norwegian, and Swedish Sign Language. In M. Vermeerbergen, L. Leeson, & O. Crasborn (Eds.), *Simultaneity in signed languages: Form and function* (pp. 187–216). Amsterdam, The Netherlands: John Benjamins.

Loncke, F. (1983). "Fonologische aspecten van gebaren" [Phonological aspects of signs]. In B. T. Tervoort (Ed.), *Hand over hand: Nieuwe inzichten in de communicatie van de doven* [Hand over hand: New insights in the communication of deaf people] (pp. 105–119). Muiderberg, The Netherlands: Coutinho.

Loncke, F. (1990). *Modaliteitsinvloed op Taalstructuur en Taalverwerving in Gebarencommunicatie* [Modality influence on language structure and language acquisition]. Unpublished doctoral dissertation. University of Brussels.

McDonald, B. (1982). *Aspects of the American Sign Language predicate system*. Unpublished doctoral dissertation. University of Buffalo.

Metzger, M. (1995). Constructed dialogue and constructed action in American Sign Language. In C. Lucas (Ed.), *Sociolinguistics in deaf communities* (pp. 255–271). Washington DC: Gallaudet University Press.

Morford, J. P., & Kegl, J. A. (2000). Gestural precursors to linguistic constructs: How input shapes the form of language. In D. McNeill (Ed.), *Language and gesture* (pp. 358–387). Cambridge, UK: Cambridge University Press.

Mylander, C., & Goldin-Meadow, S. (1991). Home sign systems in deaf children: The development of morphology without a conventional language model. In P. Siple & S. D. Fischer (Eds.), *Theoretical issues in sign language research, Vol. 2: Psychology* (pp. 41–63). Chicago, IL: University of Chicago Press.

Nyst, V. (2007). Simultaneous constructions in Adamorobe sign language (Ghana). In M. Vermeerbergen, L. Leeson, & O. Crasborn (Eds.), *Simultaneity in signed languages: Form and function* (pp. 127–145). Amsterdam, The Netherlands: John Benjamins.

Ochs, E. (1979). Planned and unplanned discourse. In T. Givón (Ed.), *Syntax and semantics. Vol. 12, Discourse and syntax* (pp. 51–80). New York, NY: Academic Press.

Ong, W. (1982). *Orality and literacy: The technologizing of the word.* London, UK: Methuen.

Padden, C. (1988a). *Interaction of morphology and syntax in American Sign Language.* New York, NY: Garland Publishing.

Padden, C. (1988b). Grammatical theory and signed languages, In F. Newmeyer (Ed.), *Linguistics: The Cambridge survey* (Vol. 2, pp. 250–266). Cambridge, UK: Cambridge University Press.

Perniss, P. (2007). Locative functions of simultaneous perspective constructions. In M. Vermeerbergen, L. Leeson, & O. Crasborn (Eds.), *Simultaneity in signed languages: Form and function* (pp. 27–54). Amsterdam, The Netherlands: John Benjamins.

Perniss, P., Pfau, R., & Steinbach, M. (2007). Can't you see the difference? Sources of variation in sign language structure. In P. Perniss, R. Pfau, & M. Steinbach (Eds.), *Visible variation. Comparative studies on sign language structure* (pp. 1–34). Berlin, Germany: Mouton de Gruyter.

Pizzuto, E. (1986). The verb system of Italian Sign Language. In B. Tervoort (Ed.), *Signs of life: Proceedings of the second European congress on sign language research.* Amsterdam: The Netherlands Foundation for the Deaf and Hearing-Impaired Child and the Institute for General Linguistics of the University of Amsterdam.

Poizner H., Klima E., & Bellugi, U. (1987). *What the hands reveal about the brain.* Cambridge, MA: MIT Press.

Rissanen, T. (1986). The basic structure of Finnish Sign Language. In B. Tervoort (Ed.), *Signs of life: Proceedings of the second European congress on sign language* research. Amsterdam: The Netherlands Foundation for the Deaf and Hearing-Impaired Child and the Institute for General Linguistics of the University of Amsterdam.

Sallandre, M.-A. (2007). Simultaneity in French Sign Language discourse. In M. Vermeerbergen, L. Leeson, & O. Crasborn (Eds.), *Simultaneity in signed languages: Form and function* (pp. 187–216). Amsterdam, The Netherlands: John Benjamins.

Schein, J. (1989). *At home among strangers. Exploring the deaf community in the United States.* Washington, DC: Gallaudet University Press.

Schembri, A. (2001) *Issues in the analysis of polycomponential verbs in Australian Sign Language (Auslan).* Doctoral dissertation, University of Sydney.

Schembri, A. (2003). Rethinking "classifiers" in signed languages. In K. Emmorey (Ed.), *Perspectives on classifier constructions in sign languages* (pp. 3–34). Mahwah, NJ: Lawrence Erlbaum Associates.

Schembri, A., Jones, C., & Burnham, D. (2005). Comparing action gestures and classifier verbs of motion: Evidence from Australian sign language, Taiwan sign language, and non-signers' gestures without speech. *Journal of Deaf Studies and Deaf Education, 10*(3), 272–290.

Siple, P. (1982). Signed language and linguistic theory. In L. Obler, & L. Menn (Eds.), *Exceptional language & linguistics* (pp. 313–333). New York, NY: Academic Press.

Slobin, D. I., Hoiting, N., Anthony, M., Biederman, Y., Kuntze, M., Lindert, R., Pyers, J., Thumann, H., & Weinberg, A. (2000, April). The meaningful use of handshapes by child and adult learners: A cognitive/functional perspective on the acquisition of "classifiers." Paper presented at the workshop Classifier Constructions in Sign Languages, La Jolla, CA.

Stokoe, W. (1960). *Sign language structure. An outline of the visual communication system of the American deaf.* Silver Spring, MD: Linstok Press.

Stokoe, W. (1972). *Semiotics and human sign languages.* The Hague, The Netherlands: Mouton.

Supalla, T. (1978). Morphology of verbs of motion and location in American Sign Language. In F. Caccamise & D. Hicks (Eds.), *American Sign Language in a bilingual, bicultural context: Proceedings of the second national symposium on sign language research and teaching* (pp. 27–46). Coronado, CA: National Association of the Deaf.

Supalla, T. (1982) *Structure and acquisition of verbs of motion and location in American Sign Language.* Doctoral dissertation, University of California, San Diego.

Taub, S. (2001). *Language from the body: Iconicity and metaphor in American Sign Language.* Cambridge, UK: Cambridge University Press.

Taub, S, Pinar, P., & Galvan, D. (2002). Comparing spatial information in speech/gesture and signed language. Paper presented at the "Gesture: The Living Medium" conference, Austin, Texas, June 5–8, 2002.

Tervoort, B. (1953). *Structurele analyse van visueel taalgebruik binnen een groep dove kinderen* [Structural analysis of visual language use within a group of deaf children]. Amsterdam, The Netherlands: Noord-Hollandse Uitgevers Maatschappij.

Van der Kooij, E. (2002). *Phonological categories in sign language of the Netherlands. The role of phonetic implementation and iconicity.* Utrecht, The Netherlands: LOT.

Van Herreweghe, M. (1995). *De Vlaams-Belgische gebarentaal: Een eerste verkenning,* [Flemish-Belgian Sign Language. An initial exploration]. Gent, Belgium: Academia Press.

Van Herreweghe, M., & Vermeerbergen, M. (2004). Flemish Sign Language: Some risks of codification. In M. Van Herreweghe & M. Vermeerbergen (Eds.), *To the lexicon and beyond: Sociolinguistics in European deaf communities* (pp. 111–137). Washington, DC: Gallaudet University Press.

Van Herreweghe, M., & Vermeerbergen, M. (2008, February). Referent tracking in two unrelated sign languages and in home sign systems. Paper presented at the 30th Annual Meeting of the German Linguistics Society DGfS, Bamberg, 27–29.

Van Herreweghe, M. & Vermeerbergen, M. (2010). Deaf perspectives on communicative practices in South Africa: institutional language policies in educational settings, *Text & Talk, 30*(2), 125–144.

Vermeerbergen, M. (1996). *ROOD KOOL TIEN PERSOON IN. Morfo-syntactische Aspecten van Gebarentaal.* [RED CABBAGE TEN PERSON IN. Morphosyntactic aspects of sign language] Doctoral dissertation. University of Brussels.

Vermeerbergen, M. (1997). *Grammaticale Aspecten van de Vlaams-Belgische Gebarentaal* [Grammatical aspects of Flemish-Belgian Sign Language]. Gentbrugge, Belgium: Cultuur voor Doven.

Vermeerbergen, M. (1998). The use of space in Flemish Sign Language. In S. Santi, I. Guaïtella, C. Cavé, & G. Konopczynski, G. (Eds.), *Oralité et Gestualité* [Orality and gestuality] (pp. 131–136). Paris, France: L'Harmattan.

Vermeerbergen, M. (2006). Past and current trends in sign language research. *Language & Communication, 26*(2), 168–192.

Vermeerbergen, M., & Demey, E. (2007). Sign + Gesture = Speech + Gesture? Comparing aspects of simultaneity in Flemish Sign Language to instances of concurrent speech and gesture. In M. Vermeerbergen, L. Leeson, & O. Crasborn (Eds.), *Simultaneity in signed languages: Form and function* (pp. 257–282). Amsterdam, The Netherlands: John Benjamins.

Vermeerbergen, M., Leeson, L., & Crasborn, O. (Eds.). (2007a). *Simultaneity in signed languages: Form and function*. Amsterdam, The Netherlands: John Benjamins

Vermeerbergen, M., Van Herreweghe, M., Akach, P., & Matabane, E. (2007b). Constituent order in Flemish Sign Language and South African Sign Language. A cross-linguistic study. *Sign Language & Linguistics, 10*(1), 25–54.

Wilcox, S., Shaffer, B., Jarque, M. J., Segimon i Valenti, J. M., Pizzuto, E., & Rossini, P. (2000, July). *The emergence of grammar from word and gesture: A cross-linguistic study of modal verbs in three signed languages*. Paper presented at the Seventh International Conferences on Theoretical Issues in Sign Language Research, Amsterdam.

Woll, B. (2003). Modality, universality, and the similarities among sign languages: An historical perspective. In A. Baker, B. van den Bogaerde, & O. Crasborn (Eds.), *Cross-linguistic perspectives in sign language research* (pp. 17–27). Hamburg, Germany: Signum.

Zeshan, U. (2000). Indopakistani Sign Language "classifiers": Evidence from discourse. Paper presented at the workshop *Classifier Constructions in Sign Languages*, La Jolla, CA.

Zeshan, U. (Ed.). (2006a). *Negatives and interrogatives across signed languages*. Nijmegen, The Netherlands: Ishara Press.

Zeshan, U. (2006b). Negative and interrogative constructions in sign languages: A case study in sign language typology. In U. Zeshan (Ed.), *Negatives and interrogatives across signed languages* (pp. 28–68). Nijmegen, The Netherlands: Ishara Press.

Zeshan, U. & Perniss, P., (Eds.). (2008). *Possessive and existential constructions in sign languages. Sign Language Typology Series No. 2*. Nijmegen, The Netherlands: Ishara Press.

35 Language in Autism: Pragmatics and Theory of Mind

Jennifer Barnes and Simon Baron-Cohen

It has been suggested that the skills required to interpret social interaction are the same skills necessary for understanding the fictional content of narratives (e.g., movies, books, storytelling, or theater; Mar, 2004; Mar, Oatley, Hirsh, de la Paz, & Peterson, 2006; Oatley, 1994, 1999). Although film-production and book writing are only seen in some cultures, across cultures humans engage in storytelling (Scalise Sugiyama, 1996). In this chapter, we examine narrative production and comprehension in terms of cognitive mechanisms that subserve pragmatics.

First, we review theories that look at narrative in terms of ability to empathize with and ascribe mental states to others in the social world. Then, we examine narrative comprehension and production in a clinical population with deficits in social cognition and pragmatic communication—individuals with autism spectrum conditions (ASC). Finally, we present the results of a study that examines the way that individuals with and without ASC view film clips and produce narratives about what they have viewed.

NARRATIVE, PRAGMATICS, AND SOCIAL COGNITION

NARRATIVE AND PRAGMATICS

Narratives are, by definition, created for an audience: films are made to be seen, books are made to be read, and stories are told specifically to listeners. For this reason, there is an inherent connection between the study of how we create and understand narratives and pragmatics (the study of language as used in a social context). Narrative competence—defined as the ability to both tell and understand stories—requires an understanding not only of the events and characters in a story, but also of the relationship between the person creating the narrative and the audience who will receive it. Storytellers must be sensitive to the information that their audience needs to understand and enjoy the story, while readers or listeners need to attend to the details that a narrative's creator intended to be the center of focus. For this reason, some theorists have suggested that the pleasure we derive from reading or viewing fiction is related to our interaction both with the fictional characters and with the unseen author telling the story (Carroll, 2004).

NARRATIVE AND THEORY OF MIND

Pragmatic communication, narrative competence, and everyday social functioning all require an advanced ability to consider the minds of others. This ability to
imagine the thoughts, beliefs, knowledge, emotions, goals, and desires of others is
referred to as employing a "theory of mind" (ToM; Baron-Cohen, 1995). A storyteller must "mind-read" his or her audience to know what information to provide
to guide their understanding of a story (Colle, Baron-Cohen, Wheelwright, &
van der Lely, 2007). Simultaneously, understanding a movie or book requires the
ability to ascribe mental states to the narrative's characters (Keen, 2006; Losh
& Capps, 2003; Tan, 1996; Zunshine, 2006). Here, we briefly review empirical
research that examines the connection between ToM and the ability to both produce and understand narratives in a variety of media.

NARRATIVE PRODUCTION AND THEORY OF MIND

A variety of experiments have attempted to directly examine the relationship
between ToM and the ability to produce coherent narratives. Younger children,
who generally perform poorer on tests that require conceptualizing the beliefs of
others, produce narratives that are skewed toward actions, rather than thoughts,
and narratives that integrate thoughts with actions only develop with age (Pelletier,
2004). Similarly, children with Williams syndrome, a condition marked by hyper-
sociality and associated with intact social cognition (Gosch & Pankau, 1997;
Tager-Flusberg, Boshart, & Baron-Cohen, 1998) use more narrative techniques
aimed at audience engagement than do typically developing controls (Losh,
Bellugi, Reilly, & Anderson, 2000). Consistent with the theory that ToM development is related to narrative competence, a direct correlation has been found (after
controlling for age) between the ability to pass classic mentalizing tasks and the
level of narrative sophistication (as measured by the number of techniques used
to engage a listener) in typically developing, low-income, African American preschoolers (Currenton, 2004). Among children with ASC, performance on ToM
tasks is also correlated with achievement in narrative production (Capps, Losh, &
Thurber, 2000). This body of research strongly supports the idea that the ability
to produce coherent narratives is directly related to the ability to conceptualize
the mind of the listener.

NARRATIVE COMPREHENSION AND THEORY OF MIND

Engaging in fictional narratives is often conceptualized as practicing the skills
necessary to function socially in the real world (Oatley, 1999; Zunshine, 2006).
Some have suggested that a drive toward narrative might even be the product of

evolution (Cosmides & Tooby, 2000; Scalise Sugiyama, 2003). In one experiment, Mar and colleagues (2006) found that individuals with a greater drive toward fiction (as measured by a familiarity with fiction authors) scored higher on self-reported empathy and interpersonal perception. Of interest, the drive toward fiction was correlated with performance on a test of real-world social ability, the "Reading the Mind in the Eyes" Test (Baron-Cohen, Wheelwright, Hill, Raste, & Plumb, 2001). In this task, individuals are asked to look at pictures of the eye region of the face and choose one of four multiple-choice terms to describe the emotion or mental state depicted by the expression in the eyes of the picture.

The "Reading the Mind in the Eyes" Test was developed specifically for use with populations with ASC (Baron-Cohen et al., 2001; Baron-Cohen, Wheelwright, & Joliffe, 1997). ASC are characterized in part by significant social impairments and language and communication delays (APA, 1994). Individuals with ASC have deficits in ToM (Baron-Cohen, 1995; Baron-Cohen, Leslie, & Frith, 1985) and pragmatic communication ability (Happé, 1995; Tager-Flusberg, 2000). For this reason, the study of narrative comprehension and production has been a central focus in autism research in the past decade.

NARRATIVE PRODUCTION IN AUTISM

Because ASC are characterized in part by specific deficits in ToM, which plays a key role in narrative and pragmatic communication, many experiments have investigated the abilities of children and adolescents with ASC to create spoken narratives. In one experiment, when asked to produce fictional narratives, children with ASC produced shorter narratives that contained fewer imaginative elements than neurotypical controls; however they produced real-life, event-based narratives of similar length to control children (Craig & Baron-Cohen, 2000). Other researchers have attempted to focus on narrative ability, rather than imaginative ability, by attempting to minimize the burden of creating content. Typically, these studies elicit storytelling by showing children either a wordless picture book or some kind of live action display, such as a puppet show, and ask them to retell the story they have just seen (Capps et al., 2000; Diehl, Bennetto, & Young, 2006; Losh & Capps, 2003; Loveland, McEvoy, Tunali, & Kelley, 1990; Pelletier, 2004; Tager-Flusberg & Sullivan, 1995). Participants' responses in these experiments were then coded for length, syntactic complexity, accuracy in recalling key details of the story, and the number and range of techniques used to engage the listener in the story.

Although most experiments have found no difference in the length or syntactic complexity of narratives produced by children with autism and controls, recent research has revealed important differences in the ways children with and without ASC construct narratives for their audience. For example, while children with ASC use mental state terms as frequently as controls, they are more likely to simply label mental states, rather than drawing connections between mental states and their causes or effects (Capps et al., 2000), and are less likely to organize their narratives coherently around significant story events (Diehl et al., 2006). These results suggest that in addition to providing important indices of social cognitive abilities in autism, analyzing autistic narratives may also be relevant to the weak central coherence theory of autism (Frith, 1989). This theory proposes that individuals with ASC perceive local details very well, but have difficulty seeing the global big picture. In the examples given above, narrative organization depends on an individual's ability to separate unimportant details or story events from those that define the meaning of the scene, and to recognize mental states within a larger web of social interaction. Weak central coherence might lead individuals with ASC to create narratives more grounded in detail, and less focused on key story events.

Interestingly, however, in addition to producing narratives of the same length and syntactic complexity as controls, children with ASC have been shown to have no difficulty incorporating the theme or gist of the story into their narratives (Losh & Capps, 2003; Diehl et al., 2006). A variety of researchers have interpreted this, along with the presence of mental state terms in the narratives of children with ASC, as suggesting that the differences seen in narrative production are not based on comprehension, but rather on decreased sensitivity or attention to the type of information the listener needs. Monitoring the informational needs of one's listener is, of course, an aspect of ToM (Baron-Cohen, 1988). Consistent with this ToM hypothesis, children with autism use a smaller range of evaluative techniques designed at drawing the reader into the story, such as character voices, sound effects, and intensifiers, than do typical controls (Losh & Capps, 2003).

A recent experiment with adults with high functioning autism (HFA) or Asperger syndrome (AS) also supports this claim. Colle and colleagues (2007) presented adults with HFA/AS the same wordless picture book used in the experiments described above. Participants were asked to look through the book and then tell a story based on the pictures. The results showed that while subjects in the ASC group had no impairments in general storytelling ability, they did demonstrate specific deficits with regard to using two types of phrases that take into account the listener's needs. For example, temporal adverbs and other terms that reference time provide the listener with a frame of reference in which to consider the events of the story. By using these terms, a storyteller can move the reader temporally through the story, increasing their understanding of the story events and their connections to each other. Similarly, a skilled storyteller avoids using ambiguous pronouns that might confuse their audience, but favors using pronouns in disambiguated cases to avoid the unnecessary repetition of a given noun phrase, offering the listener more variety and engaging them further in the story. In Colle et al's (2007) experiment, participants in the ASC group used fewer temporal adverbs and fewer anaphoric pronouns, while using more confusing, ambiguous pronouns than typical controls. The authors interpret these deficits as reflecting larger deficits in pragmatic communication that may partially explain difficulties that ASC individuals have with engaging others in conversation.

Taken together, the studies outlined above provide strong evidence that people with ASC show impairments in the realm of narrative production, and these deficits appear to be specific to pragmatics (Baron-Cohen, 1988). In order to tell an engaging story, you need to take into account what the listener knows (Astington, 1991) and what kind of presentation they will find interesting. Subtle deficits in ToM affect an individual's ability to do this.

NARRATIVE COMPREHENSION IN AUTISM

In exploring the social deficits that individuals with ASC show in real-world social situations, many researchers use visual or written narrative stimuli as a stand-in for the actual social world. For this reason, many studies that test social cognition in autism use narratives and may therefore be examined as testing narrative comprehension as well. For example, Happé (1994) presented children with autism or learning difficulties, and typically developing children, with a series of stories that probed the participants' understanding of literally untrue utterances (e.g., pretense, sarcasm, and deception) within a given context. For each story, participants were asked to explain why a character had said something that was literally untrue. For example, in one story, a girl named Anna is playing inside and breaks a vase. Knowing that her mother will be angry with her for breaking the vase, Anna tells her mother that the dog did it. Children with ASC were more likely than either control group to give incorrect (e.g., "Anna was joking") rather than correct (e.g., "Anna lied so that she wouldn't get in trouble") explanations. While this result certainly reflects a deficit that could affect real-world social processing and functioning, it also shows an interesting deficit in narrative comprehension—namely that individuals with ASC, in interpreting the situations incorrectly, seem to be missing out on the core meaning that the scenes are *intended* to portray.

In a related experiment (Baron-Cohen, 1997), children were asked why the experimenter produced utterances such as "This is a shoe" while he was pointing at a cup. While typically developing 2 year olds spontaneously said it was because the experimenter was *joking* or *pretending* (thus referring to his mental state), children with autism said it was because the experimenter was wrong (simply referring to the mismatch between the word and its referent). This failure to monitor mental states in communication was also evident in a test of understanding Gricean Maxims. Gricean Maxims are implicit rules that speakers follow to be cooperative in conversation (Grice, 1957), such as "Be truthful," or "Be relevant," or "Be Informative." In a related experiment, children were presented with two possible answers to a question and were asked, "Which one said something silly?" For example, in answer to the question "Where do you live?" the two answers might be "I live in England" versus "I live on the moon." Four-year-old typically developing children were much more accurate in identifying the inappropriate answer compared to young children with autism (Surian, Baron-Cohen, & van der Lely, 1996), reflecting the typically developing child's sensitivity to a speaker's *intentional* violations of a listener's *expectations*—the mental states of the interlocutors; and reflecting the deficit in this skill in children with autism.

A variety of other experiments have probed social cognition in autism using stimuli taken from television or films. Because film is a multimodal medium, these film stimuli are a closer laboratory approximation of the requirements of real-world processing than are written stories. Across experiments, individuals with ASC show deficits in their ability to ascribe the correct meaning to interactions in films. In the "Reading the Mind in Films" task (Golan, Baron-Cohen, Hill, & Golan, 2006), participants were asked to view short, 20 second film clips and were then given a multiple-choice question that asked them to choose which of four words described a character's mental state or emotion at the end of the clip. Participants with ASC performed significantly worse than controls to the extent that 90% of participants could be allocated to the correct group based on their performance on this task alone. In a similar study, Dziobek and colleagues (2006) asked participants to view a 15 minute long movie that incorporated classic tests of social cognition, including false belief, faux pas, and sarcasm, as well as ongoing narrative and character interactions. During the course of the experiment, the narrative was stopped 46 times, and participants were asked to answer open-ended questions about characters' mental states, including their emotions, thoughts, and intentions. Participants with ASC performed significantly worse than controls, showing difficulty in understanding each scene and the characters' social interactions in terms of underlying mental states. Other studies using film stimuli have obtained similar results (Heavey, Phillips, Baron-Cohen, & Rutter, 2000).

It has been argued that tasks that use dichotomous scoring, where a participant's answers are coded as either correct or incorrect, do not reflect the demands and subtlety of real-world social interaction (Klin, 2000). In line with this idea, several experiments have used more open-ended methods to investigate the way that individuals with ASC view and understand films. Klin, Jones, Schultz, Volkmar, & Cohen (2002) tracked participants' eye gaze as they viewed a clip from the film *Who's Afraid of Virginia Woolf?* and found that individuals with ASC use different scanning strategies when attempting to extract information from film narratives. Individuals in the control group tended to focus on people in the scenes, and specifically on the eye region of their face, whereas people with ASC focused more on objects. When they looked at faces, they spent less time looking at the eye region and more at the mouth. This result is particularly interesting not only in its implications for attentional scanning patterns in the real world, but also in that it reveals a further disconnect between what the scene's director presumably *intended* to communicate with this social scene, and the information that individuals with autism take from it.

The remainder of this chapter describes an experiment (Barnes, Lombardo, Wheelwright, & Baron-Cohen, 2009) that combines the narrative elicitation method used in studies of narrative production (Colle et al., 2007; Diehl et al., 2006; Losh & Capps, 2003) with the use of complex, naturalistic film stimuli similar to those used in studies of advanced social comprehension (Golan et al., 2006; Klin et al., 2002).

A TEST OF NARRATIVE PRODUCTION AND
COMPREHENSION: THE MORAL DILEMMAS FILM TASK

The vast majority of experiments in which participants with autism are asked to produce a narrative based on source material focus on narrative production rather than comprehension. For this reason, the stimuli used to elicit narratives in these experiments tend to be very simple stories, most commonly a wordless picture book about a boy who loses his pet frog and then proceeds to look for the frog in many different places. By asking participants to retell a simple story, these experiments minimize the requirements of narrative comprehension. Not surprisingly, most participants (in both the autism and control groups) show no deficits in grasping the gist of these stories, or attending to the mental states of the main character (Capps et al., 2000; Diehl et al., 2006; Losh & Capps, 2003).

In contrast, however, one previous experiment used participants' narratives to examine their understanding of a more complex film-based narrative. Klin (2000) asked participants to view a short animated movie (taken from Heider & Simmel, 1944), in which a variety of geometric shapes move and interact in ways that can be described with either purely mechanical ("the triangle moved upward") or intentional ("the triangle was being chased by the square") language. In this case, the elicited narratives revealed sharp differences in the way that people with and without ASC viewed the film's content, with individuals on the autistic spectrum tending to view the show more mechanically, producing narratives that contained fewer mental state terms than controls.

These results form an interesting contrast, with individuals with ASC showing different patterns of mental state term production in their narratives depending on the type of stimuli used to elicit narrative production. When asked to retell simple stories, people with ASC do attribute mental states to the story's characters, but they fail to do so with other kinds of stimuli such as moving geometric shapes. What is unclear from this is whether the deficit found in the Klin study reflects the fact that the autistic population under-attribute mental states to film stimuli, or whether it indicates over-attribution of mental states by typical controls.

In order to answer the question of whether these deficits would extend to narratives based on more ecological film scenes, we developed a new task, The Moral Dilemmas Film Task, in which adult participants with AS and HFA were asked to view four brief film clips and write about what they saw (Barnes et al., 2009). Their narratives were then coded for variables related to social comprehension and ToM, and their performance was compared to self-reported empathizing ability and verbal IQ. It was predicted that narratives by people with ASC would be impoverished compared to controls and focus less on mental states, and that different factors might predict spontaneous mentalizing in ASC and control populations, reflecting different strategies in the way that individuals with autism search for and represent meaning in the social world.

We tested 28 individuals with ASC and 28 neurotypical controls. The individuals in the ASC group were diagnosed with either HFA or AS. Individuals with HFA and AS have average or above average intelligence, but like others on the autistic spectrum, they have significant social impairments. AS is differentiated from autism by the absence of any delays in language acquisition and development (Schoper, 1985). The ASC and control groups were matched for age (ASC: mean = 30.29, sd = 7.78; control: mean = 30.21), sex (14 males and 14 females in each group), and Verbal IQ (ASC mean = 116.29, sd = 10.75; control mean = 116.93, sd = 8.79).

All participants were asked to complete three tasks: the empathy quotient (EQ), the verbal subtests of the Weschler Abbreviated Scale of Intelligence (WASI; Wechsler, 1999), and the film-based task designed for this experiment, the Moral Dilemmas Film Task. The EQ is a 40-question self-report questionnaire tapping cognitive and affective empathy (Baron-Cohen & Wheelwright, 2004). It asks questions geared at gauging an individual's ability to recognize and correctly respond to the emotions of others. Verbal WASI scores were used to match the ASC and control groups on verbal ability, and both Verbal IQ and EQ scores were compared to participants' performance on the Moral Dilemmas Film Task. It was hypothesized that if individuals with ASC and neurotypical individuals used different strategies to understand film narratives, the complexity of their narratives might be predicted by different factors.

THE MORAL DILEMMA'S FILM TASK

This test asks participants to view four short naturalistic film clips taken from a modern American television show (*House*) and write about what they saw. Each clip lasted between 30 seconds and 2 minutes, contained two characters (one male and one female), and depicted a self-contained story arc with a beginning, a middle, and an end. Because all four clips were taken from the same television show, they are similar in style and content, but each clip features different characters and a different moral dilemma.

We chose to use clips that featured moral dilemmas as the central conflict in an effort to encourage participants to pay attention to the characters' mental states and emotions, which play a key role in dilemmas of this kind. For example, in one scene, a bouncer at a club must decide whether or not to sneak in a homeless woman who cannot afford the entrance ticket. While the external conflict is clear (the woman says she wants to go into the club, the man demands the money and she admits to not having it), understanding the scene as a whole (particularly the outcome) requires conceptualizing the bouncer's inner debate weighing his obligation to fulfill the requirements of his job and the woman's obvious desperation. In a second clip, the external conflict exists because a young cancer patient asks her doctor to kiss her, so that she experiences what this feels like just once before she dies. In order to fully understand why the doctor eventually accedes to her request, a viewer must consider not only the external debate between the two characters, but also the doctor's internal debate about the medical ethics of the situation and his feelings about the girl's belief that she is dying and the role that plays in her request. In this way, each of the four clips required participants to pay attention to the characters mental states and emotion to fully understand the content of the scene.

Before beginning the film task, participants were asked to create a control narrative. In this condition, participants were told to write for "about five minutes" about something that they found interesting. After completing their interest narratives, participants moved on to the film portion of the task, where they were asked to watch each of the four film clips and spend "about five minutes" writing about what they saw. Ultimately, each participant produced five written narratives: one interest narrative, and four film-based narratives. We scored the following variables.

Narrative Length: All narratives were coded for length (in words). It was predicted that individuals with ASC might take less away from the highly mental scenes and therefore produce film-based narratives that were significantly shorter than controls and also impoverished compared to their own interest-based narrative.

Narrative Comprehension: Participants' four film-based narratives were coded for the number of references a participant made to either objects or a character's mental state, with a *mental state* being defined as a "cognitive, affective, perceptual, or attentional state" (Baron-Cohen et al., 2005). Because individuals with ASC have been shown to have deficits in their understanding of film-based characters' mental states (Dziobek et al., 2006; Golan et al., 2006) and have viewing patterns that are skewed toward objects, rather than people (Klin et al., 2002), we predicted that individuals with ASC would produce narratives that included fewer mental state terms and more references to objects.

Narrative Production: We were interested in examining the degree to which participants used language—and specifically adverbs—that indicated a richness in mental state understanding. In previous experiments, the use of emphatic markers has been identified as an evaluative storytelling technique, used to "pull" a reader or listener into a narrative (Reilly, Klima, & Bellugi, 1990). Here, we looked at the kinds of terms participants used to modify mental states or emotions. Specifically, we coded for the presence or absence of what we call *quantity* and *apparency* modifiers.

Quantity Modifiers were defined as any term applied to a mental state or emotion in order to indicate the degree to which that emotion was felt. For example, modifiers that indicate quantity could be applied to the term "happy" to differentiate between someone who is "really happy," "somewhat happy," "a little bit happy," "extremely happy," and "the happiest woman in the world." In this way, use of these terms allows a participant to indicate nuances of a single emotion.

Apparency Modifiers were defined as any term applied to a mental or emotional state that indicated the obviousness of that state. In other words, the terms referred to as "apparency modifiers" indicate how *apparent* it is that an individual is thinking or feeling a certain way. Words like "obviously," "clearly," and "visibly" can be applied to mental state terms to indicate the certainty with which the participant attributed a given mental state to an individual in the film. It was hypothesized that even if individuals with ASC produced narratives with equivalent numbers of mental state terms as controls, they might differ in the degree to which they used adjectives that indicated high level of confidence in those attributions.

RESULTS OF THE BARNES AND COLLEAGUES EXPERIMENT

While the neurotypical and ASC groups did not differ based on the lengths in words of narratives they produced in response to the open prompt, "Write about something that interests you," across the four film-based narratives, participants in the control group produced significantly more words than participants in the autism group (ASC: mean = 364.21, sd = 98.91; control: mean = 521.75, sd = 155.84; $t(54)$ = 4.51, $p < .001$). Additionally, while individuals in the control group generally produced film-based narratives similar in length to their response to the open prompt, the individuals in the ASC group produced film-based narratives that were significantly shorter than their responses to the open prompt (interest narrative: mean = 124.04, sd = 45.61; average film-based narrative: mean = 91.05, sd = 24.73; $t(26)$ = 3.975, $p < .001$).

Across the four film-based narratives, individuals in the control group produced significantly more total mental state terms than those in the ASC group (control: mean = 30.82, sd = 12.27; ASC: mean = 20.86, sd = 24.73; $t(54)$ = 3.096, $p = .003$), but the two groups did not differ in the frequency with which they referenced objects. In other words, while the vast majority of individuals in both groups showed a bias for talking about mental states over objects in their film-based narratives, this bias was significantly stronger in the control group control bias: mean = 25.29, sd = 12.79; ASC bias: mean = 16.79, sd = 13.65; $t(54)$ = 2.404, $p = .02$).

Twenty-four out of 28 controls used quantity modifiers, such as "really" or "a little" to indicate degrees of mental state terms, compared to only 15 out of 28 individuals in the ASC group. A two-tailed chi-square revealed that this difference was significant · $\chi^2(1, N = 56)$ = 6.842, $p = .019$). Similarly, while 20 out of 28 controls, used words like "obviously" and "clearly" to modify mental state terms in their narratives, only three individuals with ASC did so ($\chi^2(1, N = 56)$ = 21.323, $p < .001$).

Within the control group, there was no correlation between verbal IQ and any outcome measure, such as total number of mental state words in their film-based narratives. In contrast, within the ASC group, verbal IQ was correlated with the number of mental state terms included in film-based narratives($r(26)$ = .496, $p = .007$), but was not related to the length of these narratives as a whole. Conversely, while no correlation was found in the ASC group between an individual's EQ score and the total number of mental state terms produced, there was a significant correlation between these variables in the control group ($r(26)$ = .461, $p = .013$)

DISCUSSION OF THE BARNES AND COLLEAGUES EXPERIMENT

In this study, individuals with and without HFA and AS, conditions marked by social impairments, were asked to view short film narratives and to write a story retelling what they had seen. While individuals in both groups had no trouble creating narratives on a topic of their own and wrote equal amounts of text in response to the prompt "write about something that interests you," individuals with ASC created impoverished film-based narratives compared to neurotypical individuals, and compared to their own interest narratives. While ASC and control film-based narratives were equally descriptive of the objects they had seen in the film, people with ASC produced narratives that contained fewer descriptions of the characters' thoughts, beliefs, emotions, goals, or desires than controls. Further, while individuals with ASC did produce mental state terms in their narratives, they were less likely than controls to describe these mental states in rich ways by using modifiers that indicated nuance, and they were less likely to spontaneously indicate that they were sure of their mental state attributions.

Taken as a whole, these results form a striking picture of differences in the way that participants with and without autism view and understand film scenes they watch. While the content of an individual's narrative cannot be taken as comprehensive with respect to their understanding, it does provide important insight into the information that stood out in their mind—as significant enough to merit inclusion in their narratives. Just as a filmmaker makes choices about how to frame a shot, or how a particular piece of dialogue should be delivered, in producing their narratives, all participants had to decide which parts of the film they viewed were important enough to be communicated in their retelling of the scene. In producing narratives that were rich with mental state description and showing a strong bias for describing emotions over objects, the neurotypical group showed not only a proficiency at spontaneously thinking about and identifying the unseen thoughts of others, but also a predisposition for communicating that key information to an implied audience. In contrast, though the ASC group did show an overall bias for paying more attention to mental states than object, this bias was weak compared to controls, and their narratives were shorter, more impoverished, and contained less detail than both control narratives and the narratives they are capable of creating when they must only decide what to say, rather than having to decode a social scene and then recreate it on someone else's behalf.

Of particular interest, to the extent that individuals with ASC and controls did manage to extract mentalistic information from the films and include that information in their narratives, they appeared to be using different techniques with which to do so. The ASC performance on this task was directly related to verbal ability, and suggested that individuals with HFA and AS may rely strongly on verbal information—for example, spoken dialogue—to attribute meaning to the scenes, whereas performance among controls was predicted not by verbal ability but by self-reported empathy. Significantly, in the *Virginia Woolf* study described earlier (Klin et al., 2002), individuals with autism spent more time focused on the mouth region of the face than on the eyes, a region of the face thought to be very important for reading the emotions of others (Baron-Cohen et al., 2001), while individuals in the control group showed the reverse pattern. Taken together with the results on this task, it appears that people with ASC may be using verbal scaffolding to increase their mentalistic understanding of films. Viewed in the context of pragmatics, individuals with autism may be paying more attention to *what* is said than *how* it is said, a result consistent with previous findings, which catalogue ASC difficulties with sarcasm and deception (Happé, 1994).

SUMMARY AND CONCLUSION

In the previous section, we reviewed a new test of social cognition, the Moral Dilemmas Film Task. Participants with and without ASC viewed short, emotionally charged film clips that centered on moral dilemmas and were asked to write about what they saw. Neurotypical controls and individuals with ASC differed in the amount of text they produced based on the films, the degree to which they showed a bias for mental states over objects in that text, and the degree to which their performance depended on self-reported empathy and verbal intelligence. These results form an interesting complement to the results of the studies outlined in the second and third sections. By combining the methods of previous studies that have examined narrative production and narrative comprehension respectively, the Moral Dilemmas Film Task provides an important window into the way that individuals with autism view social scenes similar to those that they might encounter in real-life.

For example, individuals with ASC often have trouble identifying and responding to the emotions of others in everyday life and may fail to correctly identify the emotions of film-characters in multiple-choice paradigms within a lab setting, and their performance on the Moral Dilemmas Film Task indicates that their spontaneous representations of these scenes might be impoverished. In other words, participants may have difficulty not only because when attempting to identify mental states they often do so incorrectly, but also because they might be less predisposed to seek out this information, or to view it as significant.

While the Moral Dilemmas Film Task is a task that uses film narratives as a proxy for real-world social interactions to probe social understanding in ASC, the results also have interesting implications for the study of narrative cognition more broadly. For example, the study reported here and the experiments with ASC strongly suggest that narrative ability is inextricably tied to ToM ability. Thus, ToM turns out not only to be important for mindreading and predicting what others will do or what they might think, but also for any communicative activity, be it narrative or culture itself.

REFERENCES

American Psychiatric Association. (1994). *Diagnostic and statistical manual of mental disorders,* 4th ed. Washington, DC: Author.
Astington, J. (1991). Intention in the child's theory of mind. In D. Frye & C. Moor (Eds.), *Children's theories of mind: Mental states and social understanding.* Hillsdale, NJ: Lawrence Erlbaum Associates.

Barnes, J. L., Lombardo, M.V., Wheelwright, S., & Baron-Cohen, S. (2009). The Moral Dilemmas Film Task: A study of spontaneous narratives by individuals with autism spectrum conditions. *Autism Research, 2*(3), 148–156.

Baron-Cohen, S. (1988). Social and pragmatic deficits in autism: Cognitive or affective? *Journal of Autism and Developmental Disorders, 18*(3), 379–402.

Baron-Cohen, S. (1995). *Mind-blindness.* Cambridge, MA: MIT Press.

Baron-Cohen, S. (1997). Hey! It was just a joke! Understanding propositions and propositional attitudes by normally developing children and children with autism. *Israel Journal of Psychiatry, 34*, 174–178.

Baron-Cohen, S., Leslie, A. M., & Frith, U. (1985). Does the autistic child have a "theory of mind"? *Cognition, 21*, 37–46.

Baron-Cohen, S., & Wheelwright, S. (2004). The empathy quotient: An investigation of adults with Asperger syndrome or high functioning autism, and normal sex differences. *Journal of Autism and Developmental Disorders, 34*(2), 163–175.

Baron-Cohen, S., Wheelwright, S., Hill, J., Raste, Y., & Plumb, I. (2001). The "reading the mind in the eyes" test revised version: A study with normal adults, and adults with Asperger syndrome or high functioning autism. *Journal of Child Psychiatry, 42*, 241–252.

Baron-Cohen, S., Wheelwright, S., & Jolliffe, T. (1997). Is there a "language of the eyes"? Evidence from normal adults and adults with autism or Asperger syndrome. *Visual Cognition, 4*, 311–331.

Baron-Cohen, S., Wheelwright, S., Lawson, J., Griffin, R., Ashwin, C., Billington, J., & Chakrabarti, B. (2005). Empathizing and systemizing in autism spectrum conditions. In F. Volkmar, A. Klin, and R. Paul (Eds.), *Handbook of autism and pervasive developmental disorders* (3rd ed.). New York, NY: John Wiley and Sons.

Capps, L., Losh, M., & Thurber, C. (2000). "The frog ate the bug and made his mouth sad": Narrative competence in children with autism. *Journal of Abnormal Child Psychology, 28*(2), 193–204.

Carroll, J. (2004). *Literary Darwinism.* New York, NY: Routledge.

Colle, L., Baron-Cohen, S., Wheelwright, S., & van der Lely, H. (2007). Narrative discourse in adults with high-functioning autism or Asperger syndrome. *Journal of Autism and Developmental Disorders, 38*(1), 28–40.

Cosmides, L., & Tooby, J. (2000). Consider the source: The evolution of adaptations for decoupling and metarepresentations. In D. Sperber (Ed.), *Metarepresentations: A multidisciplinary perspective* (pp. 53–116). New York, NY: Oxford University Press.

Craig, J., & Baron-Cohen, S. (2000). Story-telling ability in children with autism or Asperger syndrome: A window into the imagination. *Israel Journal of Psychiatry, 37*, 64–70.

Currenton, S. (2004). The association between narratives and theory of mind for low-income preschoolers. *Early Education and Development, 15*(2), 124–146.

Diehl, J. J., Bennetto, L., & Young, E. C. (2006). Story recall and narrative coherence of high-functioning children with autism spectrum disorders. *Journal of Abnormal Child Psychology, 34*(1), 87–102.

Dziobek, I., Fleck, S., Kalbe, E., Rogers, K., Hassenstab, J., Brand, M., … Convit, A. (2006). Introducing MASC: A movie for the assessment of social cognition. *Journal of Autism and Developmental Disorders, 36*, 623–636.

Frith, U. (1989). *Autism: Explaining the enigma.* Oxford, UK: Basil Blackwell.

Golan, O., Baron-Cohen, S., Hill, J., & Golan, Y. (2006). The "reading the mind in films" task: Complex emotion recognition in adults with and without autism spectrum conditions. *Social Neuroscience, 1*(2), 111–123.

Gosch, A., & Pankau, R. (1997). Personality characteristics and behaviour problems in individuals of different ages with Williams syndrome. *Developmental Medicine & Child Neurology, 39*, 527–533.

Grice, H. P. (1957). Meaning. *Philosophical Review, 66*, 377–388.

Happé, F. (1994). An advanced test of theory of mind: Understanding of story characters' thought and feelings by able autistic, mentally handicapped, and normal children and adults. *Journal of Autism and Developmental Disorders, 24*(2), 129–154.

Happé, F. (1995). The role of age and verbal ability in the theory of mind task performance of subjects with autism. *Child Development, 66*, 843–855.

Heavey, L., Phillips, W., Baron-Cohen, S., & Rutter, M. (2000). The awkward moments test: A naturalistic measure of social understanding in autism. *Journal of Autism and Developmental Disorders, 30*(3), 225–236.

Heider, F., & Simmel, M. (1944). An experimental study of apparent behavior. *The American Journal of Psychology, 57*, 243–259.

Keen, S. (2006). A theory of narrative empathy. *Narrative, 14*(3), 207–235.

Klin, A. (2000). Attributing social meaning to ambiguous visual stimuli in higher-functioning autism and Asperger syndrome: The social attribution task. *Journal of Psychology, 41*(7), 831–846.

Klin, A., Jones, W., Schultz, R., Volkmar, F., & Cohen, D. (2002). Visual fixation patterns during viewing of naturalistic social situations as predictors of social competence in individuals with autism. *Archives of General Psychiatry, 59*, 809–816.

Losh, M., Bellugi, U., Reilly, J., & Anderson, D. (2000). Narrative as a social engagement tool: The excessive use of evaluation in narratives from children with Williams Syndrome. *Narrative Inquiry, 10*(2), 265–290.

Losh, M., & Capps, L. (2003). Narrative ability in high-functioning children with autism or Asperger's syndrome. *Journal of Autism and Developmental Disorders, 33*, 239–251.

Loveland, K., McEvoy, R., Tunali, B., & Kelley, M. L. (1990). Narrative story telling in autism and Down's syndrome. *British Journal of Developmental Psychology, 8*, 9–23.

Mar, R. A. (2004). The neuropsychology of narrative: Story comprehension, story production and their interrelation. *Neuropsychologia, 42*(10), 1414–1434.

Mar, R. A., Oatley, K., Hirsh, J., de la Paz, J., & Peterson, J. B. (2006). Bookworms versus nerds: Exposure to fiction versus non-fiction, divergent associations with social ability, and the simulation of fictional worlds. *Journal of Research in Personality, 40*, 694–712.

Oatley, K. (1994). A taxonomy of the emotions of literary response and a theory of identification in fictional narrative. *Poetics, 23*, 53–74.

Oatley, K. (1999). Why fiction may be twice as true as fact: Fiction as cognitive and emotional simulation. *Review of General Psychology, 3*, 101–117.

Pelletier, J. (2004). Actions, consciousness, and theory of mind: Children's ability to coordinate story characters' actions and thoughts. *Early Education and Development, 15*(1), 5–22.

Reilly, J., Klima, E., & Bellugi, U. (1990). Once more with feeling: Affect and language in atypical populations. *Development and Psychopathology, 2*(4), 367–391.

Scalise Sugiyama, M. (1996). On the origins of narrative: Storyteller bias as a fitness-enhancing strategy. *Human Nature, 7*, 403–425.

Scalise Sugiyama, M. (2003). Cultural relativism in the bush: Towards a theory of narrative universals. *Human Nature, 14*, 383–396.

Schopler, E. (1985). Convergence of learning disability, higher-level autism, and Asperger's syndrome. *Journal of Autism and Developmental Disorders, 15*, 359.

Surian, L., Baron-Cohen, S., & van der Lely, H. (1996). Are children with autism deaf to Gricean Maxims? *Cognitive Neuropsychiatry, 1*(1), 55–72.

Tager-Flusberg, H. (2000). Language and understanding minds: Connection in autism. In S. Baron-Cohen, H. Tager-Flusberg, & D. J. Cohen (Eds.), *Understanding other minds: Perspectives from autism and developmental cognitive neuroscience* (2nd ed.). Oxford, UK: Oxford University Press.

Tager-Flusberg, H., Boshart, J., & Baron-Cohen, S (1998). Reading the windows to the soul: Evidence of domain-specific sparing in Williams syndrome. *Journal of Cognitive Neuroscience, 10*, 631–639.

Tager-Flusberg, H., & Sullivan, K. (1995). Strategies for conducting research on language in autism. *Journal of Autism and Developmental Disorders, 34*, 75–80.

Tan, E. S. (1996). *Emotion and the structure of narrative film: Film as an emotion machine.* Mahwah, NJ: Erlbaum.

Wechsler, D. (1999). *Wechsler abbreviated scale of intelligence.* San Antonio, TX: Psychological Corporation.

Zunshine, L (2006). *Why we read: Theory of mind and the novel.* Columbus, Ohio: Ohio State University Press.

36 Relevance Theory and Language Interpretation

Nuala Ryder and Eeva Leinonen

INTRODUCTION

For many years now there have been reports of children and adults with difficulties with how to use language in communication. The utterances produced are generally grammatically and semantically well-formed but do not always seem to fit the conversational context. Often the listener is unable to infer what the given utterance means in a particular conversational context because of the unusual and disconnected nature of the utterance. They can be described as not always having the necessary degree of relevance with regard to the ongoing topic. Speech and language therapists have been providing therapy for individuals whose difficulties seem to lie with the understanding and/or production of connected discourse rather than linguistic structures but it was not until the 1980s that researchers (McTear & Conti-Ramsden, 1992; Rapin & Allen, 1983) began to investigate such difficulties. First referred to as "semantic-pragmatic disorders" (Bishop & Rosenbloom, 1987; Rapin & Allen, 1998; Vance & Wells, 1994), they came to be known as "pragmatic language impairments," or "pragmatic impairment" (Bishop, 2000) to reflect the primary difficulties of using language in context. It is now recognized that pragmatic impairments are a likely reflection of some underlying cognitive and social impairments (Bishop, 2000; Brook & Bowler, 1992; Hays, Niven, Godfrey, & Linscott, 2004; Linscott, 2005) and exist across a range of diagnostic boundaries such as autistic spectrum disorder (ASD) and pervasive developmental disorder not otherwise specified (PPDNOS). The relationship of such impairments experienced by children and adults on the autistic continuum has been subject to much debate (Bishop, 2000; Botting & Conti-Ramsden, 1999; Brook & Bowler, 1992; Gagnon, Mottron, & Joanette, 1997) with the outcome that the term "pragmatic impairment" is best considered a descriptive tool rather than a diagnostic entity. However, there is general agreement that, especially in children, the identification of pragmatic language impairment is important in the consideration of appropriate therapeutic and educational needs (Bishop, 2002). The remediation of children with pragmatic language impairment (PLI) continues to form a significant part of the caseload of speech and language therapists (Adams, Lloyd, Aldred, & Baxendale, 2006).

Early investigations of pragmatic difficulties were based on conversational analysis approaches where conversations involving individuals with such difficulties were analyzed for various characteristics such as turn-taking, degree of coherence, and use of cohesive devices (Bishop, Chan, Adams, Hartley, & Weir, 2000). The common communicative behaviors were identified as strategies the children used to handle a failure to understand, and focused on language production rather than comprehension. These analyses provided a useful starting point but carried with them problems associated with a lack of a rigorous theoretical framework that would generate testable predictions. Though expressive language was characterized by coherence and turn-taking, the comprehension abilities were undefined. It became clear that the cognitive nature of pragmatic understanding in relation to the social difficulties associated with inadequate pragmatic skills and weaknesses in communicative competence, was needed (Shields, Varley, Broks, & Simpson, 1996). One cognitive pragmatic approach focused on speech acts defined these as simple (direct) versus complex (indirect) according to the number or chain of inferences necessary for understanding (Airenti, Bara, & Colombetti, 1993; Bara, Bosco, & Bucciarelli, 1999). Around this time, Sperber and Wilson's (1995) Relevance Theory (RT) was being recognized as a theory of communication that defined the processes necessary for language interpretation, and went some way to explaining the dynamic nature of the generation of inferences (based on context) and how linguistic and nonlinguistic meaning were interactively achieved.

Happé (1993, 1995) found the framework of RT useful in the investigation of pragmatic language understanding and theory of mind abilities in children with autism. Leinonen and Kerbel (1999) later explored children's impairment of pragmatic comprehension within a RT paradigm. Leinonen and Ryder furthered this research (Leinonen & Ryder, 2003; Ryder & Leinonen, 2003) and found the framework useful and robust for investigating both typical development and disorders of pragmatic functioning in both English-speaking and Finnish-speaking children (Loukusa et al., 2007). The use of a framework developed on the basis of this theory has enabled rigorous and testable hypotheses to be generated that in turn has advanced our ability to study pragmatic language functioning in both normal and disordered children in a solid and systematic way.

RELEVANCE THEORY

Relevance Theory (Sperber & Wilson, 1995) is a psychological theory of communication. It details the processes of meaning interpretation in communicative situations and lends itself to empirical investigation of language impairment, especially the use of language in communication. Relevance theory supports Grice's (1989) assertion that looking at language structure alone ignores the reality of the communicative situation, where the interpretation of meaning by the hearer often involves understanding more than the meaning of the words and inferences alone. Meaning in communication is said to be derived from the context in which the communication takes place. Utterances such as "He was late again" can be produced in different contexts with different meanings. The words themselves (linguistic form and syntax) are frequently underdetermined and much of the meaning intended by the speaker is derived from intonation, gesture, eye gaze, the physical environment, and the knowledge/experience of the hearer including that of similar communicative situations. This cognitive view suggests that often, in order to interpret intended meaning, the ability to integrate relevant information is necessary and RT details the processes facilitating this. Based on the assumptions of cognition, RT argues that humans have an inborn inferential ability and a cognitive system is geared toward the processing of relevant information (governed by a principle of relevance and logical operations). They develop the ability to draw implicated conclusions from this information often necessary in communicative situations. In communication, the speakers want to be understood and therefore make their utterances as easy as possible for the hearer to understand. This results in the hearer being able to recover the intended meaning with minimum processing effort and the most accessible interpretation is therefore the most relevant one.

Pragmatic Processes

In RT's view, the processes of reference assignment, enrichment, disambiguation and implicature facilitate successful interpretation. The first three of these processes are argued to require inferences based on context. Reference assignment is the assignment of the relevant referent intended by the speaker in a communicative exchange, such as the person or thing a pronoun is used to refer to. Disambiguation refers to the meaning derived from context via inference when the expressed word has multiple meanings. For example, "rich" can mean wealthy, fertile, or calorific depending on the context. Similarly, enrichment relates to the relevant semantic meaning based on the context. When a hearer comprehends the meaning of words uttered in communication, enrichment of the linguistic meaning with other aspects of meaning are needed to form a coherent conceptualization. Inferring the meaning of words such as "enough" or "nothing" vary according to the context in which they are used. In the context of going to a party, the words in the phrase "nothing to wear" are enriched together to mean "nothing suitable or that I want to wear" rather than "nothing at all to wear." The conceptual information in memory about having "nothing to wear" to events such as parties are accessed on hearing the utterance. To constrain the possibilities of all the possible inferences from the conceptual information overloading our interpretation process, an unconscious logical operator guides access to conceptual information and a principle of relevance constrains interpretation such that the first relevant interpretation is taken as the one meant. In utterances with ambiguous words and ambiguous contexts the wrong interpretation can be reached as can and does happen in normal communication. RT suggests that in addition to these inferential processes, a process of implicature is necessary. Implicatures are not inferred, but are the result of a process of integrating previously generated inferences with perceptual information and knowledge as is necessary for interpreting the intended meaning. This process facilitates the understanding of meaning that is not inferable from the linguistic form and conceptual information alone. Implicatures are then the result of the combination of the inferences following from the linguistic form of an utterance *and* relevant contextual information. What determines whether some or all of these processes are necessary for a successful interpretation is the specificity of the utterance being interpreted (akin to how literally they can be interpreted). Utterances intended to be interpreted literally are relatively infrequent and do not necessitate recovering implicature(s). Most often in communication, the words uttered and their meanings have to be enriched and relevant contextual information integrated to understand the intended meaning. RT suggests that the result of integrating or combining information (implicated premises) leads to an implicated conclusion (an implicature). The interpretation of intended meaning reached via the process of implicature is therefore contextually based. Context in this sense refers to the information available to the hearer at the time of the interpretation including perceptual information (e.g., facial expression, gesture, nodding in the direction of something or someone), intonation, the words uttered, and knowledge and experiences in memory. Examples of meaning that depend on the generation of implicatures include the understanding of indirect answers to questions, of figurative language such as metaphor, irony, lies, sarcasm, and of understanding vague expressions.

It can be seen then that the more underdetermined a language expression, the more contextual information has to be processed (increasing cognitive effort) for comprehension. Increased cognitive effort is incurred when implicatures are recovered (unless they are very frequent or routinely processed in everyday communication). Therefore, this theory allows predictions in terms of complexity of a language expression. In RT, cognitive effort positively correlates with increased assumptions or contextual effects derived from the context necessary for successful understanding. For example, if the answer to the question "Do you know where the dog is?" is indirect as in "The back gate's open" then increased cognitive effort is incurred as the interpretation gives rise to the implication that the dog may have gone out of the gate. Whereas, a direct answer such as "It's behind the shed" does not give rise to these implications and therefore cognitive effort in interpretation is decreased. Therefore, understanding a language expression that requires inferencing (reference assignment, enrichment, disambiguation) is less demanding in terms of cognitive effort than language expressions that necessitate recovery of implicature(s). However, it is important to note that these processes are not suggested to be linear.

RT therefore lends itself to empirical investigation of the processes involved in the comprehension of language, the validity of the notion of cognitive effort (the path of least effort to successfully process the utterance) or of communicative competence and the nature of the development of pragmatic language comprehension. It provides a comprehensive account of how underdetermined language expressions can be interpreted in context. The theory has been utilized in the investigation of the notion of complexity of pragmatic language understanding in autism (Happé, 1995; Loukusa et al., 2007) in patients with right hemisphere lesions and TBI (Dipper, Bryan, & Tyson, 1997; McDonald, 1999), in young typically developing children (Papafragou & Tantalou, 2004; Ryder & Leinonen,

2003), in children with specific language impairment (SLI), and in children with PLI (Leinonen & Ryder, 2003; Ryder, Leinonen, & Schulz, 2008).

PRAGMATIC LANGUAGE COMPREHENSION

BRIDGING INFERENCES AND RIGHT HEMISPHERE BRAIN INJURY

Research into communicative disorders of patients with right hemisphere damage (RHD) suggests that they can have impaired pragmatic language abilities. Dipper et al. (1997) investigated the reduced ability of patients with RHD to draw correct inferences from texts using an RT approach. Dipper and colleagues noted that when answering questions based on a story, patients with RHD did not use the context of the story in their answers, but were able to justify their answers. The justifications revealed that the RHD participants did not appear to be aware of the contextual information but were relying on world knowledge (from memory) generating semantically related inferences rather than utilizing the story context. Dipper et al. (1997) proposed that RT provided a way of investigating the reasons for these incorrect answers. Six stroke patients with a single neurological episode resulting in unilateral RHD participated (aged 31–74 years) and there were 12 age-matched controls. The experimenters based the study on RT's predictions regarding an unconscious logical deductive system said to operate on linguistic input and the notion that concepts consist of addresses in memory that give rise to logical (e.g., or, either), encyclopedic (cutting your finger makes it bleed, etc.), and lexical information (syntactical and grammatical information). When words are heard or seen, an automatic process of meaning retrieval accesses the appropriate concept address. The participants listened and read two sentence scenarios and answered three question types that targeted three types of bridging inference. The first (textual inference) required utilizing linguistic input in order to answer correctly. The second (textually reinforced inference) targeted information generated by discourse connectives where the contextually generated inference does not require accessing encyclopedic information (RT suggests that discourse connectives are procedural and do not have encyclopedic entries). The third inference required encyclopedic information to answer correctly.

Findings revealed that RHD participants performed less well than controls on all inference types. This group relied on encyclopedic information and questions targeting linguistic deduction were problematic for this group, particularly discourse connectives. Dipper et al. (1997) suggest that if RT's view of the procedural and nonencyclopedic nature of discourse connective concepts is correct, then the brain damage suffered by RHD patients affects the deductive device. Utilizing linguistic context to infer intended meaning is therefore affected. They suggest that this inability to use linguistic information from the text in the deductive system, was coupled with an over-reliance on encyclopedic information (not a preferential use of encyclopedic information). It is interesting to note that in typically developing 4- and 5-year-old children a tendency to use their own experiential knowledge of events (rather than the information in the story) was found when answering questions requiring semantic inferencing (enrichment) in context (Ryder & Leinonen, 2003). In a similar way to the answers given by RHD patients, the ability to utilize the relevant given context was implicated.

SARCASM AND TRAUMATIC BRAIN INJURY

As mentioned, complexity in pragmatic language understanding is dependent on the cognitive effort involved in combining relevant information from context. The interpretation of irony and sarcasm for example, is effortful in the sense that an additional recognition of the speaker's emotion or intentions is required for interpretation. In patients with traumatic brain injury (TBI) difficulties in under-standing sarcasm are well-documented (McDonald, 1999). Often these patients interpret sarcastic utterances literally (where a literal interpretation is possible). McDonald (1999, p. 489) investigated the understanding of sarcasm in patients with TBI using RT to examine more closely the nature of the difficulty. In utter-ances such as "A lovely day for a picnic indeed" the interpretation depends on the hearer recognizing the echoed proposition from previously shared knowledge. That is, if previously it was suggested that it was a lovely day for a picnic and it was now cold or raining, the speaker's utterance echoes the previous utterance. Relevance theory suggests the understanding of sarcasm requires inferences about both the facts of the situation and of the mental state of the speaker (attitudes, knowledge, and intentions). In the same way that other linguistic expressions are interpreted, linguistic and contextual features are integrated but RT suggests that sarcastic comments additionally echo a prior assertion, and this echo com-municates the speaker's derogatory attitude. Patients with TBI have been shown to be better able to interpret literal sarcastic utterances than when the sarcastic utterances were intended to mean the opposite of what was said (McDonald & Pearce, 1996). Patients watched videotapes of the interaction between two peo-ple and conversations included utterances that were sincerely meant or were sar-castic. In some cases understanding the emotion of the speaker was necessary to understand that the literal utterance was not intended (the speaker does not mean what they say) but if this was not recognized a literal meaning could be comprehended. For example, patients were asked whether the speaker in say-ing "Sorry I made you come" was pleased that he made his addressee come. In another variation, the speakers utterance could not be understood literally; that is, the speaker asked the hearer if they remembered their passport and the hearer replied saying they had torn it up and thrown it away. Patients were also asked questions about the emotions of the speaker. Findings suggested that the patients had no appreciable difficulty in understanding literal utterances or the emotional tone of the speaker. They performed poorly (failed to understand sarcasm) in these verbal exchanges, particularly when no literal interpretation was possible. McDonald suggests the patients' ability to understand sarcasm was independ-ent of their ability to comprehend emotional tone and the difficulty lay in infer-ential reasoning of verbal information. In his review of studies of patients with TBI, McDonald notes that patients with TBI performed better when interpreting physically presented counterfactual sarcastic comments than verbally presented counterfactual comments. This suggests that these patients can utilize relevant visual information from context, but have particular difficulty when this information is verbal. According to McDonald (1999), RT's account of interpretation is well-founded with the exception of the notion of comprehending scornful echo. The patients with TBI were able to understand the literal meaning suggesting that they comprehended the previous assumption (and they were able to understand the speaker's emotion), but still they were unable to interpret the sarcastic intent. McDonald points out that studies (Kaplan, Brownell, Jacobs, & Gardner, 1990; McDonald & Pearce, 1996) have shown that even when the speaker's attitude is explicit (rather than inferred) patients with TBI still did not recognize the sarcastic intent. Therefore a mentalizing ability is suggested to be crucial.

MENTALIZING AND AUTISM

In a study by Happé (1993), RT's predictions of complexity of processing and notion of attributing mental states to others (understanding communicative intention) were used to examine the communicative competence of children and adults with autism (aged 9–28 years old) and children and adults with mild learning disabilities (aged 12–38 years). The participants answered questions targeting similes, metaphors, and irony. Based on RT, similes were suggested to require less processing than metaphors whereas irony was the most complex to process because of the necessity of attributing mental states to others. The ability to understand figurative language (sarcasm, metaphor, irony) develops gradually from the age of five in typically developing children (Laval & Bert-Erboul, 2005). However, in children and adults with autism this development is not seen and in addition the ability to understand other's intentions (suggested to be key in communication) and to integrate contextual information such as knowledge of the hearer during communication, appears either delayed or deviant. Happé (1993, 1995) found that in children with autism, the ability to understand the intentions of others was directly associated with the comprehension of pragmatically demanding figurative language such as metaphor and irony. There were underlying differences in the mentalizing ability of the two groups with autism, which mediated false-belief performance and utterance comprehension. Findings supported relevance theory's predictions regarding the increasing degree of mind necessary for understanding simile, metaphor, and irony.

THE DEVELOPMENT OF PRAGMATIC LANGUAGE COMPREHENSION

Dipper et al. (1997) focused on the inferential and conceptual claims of RT whereas McDonald (1999) and Happé (1995) focused on the notion of increased cognitive effort or more pragmatically demanding language expressions in relation to communication difficulties. Another approach used to investigate the use of context in pragmatic language understanding (and hence the notion of pragmatic complexity) focuses on the processes suggested to be involved in pragmatic language comprehension. These have been used to investigate the pragmatic language abilities of children with high functioning autism (HFA), Asperger syndrome (AS), SLI, and PLI. Children with autism and AS have difficulties in social interaction suggested to be linked to problems in attributing mental states to others or recognizing others' intentions. They often interpret language expressions literally. Relevance theory's outline of pragmatic language understanding suggests that understanding the intention of the speaker is linked to an inherent ability to infer, to attend to relevant information, and to process implicatures. Children with SLI have been suggested to have some problems with inferencing (Botting & Adams, 2005) and a subgroup of children with PLI have similar but more marked difficulties. Relevance theory suggests that inferencing is only one process in language understanding and this ability is necessary to assign referents (e.g. assigning meaning to pronouns) and to enrich semantic meaning in context (as in disambiguation). These processes, particularly pronoun resolution, are common in everyday communication. RT suggests that frequency can lead to automaticity of processing, which is facilitated by a logical deductive device (see Sperber & Wilson, 1995 for details). Thus, the development of pronoun resolution or reference assignment occurs early in language development (around the age of three) and is suggested to be a relatively automatic process compared to inferring semantic meaning or enriching meaning in context (loosening, broadening, or disambiguating meaning), which continues to develop between the ages of 3 and 5. Examples of reference assignment and enrichment can be seen in the following example.

Speaker A: Jane worked hard in her aerobic class.
Speaker B: The wedding's in six weeks.

In this example "Jane" is assigned to the person known as Jane to both speakers (reference assignment) and "worked hard" is enriched to mean exercising most energetically and not other meanings of "work" and "hard" that are not relevant in this context. The understanding of Speaker A's utterance is not dependent on the recovery of an implicature. Comprehension of the intended meaning of Speaker B's utterance is not achieved by inferring referents and enriching meaning alone. For speaker A to recover the meaning of "Jane is working hard at aerobics because she wants to look good at the forthcoming wedding," further processing is necessary. When the intended meaning is not recoverable from inferencing alone as in this example, previous relevant inferences, knowledge from memory, and perceptual information combine to yield implicatures. Intonation, facial expression, and world knowledge (including knowledge of these kinds of exchanges) are part of the contextual information the hearer uses to recover the intended meaning. RT suggests that this process incurs increased cognitive effort compared to the solely inferential processes of reference assignment and enrichment. Therefore, increased pragmatic demands may be associated with each of these processes (reference assignment < enrichment < implicature).

Leinonen and Kerbel (1999) explored data from three children with language impairment. The characteristic features of pragmatic impairment were examined within the RT framework. The processes detailed in RT were found to be useful in interpreting the difficulties. Communication breakdown could be attributed to difficulties in enriching meaning and in understanding implicatures. In production, the children's use of pronouns instead of naming the referent was suggested to reflect difficulty with relevance in relation to reference assignment. The seemingly irrelevant answers of the children in different communicative situations revealed that the children sometimes answered when they did not know what a word meant and on explanation of the word could then answer correctly. The children sometimes knew the meaning of a word but had difficulty in disambiguating or enriching the meaning in context. For example interpreting "hole" (in the context of planting trees) to mean a place where you put a treasure rather than a hole to plant a tree in. This interpretation was arrived at despite having discussed the context of the picture beforehand (workmen in the park using spades to dig holes, the trees ready for planting). Interpreting the children's utterance within RT's framework was suggested to be clinically useful and shows the importance of understanding the language abilities of the child in order to decide on how best to communicate meaning.

In line with RT's view of cognitive processes and cognitive effort, studies using questions targeting reference assignment, enrichment, and implicatures have supported the notion of increased pragmatic language demands of the question types, in particular those targeting implicature. A developmental trend was evident in young children when answering the three question types (based on stories or scenarios) in both English and Finnish children (Loukusa et al., 2007; Ryder & Leinonen, 2003; Ryder, Leinonen, & Schulz, 2008). Three-year-old English children were unable to answer questions targeting implicatures, a finding that was also found in Finnish 3 year olds except when answering implicature questions based on very familiar daily routines, for example, interpreting "it's dinner time" to mean a request to go inside and get ready to have dinner. At the age of four both English and Finnish children were competent at enriching semantic meaning. Although this ability is still developing and by the age of five, children were found to be still developing the ability to recover implicatures (competence is evident by the age of seven). The wrong answers of the four year olds suggest that these children tend to rely on their world knowledge when they did not recover the intended implicature. For example, they would use their own knowledge of going to a birthday party rather than the information about the birthday party given in the story context. Three year olds also used world knowledge but most frequently produced answers that were irrelevant in the given context (Ryder & Leinonen, 2003).

Comparing the typically developing children (Ryder & Leinonen, 2003) to children with SLI, a further study by Leinonen and Ryder (2003) found the children with SLI performed less well than their peers. Children with SLI are a heterogeneous group presenting with various structural language deficits. Bates (2004, p. 249) suggests the deficits in SLI manifest themselves as a result of problems in the cognitive domain during development. In this study the children with SLI performed similarly to the typically developing 4 year olds when enriching semantic meaning and generating implicatures suggesting delayed language development.

The pragmatic comprehension of a subgroup of children with SLI who had difficulties with pragmatic language understanding (whose primary difficulties are with pragmatic language meaning in the absence of autistic spectrum symptoms) was recently investigated (Ryder et al., 2008). The children, aged 7–11 years, perform significantly below their peers and children with SLI without pragmatic impairment, when answering questions targeting implicature(s) based on verbal scenarios and stories. The children with PLI could be identified from the rest of the SLI group on their performance on questions targeting implicatures. These children had particular difficulty in using the given verbal context (scenario or story). All groups were competent at reference assignment and had no appreciable difficulties on the whole with enriching semantic meaning, but wrong answers revealed that the children tended to use world knowledge in preference to the context when incorrectly answering. The tasks in the study included verbal input with and without pictures. In the with-picture task where the answer was available in the picture, the children with SLI performed similarly to their peers when answering questions targeting implicatures. However, when pictures were not available and the input was verbal only, these children appear significantly delayed in understanding implicatures. The children with PLI performed worst of all on this task, a finding that was not explained by their structural language or auditory memory abilities. RT's framework was useful in examining the role of context in interpretation and highlights the interactive nature of meaning in interpretation.

Loukusa et al. (2007) carried out a similar study of Finnish children. Typically developing Finnish children were compared with children with AS and HFA. The reference assignment, enrichment, and implicature questions in this study were asked on the basis of verbal scenarios. The youngest children with AS/HFA (7–9 year olds) had some difficulties in answering questions targeting enrichment but this was not evident in the older (10–12 year old) group. However both groups were found to have significant difficulties with questions targeting implicatures (Loukusa et al., 2007) compared to typically developing children. This finding, taken with Happé's findings (1993, 1995) indicates the difficulty in understanding implicatures as being a core deficit in children and adults in autism affecting the ability to interpret metaphor and other language expressions requiring the generation of implicatures.

The studies discussed, taken together, show that the clinical groups were competent at reference assignment (resolution of pronouns, assigning referents), a process that develops relatively early in language development as seen in the typically developing children (English and Finnish) who were competent at the age of 3–4 years and by the age of six were competent at enriching semantic meaning.

SUMMARY AND CONCLUSIONS

There had been comparatively little progress in the understanding of the nature of pragmatic language abilities compared to structural language abilities largely because of a need for a theoretical framework. RT has provided a framework with which to investigate the nature of language comprehension in disordered populations including details of the processes that may be impaired and the prediction of cognitive effort involved in communicative utterances. The studies discussed have supported RT's notion of pragmatic complexity and language development. It has also shown that instances of pragmatic language breakdown can be explained and predicted by this theory.

Relevance Theory has provided testable predictions about language impairment and the kinds of language behavior that children and adults with communication difficulties may exhibit. It has enabled us to move away from a description of the communication behaviors to a better understanding of pragmatic language difficulties including why they result in difficulties in communication and their effects on the quality of conversational interactions. RT may provide a useful tool for addressing the issue of the assessment of PLI, given that the interpretation of implicature was found to be problematic in children and adults with pragmatic language difficulties. The findings that individuals with PLI often produce irrelevant utterances/answers as do very young children (3-year-olds) suggests that the processing involved in integrating contextual information or utilizing relevant context is implicated. RT maintains that humans cannot help but interpret the relevant meaning. However, in development children may stop processing at the first relevant interpretation because they have not yet developed the ability (or do not have the knowledge) to fully interpret the speaker's perspective. It is not clear how children develop this ability, though it may be the experience of interacting and conversing that provides the knowledge that they can then use in interpretation. On this view, children with PLI might lack this knowledge because of different experiences with language use during development. However, there is currently little data to support this and more research is needed. The data from typically developing children suggests that the development of the ability to recover implicatures occurs between the ages of 4 and 7 years and therefore early intervention would be recommended. We have found that using this theoretical framework is useful in suggesting ways of facilitating interactions with pragmatically impaired individuals for example, consideration of the conceptual properties of words in relation to the context, and the context itself. The consequences of both the specificity of the verbal information used in tasks and the perceptual information/materials have consequences that ought to be considered in the assessment process.

The research has largely supported the psychological validity of the theory but further research is necessary to validate the notion of relevance. Some also refute RT's view of an unconscious deductive device operating on linguistic input and consequent automatic conceptual access said to occur during enrichment (Cummings, 1998). Similarly, McDonald (1999) casts doubt on RT's notion of scornful echo as an explanation for the comprehension of sarcasm.

The data from the studies of patients with TBI was not consistent with this explanation. However, these theoretical considerations do not alter the contribution of the theory in focusing attention on other factors besides language structure that are important in the assessment of language and communication disorders.

RT's view of communication demonstrates both the responsibilities of the speaker and the limitations of the hearer in the interactional process. The studies have shown how individuals are responsible for communicative success or breakdown and how interaction in communication is facilitated. When breakdown occurs in communication, repair depends on knowledge of the hearer's language difficulties and their developmental level. These observations have important implications for therapy in the clinical setting. Difficulties with utilizing relevant context or integrating information from both the context and memory may be addressed in the clinical setting by encouraging our understanding of how the context is relevant to the interpretation. Within this framework it is possible to explore the language of those engaging with language impaired children and consider what kinds of contributions may be most facilitative.

FURTHER READING

Cummings, L. (2009). *Clinical pragmatics*. Cambridge: CUP.

Leinonen, E., Letts, C., & Smith, B. R. (2000). *Children's pragmatic communication difficulties*. London, UK: Whurr.

Perkins, M. (2007). *Pragmatic impairment*. Cambridge, MA: Cambridge University Press.

REFERENCES

Adams, C., Lloyd, J., Aldred, C., & Baxendale, T. (2006). Exploring the effects of communication intervention for developmental pragmatic language impairments: A signal-generation study. *International Journal of Language and Communication Disorders, 41*(1), 41–65.

Airenti, G., Bara, B. G., & Colombetti, M. (1993). Failures, exploitations and deceits in communication. *Journal of Pragmatics, 20*, 303–326.

Bara, B. G., Bosco, F. M., & Bucciarelli, M. (1999). Developmental pragmatics in normal and abnormal children. *Brain and Language, 68*, 507–528.

Bates, E. A. (2004). Explaining and interpreting deficits in language development across clinical groups: Where do we go from here? *Brain and Language, 88*, 248–253.

Bishop, D. V. M. (2000). Pragmatic language impairment: A correlate of SLI, a distinct subgroup, or part of the autistic continuum? In D. V. M. Bishop & L. B. Leonard (Eds.), *Speech and language impairments in children: Causes, characteristics, intervention and outcome* (pp. 99–114). Hove, UK: Psychology Press.

Bishop, D. V. M. (2002). Speech and language difficulties. In M. Rutter & E. A. Taylor (Eds.), *Child and adolescent psychiatry*. London, UK: Blackwell.

Bishop, D. V. M., Chan, J., Adams, C., Hartley, J., & Weir, F. (2000). Conversational responsiveness in specific language impairment: Evidence of disproportionate pragmatic difficulties in a subset of children. *Development and Psychopathology, 12*, 177–199.

Bishop, D. V. M., & Rosenbloom, L. (1987). Classification of childhood language disorders. In W. Yule & M. Rutter (Eds.), *Language development and disorders*. London, UK: Mac Keith Press.

Botting, N., & Adams, C. (2005). Semantic and inferencing abilities in children with communication disorders. *International Journal of Language and Communication Disorders, 4*, 49–66.

Botting, N., & Conti-Ramsden, G. (1999). Pragmatic language impairment without autism: The children in question. *Autism, 3*(4), 371–396.

Brook, S. L., & Bowler, D. (1992). "Autism by another name?" Semantic and pragmatic impairments in children. *Journal of Autism and Developmental Disorders, 22*, 61–81.

Cummings L. (1998). The scientific reductionism of relevance theory: The lesson from logical positivism. *Journal of Pragmatics*, 29, 1–12.

Dipper, L. T., Bryan, K. L., & Tyson, J. (1997). Bridging inference and relevance theory: An account of right hemisphere inference. *Clinical Linguistics and Phonetics, 11*, 213–228.

Gagnon, L., Mottron, L., & Joanette, Y. (1997). Questioning the validity of the semantic-pragmatic syndrome diagnosis. *Autism, 1*, 37–55.

Grice, H. P. (1989). *Studies in the way of words*. Cambridge, MA: Harvard University Press.

Happé, F. G. E. (1993). Communicative competence and theory of mind in autism: A test of relevance theory. *Cognition, 48*, 101–119.

Happé, F. G. E. (1995). Understanding minds and metaphors: Insights from the study of figurative language in autism. *Metaphor and Symbol, 10*, 275–295.

Hays, S. J., Niven, B. E., Godfrey, H. P. D., & Linscott, R. J. (2004). Clinical assessment of pragmatic language impairment: A generalizability study of older people with Alzheimer's disease. *Aphasiology, 18*, 693–714.

Kaplan, J. A., Brownell, H. H., Jacobs, J. R., & Gardner, H. (1990). The effects of right hemisphere brain damage on the pragmatic interpretation of conversational remarks. *Brain and Language, 38*, 315–333.

Laval, V., & Bert-Erboul, A. (2005). French-speaking children's understanding of sarcasm: The role of intonation and context. *Journal of Speech, Language, and Hearing Research, 48*, 610–620.

Leinonen, E., & Kerbel, D. (1999). Relevance theory and pragmatic impairment. *International Journal of Language and Communication Disorders, 34*, 367–390.

Leinonen, E., & Ryder, N. (2003). The use of context in pragmatic comprehension by specifically language-impaired and control children. *Linguistics, 41*(2), 407–423.

Linscott, R. J. (2005). Thought disorder, pragmatic language impairment, and generalized cognitive decline in schizophrenia *Schizophrenia Research, 75*(2–3), 225–232.

Loukusa, S., Leinonen, E., Kuusikko, S., Jussila, K., Mattila, M. L., Ryder, N., … Moilanen, I. (2007). Use of context in pragmatic language comprehension by children with Asperger syndrome or high-functioning autism. *Journal of Autism and Developmental Disorders, 37*(6), 1049–1059.

McDonald, S. (1999). Exploring the process of inference generation in sarcasm: A review of normal and clinical studies. *Brain and Language, 68*(3), 486–506.

McDonald, S., & Pearce, S. (1996). Clinical insights into pragmatic language theory: The case of sarcasm. *Brain and Language, 53*, 81–104.

McTear, M., & Conti-Ramsden, G. (1992). *Pragmatic disability in children*. London, UK: Whurr.

Papafragou, A., & Tantalou, N. (2004). Children's computation of implicatures. *Language Acquisition, 12*, 71–82.

Rapin, I., & Allen, D. (1983). Developmental language disorders: Nosologic considerations. In U. Kirk (Ed.), *Neuropsychology of language, reading, and spelling*
(pp. 155–184). New York, NY: Academic Press.

Rapin, I., & Allen, D. A. (1998). The semantic-pragmatic deficit disorder: Classification
issues. *International Journal of Language and Communication Disorders*,
33, 82–87.

Ryder, N., & Leinonen, E. (2003). Use of context in question answering by 3-, 4- and
5-year-old children. *Journal of Psycholinguistic Research, 32*(4), 397–415.

Ryder, N., Leinonen, E., & Schulz, J. (2008). A cognitive approach to assessing
pragmatic language comprehension in children with specific language impairment.
International Journal of Language and Communication Disorders, 43(4), 427–447.

Shields, J., Varley, R., Broks, P., & Simpson, A. (1996). Social cognition in developmental language disorders and high level autism. *Developmental Medicine and Child
Neurology, 38*, 487–495.

Sperber, D., & Wilson, D. (1995). *Relevance: Communication and cognition* (2nd ed.).
Oxford, UK: Blackwell.

Vance, M., & Wells, B. (1994). The wrong end of the stick: Language-impaired children's
understanding of non-literal language. *Child Language Teaching and Therapy, 10*,
23–46.

37 Psycholinguistics and Augmentative and Alternative Communication

Filip Loncke

INTRODUCTION

Augmentative and Alternative Communication (AAC) is the term used for practices, methods, systems, and devices that are aimed at providing and supporting communication for individuals with little or no functional natural speech. AAC has developed in the last 30 years as a predominantly applied discipline with a growing target population. AAC can be considered to be the use of nonstandard communication forms as an addition or a compensation for insufficient access to standard forms. Standard forms of communication are natural speech and writing. In more recent developments within society, electronic communication forms such as cell phone communication and electronic mail (email) have also acquired the status of standard communication.

AAC *techniques* include nontech approaches such as the use of manual signs, besides low-tech solutions such as communication boards or single switch speech generators, and more complex speech-generating computer based devices at the high tech end. Within the field of AAC, new developments are predicted, reflecting more advanced technology such as brain wave directed communication.

AAC *interventions* can consist of training the individual to use the alternative communication system or device, as well as training the individual's communication partners, planning learning steps, and modifying the environment (such as routines, the curriculum, expectations, and attitudes).

AAC is primarily an applied field as it attempts to find solutions for individuals with severe limitations due to a wide range of causes, at different stages in life, and with a wide variety of social, cognitive, and linguistic skills. At the same time, however, AAC is a field that offers interesting opportunities to investigate psycholinguistic processes. In the first place, it allows observing the flexibility of language production when the output modality is altered. Besides the applied use of AAC, this chapter is primarily concerned with the underlying psycholinguistic mechanisms of AAC use. The chapter will focus on historical developments that have contributed to the emergence of AAC as an applied field (taxonomy and classifications that are relevant for psycholinguistic understanding of AAC, motor execution and access, the nature of the symbols used in AAC, and AAC processing).

HISTORICAL ROOTS OF AUGMENTATIVE AND ALTERNATIVE COMMUNICATION

It is probably no coincidence that AAC started to develop in the 1970s. In that period psycholinguistic research had developed an interest in the flexibility of the human language capacity. The discovery that sign languages of deaf communities are linguistically full-fledged languages (Klima & Bellugi, 1979) stands as an example of this renewed and refreshed look at communication and language (Vermeerbergen & Van Herreweghen, Chapter 34 of this volume). Although speech is clearly and without doubt the preferred modality for direct linguistic communication, other modalities function as alternatives.

The discovery of language in the gestural modality also led to exploring the transitions and the dividing lines between nonlinguistic communication and linguistic communication. This is exemplified in the description of gestures versus manual signs: gesturing is typically a phenomenon that is co-occurring with speech (McNeill & Duncan, Chapter 32 of this volume) with which it has a dynamic relation. In many instances, gestures do not have any meaning as such but serve as a psychomotor underpinning—or reinforcement—of the speech process. Gesturing can move to the foreground by assuming meaning through the use of conventionalized or semi-conventionalized forms. Deaf children of hearing parents with limited contact to sign language users have been described to develop "home signs," gestures that have taken on a meaning that is understood by a limited number of individuals with whom the person interacts. For example, pointing to the chin may be sign that refers to a specific person (e.g., a neighbor) who has a small beard (Vermeerbergen & Van Herreweghen, Chapter 34 of this volume). Gestures can also become more prevalent in situations of processing difficulties in speech. One example is lexical access. An increasing number of studies shows that gesturing facilitates in cases of word finding (Ravizza, 2003), possibly as a result of both iconic facilitation and neurological activation.

As linguistic processing in the spoken modality becomes less available, gesturing tends to overtake language role. Goldin-Meadow's (1998) research has shown how gesture assumes linguistic value in instances where a developing person does not have sufficient exposure to spoken language. Gestural applications within AAC capitalize on this principle. Gesturing and manual signing have been forms of AAC since the earliest days and remain in use until today. Since the 1970s sign language has regained recognition as full-fledged languages and manual signs are considered being powerful linguistic elements that will foster communication. In the past, educators often feared that signing would impede the development of natural speech. Although some of these fears still subsist, manual signing is now often used as a complement, a replacement, or as a trigger for speech. The (in)compatibility hypothesis will be discussed later in this chapter.

In the late 1960s, there was a growing interest in whether animals could learn and use manual signs. The studies and reports of the Gardners (1969), Fouts (1987), and others raised the possibility of the communicative potential of non-speech signs for individuals deprived of speech. Bonvillian and Nelson (1976) were among the first to explore the possibilities of manual signing with non-speaking developmentally disabled individuals. Since then, the use of manual signing has become common practice and a typical component in the intervention of nonspeaking children (and adults) with severe expressive limitations (Snell & Brown, 2006). Several explanations have been proposed for the success of manual signing in children with autism. Authors often refer to the iconic nature of many of the basic manual signs. Iconicity is the term used to indicate that a symbol bears a physical resemblance to its referent. Klima and Bellugi (1979) propose two degrees of iconicity: transparency and translucency. A symbol is transparent if the meaning is readily available to the observer. Translucency refers to situations where the observer can understand the link with the referent once this connection is made explicit. For example, the meaning of the American Sign Language (ASL) sign BALL (curving the hands around an imaginary ball) is likely to be understood, while the sign GIRL (tip of extended thumb slides down the cheek) can only be grasped after one explains that it refers to the string of the bonnet that girls and women used to wear in the late eighteenth century in France (the time of heightened interest in signing, and a time that signs were recorded onto books).

This early development coincided with an increased interest in presymbolic and prelinguistic communication. What are the mechanisms and dynamics between birth and the first expressed word that move a child into the use of a symbolic system? Several indications point to the fact that gestures provide a bridge between primarily sensorimotor functioning in the first months of life toward symbolic conceptualization and language use. A major part of AAC-practice is focused on facilitating communication through the systematic use of external symbols or referents, as well as attempts to help transition a person to symbolic and/or linguistic communication. For example, low functioning children with autism may be taught to use an object (e.g., a cereal box) as a tangible referent for breakfast. The object becomes part of a ritualized routine sequence in which it assumes the function of a signal or a presymbol. Systematic use of presymbols is reinforced and shaped toward genuine symbolic and linguistic functioning. This type of intervention usually is part of a concept of trainability through stages toward internalized symbol use (Taylor & Iacono, 2003).

In short, the breakthrough of AAC practice has been facilitated by the recognition that nonspeech modalities can be communicative and linguistic. The potential of modalities other than speech was also explored through the use of graphic symbols such as Blissymbolics (see discussion below) or pictures that were used on a communication board (Archer, 1977) to function as lexical elements, replacing spoken words or spoken messages. The development of synthetic and computer generated speech in the past 30 years made it clear that natural articulation can be substituted by machine-generated speech.

It is impossible to draw a strict distinction between AAC and standard forms of communication. As electronic forms of communication have become common, the distinction between standard communication and AAC tends to become less clear. For example, cell phone technology and email communication are increasingly used as assistive devices or techniques (McNaughton & Bryen, 2007). Applied applications are reflected in identifying the aids that will help a person and his/her communication environment to interact.

In present-day's speech language pathology intervention, in special education, and in rehabilitation, AAC plays an increasing role in assessing a person's communication skills and communication potential (Huer, 1997), enhancing learning and development (Von Tetzchner, Brekke, Sjothun, & Grindheim, 2005), promoting literacy development (Sturm & Clendon, 2004), and social networking (Blackstone & Hunt Berg, 2003).

AUGMENTATIVE AND ALTERNATIVE COMMUNICATION: TAXONOMY AND TYPOLOGY

AAC-solutions can vary from nontech adaptations (e.g., manual signing) over low tech (e.g., picture communication) to high tech (e.g., speech-generating devices that are part of a computer). New applications for the future may include the use of implanted electrodes that help to steer communication devices along with other assistive technology through a brain–computer interface (BCI; Birbaumer & Cohen, 2007). These new developments offer exciting avenues to compare typical and atypical language processing, as they attempt to bypass the muscular system of the person. The computer may respond to the EEC pattern of a person "thinking" to move the cursor up or down.

AIDED AND UNAIDED COMMUNICATION

One distinction that is often made (Fuller, Lloyd, & Schlosser, 1992) is that between aided and unaided communication. Unaided communication requires no aid external to the person's body. Besides natural speech, gesturing, manual sign use, pointing, body posturing, and so forth are forms of unaided communication. Aided communication implies that the user relies on a device, a communication board, a pictures set, or other piece of equipment or material that is external to the body. The distinction is less trivial than it might seem. It raises the question of how much of the communication system is "internalized" and how much is part of an externally made up list. For example, one of the main discussions within the field of AAC practice is how to decide on the first (and growing) vocabulary of an AAC user. It is often the clinician or another communication partner that provides the words (symbols). In typical language and communication development, the lexicon grows spontaneously within the mind of the user, in interaction with the environment. The environment does not "decide" on a vocabulary, while caregivers often exert a controlling and restricting influence on the lexicon that is available to individuals who use AAC.

Another characteristic of aided communication is that it may limit face-to-face communication. Communication partners are drawn toward the aided communication tool. An aided technique that is commonly used for individuals with autism spectrum disorders (ASD) is Picture Exchange Communication System (PECS; Bondy & Frost, 2001). The users of the system literally materialize the exchange of messages in the form of picture symbols on cards that are handed to the communication partner. The partner "reads" the message from the card, interrupting the face-to-face interaction with the communicator, whereas the use of speech or manual signing encourages facial contact. Pragmatically, users of aided communication and their partners need to develop specific strategies to monitor attention of the partner while the message is constructed. The use of speech-generating communication devices may lead to similar differences with natural face to face communication. While the communicator is "entering" the message on the device, eye contact with the interlocutor is interrupted. At present, there is little research that indicates how the aided AAC user monitors the attention of the communication partner.

THE USE OF GRAPHIC SYMBOLS

Communication boards, displaying graphic symbols were among the very first low-tech forms of AAC (McDonald & Schultz, 1973). Since then, developers and practitioners are faced with a number of questions that all touch on important psycholinguistic issues: (1) What exactly should be put on the board? (2) How can an ergonomic use of the board be assured? (3) How can one maximize the number of messages that can be generated? (4) Can and will users of the board combine the elements into more complex messages? The same questions apply to the use of electronic speech-generating devices displaying symbols on screens.

A wide variety of graphic symbols are in use. Sometimes, clinicians use photographs of the AAC users' relatives, their home environment, and their personal topics of interest. Besides these personal symbols, a wide range of graphic symbols have become available, increasingly in electronic format. The use of these symbols raises a number of interesting psycholinguistic questions.

Fuller et al. (1997) propose a distinction between sets and systems. A set of symbols is mainly a more or less loose collection of graphic representations without a systematic organization as such. A *system* is a collection of symbols that are constructed based on design and combination principles. For example, concepts that are semantically related may be represented in a specific color. Nouns and verbs can be coded in specific ways. And "complex" concepts can be represented by a combination of more basic symbols. Often, systems include markers such as arrows to indicate direction, movement, size, or time.

Graphic symbols differ in their degree of abstractness. Several studies have focused on the learnability of graphic symbols. The iconicity continuum from high transparent to low translucent symbols that was proposed for manual signs, is also valid here (Lloyd, Loncke, & Arvidson, 1999).

Blissymbolics is a graphic symbols system that is based on a proposed visual-iconic communication system proposed by Charles Bliss (1965). Bliss's system was originally not designed for individuals with communication limitations, but was meant as an attempt to make intercultural communication more transparent and less ambiguous. In the early 1970s, the use of Blissymbolics was first introduced for children with cerebral palsy who had no functional speech (Bliss & McNaughton, 1976). Contrary to most other graphic symbols systems, a sublexical level can be distinguished in most of the symbols used in Blissymbolics. There are about a hundred basic symbols that are combined into new symbols. The symbols can be broken down into subcomponents, which, in turn, can be recombined into another symbol. The system is meant to be similar to a natural language where the combinatorial principle allows thousands of words to be formed with a limited number of phonemes.

How do users of Blissymbolics process the symbols? It is tempting to think that the most effective users store and process the basic symbols in a way that is equivalent to the use of morphemes. Koul and Lloyd (1998) found that individuals with aphasia can learn to use translucent symbols of the system. Raghavendra and Fristoe (1995) found that 3-year-old children learn the symbols better if some of the visual characteristics are visually enhanced. From a psycholinguistic viewpoint, it would be interesting to know if the users effectively process symbols as combinations of sublexical recurring elements. In other words, how "linguistic" is a system such as Blissymbolics? Although the question may appear largely academic, it has some interesting applied aspects. The system, in its workings, functions largely in connection with another spoken or written language; that is, the symbols are paired with written words and its use (both in clinical situation and in direct communication) is often a form of simultaneous communication. The user is encouraged to point to the symbols that are conceived to be substitutes of the spoken words. But can the system function alone without being paired to words from a spoken language? We are not aware of research that looks into this fascinating question. One hypothesis could be that users will tend to invest linguistic value into the graphic system, much like children create a Creole language (Bickerton, 1999). Soto and Toro-Zambrana (1995) analyzed the morphosyntactic structures of three native Spanish speakers using Blissymbolics. They observed that the participants produced morphosyntactic structures that were not always congruent with those of Spanish. However, these structures do have an inherent consistent pattern. Such research should observe how the use of these symbols would evolve through dialogues without a linkage to speech or written language

THE REPRESENTATIONAL NATURE OF GRAPHIC SYMBOLS

Another issue is the representation itself, which entails a whole view of semantics. What exactly does the graphic stand for: a word or a concept?—the selection of the symbols is typically based on an intuitive connection, between a word and a graphic representation. In most cases, the chosen representation appears to reflect a perspective of the adult developer of the system, taken the approach that pictures can match the semantic field that is covered by a lexical entity. Adult language users can easily make abstraction of the accidental characteristics of the picture, especially if the printed word is displayed along with the symbol. However, it is not clear that this will be the path taken by preliterate children without functional speech. DeLoache's (1995) research has shown that the understanding of picture symbols is a complex developmental process. Their linkage to words and their semantic fields requires an understanding of external representation of a concept—"a model of a model." It is not clear how the acquisition of speech contributes to this developmental process. This is all the more the case for nonspeaking children.

Moreover, it is questionable that the symbols that are used in practices reflect, in fact, the way individuals build internal representations. Light, Page, Curran, & Pitkin (2007) demonstrated an impressive discrepancy between the way words are represented in iconic systems and the way children intuitively conceptualize these words.

The problem of representation through pictures is complex. Several researchers have attempted to compare the "guessability" of graphic symbol systems (e.g., Bloomberg, Karlan, & Lloyd, 1990). However, these guessing rates almost always refer to identification of a word, not a concept. The meaning of verbs and abstract words are virtually impossible to catch in a picture. For example, in one symbol system (Picture Communication System, PCS), "Walking" is differentiated from "Running" by a different body posture of a cartoon-like little man. Perception and interpretation research across ages and cultures can help understand how universally these meanings are grasped.

PERCEPTION, ACCESS, AND MOTOR EXECUTION

The use of AAC implies that at least one of the main components in the sender-message-receiver chain has been modulated. Most forms of AAC entail a visual component (the symbols on the screen or on the communication board, as well as manual signs) along with auditory information.

Speed of access and processing is the main reason why research is needed to understand how these components of communication interact in AAC. While typical natural speech is easily produced at a rate of two or three words a second (Levelt, 1993), it is not unusual that AAC users only produce a very limited number of words in the time of one minute, due to a combination of motor-perceptual limitations as well as challenges for navigating or handling a communication board or a device. One of the challenges of AAC-users is to match speed of motor execution with the message that needs to be conveyed. Because generating a message takes more time, AAC-users tend to develop strategies such as shortening the message, leaving out function words, and employing prestored phrases or entire messages (Hoag, Bedrosian, McCoy, & Johnson, 2004). Rate enhancement is a major objective of AAC intervention as it is often considered to be the only way to prevent the user from device abandonment (Johnson, Inglebret, Jones, & Ray, 2006).

The fact that the visual modality plays a more dominant role has been suggested to be one of the possible explanations why AAC can work in conditions where typical communication is beyond reach. Visual symbols allow the user more processing time than the auditory information, which can be a key factor for individuals with developmental limitations (Lloyd & Karlan, 1984).

Clinicians and developers of communication devices generally try to organize the symbols on the screen in a way that is felt to be conducive to processing. Most of the communication boards and devices have the symbols arranged by the caregivers or the manufacturing company. These adult-generated displays may not always reflect the ways developing children organize their developing semantic networks (Fallon, Light, & Achenbach, 2003). In the past decade, technology has made it easier to customize boards and device displays, according to a person's processing preferences. Jagaroo and Wilkinson (2008) argue that AAC clinicians should tap into the growing knowledge and understanding of neurocognitive sciences for decisions on how to present AAC symbols on screens. The use of communication devices and board displays also hold the promise of an interesting avenue to investigate lexical and semantic organization in a variety of populations.

Beside considerations related to vocabulary organization, developers need to pay attention to the ergonomic aspects of communication board and device use. Blackstone, Williams, and Wilkins (2007) identify ergonomics as a key to successful communication. It appears that ergonomics will also play a decisive role in effective processing; that is, whether lexical items are accessed within processable time limits and if syntactic combinations can be activated. Motor access, planning, and coordination also make AAC distinct from typical speech communication. The use of communication boards and screens can be compared to the use of a typical keyboard. Dynamic screen use is comparable to navigating folders and windows on a computer. The use of dynamic screens that allow the user to navigate through a number of screens, raises interesting questions concerning the use of memory and planning, similar to questions related to the issue of lexical access by typical language users. One of the criteria presently used to compare efficacy in use of communication devices is related to speed of access (motor execution and coordination) and learnability of motor patterns. Stuart and Ritthaler (2008) discuss case studies that illustrate that learning symbol locations on a screen are facilitated if intervention is geared at learning combinatory motor patterns.

Access

AAC-literature has contributed a major part to the discussion of how to build a vocabulary for AAC users. This problem is most prevalent in the use of aided communication. The AAC user needs to learn to perform a limited number of actions to produce a communicative output. These include touching symbols on a screen, pointing to symbols, eye gazing at symbols, scanning a barcode, or respond to a sequence of symbols that light up (scanning).

AAC and Assistive Technology attempt to accommodate the person's best abilities to control a message output. Individuals often need AAC because of limitations in motor speech production. A major characteristic of many AAC solutions is the accommodation or compensation for motor execution. Manual signs are generally easier to produce than articulated speech because manual signs use more peripheral musculature than natural speech and do not require the same speed of coordination.

The use of communication boards, where the person is only required to point to graphic symbols (pictures or words) is among the most widespread. It was first used with children and adults with cerebral palsy who have normal or near-normal cognitive and linguistic skills, but are limited in natural speech execution. Besides pointing, alternative access forms have been successfully implemented, increasingly accommodating individuals with limited motor functions, including persons with locked-in syndrome. Switch technology, visual scanning, eye-gaze response systems, and more recently new developments in Brain-Computer Interaction continue to raise expectations and open possibilities for individuals with expressive motor limitations.

However, access is more than just the physical action of somehow activating a symbol or message on a board or a screen. Higginbotham, Shane, Russell, and Caves (2007) make a strong case that access cannot be seen separately from memory, internal representation, and planning. Time and cognitive effort needed for planning and executing the expression of a single word will reduce the potential for longer utterances. Developers and manufacturers of technological solutions are challenged to find ways to reduce mental-linguistic efforts.

PROCESSES AND CHALLENGES AUGMENTATIVE AND ALTERNATIVE COMMUNICATION

The practice of AAC targets the facilitation of a number of processes involved in generating messages. These processes can include: (1) accessing the elements; (2) internally planning and monitoring the message execution; and (3) activating the sequence into overt expression.

AAC system and device developers have been trying to grasp a model that can serve as a framework to understand and facilitate the processes. The model that is underlying most approaches seems to be that of matching of spoken (linguistic) elements with elements in an alternative mode. However important issues remain concerning the level of message construction, characteristics of the lexicon that is made available to the user, navigation through the system, multimodality and compatibility of modalities, and the role of internal speech.

THE LEVEL OF MESSAGE CONSTRUCTION

What is the level at which selection should occur? Many AAC systems assume that users will do one of the following (or combine them in some ways): (1) select sublexical elements (letters or graphic symbols); (2) select symbols at the word-level; or (3) select phrases. Each of these strategies requires a different configuration of mental operation as well as operational skills. Combining letters allows the generation of an infinite number of messages but requires literacy skills as well as speed in motor production. Accessing symbols at the lexical level requires symbolic representational skills and poses storage problems. Many present-day AAC devices allow for a personalized set up accommodating the person's best strategies. Higginbotham, Kim, & Scally (2007) summarize research indicating that AAC-users employ a multitude of strategies, motivated by the best tradeoff between message accuracy and speed. Todman, Alm, Higginbotham, and File (2008) argue that whole-utterances approaches in AAC with present-day devices may prove more functional in establishing a higher rate than a word construction approach, without losing precision.

MinSpeak™ is a combined access and coding system developed by Baker (Baker, 1982; Baker & Erickson, 1996). The user works with a limited number (e.g., 84) of graphic symbols (called icons) that assume different meanings depending on how they are combined. For example, the meaning "to read" requires the icon sequence "Shakespeare" and "Activity," the meaning "to eat" the sequence "Apple" and "Activity," and the meaning "Early" is called up by sequencing the "Wristwatch" icon with the "Rising Sun" icon.

In the past few years, several alternatives have been discussed for presenting communication symbols. Instead of presenting discrete de-contextualized symbols in a board format, the use of visual scene displays has been tried out and implemented. These displays are boards displaying a whole scene (e.g., a living room) where hot spots can be activated either to produce a speech-out message, or to navigate to another scene. Fundamentally, the efficacy of these displays is largely affected by cognitive effort in mentally using the boards to internally activate message patterns (Wilkinson & Jagaroo, 2004). The use of visual scene displays has been especially explored with individuals with aphasia (McKelvey, Dietz, Hux, Weissling, & Beukelman, 2007). An interesting other form of access is the use of a speech-generating barcode reader (Loncke, Alves, & Meyer, 2006a) that allows generating messages through pointing the device at labels attached to the environment.

THE LEXICON

One of the challenges of AAC developers is to determine the lexicon to be made available to the user. Contrary to natural language use, access is most often dependent on words that have been entered in the device. This poses a major challenge for the caregiver as vocabulary growth can be hampered or facilitated by accessibility of words.

One major discussion among AAC clinicians is how the number of available words as well as the type of words relates to a person's ability to generate message and participate in communication. The discussion centers around the use of core vocabulary with a limited number of easily accessible words (and phrases) versus fringe vocabulary with less frequent but, dependent on the context, more precise words. Again, speed of access is crucial. If finding the word takes too much of an effort, the user will shorten the message, or not feel encouraged to communicate at all. It is easy to see how improved access through improved technology leads to better pragmatics. Conversely, painstaking efforts lead to frustration both for sender and receiver, and may cause device abandonment.

Hill (2004) defends the position that easy and fast access and training to use a core vocabulary effectively is preferable over focusing on fringe vocabulary. Users can learn effective core-vocabulary strategies to maximize the communicative output without losing precision.

NAVIGATING OR ENCODING

The number of messages, phrases, or words that can be stored in today's communication devices is virtually infinite. A typical approach is to organize icons on screens in such a way that they are connected to each other through links, much as computer software allows a person to organize information in folders and subfolders. In order to combine two symbols into one utterance, the user of the system will need to find a path from one screen to another.

The use of navigation obviously requires memory and planning. For example, if a user wants to combine the phrase "My briefcase" with "is in" and "the kitchen," she may have to identify each of the phrases on different pages within the device. This requires remembering where the words or phrases are stored and how to navigate to them. Besides the memory constraint, users have a timing problem: even if navigation will require less mental effort from an experienced use, it will still take time to link one page to another.

COMBINING MESSAGES

How do lexical elements combine into utterances, and do these utterances have a sentence-like status? In the early years of sign language research, this question had been raised concerning ASL and other signed languages (e.g., Bellugi & Fischer, 1972). The issue was raised by scholars who wondered if a visual and partially iconic (e.g., Tervoort, 1973) based system would lend itself to language. At present, linguists agree that sign languages are indeed governed by linguistic rules, which must have developed in accordance to visual processing demands and restrictions, just as sentence structures of spoken languages are influenced by the acoustic processing principles.

As for graphic symbols, their use may be influenced by two different principles, on the one hand graphic symbols can be combined following the syntactic rules of an internalized spoken language. For individuals in an English speaking environment, it would be expected that most utterances would have the S-V-O structure. Often this "spoken language combinatorial principle" is encouraged by clinicians and is reinforced by simultaneous use of speech and graphic symbols. On the other hand, it may be that the visual or iconic nature of the symbols guide the users to a different sequential strategy. Smith (1996) did find that "the medium is the message"; that is, that children are influenced by the visual-graphic nature of the symbols in organizing the information. Trudeau, Sutton, Dagenais, de Broeck, and Morford (2007) and Sutton, Trudeau, Morford, Rios, and Poirier (2009) found indications that typical children older than 7 and typical adults are in fact guided by the syntactic rules of their internalized spoken language knowledge, while younger children follow a more visually based strategy.

COMPATIBILITY

An issue that is frequently raised by caregivers is the compatibility of expressive modalities. Parents and teachers often wonder whether the use of an alternative to speech will lead to extinction of all speech behavior.

Millar, Light, and Schlosser (2006) conducted a meta-analysis of clinical studies and reports on the effects of the use of AAC on natural speech. Although it is not possible to make a conclusive statement about the relation between AAC use and natural speech, they report that "the best evidence indicates that AAC interventions do not have a negative impact on speech production" (p. 257). A number of hypotheses on the relationship between natural speech and alternative modes have been proposed. Most hypotheses assume a mutual reinforcing effect of the nonspeech modality on natural speech. Romski and Sevcik (1993) state that "the consistency of the synthetic speech output preserves dimensions of the auditory signal that permit the listener to segment the stream of speech more easily" (p. 283). Along the same lines and more specifically, Blischak (1999) observes that "the synthetic speech output may activate or strengthen the phonologic code, which may then focus the child's attention on the phonological characteristics of the words.

AAC users illustrate how internal representations of speech are connected with acoustic output without speech articulation.

Binger, Berens, Kent-Walsh, and Taylor (2008) analyzed data of two studies with a total of six children in single subject, multiple baseline, studies across participant research designs. The authors' data include some of the few that directly track the relation between the use of a speech-generating device (SGD) and natural speech. Their analysis indicates that the use of the devices does not have a negative impact effect on speech (p. 109).

INTERNAL SPEECH

One of the most prominent characteristics of AAC is the use of a nonspeech modality for linguistic expressions. For example, SGD provide an alternative for natural speech to individuals with complex communication needs (CCN). From a psycholinguistic perspective, the use of SGDs provides an opportunity to explore underlying processes in message generating.

Does the use of an SGD mirror the use of natural speech? Or, knowing that natural speech is the outcome of a micro-genesis of processes including syntactic planning, lexicalization, and phonetic planning, will we be able to identify the same subskills and processes in the use of an SGD? One candidate that might provide a difference between natural speech and the use of SGDs are processes that are related to internal phonological representations and phonetic actualizations. These processes are often referred to as internal speech (or inner speech).

Loncke et al. (2008) conducted a study in which they presented 60 nondisabled adults with 40 written pseudowords. Forty of the participants were native English speakers in the United States, and 20 were native French speakers in France. The words differed in phonological complexity (two-syllabic and three- or four-syllabic). Each word was associated with a picture of a common object (e.g., a strawberry, a key). Half of the words were presented along with auditory feedback through a speech-generating barcode reader. The hypothesis that words with auditory feedback would strengthen an internal phonological representation and be more likely remembered. The results showed that this was significantly the case for the complex three or four syllable words, but not for the simpler two-syllable words. The results were similar for the French and for the English speakers, indicating that the feedback effect works across languages.

The results of the study indicate that all participants did make significant learning gains in all conditions—at the fourth probe, many of the participants had learned all the words. The results showed an advantage of the speech-generated auditory feedback. This advantage is more pronounced for the phonologically complex word (four-syllables) than the less complex words. The more challenging the structure of the word is, the more the learner seems to benefit from acoustic-phonological information. Initial inspection of the results indicates that there is no significant effect of the phonology of the participants' native language (English vs. French). These limited data favor the hypothesis that an internal phonological representation can be built based on the auditory feedback from the device.

SUMMARY AND CONCLUSIONS

Augmentative and Alternative Communication presents itself as a field with fascinating psycholinguistic questions. AAC as a discipline is built on the presupposition that nonfunctional speech can be compensated by replacing articulated speech with alternative forms of motor expression, by adding new modalities such as graphic symbols, or reinforcing nonverbal modalities such as gestures.

Replacing natural speech with alternative expressive modes helps to gain insight into how natural speech articulation processes are linked to internal phonology, utterance planning, working memory, and the rate of production. Furthermore, AAC provides an avenue for research in multimodality, graphic symbol representation, and lexical access strategies. The efficacy of the use of communication boards and devices is most likely dependent on how the tools favor and reinforce semantic organization. Brain–Computer Interaction applications will provide us with information on how mental strategies are best modeled by the computer.

These are areas that require and merit more research. Ultimately, we will want to know how better psycholinguistic strategies yield to better and less cumbersome message generating, and better communicative pragmatics.

REFERENCES

Archer, L. A. (1977). Blissymbolics: A nonverbal communication system. *Journal of Speech & Hearing Disorders, 42*(4), 568–579.

Baker, B. (1982). Minspeak: A semantic compaction system that makes self-expression easier for communicatively disabled individuals. *Byte, 7*(9), 186–202.

Baker, B., & Erickson, K. (1996). Language, literacy, and semantic compaction. Proceedings of the 7th Biennial Conference of the International Society for Augmentative and Alternative Communication (ISAAC). (pp. 214–215).Vancouver, Canada.

Bellugi, U., & Fischer, S. (1972). A comparison of sign language and spoken language. *Cognition, 1*(2), 173–200.

Bickerton, D. (1999). Creole languages, the language bioprogram hypothesis, and language acquisition. In W. C. Ritchie, T. K. Bhatia, W. C. Ritchie, & T. K. Bhatia (Eds.), *Handbook of child language acquisition* (pp. 195–220). San Diego, CA: Academic Press.

Binger, C. (2008). Grammatical morpheme intervention issues for students who use AAC. *Perspectives on Augmentative and Alternative Communication, 17*, 62–68.

Binger, C., Berens, J., Kent-Walsh, J., Taylor, S. (2008). The effects of aided AAC interventions on AAC use, speech, and symbolic gestures. *Seminars in Speech and Language, 29*(2), 101–111.

Binger, C., Berens, J., Kent-Walsh, J., & Hickman, S. (2008). The impacts of aided AAC interventions on AAC use, speech, and symbolic gestures. *Seminars in Speech and Language, 29*(2), 101–111.

Birbaumer, N., & Cohen, L. G. (2007). Brain-computer interfaces: Communication and restoration of movement in paralysis. *The Journal of Physiology, 579*, 621–636.

Blackstone, S., & Hunt Berg, M. (2003). *Social networks: A communication inventory for individuals with complex communication needs and their communication partners.* Manual. Monterey, CA: Augmentative Communication, Inc.

Blackstone, S. W., Williams, M. B., & Wilkins, D. P. (2007). Key principles underlying research and practice in AAC. *Augmentative and Alternative Communication, 23*(3), 191–203.

Blischak, D. M. (1999). Increases in natural speech production following experience with synthetic speech. *Journal of Special Education Technology, 14*(2), 44–53.

Bliss, C. K. (1965). *Semantography (Blissymbolics).* Sydney, Australia: Semantography Press.

Bliss, C. K., & McNaughton, S. (1976). *The book to the film Mr. Symbol man.* Sydney, Australia: Semantography-Blissymbolics.

Bloomberg, K., Karlan, G., & Lloyd, L. (1990). The comparative translucency of initial lexical items represented in five graphic symbols systems and sets. *Journal of Speech and Hearing Research, 33*, 717–725.

Bondy, A., & Frost, L. (2001). The picture exchange communication system. *Behavior Modification, 25*(5), 725–744.

Bonvillian, J. D., & Nelson, K. E. (1976). Sign language acquisition in a mute autistic boy. *Journal of Speech & Hearing Disorders, 41*(3), 339–347.

DeLoache, J. S. (1995). Early understanding and use of symbols: The model model. *Current Directions in Psychological Science, 4*(4), 109–113.

Fallon, K. A., Light, J., & Achenbach, A. (2003). The semantic organization patterns of young children: Implications for augmentative and alternative communication. *Augmentative and Alternative Communication, 19*(2), 74–85.

Fouts, R. S. (1987). Chimpanzee signing and emergent levels. In G. Greenberg & E. Tobach (Eds.), *Cognition, language and consciousness: Integrative levels* (pp. 57–84). Hillsdale, NJ/England, UK: Lawrence Erlbaum Associates, Inc.

Fuller, D. R., Lloyd, L. L., & Schlosser, R. W. (1992). Further development of an augmentative and alternative communication symbol taxonomy. *Augmentative and Alternative Communication, 8*(1), 67–74.

Gardner, R. A., & Gardner, B. T. (1969). Teaching sign language to a chimpanzee. *Science, 165*(894), 664–672.

Goldin-Meadow, S. (1998). The development of gesture and speech as an integrated system. In J. M. Iverson, S. Goldin-Meadow, J. M. Iverson, & S. Goldin-Meadow (Eds.), *The nature and functions of gesture in children's communication* (pp. 29–42). San Francisco, CA: Jossey-Bass.

Higginbotham, D. J., Kim, K., & Scally, C. (2007a). The effect of the communication output method on augmented interaction. *Augmentative and Alternative Communication, 23*(2), 140–153.

Higginbotham, D. J., Shane, H., Russell, S., & Caves, K. (2007b). Access to AAC: Present, past, and future. *Augmentative and Alternative Communication, 23*(3), 243–257.

Hill, K. (2004). Augmentative and alternative communication and language: Evidence-based practice and language activity monitoring. *Topics in Language Disorders, 24*(1), 18–30.

Hoag, L. A., Bedrosian, J. L., McCoy, K. F., & Johnson, D. (2004). Trade-offs between informativeness and speed of message delivery in augmentative and alternative communication. *Journal of Speech, Language, and Hearing Research, 47*(6), 1270–1285.

Huer, M. B. (1997). Culturally inclusive assessments for children using Augmentative and Alternative Communication (AAC). *Communication Disorders Quarterly, 19*(1), 23–34.

Jagaroo, V., & Wilkinson, K. (2008). Further considerations of visual cognitive neuroscience in aided AAC: The potential role of motion perception systems in maximizing design display. *Augmentative and Alternative Communication, 24*(1), 29.

Johnson, J. M., Inglebret, E., Jones, C., & Ray, J. (2006). Perspectives of speech language pathologists regarding success versus abandonment of AAC. *Augmentative and Alternative Communication, 22*(2), 85–99.

Klima, E., & Bellugi, U. (1979). *The signs of language.* Cambridge, MA: Harvard University Press.

Koul, R. K., & Lloyd, L. L. (1998). Comparison of graphic symbol learning in individuals with aphasia and right hemisphere brain damage. *Brain and Language, 62*(3), 398–421.

Levelt, W. (1993). *Speaking. From intention to articulation* (2nd ed.). Cambridge, MA: MIT Press.

Light, J., Page, R., Curran, J., & Pitkin, L. (2007). Children's ideas for the design of AAC assistive technologies for young children with complex communication needs. *Augmentative and Alternative Communication, 23*(4), 274.

Lloyd, L. L., & Karlan, G. R. (1984). Non-speech communication symbols and systems: Where have we been and where are we going? *Journal of Mental Deficiency Research, 28*(1), 3–20.

Lloyd, L. L., Loncke, F., & Arvidson, H. (1999). Graphic symbol use: An orientation toward theoretical relevance. In F. Loncke, J. Clibbens, H. Arvidson, & L. Lloyd (Eds.), *Augmentative and alternative communication. New directions in research and practice* (pp. 161–173). London, UK: Whurr.

Loncke, F., Alves, M., & Meyer, L. (2006a). B.A.Bar™: The speaking barcode reader. *Closing the gap,* February–March, 21–22.

Loncke, F., Crato, D., Canty, T., Goldkamp, J., Leconte, C., & Marichez, D. (2008, November 20). *Are users of speech generating devices using an internal phonology?* Presentation at the Annual Convention of the American Speech-Language and Hearing Association (ASHA). Chicago, IL.

McDonald, E., & Schultz, A. (1973). Communication boards for cerebral-palsied children. *Journal of Speech and Hearing Disorders, 38*(1), 73–88.

McKelvey, M. L., Dietz, A. R., Hux, K., Weissling, K., & Beukelman, D. R. (2007). Performance of a person with chronic aphasia using personal and contextual pictures in a visual scene display prototype. *Journal of Medical Speech-Language Pathology, 15*(3), 305–317.

McNaughton, D., & Bryen, D. N. (2007). AAC technologies to enhance participation and access to meaningful societal roles for adolescents and adults with developmental disabilities who require AAC. *Augmentative and Alternative Communication, 23*(3), 217–242.

Millar, D. C., Light, J. C., & Schlosser, R. W. (2006). The impact of augmentative and alternative communication intervention on the speech production of individuals with developmental disabilities: A research review. *Journal of Speech, Language, and Hearing Research, 49*(2), 248–264.

Raghavendra, P., & Fristoe, M. (1995). "No shoes; They walked away?": Effects of enhancements on learning and using blissymbols by normal 3-year-old children. *Journal of Speech & Hearing Research, 38*(1), 174–186.

Ravizza, S. (2003). Movement and lexical access: Do noniconic gestures aid in retrieval? *Psychonomic Bulletin & Review, 10*(3), 610–615.

Romski, M. A., & Sevcik, R. A. (1993). Language comprehension: Considerations for augmentative and alternative communication. *Augmentative and Alternative Communication, 9*(4), 281–285.

Smith, M. (1996). The medium is the message: A study of speaking children using communication boards. In S.Von Tetzchner & M.H. Jensen (Eds.). *Augmentative and alternative communication: European perspectives* (pp. 119–136). London: Whurr Publishers.

Snell, M., & Brown, F. (2006). *Instruction of students with severe disabilities.* Upper Saddle River, NJ: Pearson/Merrill/Prentice Hall.

Soto, G., & Toro-Zambrana, W. (1995). Investigation of blissymbol use from a language research paradigm. *Augmentative and Alternative Communication, 11*(2), 118–130.

Stuart, S., & Ritthaler, C. (2008). Case studies of intermediate steps/Between AAC evaluations and implementation. *Perspectives on Augmentative and Alternative Communication, 17*(4), 150–155.

Sturm, J. M., & Clendon, S. A. (2004). Augmentative and alternative communication, language, and literacy: Fostering the relationship. *Topics in Language Disorders, 24*(1), 76–91.

Sutton, A., Trudeau, N., Morford, J., Rios, M., & Poirier, M.-A. (2009). Preschool age children have difficulty constructing and interpreting simple utterances composed of graphic symbols. *Journal of Child Language, 37* (1), 1–26.

Taylor, R., & Iacono, T. (2003). AAC and scripting activities to facilitate communication and play. *Advances in Speech Language Pathology, 5*(2), 79–93.

Tervoort B. (1973). Could there be a human sign language? *Semiotica, 9*(4), 347–382.

Todman, J., Alm, N., Higginbotham, J., & File, P. (2008). Whole utterance approaches in AAC. *Augmentative and Alternative Communication, 24*(3), 235–254.

Trudeau, N., Sutton, A., Dagenais, E., de Broeck, S., & Morford, J. (2007). Construction of graphic symbol utterances by children, teenagers, and adults: The effect of structure and task demands. *Journal of Speech, Language, and Hearing Research, 50*(5), 1314–1329.

Von Tetzchner, S., Brekke, K. M., Sjothun, B., & Grindheim, E. (2005). Constructing preschool communities of learners that afford alternative language development. *Augmentative and Alternative Communication, 21*(2), 82–100.

Wilkinson, K. M., & Jagaroo, V. (2004). Contributions of principles of visual cognitive science to AAC system display design. *Augmentative and Alternative Communication, 20*(3), 123–136.

Epilogue

Jackie Guendouzi, Filip Loncke, and Mandy Williams

RELEVANCE OF THEORIES AND MODELS TO THE STUDY OF COMMUNICATION DISORDERS

For the student or researcher new to this field, there are some key issues that we hope this text has raised, in particular the notion that language is a phenomenon that results from an interaction between several cognitive systems and in particular the following: attention, memory, the motor system, gesture and other non-verbal cues, the auditory system, the lexicon(s), the morphosyntactic system and the phonological system. Current models consider language processing in terms of how one part of the system affects the another part of the system, for example, the question of whether syntax uses procedural memory systems and is therefore more "automatic" than semantic aspects of language. Considering language in terms of storage capacity and processing trade-offs may better explain many questions that have driven research over the past two decades.

This is an important volume for researchers in the field of both communication disorders and language processing, however, it is equally important to the practicing clinician. Clinicians rely on research to inform their clinical practice; indeed, good practice should always be grounded in both evidence-based practice and theory. Thus the endpoint of theoretical and experimental research is of great relevance to speech language pathologists and audiologists. While to some degree work in psycholinguistics and cognitive neurosciences have been viewed separately, the field of communication disorders is a natural meeting point for both the physiological, psychological, and linguistic approaches to language processing. Certainly, clinical populations have been of interest to a variety of researchers when looking for data to support theories and models. When communication breaks down due to developmental problems or acquired traumatic injury, it provides clues to the ways in which language and cognitive systems both function and interact.

Communication disorders is a field that has more than a vested interest in "finding" a theory that explains, the language deficits that present in clinical populations, or the delays some children experience in acquiring language. Within the health sciences, rather like attempts in physics to find a central unifying "theory of everything," there has been a tendency to want to find "the" definitive cure or answer to the problem. However, even if such a theory or explanation exists it will ultimately be the result of considering many competing theoretical approaches and testing models against data collected from both normal and atypical populations.

779

This process starts with theories that hypothesize what might be happening in the brain when we speak, listen, read, or write. We then need to build models with a goal for testing data that will prove a particular theory (see Roelofs, Chapter 9). The results of model building help us to prove or falsify particular claims that in turn help us to revise both our models and theories. This is an ongoing process not unlike the Socratic tradition of rhetorical argument, and it is competing research paradigms that drive this process. For students who are invariably primed to want to know "the" correct explanation or theory for a problem the research process can be an uncomfortable experience, but it should be embraced rather than feared. It is important that a good theoretical text should raise as many questions as it provides answers for its readers, thus the differences in approaches represented here represent a strength in the field rather than weakness, moreover the authors have provided a range of perspectives that we hope will inspire those studying this field to utilize in further investigating problems in the field of communication disorders.

Author Index

Subject Index